ACUTE NURSING CARE

Visit the *Acute Nursing Care: Recognising and Responding to Medical Emergencies,* Companion Website at
www.routledge.com/cw/peate-9780273743712/
to find valuable **student** learning material including:

- Interactive case studies presenting patient care scenarios
- Multiple choice questions to test and develop your knowledge
- Flashcards to help you revise key terms and concepts
- Searchable glossary of terms

ACUTE NURSING CARE

Recognising and Responding to Medical Emergencies

Ian Peate

EN(G), RGN DipN (Lond), RNT, BEd (Hons), MA (Lond), LLM

Professor of Nursing

Editor in Chief, *British Journal of Nursing*

Helen Dutton

MSc BA, RNT, RGN

Senior Lecturer

School of Nursing Midwifery and Healthcare

University of West London

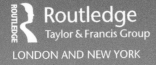 Routledge
Taylor & Francis Group

LONDON AND NEW YORK

First published 2012 by Pearson Education Limited

Published 2013 by Routledge
2 Park Square, Milton Park, Abingdon, Oxon OX14 4RN
711 Third Avenue, New York, NY 10017, USA

Routledge is an imprint of the Taylor & Francis Group, an informa business

ISBN 13: 978-0-273-74371-2 (pbk)

British Library Cataloguing-in-Publication Data
A catalogue record for this book is available from the British Library

Library of Congress Cataloging-in-Publication Data
A catalog record for this book is available from the Library of Congress

Typeset in 10.5/13pt Minion by 35

Brief contents

Contents

Chapter 10
The patient with acute gastrointestinal problems

Julian Howard and Angela Morgan

Chapter 11
The patient with acute endocrine problems

Angela Morgan, Julian Howard and
Margaret Kirkby

Chapter 12
The immune and lymphatic systems, infection and sepsis   283

Andrea Blay, Jacqui Finch and Helen Dutton

Chapter 13
The safe transfer of acutely ill patients   313

Jacqui Finch

Supporting resources

Visit www.routledge.com/cw/peate-9780273743712/

Companion Website for students

- Interactive case studies presenting patient care scenarios
- Multiple choice questions to test and develop your knowledge
- Flashcards to help you revise key terms and concepts
- Searchable glossary of terms

For instructors

- PowerPoint slides containing all key diagrams from the text

Also: The Companion Website provides the following features:

- Search tool to help locate specific items of content
- E-mail results and profile tools to send results of quizzes to instructors
- Online help and support to assist with website usage and troubleshooting

List of figures and tables

Figures

Tables

Guided tour

This user-friendly text uses various integrated resources to enable and encourage you to apply the content to contexts in which you find yourself. These features have been specially designed to benefit both your understanding and practice, to help you become a better practitioner.

Aims

This chapter aims to provide the reader with insight and understanding concerning the vulnerable adult in the acute care setting and those whose health is at risk of deterioration.

Each chapter contains a specific set of **Aims**. These help to précis what you will learn about within the chapter.

Objectives

After reading this chapter you will be able to:

→ Describe key terms

→ Understand the rights of vulnerable adults in acute care situations

→ Examine the health and social policy provisions for vulnerable people

→ Ensure that the voice of the vulnerable adult is heard and acted upon

→ Outline some of the ethical considerations relevant to the care and treatment of vulnerable people in the acute care setting

→ Provide safe and effective care to vulnerable people in acute care settings or those whose health is at risk of deterioration

All chapters list the **Learning Objectives** you should attain after reading the chapter and undertaking the various activities within. You can check your progress by confirming which of the learning objectives you understand and which you still need to learn.

Drugs associated with hyponatraemia

- Diuretics (especially loop and thiazide diuretics)
- Anticoagulants (heparin)
- Anticonvulsants (carbamazepine)
- Desmopressin acetate (DDAVP)
- Recreational (MDMA, ecstasy)
- Antidepressants and antipsychotics (fluoxetine sertraline, SSRIs)
- Antineoplastics (cyclophosphamide and vincristine).

Hyponatraemia

Hyponatraemia is the most common electrolyte imbalance in hospitalised patients and refers to a serum sodium

Clinical Alert boxes spread throughout the text help to highlight particular aspects of clinical practice and important information. These practical resources can help you to improve your understanding and capability in the clinical setting.

CASE STUDY 11.1 Mr Richards, type I diabetic: hypoglycaemic secondary to chest sepsis - Part 1

INITIAL ASSESSMENT

Mr Richards, 61 years old, is brought to A&E with shortness of breath and a temperature. He has a past medical history of type I diabetes. He is a coach driver and appears overweight.

Airway/breathing

On assessment, his nurse notes he is able to speak a sentence but is very short of breath. He is drowsy and says he feels unwell. He has a respiratory rate of 23/minute on 4L oxygen via a non-fixed-performance Hudson mask with oxygen saturations of 93%, suggesting he is hypoxic as this is below his target saturation of 94–98%. The nurse requests an arterial blood gas sample. He is using accessory muscles with poor respiratory excursion. He has bilateral air entry with coarse crackles at the lung bases and is

daily long-acting insulin). It is now 1800h. He has his evening dose and she checks he eats supper.

Exposure

Mr Richards looks flushed and feels clammy. The nurse reads his notes and finds that his BMI is 40, confirming obesity. His abdomen is large but soft. He is splinting his diaphragm which will contribute to his shortness of breath, so she sits him up. He has bowel sounds, is not constipated and is pain free. His nurse notices nicotine stains on his fingers and asks if he smokes. He says he has smoked about 20 cigarettes a day for the last 45 years.

Diagnosis

Given his history and presentation, a provisional diagnosis is made of sepsis secondary to a chest infection.

Detailed and realistic **Case Studies** are included throughout each chapter, helping to relate theory to practice. Based on real life scenarios, the case studies will help prepare you for the realities of clinical practice.

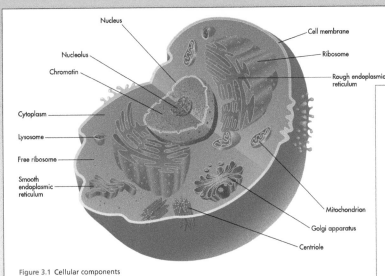

Figure 3.1 Cellular components

(Labels: Nucleus, Nucleolus, Chromatin, Cytoplasm, Lysosome, Free ribosome, Smooth endoplasmic reticulum, Cell membrane, Ribosome, Rough endoplasmic reticulum, Mitochondrion, Golgi apparatus, Centriole)

The text is illustrated with full colour **diagrams and pictures** throughout, relating to core systems and good practice.

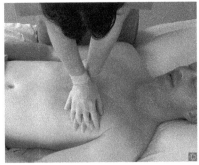

Figure 7.11 Chest compressions
Source: Resuscitation Council UK (2011) *Advanced Life Support.* Photograph reproduced with kind permission by Michael Scott and the Resuscitation Council (UK).

Glossary

Adrenaline Naturally occurring hormone, also known as epinephrine, given during cardiac arrest to increase coronary and cerebral perfusion.

Agonal breathing Deep sighing, irregular gasping breathing, also known as Cheyne–Stokes breathing, which occurs at the end of life.

Algorithm Step-by-step procedure for problem-solving, often expressed as diagram or flow chart.

Asystole Complete absence of electrical and mechanical activity in the heart.

Bag valve mask A device used to provide artificial ventilation which consists of a manual compressible chamber with an oxygen reservoir at one end and a one-way valve and mask at the other.

Basic life support See cardiopulmonary resuscitation.

Cardiopulmonary arrest The sudden cessation of breathing and effective cardiac output.

Hyperkaleamia High level of potassium in the blood.

Hypokalaemia Low level of potassium in the blood.

Hypothermia Abnormally low temperature.

Hypovolaemia Low circulating blood volume.

Hypoxia Low levels of cellular oxygen.

Intraosseous The inside of a bone.

Intravenous The inside of a vein.

Pulmonary embolism The blockage of a pulmonary artery by a blood clot, fat or air.

Key terms are highlighted in the text and definitions are included in the **Glossary** at the end of each chapter. A comprehensive Glossary appears listing all key terms and definitions appears at the end of the book.

Check your understanding by attempting the **Test Yourself** self-assessment tests provided at the end of each chapter. Answers are available in the appendix.

Test yourself

1 The nephron is the functional unit of the kidney. Which of the following structures is not part of the tubular area?

a. glomerulus
b. proximal convuluted tubule
c. loop of Henlé
d. vasa recta
e. distal convuluted tubule
f. collecting duct

2 The ureters and bladder have three layers, name them:

the tunica _____
the tunica _____
the tunica _____

5 What is the average glomerular filtration rate for an adult male?

a. 125ml per minute
b. 160ml per minute
c. 180ml per minute

6 Which substance regulates water reabsorption or excretion in the body?

a. renin
a. erythropoietin
c. vasopressin

7 Which of the following is not a usual symptom of a urinary tract infection?

a. pyrexia

References

Bickley, S. (2007) *Bates' Guide to Physical Examination and History Taking.* London: Lippincott, Williams & Wilkins.

British Thoracic Society Standards of Care Committee Pulmonary Embolism Guideline Development Group (2003) British Thoracic Society guidelines for the management of suspected acute pulmonary embolism. *Thorax* 58, 470–84.

Coons, J. and Seidl, E. (2007) Cardiovascular pharmacotherapy update for the intensive care unit. *Critical Care Nursing Quarterly*

Priori, S. G. and Swedbergm, K. (2008) ESC guidelines for diagno and treatment of acute and chronic heart failure. *European Heart Journal* 29, 1682–8.

ESC (2010) *Guidelines for the Management of Atrial Fibrillation.* The Task Force for the Management of Atrial Fibrillation of the European Society of Cardiology (ES contribution of the European Heart Endorsed by the European Associati (EACTS). *European Heart Journal* 31 http://www.escardio.org/guidelines- GuidelinesDocuments/guidelines-afi

Further reading

Mills, A. (2011) *Gastrointestinal Emergencies.* London: Saunders.

Norton, C. (2008) *Oxford Handbook of Gastrointestinal Nursing.* Oxford: Oxford University Press.

Tham, T. C. K., Collins, J. S. A. and Soetikno, R. (2008) *Gastrointestinal Emergencies*, 2nd edn. Oxford: Wiley-Blackwell.

The latest **References** are included for each chapter of the text, ensuring an evidence-based practice approach to acute care.

To help you take the subject further, extra resources are listed in the **Further Reading** sections at the end of each chapter.

Preface

Ian Peate and Helen Dutton

This text will meet the needs of a range of health care workers including student nurses working towards graduate status and professional registration, those returning to practice as well as the newly qualified practitioner who has chosen to begin their professional career in the acute care setting.

There have been and will continue to be changes in the delivery of health care, demonstrating that a larger proportion of care will take place outside of traditional settings. This strategic shift for nursing – from hospital to community – focuses on prevention and with patients and the public as the drivers of their care. Nurses have to be aware of the changing needs of the health care settings and the communities they provide services to, responding to both current and future need. The need to care for and respond appropriately to people who are experiencing medical emergencies is also changing and is ongoing as the technological support provided to those people advances. Medical advances and major developments in technology mean that the nurse of the future must be prepared to work safely and confidently in a number of care environments, providing care that is compassionate and effective. The knowledge base provided here is one that is rooted in applied physiology and some of the disorders that may give rise to a medical emergency.

The Nursing and Midwifery Council (NMC) (NMC 2010a) have issued new standards that must be achieved prior to registration with the NMC to practise as a nurse. The standards lay out what must be achieved when the student is at the point of registration. This text was written with those standards in mind in helping you to achieve the competencies required within the sphere of medical emergencies. The practice of delivering nursing and midwifery care involves a capacity not only to participate actively in care provision, but also to accept responsibility for the effective and efficient management of that care, practised within a safe environment. This involves:

- the capacity to accept accountability;
- taking responsibility for the delegation of aspects of care to others;
- effectively supervising and facilitating the work of such carers;
- the capacity to work effectively within the nursing, midwifery and wider multidisciplinary team;
- accepting leadership roles, where appropriate, within such teams and demonstrating overall competency in care and case management.

As well as being competent practitioners nurses must also be concerned with the environment of care and the interest and safety of people in their care. The nurse must make concerns about failing standards of public protection known to the NMC, and do this through the *Code of Conduct* (NMC 2008). Nurses have a duty to protect the vulnerable in society. The *Code* makes clear what is expected of the nurse and is a vital tool in delivering effective public protection. While the student nurse is not subjected to the *Code of Conduct*, she should strive to meet those standards under the auspices of a registered nurse.

The student must work towards the guidance produced by the NMC for professional conduct as nursing student (NMC 2010b) and the content in this book will advance this. This text will help you become a competent nurse as well as encouraging you to uphold the reputation of the profession.

It is the student nurse who will become the dynamic responsive nurse of tomorrow, with the ability to adapt to meeting the needs of the public in a variety of situations and settings. This text provides you with the principles on which to offer effective, safe, acute medical care to adults in a hospital setting. The nurse works with other highly skilled health care professionals and this interdisciplinary role will be emphasised throughout. As the move towards an all-graduate nursing profession gathers momentum and becomes a reality there is need for you to be able to demonstrate that you have the skills associated with higher level decision-making, become an autonomous practitioner and have at the heart of all you do the safety of the people you have the privilege to care for. According to the NMC (2010a) degree-level nurses will be able to:

- be more independent and innovative, making use of higher levels of professional judgement and decision-making when working in increasingly complex care environments;

- make available evidence-based care with confidence;
- assess the evidence base when applying this to care provision;
- work as a member of the multidisciplinary team and where appropriate lead those teams;
- provide leadership, sustain change and develop service provision.

The next five years will see a change in the way health and social care is delivered, with a focus upon the need to maximise the contribution nurses make to the demands placed upon the health service by society, government and technological changes.

You will have to be able to respond effectively to medical emergencies and this text will enable you to learn the fundamentals in order to do this as you learn to become a practitioner of the future. There is a clear need for change to enable nurses to meet the demands arising from a modernised health service: being aware of this and honing the skills required to make that change and to be an effective member of health and social services are prerequisites.

Future career frameworks will take into account nurses from all fields providing five broad categories of service delivery. The one category that is particularly pertinent to this text (but not exclusively) is acute and critical care, other categories, for example, the first contact, access and urgent care and managing long-term conditions, are also worthy of consideration.

Care provision is becoming more complex. An ageing population, shorter length of stay and higher consumer expectations will result in the provision of a higher level of care than has been previously offered. You will therefore need to be equipped with the skills to recognise and manage deterioration in the patient in a competent and confident manner.

Recommendations made by the National Institute for Health and Clinical Excellence (NICE 2007) have been formulated in response to a strong body of evidence produced by the National Patient Safety Agency (NPSA 2007), who have determined that delays in recognising deterioration in a patient's condition and treating and managing that condition appropriately can and does result in avoidable admission to intensive care units and in some cases unnecessary deaths. This text will help you improve and develop competence and confidence when caring for the acutely ill patient.

The level at which the information contained in this book is presented makes this a unique text. A fundamental approach is used to enable and encourage you to apply the content to contexts that you may find yourself in, it adopts a user-friendly approach. There are a number of features in the book that help this process happen.

In order to apply theory to practice, each chapter provides a range of teaching features, for example, the inclusion of case studies that can make the understanding and application of some complex concepts easier to come to terms with and assimilate. The case studies will 'set the scene' for the application of chapter content to (as near as possible) clinical practice. There are aims and objectives that provide you with structured, guided learning. Key terms are highlighted in the text in red and a glossary of terms at the end of each chapter is provided to help you to develop your nursing and medical vocabulary even further. A full Glossary also appears at the end of the book.

The chapters within the text provide you with links to relevant and related websites to help guide and support learning, links to professional and statutory websites such as the Department of Health (DH), National Institute for Health and Clinical Excellence (NICE) and the Scottish Intercollegiate Guidelines Network (SIGN). A bank of multiple-choice test questions is provided with the aim of reinforcing your learning.

The use of illustrations is key to this text, providing you with visual stimulation which promotes learning and aids retention. Simple line drawings are used and outlines of diagnostic and investigatory tests and procedures provided. Where appropriate the provision of diagnostic test outcomes will be supplied to demonstrate the 'normal' and 'abnormal', for example, a 'normal' electrocardiograph (ECG) and an 'abnormal' ECG depicting a cardiac arrhythmia.

The text includes a range of 'normal' values. A word or two on normal values is important. There are a variety of techniques that those who analyse blood, for example, use in the laboratory to identify the various components. These techniques may differ from laboratory to laboratory, and it is essential that when assessment of blood results is carried out referral to the local laboratory's normal values is made. The values provided here are related to a full blood count and are offered only as a guide rather than a fixed indicator of limits. Variation occurs across the UK, Europe and globally.

These variations will also occur with a person's age, gender and co-morbidity. Any variation has the potential to artificially alter a situation, triggering a response that may be not be appropriate when the person is stable and not in danger. Duckitt *et al.* (2007), for example, note that adults under 55 years will have an average respiratory rate of 18 breaths per minute, however those who are older may have a respiratory rate in excess of 20 breaths per minute and this respiratory rate is seen as their norm. The person's age and their current medications will also have an effect on the 'normal' observations and the 'normal' blood value. According to Creed *et al.* (2010), these factors should be taken to into account as opposed to relying purely upon the numerical values allocated the blood or other physiological measurements.

The overarching aim of the text is to help you better understand the fundamental aspects associated with a number of acute medical conditions in order to provide skilled and effective care to patients in various situations. The use of a contemporary evidence base will encourage safe and effective practice.

It is hoped that you will develop your caring skills with a sound knowledge base underpinning the delivery of care – preparing you for registration with the NMC. This book is based upon the principles of care and is a foundation text that will encourage you to grow and develop.

The structure promotes the concept of lifelong learning, supporting you and encouraging you to delve deeper and discover further. Referral to the *Code* (NMC 2008) encourages you to practise ethically and morally, with the patient's best interests at heart at all times.

The text is designed to be used as a reference text in either the clinical setting, the classroom or at home, and is not intended to be read from cover to cover in one sitting. It will provide you with the help you need to respond in a confident and competent manner to a variety of medical emergencies you may come across.

We have enjoyed writing this book and we very much hope that you will find it useful and enjoyable. It is our wish that by using this book, and applying the principles within it to the care that you give the people you nurse, you will be able minimise their distress and the anxieties that are associated with acute illness and critical care.

References

Creed, F., Dawson, J. and Looker, K. (2010) Assessment tools and track-and-trigger systems. In Spiers, F. and Creed, S. (eds) *Care of the Acutely Ill Adult*, Oxford: Oxford University Press, pp. 338–61.

Duckitt, R. W., Buxton, R., Walker, J. and Cheek, H. (2007) Worthing Physiological Scoring Stem: Derivation and validation of a physiological warning score for medical admissions. *British Journal of Anaesthesiology*, 98(6), 769–74.

NICE (National Institute for Health and Clinical Excellence) (2007) *Acutely Ill Patients in Hospital. Recognition and Response to Acute Illness in Adults in Hospital.* London: NICE.

NPSA (National Patient Safety Agency) (2007) *Recognising and Responding Appropriately to Early Signs of Deterioration in Hospitalised Patients.* London: NPSA.

Nursing and Midwifery Council (2008) *The Code: Standards of Conduct, Performance and Ethics for Nurses and Midwives.* London: NMC.

Nursing and Midwifery Council (2010a) *Standards for Pre-registration Nursing Education.* London: NMC. Available from http://standards.nmc-uk.org/PublishedDocuments/Standards%20for%20pre-registration%20nursing%20education%2016082010.pdf, last accessed June 2011.

Nursing and Midwifery Council (2010b) *Guidance on Professional Conduct for Nursing and Midwifery Students.* London: NMC.

Contributors

Liz Allibone
RGN, BSc, PGCTLCP, FEA, ENB 294

Head of Clinical Education and Training
Royal Brompton and Harefield NHS Foundation Trust

Liz leads Royal Brompton and Harefield NHS Foundation Trust's in-house education programmes for nursing staff. With an active interest in learning and teaching, she is responsible for developing clinical knowledge and skills at the Trust. Liz also works closely with partner universities to support learning and mentoring of student nurses on clinical placements. Simulation and training in the clinical environment is a key focus of her management of the Trust's Resuscitation Team. Liz has extensive experience of the clinical and academic demands of cardio-respiratory nursing from her career in both the UK and the United States.

Andrea Blay
MSc, RGN ENB100

Consultant Nurse, Critical Care

Andrea trained at St. Bartholomew's Hospital qualifying as a nurse in 1987. She started her foray into intensive care at the Homerton hospital, this was followed by a further 16 years working in intensive care at various hospitals including, The Royal London, Kings College, Newham General, The Brook, St Helier and Chelsea & Westminster undertaking a Sister's post. A new challenge came as a lecturer practitioner at Kings College University and Kings College Hospital where she was responsible for delivering the Biological Science courses, contributing to the intensive care course and overseeing the educational and training needs over a hundred nurses.

In 2001 Andrea rejoined C&W as nurse consultant in critical care and set up the critical care outreach team. She held an honorary lecturer post at Imperial College developing and teaching on the Masters programmes.

Her main clinical and research interests are the use of high flow oxygen therapies, concept of level one care, new organisational systems, the recognition of early deterioration through development of our own EWS.

Helen Dutton
MSc BA, RNT, RGN

Senior Lecturer
School of Nursing Midwifery and Healthcare
University of West London

Helen completed her RGN at Addenbrooke's Hospital Cambridge. After gaining experience in medical and surgical nursing she moved to St Thomas' Hospital London to work in intensive care, then progressing to become a Sister in Cardio-thoracic Intensive Care at the Royal Brompton and Harefield NHS Trust. Her education career started at the Royal Brompton and she is now currently employed as a Senior Lecturer at the University of West London. Intensive and critical care nursing have been her main areas of interest, teaching both pre- and post-qualifying nurses. Currently her main interests are centred on ward-based critical care and the early recognition and treatment of critical illness.

Sharon Elliott
MSc, BA (Hons) RCNT, RN

Sharon qualified as a nurse at the Royal London Hospital and worked in trauma and then critical care. She entered education as a clinical teacher, working in ICU and subsequently as Course Tutor to the ENB 100 course. Currently she works at the University of West London as a senior lecturer specialising in clinical skills and simulation, with a particular interest in the integration of this approach to teaching and learning into curricula. Sharon continues to work part-time in adult critical care.

Jacqui Finch
MSc, BSc (Hons), RGN, RM, ENB 100, Cert Ed, RNT

Senior Lecturer/Practitioner in Intensive Care Nursing
School of Nursing, Midwifery and Healthcare
University of West London and the North West London NHS Trust

Jacqui began her nursing career at the Royal Free Hospital in London, qualifying as a registered nurse in 1984 and then as a registered midwife in 1986. Progressing from junior to senior positions, she has worked in a variety of intensive care settings including general, cardiothoracic, neurosurgical, paediatric and neonatal. Her career in nurse education started in 1989 as a clinical teacher and she currently holds a joint post with the University of West London and an NHS Trust delivering intensive care education for nursing and junior medical staff. Her particular interests are outreach services and the recognition of deteriorating patients, critical care transfer and the care of level 3 patients with multiple organ dysfunction.

Julian Howard
MA, MRCP, FRCA, FFICM

Consultant Intensive Care and Anaesthesia
Educational Board Tutor for Intensive Care Medicine
Royal Free Hospital, London

Julian trained at Oxford University and the Middlesex Hospital, qualifying in 1982. Initially, he worked in general medicine and later in anaesthesia and intensive care, including a year in Australia. He has been in his current post since January 1998.

Margaret Kirkby
RGN, BSc (Hons)

Clinical Nurse Specialist: Patient at Risk and
Resuscitation Team
Royal Free Hospital, London

Margaret trained at University College Hospital, London and
qualified in 1981. Her intensive care career began as a Staff
Nurse at Kings College Hospital, London in 1983. She transferred to the Royal Free Hospital ICU in 1985 and became a
Sister in 1986. In 2001, following periods as Acting Clinical
Nurse Manager in ICU, she helped set up the Critical Care
Outreach Team which combined with the Resuscitation Team in
2005 to become the PARRT. Her key areas of interest are the
management of the acutely unwell ward patient and rehabilitation after critical illness.

Carl Margereson
MSc, BSc (Hons), DipN (Lond) RNT, RGN, RMN

Senior Lecturer/Teaching Fellow
College of Nursing, Midwifery and Healthcare
University of West London

Carl gained clinical experience both in the UK and overseas. He
has worked for a number of years in nurse education with initial
teaching experience gained in Nottingham and Sheffield. On
moving to London in 1985, he returned to clinical practice and
worked in cardiothoracic nursing both at the London Chest
Hospital and the Royal Brompton Hospital. Resuming his career
in education, Carl taught at the Royal Brompton Hospital for
many years before moving into higher education. He currently
teaches on a number of courses at both graduate and postgraduate level.

John Mears
MSc, BSc (Hons), Dip N (Lond), Cert ED, RNT, RGN

Senior Lecturer
School of Nursing, Midwifery and Healthcare
University of West London

John trained at St George's, undertaking the two-year graduate
2+1 course. He was a staff nurse on a cardiac unit at St George's
Hyde Park Corner, later taking on a charge nurse role on an
orthopaedic ward. He undertook the Cert Ed course after a brief
secondment to the school of nursing and having undertaken the
Diploma course at the Royal College of Nursing. He has been in
nurse education since 1982, undertaking tutor and senior tutor
roles before becoming a senior lecturer. During his time at the
university he has worked in the Centre for Research and
Implementation of Clinical Practice teaching and researching in
tissue viability and wound care. He also teaches physiology and
pathophysiology at all levels.

Angela Morgan
RGN, MSc, BSc (Hons), PGCEA

Senior Educator: Intensive Care
St Mary's Hospital, London

Angela trained at the Middlesex Hospital, London, and qualified
in 1982. Following a period as a staff nurse, and then Ward

Sister, she transferred to the Royal Free Hospital, London to
begin her career in intensive care in 1987. She has always
been passionate about teaching and following a year as a
Teaching Sister in intensive care, then spent 10 years as a joint
appointment between St Mary's Hospital, London Intensive
Care Unit and Thames Valley University as a Senior Lecturer
teaching intensive care and introduction to critical care
(high-dependency) nursing. She is currently Senior Educator
for intensive care at Imperial NHS Trust with responsibility
for cross-site education at St Mary's, Charing Cross and
Hammersmith Hospitals.

Ian Peate
EN(G), RGN DipN (Lond), RNT BEd (Hons), MA (Lond), LLM

Professor of Nursing
Editor in chief, *British Journal of Nursing*
Integrating Healthcare Solutions

Ian began his nursing a career in 1981 at Central Middlesex
Hospital, becoming an Enrolled Nurse working in an intensive
care unit. He later undertook three years student nurse training
at Central Middlesex and Northwick Park Hospitals, becoming
a Staff Nurse then a Charge Nurse. He has worked in nurse
education since 1989. His key areas of interest are nursing practice and theory, men's health, sexual health and HIV/AIDS.
Ian has published widely; he is a Professor of Nursing and
Independent Healthcare Consultant and Editor in chief, *British
Journal of Nursing*.

Andrew Sargent
RN, BSc (Hons), PGDip (Learning and Teaching), PGCert
(Research), PhD student

Andrew is a Tutor in Critical Care Nursing in the Florence
Nightingale School of Nursing and Midwifery at King's College
London. His clinical background is in Cardiology, Coronary
Care and Cardiac Intensive Care nursing. He has contributed
to the *British Journal of Cardiac Nursing* and is co-author of
The ECG Workbook. Andrew lives in London with his wife and
two children.

Katie Scales
PG Dip Healthcare Ethics, HDQC Physiology, BEd (Hons)
Nurse Teachers, DPSN, Law Certificate Expert Witness,
ENB 400, ENB 100, ENB 998 RNT RN

Consultant Nurse Critical Care
Imperial College Healthcare NHS Trust

Katie trained at St Thomas' Hospital, London and has an extensive career in critical care nursing including neonatal ITU,
intensive overnight recovery, adult general and cardiac ITU as
well as cardiothoracic ITU with transplantation. In 1989 Katie
became Tutor to the ITU course at St Thomas' Hospital, London
and was a Lecturer in Intensive Care Nursing and Biological
Sciences with the Nightingale Institute. In 1995 she returned to
clinical practice as a Senior Nurse for Practice Development
in the ITU at Harefield Hospital, Middlesex. In 1997 Katie
joined Hammersmith Hospitals NHS Trust as Assistant Director
of Nursing and became a Consultant Nurse in 2000. Katie is
currently a Consultant Nurse in Critical Care at Charing Cross

Hospital, part of Imperial College Healthcare NHS Trust. Katie leads the Outreach critical care service providing support for critically ill patients and their families in ward areas.

Sarah Withey
RGN, ENB 100, ENB 998, City and Guilds Teaching and Assessing, MA

Sarah qualified as an RGN in 1987 and has specialised in Intensive and Critical Care since 1989. After working in Intensive Care at St Thomas', she worked within Cardiothoracic services at The Royal London; managing a cardiothoracic surgical ward before setting up a High Dependency and Fast Track Unit within the trust. Sarah then moved to Guy's and St Thomas' where she designed and delivered the teaching programme across High Dependency Services throughout the trust. In 2001 she became a Clinical Teacher for the Introduction to Critical Care Course (ICCC), she went on to become the Clinical Lead on the ICCC, which is delivered across 12 hospitals within North West London.

Acknowledgements

Ian would like to thank his partner, Jussi Lahtinen, for his continued support and to Helen Dutton for agreeing to co-edit this text.

Helen would like to thank her academic and clinical colleagues for their support and enthusiasm with the preparation of this book. All comments and suggestions have been constructive and gratefully received. She would also like to thank Geoff, Emma and Mike for their love, patience and encouragement during this project.

Publisher's acknowledgements

We are grateful to the following for permission to reproduce copyright material:

Figures

Figures 3.1, 3.7, 3.8, 3.10, 3.12, 3.13, 3.14, 3.15, 4.3, 5.2, 5.3, 6.1, 6.2, 6.4, 6.11, 6.13, 6.14, 6.15, 6.16, 6.17, 8.1, 8.2, 8.3, 8.4, 8.6, 8.7, 9.2, 9.3, 9.6, 9.7, 9.8, 9.10, 9.11, 9.12, 9.13, 9.14, 10.1, 10.2, 10.3, 11.1, 11.2, 11.3, 11.5, 12.1, 12.2, 12.3, 12.4, 12.5 and 12.9 from *Anatomy & Physiology for Health Professionals: An Interactive Journey*, 2nd ed., Pearson Education, Inc. (Colbert, B.J., Ankney, J. and Lee, K.T., 2011), copyright © 2009. Printed and electronically reproduced by permission of Pearson Education, Inc. Upper Saddle River, New Jersey;

Figure 1.1 from *Critical Care Beds: Critical Care Beds Time Series 1999–2011*, Department of Health (www.dh.gov.uk/en), © Crown copyright. Public sector information licensed under the Open Government Licence (OGL) v1.0 (www.nationalarchives.gov.uk/doc/open-government-licence/open-government licence.htm); Figure 1.3 from In-hospital cardiac arrest: is it time for an in-hospital 'chain of Prevention', *Resuscitation*, 81(9): 1209–11 (Smith, G.B., 2010), copyright © 2010, Elsevier; Figure 2.1 from *Motivation and Personality*, 3rd ed., Pearson Education, Inc. (Maslow, A.H., Frager, R.D. and Fadiman, J. (eds), 1987), copyright © 1987. Printed and electronically reproduced by permission of Pearson Education, Inc. Upper Saddle River, New Jersey; Figure 2.2 from *Raising and Escalating Concerns: Guidance for Nurses and Midwives* (Nursing and Midwifery Council, 2010), pp. 12–13. Reproduced with permission. Available at www.nmc-uk.org/Publications/Guidance; Figure 3.2 from *Essentials of Anatomy and Physiology*, 5th edition, Pearson Benjamin Cummings (Martini, F.H. and Bartholomew, E.F., 2009), Figure 3.3, p. 63, copyright © 2010. Reprinted and electronically reproduced by permission of Pearson Education, Inc., Upper Saddle River, New Jersey; Figure 3.3 from *Human Anatomy and Physiology*, 8th ed., Pearson Education Inc. (Marieb, E.N. and Hoehn, K., 2010), Figure 3.7, p. 69, copyright © 2010. Printed and electronically reproduced by permission of Pearson Education, Inc., Upper Saddle River, New Jersey; Figure 6.3 from *Essentials of Anatomy and Physiology*, 5th ed., Pearson Benjamin Cummings (Martini, F.H. and Bartholomew, E.F., 2009), Figure 12.7, p. 414, copyright © 2010. Reprinted and electronically reproduced by permission of Pearson Education, Inc., Upper Saddle River, New Jersey; Figure 6.14 from *Handbook of Transfusion Medicine*, 4th ed. (McClelland, D.B.L. (ed), 2007), Figure 10, p. 61, copyright © Joint UKBTS/HPA Professional Advisory Committee (JPAC), NHS Blood and Transplant; Figure 6.22 adapted from *A Nurse's Survival Guide to Acute Medical Emergencies*, 3rd Edition, Churchill Livingstone (Harrison, R. and Daley, L., 2011), copyright © Elsevier 2011; Figures 6.25 and 6.27 from *2010 Resuscitation Guidelines* (Resuscitation Council (UK), 2010), pp. 83, 88. Reproduced with the kind permission of the Resuscitation Council (UK); Figure 7.1 from Adult choking treatment algorithm, 2010 Resuscitation Guidelines (www.resus.org.uk/pages/achkalgo.pdf). Reproduced with the kind permission of the Resuscitation Council (UK); Figure 7.7 from Chain of survival, *Resuscitation*, 71: 270–1 (Nolan, J., Soar, J. and Eikeland, H., 2006), copyright © 2006, Elsevier; Figure 7.8 from *2010 Resuscitation Guidelines* (Resuscitation Council (UK), 2010), p. 49. Reproduced with the kind permission of the Resuscitation Council (UK); Figures 7.9, 7.10a,b and 7.11 from *Advanced Life Support*, 6th ed., (Resuscitation Council (UK) 2011). The photographs on pages 168 and 169 are reproduced with kind permission by Michael Scott and the Resuscitation Council (UK); Figure 7.14 from *2010 Resuscitation Guidelines* (Resuscitation Council (UK) 2010), p. 60. Reproduced with the kind permission of the Resuscitation Council (UK); Figure 9.4 adapted from Essentials of Anatomy & Physiology, 5th edition, Pearson Benjamin Cummings (Martini, F.H. and Bartholomew, E.F., 2009) Figure 8.5, p. 252, copyright © 2010. Reprinted and electronically reproduced by permission of Pearson Education, Inc., Upper Saddle River, New Jersey; Figure 12.8 adapted from WHO Guidelines on Hand Hygiene in Health Care (revised Aug 2009), Figure 1.21.5b, p. 131, http://whqlibdoc.who.int/publications/2009/9789241597906_eng.pdf, copyright © World Health Organization, 2009; Figure 12.10 from *Emergency Treatment of Anaphylactic Reactions: Guidelines for Healthcare Providers* (Resuscitation Council (UK), 2008), Figure 3, p. 20, Reproduced with the kind permission of the Resuscitation Council (UK); Figure 13.2 from Treating hypovolaemia, NWL Critical Care Network, by Dr J. Handy. Reproduced by kind permission.

Tables

Table 1.2 from Classification of severity of illness (Department of Health, 2000), © Crown copyright; Table 1.3 from Hospital episode statistics data comparing admissions from 1998–9 with 2009–10 (www.hesonline.nhs.uk) (Department of Health, © Crown copyright; Tables 3.1, 12.1 from *Anatomy and Physiology for Nursing and Health Professionals*, Pearson Education (Bruce Colbert, Jeff Ankney, Karen Lee, Martin Steggall and Maria Dingle, 2009) copyright © 2009. Printed and electronically reproduced by permission of Pearson Education, Inc. Upper Saddle River, New Jersey; Table 12.3 adapted from Shock, systemic inflammatory response syndrome and multiple organ dysfunction syndrome, in *Critical Care Nursing: A Holistic Approach*, 9th ed. (Johnson, K. and Henry, K., Morton, P. and Fontaine, D. (eds), 2009). Reproduced with permission from Lippincott, Williams and Wilkins; Table 12.4 from High impact intervention: Central venous catheter care bundle (Department of Health, 2011), pp. 2–3 (http://hcai.dh.gov.uk/files/2011/03/2011-03-14-HII-Central-Venous-Catheter-Care-Bundle-FINAL.pdf), © Crown copyright; Table 12.6 from Surviving sepsis campaign: international guidelines for the management of severe sepsis and septic shock, in *Critical Care Medicine*, 36(1): 296, 327 (Dellinger, R., Levy, M., and Carlet, J. et al., 2008), copyright © 2008, Wolters Kluwer Health. Permission conveyed through Copyright Clearance Center.

In some instances we have been unable to trace the owners of copyright material, and we would appreciate any information that would enable us to do so.

dical emergency, cardiopulmonary arrest,
cus of education and training of health
Resuscitation teams were formed as early
wever it was not until 1966 that the first
y resuscitation (CPR) guidelines were
er et al. 2006 b). Guidance on CPR con-
dated (Resuscitation Council UK 2010),
rdiopulmonary arrest are improving but
disappointing with survival rates to dis-
ospital arrests varying from 14.7–20.6%
2008). Traditionally, much attention has
after-arrest care, more recently however
s been shifting towards recognising those
e at risk of arrest or deterioration, with
enting the medical emergency occurring.
the form of medical emergency teams
f outreach services is now a key feature
rusts. Their aims are to prevent deteriora-
ulmonary arrest, averting the medical

teriorate and present as a medical emer-
quire critical care. Whatever the cause or
ctor of a medical emergency, the physio-
ences for the patient are similar. Medical
ect oxygen delivery to cells, tissues and
is essential for glucose metabolism and
spate (ATP) production: without oxygen
gan dysfunction, failure and death will
e. Prompt responses are required to sup-
ans until recovery or death and this often
port of critical care services.
studies in the late 1990s highlighted prob-
cognition and management of the acutely
on adult wards. The evidence indicated
vho deteriorate do not normally do so
e' but have abnormal clinical parameters
rs before the presentation of a medical
dhill et al. (1999) looked over a 13-month
ts admitted from the ward to the intensive
patient group had been in hospital for a
4 hours, and were at least 24 hours after
ysiological variables at 0–6hrs, 6–12hrs
efore admission were recorded. Goldhill

et al. (1999) surmised from their data that abnormal respiratory rate, heart rate and adequacy of oxygenation were strong indicators that a patient was at risk of clinical deterioration. Many critically ill patients had been identified by the clinical staff in this study, monitoring had been increased and interventions such as oxygen therapy and continuous positive airway pressure (CPAP) had been commenced in some. Despite these efforts though, cardiopulmonary arrests were not averted. Schein et al. (1990) highlighted the importance of respiratory rate in their study, finding in the 64 arrests that occurred, the average respiratory rate prior to arrest was between 28–30 breaths per minute. Only 5% of these patients survived CPR to discharge. The conclusion drawn from these and other studies was that if the patients had been identified and treated appropriately earlier, it was likely that the arrests may have been prevented.

Early identification

Although most people in hospital are unlikely to become seriously unwell, a significant number will require interventions in order to prevent or treat a medical emergency. Individuals move from experiencing minor physiological derangements, through a period of deterioration and more serious illness, which, if left undetected and untreated may progress to a life-threatening medical emergency, culminating in cardiopulmonary arrest. As people move along this continuum of wellness to the stage where death is imminent, they will be experiencing major physiological changes. The body will be attempting to restore homeostasis by the activation of compensatory mechanisms, such as increasing rate of breathing or heart rate. These compensatory mechanisms in themselves require additional energy, placing extra physiological demands on the individual. In the early stages of acute illness, these mechanisms may be sufficient to meet the extra demands, healing may occur and the problem resolve. However, if the underlying problem remains untreated, or is unresponsive to treatments, deterioration will continue. There may be a rapid progression of severity of illness resulting in cardiac arrest. Examples of acute illnesses that may or may deteriorate to a medical emergency are included in Table 1.1.

Understanding that signs of compensation may be indicative of acute illness with possible rapid deterioration should mean that if these clinical variables are recorded they can be addressed early in the continuum and the medical emergency averted. Unfortunately, this is not always the case, and when problems are recognised the appropriate treatment and management is not followed.

1

Assessment and reco
emergencies in acute

Helen Dutton

Aims

This chapter aims to give the reader an insight into
identification of risk of clinical deterioration and t
care in an appropriate and timely manner.

Objectives

After reading this chapter you will be able to:

→ Give an overview of the national and internatio
aimed at supporting the adult who has the pot

→ Understand that there are clinical signs of deter
most life-threatening events

→ Perform, analyse and interpret a rapid clinical a
risk of deterioration/medical emergency

→ Use early warning systems as a tool to calculate
familiar with interdisciplinary communication to

→ Understand how a 'chain of prevention' can be
detect patient deterioration

→ Have a context on which to base future chapter
Recognising and Responding to Medical Emerge

Introdu

The ultimate
has been th
care profess
as the 1930
cardiopulme
published ((
tinues to b
techniques i
results rema
charge for
(Peberdy et
been placed
the emphasi
patients wh
the aim of p
Expert advic
(MET) and/o
in many acu
tion to care
emergency.

Recogn

Patients who
gency often
precipitating
logical conse
emergencies
organs. Oxy
aderosinetrip
cellular and
inevitably en
port failing c
requires the s

A number
lems with the
unwell patie
that patients
'out of the b
often some
emergency. G
period at pati
care unit. Th
minimum of
surgery. The
and 12–24hr

Table 1.1 Examples of acute illnesses that may lead to a medical emergency. Note how compensatory mechanisms of increased RR, HR and decreased adequacy of oxygenation are a feature of most of the above.

Example of acute illness	Physiological derangements	Signs of compensation that may be evident
Airway swelling	Airway obstruction Hypoxeamia, hypercarbia	Raised heart rate (HR) and blood pressure
Acute asthma	Hypoxeamia Bronchoconstriction causing increased work of breathing	Raised respiratory rate, HR, BP Use of accessory muscles
Pneumothorax	Presence of air in the pleural space Pain Hypoxeamia	Sensation of breathlessness Use of accessory muscles increasing respiration rate (RR), HR and BP
Myocardial infarction	Death of myocardium due to blockage of a branch of a coronary artery Pain	Raised RR, HR BP, peripheral vasoconstriction
Acute left ventricular failure	Failure of the left ventricle to pump blood effectively into the aorta and round the body Pulmonary venous pressures rise and lead to the development of pulmonary oedema Hypoxaemia Frothy sputum	Raised RR, HR Use of accessory muscles, peripheral vasoconstriction
Hypovolaemic shock	Reduction on amount of blood/fluid in the circulation Hypoxaemia	Raised RR, HR BP lowered, peripheral vasoconstriction
Severe sepsis	An inflammatory response to infection causing vasodilation Raised central temperature	HR, RR, raised Warm with peripheral vasodilation Lowered BP

Suboptimal treatment

McQuillan et al.'s (1998) confidential enquiry into quality of care before admission to intensive care identified problems with the management of patients in whom deterioration had been recognised. Some 100 consecutive adult emergency admissions between two intensive care units were prospectively reviewed. The management of the ward patients prior to their admission to intensive care was found to be suboptimal in over 50% of the acute emergency adult patients. Alarmingly, the majority of problems identified were with airway management, oxygen therapy, breathing and circulation, the very basics of acute care management. Patients who received poor-quality care before admission to the intensive therapy unit (ITU) were 20% more likely to die than those that received optimal care (McQuillan et al. 1998).

Adverse events in acute care are not only an issue for the UK, but are part of an international problem. An Australian retrospective review of 12 months of medical records of patients prior to development of medical emergencies revealed a failure of health care professionals to appreciate the urgency of clinical changes (Buist et al. 1999). Franklin and Matthew (1994) in their USA study reported a failure of communication between nurses and physicians, a failure of physicians to act appropriately, and failure of the ITU team to stabilise the patient prior to transfer to ITU. Another Australian project, the Medical Early Response Intervention and Therapy (MERIT) study, randomised 23 hospitals to either use a medical emergency team, or to continue as usual (Merit Study Investigators 2005). This large study failed to demonstrate a direct effect of MET on unplanned emergency admissions to ITU or unexpected deaths: 50% of calls were made to the arrest team, without a cardiac arrest (non-MET group). This is in stark contrast to the UK where arrest teams are only summoned after the event. Interestingly, the cardiac arrest and unexpected death rate fell in both groups of hospitals during the study period.

The changing nature of acute care and acute care delivery

The profile of patients admitted to hospital has changed over the last few decades as the emphasis moves towards managing health care in the primary sector. The growing proportion of older people in the population combined with advances in management of many chronic illnesses has given rise to increasing number of admissions of older people, many of whom have several co-morbidities (Margereson 2010). This increase in the elderly population contributes to greater seasonal variations in admissions, which culminated in the 'winter bed crisis' of 1998–9, when patients died due to lack of appropriate care facilities (Lipley 2000).

National initiatives in acute and critical care

The Audit Commission's report in 1999, closely followed by the Department of Health (DH) publication *Comprehensive Critical Care – A review of adult critical care services* (DH 2000) recommended that patients should be classified according to their illness, and the appropriate care with necessary resources brought to them, expanding critical care provision and meeting seasonal surges in demand. The now familiar four levels of care (level 0–level 3) were identified, and have more recently been clarified with more detailed examples by the Intensive Care Society (2009) (see Table 1.2).

An expansion of critical care beds outside the 'four walls' of intensive care was recommended (DH 2000). Spreading critical care beyond the boundaries of ITU allows more flexible use of beds as they can be used by

Table 1.2 DH (2000) classification of severity of illness. Level 1 patients are usually cared for in acute wards, level 2 in acute wards or a high-dependency unit (HDU), level 3 usually cared for in ITU or some HDUs.

	DH (2000)	ICS (2009) A selection of specific examples
Level 0	Patients whose needs can be met through normal ward care in an acute hospital	Intravenous therapy Observations required less frequently than 4-hourly
Level 1	Patients at risk of their condition deteriorating, or those recently relocated from higher levels of care whose needs can be met on an acute ward with additional advice and support from the critical care team	Requiring a minimum of 4-hourly observation on the basis of clinical need Patients requiring continuous oxygen therapy Epidural analgesia or patient-controlled analgesia in use Postoperative surgical patients who are still requiring 4-hourly observations Diabetic patients receiving a continuous infusion of insulin Abnormal vital signs but not requiring a higher level of critical care
Level 2	Patients requiring more detailed observation or intervention including support for a single failing organ system or postoperative care, and those stepping down from higher levels of care	Basic respiratory support e.g. requiring 50% oxygen or supported ventilation by face mask, e.g. CPAP, non-invasive ventilation (NIV) Basic cardiovascular support treatment of circulatory instability Use of a central venous pressure (CVP) line for basic monitoring or central venous access to deliver therapeutic agents Use of an arterial line for basic monitoring of the arterial pressure and/or sampling of arterial blood Single intravenous vasoactive drug used to support or control arterial pressure, cardiac output or organ perfusion
Level 3	Patients requiring advanced respiratory support alone or basic respiratory support together with support of at least two organ systems. This level included all complex patients requiring support for multi-organ failure	As per DH (2000)

Sources: DH (2009) and ICS (2009).

The changing nature of acute care and acute care delivery 5

patients of varying degrees of illness at times of peak demand. This, however, has implications for the education, training and numbers of ward staff. Critical care outreach teams and the use of early warning scores were identified as central to the development of ward-based critical care, to support and equip health care professionals with the necessary skills to move care forward in a timely manner (DH 2000).

In the 10 years or so since the publication of *Comprehensive Critical Care* there has been a continued upward trend in number of admissions, mean age and proportion of emergency admissions but with a decreasing mean length of stay (Table 1.3). Even though the overall number

of patients in hospital is reduced, the number of patients treated has increased. The complexity of care is growing, impacting on acute care services (NCEPOD 2005).

The provision of level 2 beds has increased since *Comprehensive Critical Care*, from 720 in 1999, to 1,672 in 2011 (DH 2011) (Figure 1.1), providing a greater number of facilities for close monitoring and support therapies such as non-invasive ventilation (NIV). Interestingly, the number of level 1 beds are not recorded in this dataset. Many level 1 patients have potential to become seriously unwell and deteriorate to a medical emergency. This level of care is important to facilitate early detection and appropriate care escalation.

Table 1.3 Hospital episode statistics data comparing admissions from 1998–9 with 2009–10

	Total admissions	Mean age	Average of 75+	Emergency admissions	Mean length of stay (LOS)	Median LOS
1998–99	11 016 652	45 years	2 220 820 20%	3 784 954 34%	8.4	2
2009–10	14 537 712	51 years	3 837 988 26%	5 177 887 36%	5.6	1

Source: Hospital Episode Statistics Headling Figures 1998–99 and 2009–10 (www.hesonline.nhs.uk).

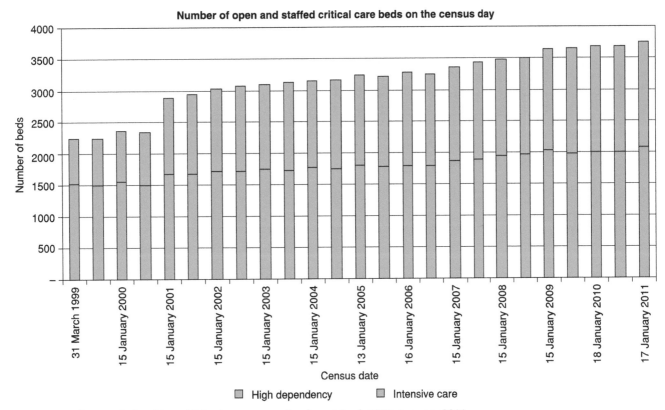

Figure 1.1 Changes in level 2 and 3 beds on census day from March 1999–January 2011

Source: Department of Health, Critical care beds: critical care beds timeseries 1999–2011 (Available from http://www.dh.gov.uk/en/Publicationsandstatistics/Statistics/Performancedataandstatistics/Beds/DH_077451).

Where are we now?

Disappointingly, five years after *Comprehensive Critical Care*, the problems of recognising and responding appropriately to prevent clinical deterioration had not been eradicated. The National Enquiry into Confidential Deaths (NCEPOD, 2005) presented their report into the management on acutely unwell medical patients, 1677 of whom were reviewed over 226 hospitals. Early warning scores (EWS) were used in only 73% of the patients, 44% of hospitals in the study did not provide outreach services. Pre-ITU medical review was deemed not acceptable in 10% of ITU admissions, and only 58% of patients received prompt and appropriate interventions. Respiratory rate monitoring was poor and written requests regarding the type and frequency of observations, rare (NCEPOD 2005). The National Patient Safety Agency (NPSA, 2007a) found further evidence that suboptimal care was continuing to contribute to preventable deaths. The National Institute for Health and Clinical Excellence (NICE) considered the evidence for physiological track and trigger systems and care escalation strategies. They published *Clinical Guideline 50* to give recommendations regarding the recognition of and response to acute illness in adults in hospital (NICE 2007). Support publications from the DH analyse the role of outreach services (DH 2007), and the role of the health care team in a chain of response DH (2009) (see Figure 1.2).

Core components of the chain of response are the ability to recognise (recogniser) and respond to (primary responder) signs of deterioration in the patient. The individuals performing these roles may vary, but recogniser and aspects of responder roles are likely to fall within the nurses' domain of care (DH 2009). Additional training may be necessary for aspects of the primary responder role but assessment and interpretative skills are essential for the competent execution of both these roles. Key clinical signs of deterioration such as tachypnoea, tachycardia, hypotension and altered level of consciousness (Resuscitation Council UK 2010) need to be interpreted in the context of a comprehensive and systematic approach to patient assessment.

> It is essential that nurses develop good assessment skills and the ability to interpret signs within the clinical context, in order to fulfil the roles of recogniser and primary responder.

Assessment priorities – the ABCDE approach

In order to prevent medical emergencies nurses must understand the clinical priorities of potentially life-threatening problems to enable them to respond to and treat problems in the correct order. Patients with serious abnormal signs are a medical emergency and require prioritised interventions using the ABCDE approach, with an appreciation of the level of urgency. Less severe

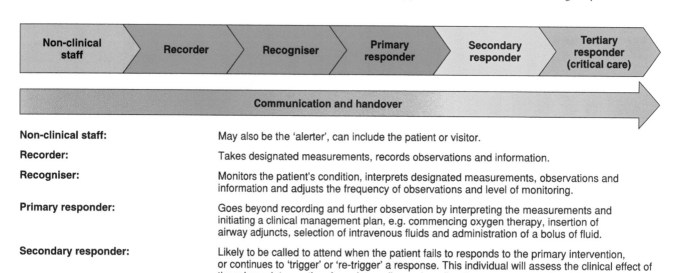

Non-clinical staff: May also be the 'alerter', can include the patient or visitor.

Recorder: Takes designated measurements, records observations and information.

Recogniser: Monitors the patient's condition, interprets designated measurements, observations and information and adjusts the frequency of observations and level of monitoring.

Primary responder: Goes beyond recording and further observation by interpreting the measurements and initiating a clinical management plan, e.g. commencing oxygen therapy, insertion of airway adjuncts, selection of intravenous fluids and administration of a bolus of fluid.

Secondary responder: Likely to be called to attend when the patient fails to responds to the primary intervention, or continues to 'trigger' or 're-trigger' a response. This individual will assess the clinical effect of the primary intervention, formulate a diagnosis, refine the management plan, initiate a secondary response and will have the knowledge to recognise when referral to critical care is indicated.

Tertiary responder (critical care): This role will be undertaken by staff possessing appropriate critical care competences such as advanced airway management, resuscitation, and clinical examination and interpretation of critically ill patients.

Figure 1.2 Chain of response

Source: Adapted from Department of Health (2009) *Competencies for Recognising and Responding to Acutely Ill Patients in Hospital*, Fig. 1, p. 9.

> **A** assess **airway** and treat if needed.
> **B** assess **breathing** and treat if needed.
> **C** assess **circulation** and treat if needed.
> **D** assess **disability** and treat if needed.
> **E** **expose** and **examine** patient fully once ABCD are stable.
>
> (Cooper *et al.* 2006a)

problems, recognised, responded to and escalated in a timely manner, should prevent the medical emergency occurring. The use of ABCDE is a recurring theme in each of the chapters of this book. This simple mnemonic was first used in cardiopulmonary resuscitation, but is now also recommended for acute care patients because it supports a rapid assessment of the patient at risk of deterioration (NCEPOD 2005, NICE 2007, Resuscitation Council UK 2010). Used in combination with track and trigger tools, good communication and care escalation, early interventions to treat clinical problems is aided. A systematic assessment is an expansion of what may be seen as the 'task' of filling in observation charts, which is often delegated to health care assistants. Using information from what you see (look), what you hear (listen), what you feel, what can be measured (measure) and additional information required in the form of investigations (investigate) ensures that all the senses are used to gather information that informs the interpretation of vital signs. The approach to a rapid ABCDE assessment will be discussed (see Figure 1.3 for a summary), but please note that further chapters contain detailed discussion of assessment, focusing on each of the main systems.

> A comprehensive approach to assessment should include:
>
> - **Look (inspect)**
> - **Listen (auscultate)**
> - **Feel (palpate/percuss)**
> - **Measure**
> - **Investigate.**

Assessment approach

When initially approaching the patient, notice their appearance, whether they are collapsed, in obvious respiratory distress, or unable to talk coherently. This immediate observation will give you an indication of the urgency of the assessment.

> Patient collapsed, with no response and showing no signs of life, necessitates a call for help and CPR (see Chapter 7).

Airway

Airway patency and adequacy of cerebral perfusion can be if assumed if a patient is engaging in a conversation, demonstrating understanding and awareness. However, partial airway obstruction is not always immediately obvious so should always be specifically excluded by ensuring that any increased respiratory effort, abnormal sounds such as stridor, grunting, gurgling and wheezing are observed for (Subbe 2006). Any of these signs require immediate management. They are covered fully in Chapter 7 and should be treated prior to moving on to assessment of breathing. Asking a patient to demonstrate an effective cough can give insight into risks of aspiration, and forms part of airway assessment.

Breathing

Changes in respiratory status can occur due to respiratory, metabolic, neurological and cardiovascular compromise, and is therefore a sensitive indicator of deterioration. Respiratory assessment is covered in detail in Chapter 5. Respiratory pattern should be determined, looking for patient indicators of distress such as use of accessory muscles, paradoxical breathing, position and difficulty in taking in complete sentences. Central cyanosis, a late sign of hypoxeamia, should be excluded. Palpation to assess equal chest expansion can exclude medical emergencies such as pneumothorax, and auscultation can identify adventitious sounds indicative of respiratory deterioration. The importance of respiratory rate cannot be overemphasised, with over 20 breaths per minute a cause for concern, and 30 breaths per minute or more indicating significant pathology necessitating immediate action (Subbe 2006). Pulse oximeters can give valuable information regarding oxygen saturations, enabling hypoxeamia to be detected. O'Driscoll *et al.* (2008) refer to SaO_2 as the 'fifth vital sign' and NICE (2007) consider SaO_2 an important addition to early warning scores. However, care must be taken when interpreting SaO_2 levels within the normal range: other factors such as inspired oxygen percentage, respiratory rate and work of breathing must be taken into account. SpO_2 monitoring will not detect hypercapnea, which can only be ascertained from arterial blood gas (ABG) analysis. The British Thoracic Society has published guidelines on oxygen therapy (O'Driscoll *et al.* 2008) and recommends that patients with an SpO_2 of below 94% should have ABG checked to assess for acid-base balance and hypercapnea. If medical emergencies such as tension pneumothorax or acute severe asthma are present you should call for help to get these treated before completing a detailed cardiovascular assessment. Recording measurements on the observation chart and noting any triggers on the early warning score (EWS) alerts the nurse to a potential medical emergency.

> When using pulse oximetry always record the amount of oxygen the patient is receiving and the flow device.
>
> Pulse oximetry does not detect hypercapnea.
>
> In patients whose SpO_2 falls below 94% ABG analysis should be considered, to check for hypercapnea and metabolic problems.
>
> (BTS 2008)

Circulation

The circulatory system is the transport mechanism by which the oxygenated blood is propelled to the tissues. A detailed cardiovascular assessment is discussed in Chapter 6. Looking at the patient should reveal any obvious massive blood loss, though internal bleeding is not readily apparent. Patient pallor as a result of sympathetic nervous system mediated vasoconstriction is an indicator of poor cardiac output. A grey sweaty patient is extremely unwell and expert help should be sought immediately.

Palpation of pulses aids assessment of the circulation. A weak and thready pulse or one with a low pulse volume is associated with low cardiac output; this is most likely to be due to hypovoleamia, though cardiac failure/shock also needs to be considered. A strong and bounding pulse is associated with the vasodilation of sepsis or anaphylaxis. Peripheral temperature tends to be cooler (feel hands and feet to see if they are cool, or warm) if cardiac output is reduced, and capillary refill time prolonged. Pitting oedema can alert the nurse to possible cardiac, renal and fluid balance problems. A normal heart rate varies from 60–100 beats per minute, values outside the range will cause an EWS to trigger. An irregular pulse should be followed up by a 12-lead ECG, to identify and enable treatment of arrhythmias such as atrial fibrillation. Guidelines for immediate treatments of tachyarrhythmia or bradyarrhythmia have been formulated by the Resuscitation Council UK (2010) and should form the basis of clinical decision-making (see Chapter 7). Rates above 150 or below 40 are unlikely to be consistent with adequate cardiac output, so expert help is required immediately.

> **Has your patient got an irregular pulse?**
> - Perform a 12-lead ECG.
> - Check that serum electrolytes, K^+ and Mg^{++} are within normal range.

Record the central temperature, and note that above 38° Centigrade could indicate infection, and would trigger on the observation chart. Check trust policy for performing a septic screen to help identify possible pathogens.

> On the observation chart, if the **heart rate** is **higher** than the **systolic blood pressure**, this is a cause for concern.

Blood pressure measurements vary with age, but systolic values range from 90–140mmHg. A drop of more than 40mmHg in the systolic pressure is a cause for concern, even if the value remains above 100mmHg. Changes in blood pressure are often a late sign of deterioration as the sympathetic response of vasoconstriction and increased force of myocardial contraction tend to compensate in the earlier stages of shock. The diastolic pressure reflects the degree of vasoconstriction, and is usually greater than 60mmHg. Vasoconstriction (as in hypovolaemia or cardiogenic shock) will raise the diastolic pressure, and narrow the pulse pressure. Vasodilation will reduce the diastolic pressure (as in sepsis or anaphylaxis) and raise the pulse pressure.

> **What is pulse pressure?**
> The difference between systolic and diastolic blood pressure.
> Normal range 35–45mmHg.

The average pressure throughout the cardiac cycle (mean arterial pressure) needs to be adequate to maintain organ perfusion. Indicators of good organ perfusion would be a urine output of more than 0.5ml/kg/hour and an alert orientated patient. Fluid balance is integral to the circulatory assessment and would normally be about 500mls positive over a 24-hour period.

> **Mean arterial pressure (MAP)**
> MAP = 1/3 pulse pressure + diastolic pressure.
> MAP reflects organ perfusion, and should be above 70mmHg.

After completing assessment of circulation record the observations, and note the parameters that trigger on the observation chart. Consider if expert help is needed immediately, and/or if concern is sufficient to require that the patient is cannulated with large bore cannula (12–14 French gauge) to enable rapid fluid resuscitation as necessary. If the patient is sufficiently stable, move on to assessment of disability.

Disability

In your initial approach, you will have noted whether your patient is talking to you. This can be used as part of the assessment of level of consciousness, using the AVPU – alert, voice, pain, unresponsive – method of assessment. If the level of consciousness is reduced, then the Glasgow Coma Scale (GCS) is a useful tool to assess neurological response. For a detailed neurological assessment please see Chapter 9. A GSC of 8 or less is a particular cause for concern, the patient needs positioning to protect the airway and expert help may be required. Blood glucose level needs to be assessed as both hyper- and hypoglycaemia can present as a medical emergency requiring urgent treatment. Hypotension or hypoxia as a cause of altered neurological status must be considered, and treated as a matter of priority. Record neurological status, and score on the observation chart as appropriate.

AVPU classification

A = alert.
V = responds to voice.
P = responds only to pain full stimuli.
U = unresponsive to all stimuli.

Resuscitation Council UK (2010)

Exposure

A head-to-toe examination is necessary to ensure every detail is considered (Smith 2003). Signs such as urticaria may signify an allergic reaction, an inflamed area on the buttock may indicate a source of sepsis and rashes indicative of meningitis are examples of clinical signs that can aid diagnosis and treatment. In addition to considering initial interventions a full review of patient charts, looking for trends, requests and reviews of relevant investigations, and decisions regarding the level of care required should be considered.

Table 1.4 Checklist for a rapid ABCDE assessment

Professional behaviour	• Be respectful and non-discriminatory at all times (NMC 2008) • Ensure comfort and dignity of patient • Demonstrate professional behaviour throughout (NMC 2008)
Preparation	• Wash hands/apply hand gel/universal precautions as appropriate
Communication skills	• Introduce self to patient, make clear requests, communicate effectively with patient and seek consent • Note appropriateness of response: orientated, vague or confused
Perform a quick systematic (ABCDE) assessment, accurately recording assessment findings, taking action as appropriate at each stage	
AIRWAY	**Assess patency** • Look for signs of airway obstruction such as paradoxical breathing, central cyanosis • Listen for signs of decreased patency such as stridor, snoring, crowing, wheezing, or gurgling • Note ability to cough and clear airway secretions • Feel for moving air as necessary *Action appropriately* Positioning, simple suction, nasopharyngeal/Guedel airway insertion. *Call for help if required*
BREATHING	Observe patient colour and position: • Centrally – lips and oral mucosa for cyanosis • Peripherally – fingers for cyanosis/clubbing • Use of accessory muscles • Assess oxygen saturations, check that acceptable ranges for patient have been recorded by medical staff • Note oxygen percentage and delivery method • Listen to what patient is saying and the ease with which they are talking • Listen and observe patient's breathing for one full minute, noting rate • Listen to breath sounds using a stethoscope • Check that the trachea midline • Look and feel for bilateral chest expansion, note depth and rhythm of breathing *Action appropriately* Position and increase oxygen as necessary according to BTS (O'Driscoll 2008) guidance to maintain target saturations. *Call for help if required*

→

Table 1.4 (*continued*)

CIRCULATION	• Look at colour/pallor
	• Look for obvious signs of blood loss
	• Feel limbs noting warmth and perfusion
	• Note temperature change along all limbs
	• Palpate pulse (radial) for 30 secs if regular (60 secs if irregular) noting rate, rhythm and characteristics
	• Assess capillary refill in finger (apply pressure for 5 seconds with finger above heart level)
	• Palpate with thumb for 5 seconds for signs of pitting oedema
	• Record temperature
	• Record blood pressure. Calculate pulse pressure and mean arterial pressure (MAP) as appropriate
	• Measure urine output at > 0.5mls/k/hour
	• Assess fluid balance
	Action appropriately. Call for help if required
	Insert a large bore cannula (12–14fg) if you think shock is present or likely
DISABILITY	• Uses AVPU to correctly assess level of wakefulness
	• Check blood glucose level
	Action appropriately. Call for help if required
EXPOSURE	• Inspect wounds/drains
	• Skin for rashes/erythema
	• Check invasive lines for phlebitis
Investigations	Identify and interpret relevant information gained from simple initial investigations such as:
	• Hb, urea, creatinine electrolytes (K^+ and Na^+, Mg^{++})
	• 12-lead ECG
	• White blood cell count (WBC), C-reactive protein (CRP)
	• Chest x-ray (CXR)
	• Simple arterial blood gas analysis: acid-base status hypoxeamia, hypercarbia, BE, lactate
Care escalation	• Complete observations on chart
	• Calculate track and trigger, escalate care appropriately using Situation, Background, Assessment, Recommendation (SBAR) or Reason–Story–Vital Signs–Plan (RSVP) as a communication tool

Early warning scores (EWS) as an aid to detect deterioration

NICE (2007) recommended that physiological track and trigger scoring systems should be utilised in monitoring all patients in acute care settings, with every patient being monitored at least every 12 hours. Six physiological parameters were identified as essential by NICE (2007). Deviation from the normal range of one or more of the parameters can be used to generate an early warning score (EWS). Urine output was not included as a core parameter as all patients are not catheterised, but this and other variables such as pain assessment, lactate, blood glucose, arterial pH and base deficit are considered important parameters to be considered in assessment of patient stability.

Track and trigger systems should include:

- Respiratory rate
- Oxygen saturations
- Heart rate
- Systolic blood pressure
- Temperature
- Level of consciousness.

NICE (2007)

Table 1.5 Example of a graded response strategy

EWS score	Clinical risk	Action
Total score 0–2		Minimum 12-hourly obs
Total score 3–5	Low	Alert nurse in charge. Escalate care if needed Increase frequency of observations to 4-hourly
Total score 6	Medium	Alert nurse in charge and doctor • Doctor: to attend within 1 hour • Patient's primary medical team and outreach to be informed Increase frequency of observations to 1–2-hourly
Total score 7–8	Medium/high	Alert nurse in charge and doctor • Doctor to attend within 30 mins • Patient's primary medical team informed • Doctor to discuss with senior doctor and/or outreach team Frequency of observations at least hourly; consider continuous monitoring
Total score 9 or more	High	Alert nurse in charge and doctor. Doctor to attend within 15 minutes. Doctor to discuss with: • Senior doctor • Emergency/ICU team with critical care competencies, diagnostic skills, advanced airway management and resuscitation skills Continuous monitoring

Source: Adapted from Resuscitation Council UK (2011) *Immediate Life Support*, 3rd ed. London: Resuscitation Council (UK).

Classification of track and trigger systems

Track and trigger systems can be categorised into single-parameter systems, multi-parameter early warning systems, and aggregated weighted scoring systems (DH and Modernisation Agency 2003). Single-parameter systems will trigger on one extreme observation value. These are simple to use, but do not allow a graded response strategy. Smith *et al.* (2008) suggest that the sensitivity of these systems is too low, meaning that some patients at risk may not be identified. More commonly used in the UK are multi-parameter systems, and aggregate weighted track and trigger systems (AWTTS). With these systems a score is obtained by adding together points that are assigned to deviation from normal observations, thus generating an EWS. The benefit of calculating an EWS is that it allows for monitoring of clinical progress. The EWS can identify patients in low-, medium- and high-risk groups and form part of a graded response strategy (NICE 2007) (Table 1.5).

AWTTS allocate points to disordered physiological parameters in a weighted manner, and these points are added to generate the early warning score. Low-, medium- and high-risk categories are identified within score bands, and specific actions are required according to the score

obtained. Unfortunately, more complex EWS systems are prone to calculation errors, though the development of computed bedside systems may enhance the accuracy and speed of calculations (Prytherch *et al.* 2006).

Working towards an NHS Early Warning Score (NEWS)

Currently a variety of approaches to track and trigger are being used in clinical practice. The Acute Medicine Task Force (ATMF) recognised that this lack of standardisation of EWS across the NHS prevents it becoming part of routine training for all health care professionals (Royal College of Physicians 2007). Caution is needed when using EWS as not all systems are validated. The development of a national validated NHS Early Warning Score (NEWS) could provide benefits of clarity and consistency, thereby reducing user error, and is currently under development (Royal College of Physicians 2007, National Outreach Forum 2011). Prytherch *et al.* (2010) have developed and validated a paper-based simple AWTTS, an adaption of which is shown in Table 1.6. They suggest that this system could form a template for NEWS, and work is continuing in this area.

Table 1.6 Example of an aggregate weighted track and trigger system

Score	3	2	1	0	1	2	3
Pulse rate		< 40	41–50	51–90	91–110	111–130	> or = 131
Breathing rate	< 8		9–11	12–20		21–24	> or = 25
Temperature	< or = 35°C		35.1–36.0	36.1–38	38.1–39	> or = 39.1	
SBP	< or = 90	91–80	81–100	111–249	> 250		
Oxygen saturations	< 88%	92–93%	94–95%	> 96% air		Any O_2	
Central nervous system use AVPU scale				A Alert			V P U

Sources: Adapted from Prytherch *et al.* (2010) and Resuscitation Council UK (2011).

CASE STUDY 1.1 Joseph Ryan – Part 1

It's 14.30 and you are caring for Joseph Ryan, aged 63, admitted earlier that morning with a 3–4 day history of a productive cough, with expectoration of green sputum. He was previously fit and healthy and has been treated initially by his GP with a course of antibiotics. He has failed to improve and is now extremely breathless.

On approaching Joseph you notice that he is sitting upright and looks in some respiratory difficulty. You introduce yourself to him, as you wash your hands and apply hand gel. The screens are pulled round and you ask Joseph if he is happy for you to perform an assessment. Joseph replies that he is happy for you to examine him, but not to ask too many questions as he is very tired. You note that he appears orientated but has some difficulty in continuing the conversation.

Airway

You assess his airway as clear, but listen carefully for stridor or gurgling that may indicate partial airway obstruction. You ask him to cough, which he is able to do effectively and so you surmise that he has a low risk of aspiration. As he is in no immediate danger you continue with your assessment.

Breathing

Joseph's lips and oral mucosa show no evidence of central cyanosis, but Joseph's use of accessory muscles indicates respiratory distress. Peripherally his fingers look a little pale. You attach the oxygen saturation probe to obtain a reading of 92% on 2L of oxygen, which he is receiving via nasal specs. You check his admission sats and note that they have fallen from 96%. This is outside the target saturation of 94–98% which has been set by your medical colleagues.

You are aware of the BTS guidance (O'Driscoll *et al.* 2008) so you increase the oxygen flow to 4L, making a mental note to recheck the saturation in a few minutes. You are concerned that he is mouth breathing and think that a face mask may be more appropriate for him. After counting his respiratory rate at 29 breaths per minute, you record this on the observation chart and note that it is in the red area of the chart, which will score 3 on the early warning score. His reduced SpO_2 and the fact he is receiving oxygen therapy also trigger on the EWS.

After seeking Joseph's consent you auscultate his lungs. You think you hear some crackles on inspiration, but as this is a skill that you are just developing you decide to ask the medical staff to confirm your findings.

On palpation you note equal lung expansion and that the trachea is midline, but his breathing is shallow and laboured.

Your recheck the oxygen saturations and note they have increased to 94% (which scores 1 on the EWS) despite his mouth breathing. You are reassured that there has been some response to this initial intervention, but plan to ask the medical staff to take an arterial blood gas sample to evaluate acid-base status. You feel that he is stable enough for you to continue your assessment.

Circulation

Joseph looks a little pale, but there is no obvious blood loss, and his radial pulse is easy to palpate, with a good pulse pressure. His wrist feels warm, and the pulse is regular, but tachycardic at 108 beats per minute. Capillary refill is at 2 seconds, and his blood pressure is 125/85. You note the normal pulse pressure, but do not calculate the mean

.7 Examples of systems for communication of deterioration in hospitals: SBAR and RSVP

		RSVP	
tion	Identify yourself and from where you are calling Identify patient by name, consultant, location resuscitation status and reason for concern	The reason	State identity of caller Check you are talking to the right person State patient's name, location, and reason for call
ground	Reason for admission, date, PMH, medications allergies, pertinent results	Story	Background information about patient Reason for admission, past medical history (PMH), resuscitation status
sment	Vital clinical signs Think ABCDE assessment	Vital signs	Vital signs Temperature PR and rhythm, blood pressure, respiratory rate, conscious level, cap refill, SaO_2, FiO_2, urine output EWS
mmendation	Be specific about what you need, make suggestion, clarify expectations Ask if there is anything else you should do Repeat instructions to ensure accuracy	Plan	My plan is . . . What is your plan? What do you want me to do?

SBAR adapted from IHI (2008); RSVP (Featherstone et al. 2008). Available at http://www.institute.nhs.uk/quality_and_service_improvement_tools/
and_service_improvement_tools/sbar_-_situation_-_background_-_assessment_-_recommendation.html

dditional considerations when sessing risk

st EWSs are helpful in identifying the patient at risk, vise to consider a comprehensive patient assessment g into account the individual. For example a patient be displaying trends over a period of time on one or nber of variables, moving towards a trigger point. ient with a normal heart rate of 60 beats per minute, e rate increases by 5 five beats per minute progres- over the day, is demonstrating a trend of deteriora- It may be wise to seek advice before the trigger point hed, as this could be a sign of acute illness. It should membered that the patient's normal medication influence the physiological response to illness. For ple in a patient taking beta-blocker medication, the al sympathetic response is blunted and signs such as ased heart rate may not be readily apparent. Another or consideration is that if just one physiological vari- noves to the extreme such as a heart rate of 150 beats ninute, or perhaps a respiratory rate of 35 breaths ninute, the points generated may not be sufficient to r to the medium risk category. The nurse in charge reviewing this patient should consider if a patient one such extreme physiological variable is in need medical review and whether it would be unwise to or other physiological variables to reach the point to the medium risk category.

The frequency of observations needs to be increased with the level of risk, in order to capture significant clinical changes in a timely manner and escalate care appropri- ately. NICE (2007) recommend a minimum of 12-hourly observations, but patients who are scoring at even a low level of risk should be monitored more frequently. Local policy will influence practice, but increasing frequency of observations to 4-hourly for a low-risk patient, hourly for a medium-risk patient, and every 15 minutes for a high-risk patient may be appropriate.

Track and trigger
- Check that you have correctly calculated the early warning score!
- Recheck the score after each intervention, and use it to track progress.
- If the score stays the same or increases after interventions, your patient is deteriorating: seek appropriate help immediately.

Moving care forward

The chain of response (DH 2009) does not stop with the arrival of outreach or the patient's primary medical team. Suboptimal care is still possible and teamwork is required to move care forward. It is important that nurses have a clear understanding of the physiological basis of deteriora- tion, in order to monitor the response to the interventions

CASE STUDY 1.1 Joseph Ryan – Part 1 (continued)

arterial pressure at this point. His temperature is raised at 38.0°C. You record this observation and note that the heart rate (HR) falls in the orange band, generating an additional score of 1.

Joseph explains that he passed urine before being admitted 2 hours ago and has no desire to go again. He has no signs of pedal oedema, but skin turgour is poor and his mouth appears dry, so you are concerned about his fluid status, knowing that his raised respiratory rate and temperature can lead to increased insensible losses. You decide to commence a record of his intake and output on a fluid balance chart.

Disability
The Glasgow Coma Scale (GCS) is 15/15 (E4, V5, M6). Neurological status is important as this can be affected by

hypoxaemia and hypercapnia. The blood ɡ checked as you are aware that this can ris sympathetic activation, but it is within nor 5mmols/L.

Exposure
You complete a quick head-to-toe examin no abnormalities. You calculate his EWS sc which places him at medium/high risk. A l observation chart indicates as upward trer rate and heart rate, and a downwards trer saturation, with increasing oxygen therapy

The track and trigger tool on your ward re call the patient's primary medical team for patient, and so you make some quick prep bleeping his doctor.

Escalating care

The recording of assessment findings, calculation of EWS score and using this to assess the appropriate response is key to the recognition of the patient at risk of deterioration or medical emergency. The next step of care escalation requires that the nurse's concerns are communicated to the health care team in a clear and coherent manner. NPSA (2007b) identified failure of communication as the biggest problem area with the deteriorating patient. Nurses do not always use the same language as their medical colleagues when talking about patients at risk of deterioration, which may cause confusion and misunderstandings. Tait (2010) found that nurses were often alerted to the acutely unwell patient by the feeling that 'something was wrong'. This 'feeling of concern' is incorporated into some EWSs as an additional trigger factor. However, a nursing observation that 'the patient looks pale and cold' may not enable doctors to appreciate the urgency of a situation as

clearly as 'the patient is peripherally va an increased capillary refill time'.

Nurses who pick up early signs of have difficulty in convincing the doc due to problems in articulating concerr is clearly understood by the doctor. Ea can help overcome these barriers by p calling criteria. More information tha needed, however. Medical staff may co of patients in differing geographical lc to prioritise their workload and infc them needs to enable this process. In communication a couple of moments o can be beneficial. The patient at risl needs that information to be commu clarity, so that the person being call aware of the impending emergency, start helping with the clinical decisio Systems such SBAR (Situation, Backgrc Recommendation) (NHS Institute to Improvement, 2008) or RSVP (Reason-Plan) (Featherstone et al. 2008) ensures the recipient are familiar with the structu giving (see Table 1.7). For senior studer nurses and health care professionals the of a patient who is deteriorating can c completely blank and the security of a system can help allay anxiety and ensu comprehensive request for help is achic

Tips when escalating care
- Ensure you are contacting the appropriate health care professional.
- Stand by the phone if possible to receive response to the bleep.
- Have patient's chart and notes to hand.
- Use SBAR or RSVP to guide the conversation.

CASE STUDY 1.2 Joseph Ryan – Part 2

Joseph has been admitted with community-acquired pneumonia (CAP) and after an assessment at 14.35, you are concerned that he is deteriorating as he has triggered on the EWS. His heart rate and respiratory rate have a rising trend, indicating an increased level of compensation, and deteriorating status. Mr Ryan is at risk of becoming a medical emergency.

You check that you know which team Joseph is under the care of, that you have the charts and notes with you. You make sure that Joseph is comfortable and hand him the call bell, whilst you bleep the doctor. Your ward uses the SBAR system as a communication tool and when the doctor responds to his bleep you give the following information.

SITUATION

'Hello Dr Jones, thanks for calling back so promptly. This is S/N Jane Wills from 2 South and I am calling because I am concerned about Joseph Ryan, a 63-year-old gentleman your team admitted earlier today. Joseph has an EWS of 8, he is triggering on respiratory rate which is 29, and oxygen saturations which dropped to 92% and are now 94% after I have increased his oxygen from 2–4L. He is becoming more tachycardic and his temperature remains elevated at 38°C. His work of breathing appears to have increased, he is using accessory muscles and is too tired to talk much.'

BACKGROUND

'Joseph Ryan was admitted at 10.30 this morning with community-acquired pneumonia. He had a history of a cough which was productive with green sputum and he has become increasingly breathless. His chest X-ray showed some consolidation and he was started on antibiotics and 2 L of oxygen via nasal specs. His past medical history includes hypertension for which he is taking Candasartan 16mg and Bisoprolol 5mg.'

ASSESSMENT

'His airway remains clear. His oxygen saturations had dropped to 92% but are now increased from 92% to 94% on increasing oxygen from 2–4L. His respiratory rate has gone up to 29 and he looks distressed. I think I heard some new crackles on auscultation, but I am not confident, so I would like you to check. His blood pressure is 135/95, and his capillary refill is 2 seconds. His heart rate has increased from 92 to 109 over the last couple of hours. I am worried that his respiratory failure is worsening, and that he may deteriorate quickly.'

RECOMMENDATIONS

'I need you to come and assess him as he may need an arterial blood gas sample taken, some intravenous antibiotics, and maybe IV fluids. Would you like me to organise a repeat chest X-ray and chase up the blood results? I was also thinking of cannulating him for IV access.'

'When will you be able to get here?'

'Is there anything else you would like me to do?'

'So can I just confirm that you would like me to cannulate him and arrange a chest X-ray? Thanks, see you in about 15 minutes.'

You go back to Joseph to explain that his doctor is coming to review him, and notice that his oxygen saturations have slipped back down to 92%. You repeat his observations and note that his respiratory rate has increased to 32, and his heart rate to 112. He can not complete sentences in one breath and is still finding it hard work to breathe. You decide to place him on a non-rebreathe mask at 15L oxygen whilst you are waiting for the doctor to attend, his oxygen saturation increases back to 94%, you are pleased that they arrive promptly. You note his EWS has now increased to 9, in the high-risk category.

Dr Jones arrives reviews Joseph noting his deteriorating clinical status. His oxygen saturations have increased to 94% on 15L of oxygen, and an arterial blood gas reveals a Ph 7.35, PaO_2 8.2kPa, and a $PaCO_2$ of 3.6kPa. Base excess (BE) and HCO_3^- are within normal range; type one respiratory failure is confirmed. His repeat CXR reveals a worsening of consolidation. Dr Jones asks you to call outreach with a view to commencing CPAP as his response to oxygen therapy is limited, and considers moving Joseph to a higher level of care. He is cannulated and after blood cultures and sputum specimen have been obtained, commenced on IV Augmentin 1.2g and Clarithromycin 500mg. 1 litre of IV normal saline is started, to run over 8 hours.

Outreach arrive and commence CPAP on 50% oxygen with a positive end-expired pressure (PEEP) of 5cmH$_2$O. The critical care team is consulted, and it is agreed that the response to CPAP will be assessed. Within 30 minutes there are signs of clinical improvement. Joseph appears more comfortable, with less evidence of accessory muscle use. His respiratory rate reduces to 24 breaths/minute and his oxygen saturations rise to 96%. Heart rate is reduced to 98 beats/minute as his work of breathing decreases. His EWS has reduced into the medium category and outreach stay with Joseph until he is stable enough for transfer to a level 2 bed, where he will be with nurses who are able monitor arterial blood gasses, have competence in caring for a patient requiring CPAP, and have sufficient staff to increase the frequency of observations as required.

After 48 hours Joseph returns back to your ward and he is discharged home 2 days later.

prescribed. Interventions need to be appropriate and timely, and should result in improvements in clinical status, reflected in a reduction of the early warning score. Newly qualified doctors and nurses may feel unsure in the management of the deteriorating patient, and education, advice and support from outreach services, the supervising consultant and ITU should be utilised (NCEPOD 2005). The chain of response will involve secondary, and maybe a tertiary responder, who will have competencies in critical care (DH 2009). Early advice should be sought if the patient does not respond to initial therapies, or requires continuing therapy to retain stability, as admission to a higher level of care may be appropriate.

Chain of prevention

Recognising and responding appropriately to patient deterioration requires complex skills, effective multidisciplinary education and team work. The 'chain of prevention' (Smith 2010) is an illustration of the components necessary to promote safe and effective care in the acute hospital setting (see Figure 1.3). Many rings of the chain have been considered in this chapter, and the themes of assessment (monitoring) recognition, asking for help, and appropriate response, are evident in subsequent chapters in this book. Every link in the chain needs to be strong, as it is only as strong as the weakest link.

'Education', the first link of the chain, is essential to ensure competence of the health care professional in patient assessment, recording and interpreting vital signs, calculating EWS, and escalating care appropriately. The NMC (2010) *Standards for Pre-registration Nursing Education* reflect this need, acknowledging that all nurses (in each of the four fields) must be able to recognise and interpret signs of normal and deteriorating mental and physical health and respond promptly. Adult nurses are

further required to recognise the early signs of illness, making accurate assessments and starting appropriate and timely management of those who are acutely ill, at risk of clinical deterioration, or requiring emergency care NMC (2010). Multidisciplinary courses such as ALERT, post-registration courses for nurses in assessment and recognising the deteriorating patient contribute to a growing level of competence in this area. The quality of 'monitoring', frequency, completeness and the recording of observations forms the second link. Qualified nurses are accountable for their practice and must ensure that, if observations are delegated to students or health care assistants, they are competently performed and regularly reviewed. The third link of the chain, 'recognition', is supported by the use of early warning systems, and the development of an NHS early warning system has potential to standardise calling criteria to assist health care professionals in the early recognition of deterioration. The 'call for help' is the fourth link of the chain. Organisational culture should be supportive and not criticise staff for calling for help. The use of tools such as SBAR and RSVP may improve the quality of communication tools both within and between disciplines. The final link in the chain, 'response', considers the functioning of teams such as critical care outreach services (CCOS), a dedicated team with specific skills in managing the acutely ill patient and medical emergency teams. The speed of response and level of support provided by these teams are crucial to moving patient care forward.

Conclusion

The problem of early recognition of acute illness, with appropriate and timely response to prevent medical emergencies occurring, is not a new one. National strategies have been implemented to support the organisation of acute care services, opening up critical care expertise

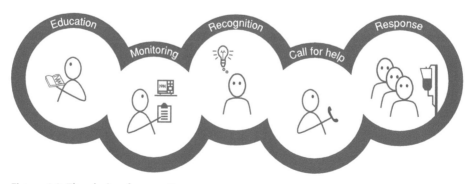

Figure 1.3 The chain of prevention

Source: Smith, G. B. (2010) In-hospital cardiac arrest: Is it time for an In-hospital 'chain of prevention'? *Resuscitation,* 81(a), 1209–1211.

and critical care beds outside the ITU environment. Education of the multidisciplinary team in the identification and management of the acutely unwell patient is ongoing. Early warning scores continue to be developed to enhance validity and refine sensitivity, and systems such as SBAR and RSVP enhance multi- and intradisciplinary communications. However, the early detection of an impending medical emergency is largely reliant on nurses performing a comprehensive patient assessment and accurately recording abnormal vital signs. Nurses need to understand the physiological basis of deterioration and have the competence and confidence to use EWS appropriately to escalate care. Critical care outreach teams and medical staff are dependent on nurses assessing their patients and adhering to the EWS criteria. Caring for patients at risk of becoming acutely unwell can be challenging, but ultimately rewarding. Expanding knowledge and expertise in recognition and response to medical emergencies is a good step forward in improving the quality of care for those at risk of becoming acutely unwell.

Glossary

Aggregated weighted track and trigger system (AWTTS) AWTTS allocate points in a weighted manner (e.g. the more the parameter has deviated from normal, the higher the score generated) and these points are added to generate the early warning score. AWTTS allow the generation of low-, medium- and high-risk categories as recommended by NICE (2007).

Care escalation Care moved forward in order that a set of timely appropriate interventions prescribed by clinicians with competence in critical care, aimed at treating/preventing acute deterioration, are commenced. May involve advice from critical care outreach, ITU, and transfer to a higher level of care.

CPAP (continuous positive airways pressure) A respiratory support therapy in which continuous positive pressure is delivered via a face mask, nasal mask or mouth piece. Positive end-expired pressure (PEEP) is achieved through a PEEP valve. This increases the lung functional residual capacity and aids oxygenation.

CPR Cardiopulmonary resuscitation (CPR) is an emergency procedure used to manually support the circulation, thereby preserving blood flow to the brain.

Critical care outreach A team, often multi-professional, that provides clinical and educational support in the recognition and treatment at the onset of deteriorating health of adult patients on general wards. It also provides for patients after a period of critical illness when they are discharged back to a lower level of care on the general wards.

EWS (early warning score/system) *System*: a process by which objective criteria are used to generate a score, which is used as an indicator for 'calling for help'. *Score*: each of six physiological variables generates a number as it deviates from acceptable ranges. The EWS is the sum of those numbers.

Hypoxaemia Low level of oxygen in the blood.

Medical emergency An acute life-threatening event, usually preceded by a period of physiological deterioration and changes in vital signs.

Medical emergency teams (MET) A team of health care professionals who have advanced life support skills, who are able to respond to patients who have abnormal physiological signs indicative of clinical deterioration. MET were first used in Australia.

Multi-parameter early warning system Multi-parameter systems trigger on two or more physiological variables that fall outside a predetermined range.

NHS Early Warning Score (NEWS) A proposed national early warning system to be used by the NHS, currently under development.

Non-invasive ventilation (NIV) A process that enables different pressures to be delivered during inspiration and expiration and providing ventilatory support. NIV is delivered via face or nasal mask, does not require intubation and is most commonly used for patients with type 2 respiratory failure.

Physiological variable A clinical measurement such as heart rate, respiratory rate, that varies over time.

RSVP Reason–Story–Vital Signs–Plan System used in acute life-threatening events recognition and treatment (ALERT) course. An easy to remember tool including essential information to be used in an emergency, to enable medical staff to respond appropriately.

SBAR Situation, Background, Assessment, Recommendation. An easy to use mechanism used to structure communication, to communicate accurately what requires a clinician's immediate attention.

Single-parameter early warning system Single-parameter systems trigger on one extreme physiological observation value.

Track and trigger tool A set of predetermined objective criteria used as indicators for 'calling for help' in the management of a patient at risk of clinical deterioration.

Test yourself

1 Patients who have a cardiopulmonary arrest:
   a. can often do so when there are no signs of anything being wrong with them
   b. usually collapse within an hour of developing a temperature
   c. often have abnormal vital signs in the 24 hours before arrest
   d. always have low oxygen saturation 6 hours before the arrest

2 The six physiological parameters that should be included in a track and trigger system are:
   a. heart rate, respiratory rate, central venous pressure, urine output, temperature and peak expiratory flow rate
   b. heart rate, respiratory rate, blood pressure, urine output, temperature and level of consciousness
   c. heart rate, oxygen saturations, blood pressure, temperature, systolic blood pressure and respiratory rate
   d. heart rate, oxygen saturation, respiratory rate, systolic blood pressure and urine output

3 Which of the following does not form part of a compensatory mechanism to acute illness?
   a. respiratory rate
   b. blood pressure
   c. heart rate
   d. hypoxaemia

4 Patients who do not trigger on the observation chart:
   a. need to have the six physiological parameters measured at least every 12 hours and their early warning score calculated
   b. need to have the six physiological parameters measured only if they say they do not feel well
   c. can be taught how to measure their own respiratory rate, heart rate, temperature, blood pressure and oxygen saturations
   d. need only to have temperature, heart rate, respiratory rate and blood pressure measured 4-hourly

5 You are with a qualified nurse and you assess a young man admitted with abdominal pain. He has a respiratory rate of 24, and oxygen saturations of 92% on room air and appears distressed. What should be done?
   a. carry on with an ABCDE assessment to calculate an early warning score
   b. draw round the screens and pull the emergency bell
   c. tell the doctor the next time they are on the ward
   d. commence oxygen at 2L/min via nasal specs, then continue to complete an ABCDE assessment and early warning score calculation

6 SBAR is a communication tool that does which of the following:
   a. gives a simple structured well-understood system for conveying information regarding a deteriorating patient to health care professionals
   b. is a tool for telling the doctor that they have to come and see your patient immediately
   c. is a mnemonic for situation, background, airway, response, which enables communication across the health care team
   d. is used to summon the cardiac arrest team when a patient collapses

7 Qualified nurses may fulfil which roles in the 'chain of response' (DH 2009)?
   a. recorder and recogniser only
   b. recorder, and secondary responder, if they have been qualified for two years
   c. recorder, recogniser, and in the areas in which they have received training and have appropriate competencies, primary responder
   d. can perform the role of primary and secondary responder if the matron says that is now part of their role

8 The problem of early recognition of acute illness, with appropriate and timely response to prevent medical emergencies occurring is:
   a. not a new problem, has been recognised since the 1990s
   b. only been a problem since everybody started using early warning scores
   c. only a problem in the United Kingdom
   d. a product of an increasing number of patients in hospital at any one time

9 The accurate measurement and recording of respiratory rate is:
   a. best done whilst talking to the patient so they relax and it is not falsely elevated
   b. quickly and accurately calculated by counting the breaths over 15 seconds and multiplying by 4
   c. not an important part of the ABCDE assessment if the patient is monitored for SpO_2
   d. counted over 1 full minute as even small deviations can be clinically significant

10 Many acute trusts have developed a critical care outreach service. The primary role of outreach is:
   a. to use specific skills in managing the acutely ill patient to support and advise nurses and medical staff in the immediate management of the deteriorating patient
   b. to look after patients who are not well and transfer them to the intensive care unit as necessary
   c. to teach doctors skills of advanced life support
   d. to support relatives whose loved ones have died whilst receiving critical care

References

Audit Commission (1999) *Critical to Success. The place of efficient and effective critical care services within the acute hospital*. London: Audit Commission. Available from http://www.auditcommission.gov.uk/SiteCollectionDocuments/AuditCommissionReports/NationalStudies/CriticalToSuccess.pdf.

Buist, M., Jarmolowski, E., Burton, P., Bernard, S., Waxman, B. and Anderson, J. (1999) Recognising clinical instability in hospital patients before cardiac arrest or unplanned admission to intensive care. A pilot studying a tertiary-care hospital. *The Medical Journal of Australia* 171 (1), 22–5.

Cooper, J., Cooper, D. and Cooper, J. (2006b) Cardiopulmonary resuscitation: History, current practice and future direction. *Circulation* 114, 2839–49.

Cooper, N., Forrest, K. and Cramp, P. (2006a) *Essential Guide to Acute Care*. London: BMJ Books, Blackwell Publishing.

DH (Department of Health) (2011) *Critical Care Beds*. Available from http://www.dh.gov.uk/en/Publicationsandstatistics/Statistics/Performancedataandstatistics/Beds/DH_077451.

DH (Department of Health) (2009) *Competencies for Recognising and Responding to Acutely Ill Patients in Hospital*. London: DH.

DH (Department of Health) (2000) *Comprehensive Critical Care: A review of adult critical care services*. London: The Stationery Office.

DH (Department of Health and Modernisation Agency) (2003) *The National Outreach Report 2003*. Available from http://www.dh.gov.uk/en/Publicationsandstatistics/Publications/PublicationsPolicyAndGuidance/DH_4091873.

Featherstone, P., Chalmers, T. and Smith, G. (2008) RSVP: A system for communication of deterioration in hospital patients. *British Journal of Nursing* 17 (13), 860–4.

Franklin, C. and Matthew, J. (1994) Developing strategies to prevent in-hospital cardiac arrest: Analysing responses of physicians and nurses in the hours before the event. *Critical Care Medicine* 22 (2), 224–7.

Goldhill, D., White, A. and Summer, A. (1999) Physiological values and procedures in the 24-h before ICU admission from the ward. *Anaesthesia* 54, 529–34.

Hospital Episode Statistics, inpatient data headline figures.

Available from http://www.hesonline.nhs.uk/Ease/servlet/ContentServer?siteID=1937&categoryID=193

ICS (Intensive Care Society) (2009) *Levels of Critical Care for Adult Patients*. London: Intensive Care Society.

Lipley, N. (2000) Government takes early action to avert another NHS winter of chaos. *Nursing Standard* 14 (37), 4–5.

Margereson, C. (2010) *Trajectory and Impact of Long-term Conditions*. In Margereson, C. and Trenoweth, S. (eds) *Developing Holistic Care for Long-term Conditions*. London: Routledge, pp. 18–33.

McQuillan, P., Pilkington, S., Allan, A., Taylor, B., Short, A., Morgan, G., Nielson, M., Barret, D. and Smith, G. (1998) Confidential enquiry into quality of care before admission to intensive care. *British Medical Journal* 316, 1853–8.

MERIT Study Investigators (2005) Introduction of the medical emergency team (MET) system: A cluster randomised controlled trial. *Lancet* 365, 2091–7.

NCEPOD (2005) *An Acute Problem? National Confidential Enquiry into Patient Outcome and Death*. London: NCEPOD.

NHS Institute for Innovation and Improvement (2008) SBAR-Situation-Background-Assessment-Recommendation.

Available from http://www.institute.nhs.uk/quality_and_service_improvement_tools/quality_and_service_improvement_tools/sbar_-_situation_-_background_-_assessment_-_recommendation.html.

NICE (National Institute for Health and Clinical Excellence) (2007) GC50 *Acutely Ill Patients in Hospital*. London: NICE.

NMC (Nursing and Midwifery Council) (2008) *The Code. Standards of conduct, performance and ethics for nurses and midwives*. London: NMC.

NMC (Nursing and Midwifery Council) (2010) *Standards for Pre-registration Nursing Education*. Available at http://standards.nmc-uk.org/PublishedDocuments/Standards%20for%20pre-registration%20nursing%20education%2016082010.pdf.

National Outreach Forum (NOrF) (2011) *NOrF Members Forum NHS Early Warning Score*. Available from http://www.norf.org.uk/NOrF_members_forum?mode=MessageList&eid=558305, accessed 2 May 2011.

NPSA (National Patient Safety Agency) (2007a) *Safer Care for the Acutely Ill Patient: Learning from serious incidents*. London: NPSA.

NPSA (National Patient Safety Agency) (2007b) *Recognising and Responding Appropriately to Early Signs of Deterioration in Hospitalised Patients*. London: NPSA.

O'Driscoll, B. R., Howard, L. S. and Davison, A. G. (2008) *BTS Guideline for Emergency Oxygen Use in Adult Patients*. London: British Thoracic Society. Available at http://www.brit-thoracic.org.uk/Portals/0/Clinical%20Information/Emergency%20Oxygen/Emergency%20oxygen%20guideline/THX-63-Suppl_6.pdf.

Peberdy, M., Ornato, J., Larking, G., Braithwaite, R., Kashner, T., Carey, S., Meany, P., Cen, L., Nadkarni, V., Praestgaard, A. and Berg, R. (2008) Surviving in-hospital cardiac arrest during nights and weekends. *JAMA* 299 (7), 785–92.

Prytherch, D., Smith, G., Schmidt, P. and Featherstone, P. (2010) ViEWS – towards a national early warning score for detecting inpatient deterioration. *Resuscitation* 81, 932–7.

Prytherch, D., Smith, G., Schmidt, P., Featherstone, P., Stewart, K., Knight, D. and Higgins, B. (2006) Calculating early warning scores – a classroom comparison of pen and paper and hand-held computer methods. *Resuscitation* 70, 173–8.

Resuscitation Council UK (2011) *Immediate Life Support*, 3rd edn. London: Resuscitation Council (UK).

Resuscitation Council UK (2010) *Resuscitation Guidelines 2010*. London: Resuscitation Council (UK). Available from http://www.resus.org.uk/pages/GL2010.pdf.

Royal College of Physicians (2007) *Acute Medical Care: The right person, in the right setting – first time report of the Acute*

Medicine Task Force, October 2007. London: Royal College of Physicians. Available from http://bookshop.rcplondon.ac.uk/contents/pub235-b42eb97d-209b-4ecd-9127-ef95cc21c819.pdf.

Schein, R., Hazday, N., Pena, N. and Ruben, B. (1990) Clinical antecedents to in-hospital cardiopulmonary arrest. *Chest* 98, 1388–92.

Smith, G. (2010) In-hospital cardiac arrest: Is it time for an in-hospital 'chain of prevention'? *Resuscitation* 81, 1209–11.

Smith, G. (2003) *ALERT Acute Life-Threatening Events Recognition and Treatment*. Portsmouth: University of Portsmouth.

Smith, G., Prytherch, D., Schmidt, P. and Featherstone, P. (2008) Review and performance evaluation of aggregate weighted 'track and trigger' systems. *Resuscitation* 77, 170–9.

Smith, G., Prytherch, D., Schmidt, P., Featherstone, P. and Higgins, B. (2008) Review and performance evaluation of single-parameter 'track and trigger' systems. *Resuscitation* 77, 11–21.

Subbe, C. (2006) Recognition and assessment of critical illness. *Anaesthesia and Intensive Care Medicine* 8 (1), 21–3.

Tait, D. (2010) Nursing recognition and response to clinical signs of deterioration. *Nursing Management* 17 (6), 31–5.

Further reading

Benner, P. E., Hooper-Kyriakidis, P. and Syannard, D. (2011) *Clinical Wisdom and Interventions in Acute and Critical Care: A thinking-in-action approach*, 2nd edn. New York: Springer.

Harrison, R. and Daly, L. (2011) *A Nurse's Survival Guide to Acute Medical Emergencies*, 3rd edn. Edinburgh: Churchill Livingstone.

Jevon, P. (2008) *Clinical Examination Skills*. Oxford: Wiley.

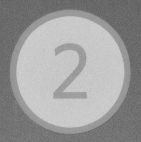

Vulnerability in the acutely ill patient

Ian Peate

Aims

This chapter aims to provide the reader with insight and understanding concerning the vulnerable adult in the acute care setting and those whose health is at risk of deterioration.

Objectives

After reading this chapter you will be able to:

→ Describe key terms

→ Understand the rights of vulnerable adults in acute care situations

→ Examine the health and social policy provisions for vulnerable people

→ Ensure that the voice of the vulnerable adult is heard and acted upon

→ Outline some of the ethical considerations relevant to the care and treatment of vulnerable people in the acute care setting

→ Provide safe and effective care to vulnerable people in acute care settings or those whose health is at risk of deterioration

Introduction

Michaels and Moffett (2008) suggest that nurses encounter vulnerability at all levels, cellular, physiological systems, mind–body, individuals, communities and societies. It is not always the case that adults can protect and care for themselves: when discussing adults in this chapter, this refers to people aged 18 years or over. Caring for vulnerable adults is a key aspect of the role of the nurse; people can be considered vulnerable for a variety of reasons.

This chapter discusses the issue of vulnerability and reminds students that they are patients' advocates and as such should always act with the patients' best interests in mind. One of the many aspects of professional practice is to ensure that those for whom you care come to no harm.

Vulnerability

A number of high-level adverse incidents have occurred over the years in hospital and social care settings that have put individuals at risk or indeed harmed them (Healthcare Commission 2009). Often in large and complex organisations such as the NHS things can go wrong, and it is essential that organisations report and learn from such incidents so that changes can be identified and they then become embedded in practice. Those people who may have a long-term condition, those who present with co-morbidities and those who have a medical emergency along with the increasingly complex nature of acute care can increase the risk of vulnerability.

Vulnerability is a multifaceted state that is not easily quantifiable. A vulnerable person can be difficult to describe, nevertheless they may be described as a person who has or may have a care need (broadly defined) arising from a mental or other disability, age or illness (Penhale and Parker 2008). Having 'a care need' means that that person needs someone to assist in caring for him or herself. The nurse is centrally placed, often as a member of a multidisciplinary team working in partnership, to assist people.

Each one of us is potentially at risk of abuse and ill treatment. Any of the following conditions have the possibility to increase vulnerability, for example:

- having a learning disability;
- experiencing mental health problems;
- having physical/sensory impairment;
- being frail or an older person;
- being acutely ill;
- having a long-term condition;

- being incarcerated;
- being homeless.

This chapter discusses the complex issue of vulnerability and how nurses can help others with their care needs, with an emphasis on the vulnerable person who may be experiencing an acute medical emergency and their significant others. Nurses must work in partnership with others to ensure that they safeguard and protect the most vulnerable and to promote high-quality care (Mencap 2007). In order to protect the public and those who are deemed vulnerable it is important to have an understanding of the moral theories and ethical frameworks that will impact on patient outcomes. This chapter will provide a very brief introduction to some of the ethical frameworks that can have an important influence on health care practice.

There has been an absence of adult safeguarding systems within the NHS that enables healthcare incidents that cause concern to be raised and addressed (Michael and the Independent Inquiry into Access to Healthcare for People with Learning Disabilities 2008, DH 2010). The Parliamentary and Health Service Ombudsman (2011) has reported on the care and treatment of 10 older people who have received care in the NHS. The report considers 10 complaints made to the Ombudsman about the standard of care these older people received. The accounts of care discussed provide a picture of an NHS that is failing to respond to the needs of older people with care and compassion. Britain has a tradition of concern for the poorest and most vulnerable in society (Equalities and Human Rights Commission 2010).

There is a need to ensure that health care professionals play a key role in the identification of abuse, harm and neglect and then put together appropriate responses to it; this will also mean that health care professionals work collaboratively with local authorities if needs be when adult safeguarding concerns arise during health care delivery (see Case study 2.1). This is what is termed an integrated process. In some areas of care new posts have been created, for example, designated nurse posts for the safeguarding of adults. These nurses have responsibility for strengthening safeguarding processes across health and social services.

Potential abuse of vulnerable adults can take many forms. Allegations can be made about physical abuse; the highest number of allegations concerning abuse is related to physical abuse, however, many people incorrectly assume that only battered people are abused, but emotional scars are just as serious as physical injuries. There are some vulnerable groups and communities that have a significantly poorer life expectancy than the general population, often as a result of their vulnerable status.

CASE STUDY 2.1 Student nurse Javelle

A third-year student nurse Javelle is on placement on an arterial high-dependency unit. She has been allocated to this placement for 12 weeks and is in her second week. She has been allocated a mentor but, unfortunately, her mentor has been off sick for most of the placement.

Javelle has been working with Sister Isharm for the last three days. They are caring for a patient with learning disabilities who is recovering from major arterial surgery but he is still too unwell to return to the general ward and requires one-to-one nursing care.

Javelle is concerned about some aspects of Sister Isharm's work style. Sister Isharm has been making derogatory, patronising and sarcastic comments about the patient, his physical appearance and also about some members of his family. She has been using offensive terms such as 'fatty'

and 'slowcoach'. Her comments are being made in an intrusive manner. Sister Isharm's actions are making Javelle increasingly uncomfortable.

Javelle has confided in another staff nurse. The staff nurse tells Janelle that Sister Isharm is the most senior nurse on the unit and is highly respected. The staff nurse told Javelle to keep her head down and she also reminds her that Sister has a lot of sway when it comes to assessing clinical practice and the completion of her practice assessment documentation.

Vulnerability and safeguarding is everyone's concern and all staff have a duty to raise and report any concerns about any aspect of care that they consider to be unacceptable. Javelle is aware of the various routes that can be taken to raise concerns and she contacts her link lecturer to discuss the issues further.

The law

The principles of protection are enshrined in various legislative and policy directives. The Human Rights Act 1998 is made up of articles, which include that no person should be subjected to any form of torture or cruel or inhumane or degrading treatment or punishment, that each person has a right to life, the right to liberty and security and security of person; there is a prohibition against discrimination. The Equality Act 2006 created the Equality and Human Rights Commission; this Commission took over the functions of the Commission for Racial Equality, the Disability Rights Commission and the Equality Opportunities Commission, bringing them all under one umbrella.

There are many more laws that can be cited when considering safeguarding and vulnerability. It is not the intention of this chapter to provide a discussion of the law, but you must be aware of the legal and professional issues that arise when you are caring for a person who is acutely ill.

vulnerable adults from abuse. The equivalent was also produced in Wales in 2000 (National Assembly for Wales 2000). In Scotland this is the Adult Support and Protection (Scotland) Act 2007 providing legislation that aims to protect vulnerable people from harm. The aim of these publications is to provide protection for those adults who are believed vulnerable in our society, those who are at risk of abuse and those who may need protection. Local authorities through the social services they provide are obliged to act and conform to the general guidance issued in the *No Secrets* publication (DH and Home Office 2000). Policy and procedures have to be in place to safeguard those who are considered at risk. *No Secrets* states that there can be no secrets and no hiding places when it comes to exposing the abuse of adults (DH and Home Office 2000).

Safeguarding Adults (DH 2009) is a review of *No Secrets*, and also provides guidance on devising and implementing multi-agency policies and procedures to protect vulnerable adults from harm. The aim of the review was to determine whether and how the *No Secrets* guidance needed to change in order to assist society in keeping adults safe from harm or abuse.

No Secrets

Guidance was produced in 2000 (in England) relating to how to develop policies and procedures to safeguard

Key terms

Guidance has been provided to help health and social care professionals to work in partnership, produce policies and ensure that appropriate procedures and practices are in place and carried out (DH and Home Office 2000, DH 2010). This guidance is derived from statute, for example, the Local Authority Social Services Act 1970, the Human Rights Act 1998 and Health Act 1999. It is not law, but the government expects that the guidance is adhered to and should only be deviated from in exceptional circumstances. The guidance covers issues of definition concerning the various and often complex terms associated with vulnerability. Other terms synonymous with vulnerability include liability, exposure and susceptibility.

It must be reiterated that regardless of the care setting (and the acute care setting is no exception) the important issue of vulnerability must be paramount for all of the people who are recipients of care. The key aim is to make sure that there are robust processes in place that ensure adult safeguarding arrangements become fully integrated into healthcare systems.

There are several terms that are used when considering adult protection issues and it is imperative that these key terms are defined. Understanding these terms can assist you when helping the people you care for.

Safeguarding

This term is associated with the need to feel safe and free from exploitation and is often seen as one of our most basic needs. Any threat to a person's safety will directly threaten their health and well-being, therefore identifying what the threat to the person's safety is and addressing it is one way of providing high-quality holistic care (De Chesnay 2008).

According to the DH (2010) safeguarding is a range of activities aimed at upholding an adult's fundamental right to be safe. This is of specific importance for those individuals who, as a result of their situation or circumstances, are unable to keep themselves safe; this would also apply to those people who are acutely ill.

Safeguarding vulnerable adults from abuse and harm is everyone's concern and this is now a significant aspect of everyday healthcare provision. In 1954 Maslow (a psychologist) postulated that humans have a hierarchy of needs, and this remains a popular theory (see Figure 2.1).

The theory suggests that each person has a hierarchy of needs and the individual must satisfy each level before they are able to move onto the next level. Five hierarchical levels are identified:

1 Physiological needs: the need for food, shelter, sexual satisfaction. These needs are required in order to survive.

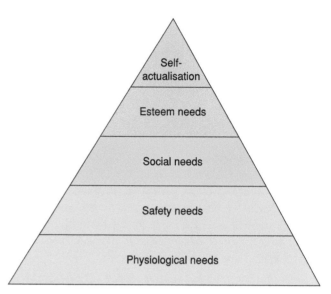

Figure 2.1 Maslow's hierarchy of needs

Source: Maslow, A. (1987) *Motivation and Personality*, 3rd ed. Upper Saddle River, NJ: Pearson.

2 *Safety needs*: we all need to feel safe within our environment. These needs also refer to emotional and physical safety.

3 *Social needs*: the need for love, friendship and a sense of belonging.

4 *Esteem needs*: the need for self-respect and recognition from others.

5 *Self-actualisation*: this is the point of reaching your full potential.

It is suggested that prior to moving onto an other level an individual must satisfy their most basic needs, hence physiological needs must be met before being able to meet safety needs and safety needs have to be met prior to being able to meet social needs and so forth.

Feeling safe and being safe, physically and emotionally, are therefore essential. If a person feels vulnerable or feels their health and well-being are at risk this may prevent them from making a full recovery. Sometimes, the health of a patient in hospital may get deteriorate suddenly and the person becomes acutely ill. There are times when this is more likely to happen, for example, if the patient is an emergency admission to hospital after surgery and after discharge from a critical care area such as a high-dependency unit. Becoming acutely ill can happen at any time during an illness and this increases a person's risk of needing to stay longer in hospital, not making a full recovery or dying. At all stages Maslow's hierarchy will need to be given consideration. Think of patients who are acutely ill and apply Maslow's model to those patients. All of those who are acutely ill are vulnerable and this may be from a physiological, emotional or psychological perspective.

Which adults are vulnerable?

Every one of us is vulnerable at some point in our lives. Penhale and Parker (2008) note that labelling a person as vulnerable can automatically assign them to a category that may be seen in a negative light. The label vulnerable may suggest a degree of weakness with no reason for this: furthermore, referring to a person as vulnerable may also ascribe victim status which may disempower the individual. The terms vulnerable and vulnerability are used in statute and policy guidance. Care must be taken when using the terms not to apportion blame; neither must we imply weakness on behalf of the person being described when using the term.

There is no formal definition of vulnerability in health care, although some people may be considered at greater risk from harm than others. This risk may have arisen as a complication of their presenting condition and their individual circumstances (DH 2010). Case study 2.2 demonstrates how a person who may be deemed low risk on admission can, because of their presenting condition and individual circumstances, be deemed high risk and subjected to increased vulnerability. This case study provides you with an idea of how a person's health status can change and their risk status can alter, making them more prone to risk and more vulnerable. Recognition of risk and appropriate responses are essential if risk and harm are to be minimised.

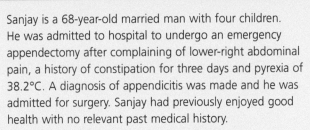

CASE STUDY 2.2 Sanjay

Sanjay is a 68-year-old married man with four children. He was admitted to hospital to undergo an emergency appendectomy after complaining of lower-right abdominal pain, a history of constipation for three days and pyrexia of 38.2°C. A diagnosis of appendicitis was made and he was admitted for surgery. Sanjay had previously enjoyed good health with no relevant past medical history.

A laparoscopic appendectomy was performed under general anaesthetic. While undergoing surgery Sanjay suffered a cardiac arrest and was resuscitated. He was returned to the intensive care unit for three days, was stabilised, made a successful recovery and was transferred to the general surgical ward area.

His abdominal keyhole incisions became infected and a methicillin-resistant *Staphylococcus aureus* was the causative organism. Two weeks later Sanjay was discharged home.

The Lord Chancellor's consultation paper 'Who Decides' (Lord Chancellor's Department, 1998) defines a vulnerable adult in broad terms as a person:

who is or may be in need of community care services by reason of mental or other disability, age or illness, and;

who is unable to take care of him or herself, or unable to protect him or herself against significant harm or exploitation.

In this broad definition, which is also used by the Department of Health in its *No Secrets* document (Department of Health and the Home Office 2000), it is important to note that community care services are broader than those services that would usually be considered community care, they will include all care services provided in any setting or context (Department of Health and the Home Office 2000). Any adult receiving any form of health care is recognised as vulnerable.

Section 80 ss 6 of the Care Standards Act 2000 describes vulnerable adults as:

a. An adult to whom accommodation and nursing or personal care are provided in a care home;
b. An adult to whom personal care is provided in their own home under arrangements made by a domiciliary care agency; or
c. An adult to whom prescribed services are provided services by an independent hospital, independent clinic, independent medical agency or National Health Service body.

The Criminal Records Bureau (CRB) (2011) describes a vulnerable adult further. A vulnerable adult is a person who is aged 18 years or older and:

- is living in residential accommodation, such as a care home or a residential special school;
- is living in sheltered housing;
- is receiving domiciliary care in his or her own home;
- is receiving any form of health care;
- is detained in a prison, remand centre, young offender institution, secure training centre or attendance centre or under the powers of the Immigration and Asylum Act 1999;

- is in contact with probation services;
- is receiving a welfare service of a description to be prescribed in regulations;
- is receiving a service or participating in an activity which is specifically targeted at people with age-related needs, disabilities or prescribed physical or mental health conditions (age-related needs includes needs associated with frailty, illness, disability or mental capacity);
- is an expectant or nursing mother living in residential care;
- is receiving direct payments from a local authority/HSS body in lieu of social care services;
- requires assistance in the conduct of his or her own affairs.

There are similarities in both definitions, but the CRB definition offers further detail. Both definitions provide meaning to this complex concept and both of them point out that services provided can expose a person to vulnerability. Vulnerability seems to be related to the provision of service.

Whether or not a person is vulnerable in the instances just described will depend upon surrounding circumstances and environment and each case must be judged on its own merits. Health care practitioners must strive to ensure that services provided are altered and amended if they are causing vulnerability, even if this is unintended, therefore practitioners need to be vigilant and aware of the potential harm that may be caused.

What constitutes abuse?

Just as it has proved a challenge to define the term vulnerability, so it is also difficult to define what is meant by abuse. All adults, irrespective of age or mental capacity, have the right to:

- live in dignity and safety, free from maltreatment of any kind;
- have their physical as well as their emotional needs met;
- make their own decisions;
- maintain autonomy (as much as possible within any health constraints).

Abuse, be it physical mistreatment and assault or an abuse that is unseen, that has emotional and psychological impact is always unacceptable. There are not and should not be any hierarchies of abuse (Penhale and Parker 2008): all forms of abuse are potentially damaging.

It may prove futile to seek a clear and delineated definition of abuse and what it is. Abuse means different things to different people in different settings; abuse is defined

by society and as such this will be different for different societies. As we generate understanding of this complex term the definition will change and reflect learning, so what constitutes abuse now will constantly change and develop: any definition is subject to change in time and place. Hence it is essential that at all times the social elements related to abuse are considered. Despite this it is important that we have a working definition of abuse in order to guide and support, with the caveat that the term abuse is subject to wide variation. A good starting point is the definition provided by the Department of Health and Home Office (2000): 'Abuse is the violation of an individual's human civil rights by any other person or persons.'

This is a broad definition and as such includes a wide range of actions that could be considered abuse. In order to make sense of the definition in a more practical way it is helpful to think of a range of types of abuse. The next section discusses the different types of abuse that can occur.

Kinds of abuse

Abuse can occur as a single act or repeated acts by a single person or a group of people. To recap, abuse may be physical, verbal or psychological, it can be an act of neglect or a failure to act or it may occur where a vulnerable person is persuaded to enter into something which they have not consented to or cannot consent to. It can range from not treating someone with dignity and respect, to extreme punishment, cruelty or torture. There are a range of types and levels of abuse and they can fall into the following categories:

- Physical abuse
- Sexual abuse
- Neglect and poor professional practice
- Institutional abuse
- Financial or material abuse
- Emotional/psychological abuse
- Discrimination.

Any list such as the one provided should be treated with caution: as time passes there may be other categories added. Table 2.1 discusses the various categories of abuse; none of the lists provided is exhaustive.

Classifying in this way can help generate discussion amongst colleagues when considering acts of abuse. When thinking about abuse it is essential that the upholding of a person's human and civil rights are taken into account – these rights are paramount. Case study 2.3 discusses the case of a patient who develops a pressure sore whilst in hospital.

Table 2.1 Types of abuse

Form of abuse	Description
Physical	This list gives what may be indicators of a number of different problems. Some of the indicators of physical abuse could be as follows: • History of falls that are difficult to explain • Unexplained bruising and injuries • Bruising in different stages of healing • Teeth indentations • Unexplained burns in unusual locations • Unexplained fractures to any part of the body • Unexplained lacerations or abrasions • Slapping, kicking, punching or finger marks • Injury shape similar to an object, for example the buckle of a belt • Untreated medical problems • Weight loss due to **malnutrition** or dehydration • Misuse of medications • Restraint or inappropriate sanctions • Deference, becoming passive
Sexual	Sexual abuse occurs when adults are involved in sexual activities which they do not fully understand, to which they are unable to give their consent, either verbally or by their behaviour, to which they object or which may cause them harm. They may have been coerced into the activity. This list may indicate a number of different problems. Some of the indicators of sexual abuse could be: • Sudden change in the person's behaviour • Sudden onset of confusion • Incontinence • Withdrawal • Overt sexual behaviour and inappropriate use of sexual language by the vulnerable adult • Self-inflicted injury • Disturbed sleep pattern and periods of poor concentration • Difficulty in walking or sitting • Torn, stained underwear • Love bites • Pain or itching, bruising or bleeding in the genitalia or anal regions • Sexually transmitted infection • Urinary tract infection • Vaginal infection (there may be discharge) • Bruising to upper thighs and arms • Severe upset or agitation when being bed bathed or bathed • Pregnancy in a person who is unable to consent
Neglect and poor professional practice	A person may suffer neglect because their physical and/or psychological (emotional) needs are being neglected by a carer. Failing to keep someone warm, clean and well nourished or neglecting to give prescribed medication could be deemed neglect. Neglect can also include a failure to intervene in situations that are dangerous to the person, particularly when the person lacks the mental capacity to assess risk. The following list may be indications of many different problems, they may also be indicators of neglect: • Poor environmental conditions • Inadequate heating and lighting • Poor physical condition of the individual • Person's clothing is ill fitting, unclean and in poor condition • Malnutrition • Failure by the carer to give prescribed medication correctly • Failure to provide appropriate privacy and dignity • Inconsistent or reluctant contact with health and social care agencies • Isolation – denying access to callers or visitors • Ignoring nursing care/medical needs • Isolated incidents of poor or unsatisfactory professional practice • Perverse ill-treatment • Professional misconduct

Table 2.1 (*continued*)

Form of abuse	Description
Institutional	Institutional abuse is concerned with who abuses and how that abuse comes to pass, as opposed to types of harm. Abuse can occur in a relationship, family, service or institution and it can be carried out by an individual or more collectively, by a regime. The following may be possible indicators of institutional abuse: • No flexibility in bedtime routine and/or deliberate waking • People left on the commode or toilet for longer periods of time than needed • Inappropriate care of a person's possessions, clothing and living area • Lack of personal clothes and belongings • Unhomely or stark living environments • Deprived environmental conditions and lack of stimulation • Inappropriate use of medical procedures e.g. enemata, catheterisation • Lack of individual care plans/programmes • Illegal confinement or restrictions • Inappropriate use of power or control • People referred to or spoken to with disrespect • Inflexible services based on convenience of the provider rather than the individual receiving services • Inappropriate physical intervention • Service user removed from the home or establishment, without discussion with other appropriate people or agencies, because staff are unable to manage their behaviours • Inability to make choices
Financial	There are many forms in which financial or material abuse can occur, for example, **fraud**, theft or using the person's property without their permission. This may involve large sums of money or even small amounts from a pension or allowance each week. It is important not to jump to the wrong conclusions too quickly. Nevertheless, the following may be possible indicators of financial abuse: • A person's sudden inability to pay bills, particularly after benefits day • Unexpected withdrawal of money from an account • The individual lacks belongings that they can clearly afford • Power of attorney obtained when the person is unable to understand what they are signing, pressure in connection with wills • Extraordinary interest by family members in the person's assets • Recent change of deeds for property • Misuse or misappropriation of property, possessions or benefits • Carers main interest is financial with scant regard for the health and welfare of the vulnerable adult • The person managing the finances is evasive and uncooperative • Reluctance to accept care services • Purchase of items that the individual does not require or use • Objects of value and personal items going missing • Unreasonable or inappropriate gifts
Emotional/ psychological	Emotional/psychological abuse can include intimidation, humiliation, shouting, swearing, emotional blackmail and denial of basic human rights. Using racist language, preventing someone from enjoying activities or meeting friends are all potential indications of emotional/psychological abuse. The following list provides other indicators: • Ambivalence about carer • Fearfulness, cowering, avoiding eye contact, flinching on approach • Deference • **Insomnia** or need for excessive sleep • Change in appetite • Unusual weight loss/gain • Tearfulness • Unexplained **paranoia** • Low **self-esteem** • Confusion, agitation • **Coercion** • Possible violation of human and civil rights • Isolation – no visitors or phone calls allowed • Inappropriate clothing

Table 2.1 (*continued*)

Form of abuse	Description
	• Sensory deprivation • Restricted access to hygiene facilities • Lack of personal respect • Lack of recognition of an individual's rights • Carer does not offer personal hygiene, medical care, regular food/drinks • Use of furniture to restrict movement • Withdrawal from services or supportive networks • The person's choices, opinions and wishes are neglected • Failure to allow the person to follow their own spiritual and cultural beliefs or sexual orientation
Discrimination	These indicators might include: • Racism • Sexism • Slurs • Harassment • Discriminatory abuse based on a person's disability or age • Low self-esteem • Withdrawal • Fear • Anger • Depression

Sources: Adapted from Department of Health and Home Office (2000); DH (2009, 2010); NMC (2009, 2010).

CASE STUDY 2.3 Mrs Ramnath

Mrs Ramnath, 68 years of age, a widower who is partially sighted was admitted to hospital with crushing chest pain. Mrs Ramnath presented with a history of severe crushing chest pain lasting for approximately one- and a-half hours. Her ECG showed changes consistent with an acute anterior myocardial infarction. Plans were made to transfer Mrs Ramnath to the cardiac care unit, however no bed was available and she was transferred to a medical ward in the hospital at 02.45h.

Analgesia for pain and other essential medications were given 30 minutes after admission to the ward. She was pain-free but anxious, it was difficult to contact her only daughter as she was abroad. A full blood count was taken and assessment was made of her urea and electrolytes, blood glucose, renal, hepatic and thyroid function – all were normal.

Mrs Ramnath has a history of asthma, she uses a salbutamol inhaler occasionally and the condition is well controlled. She is deaf in the left ear and has poor hearing in the right ear; she speaks little English.

Her father died of a myocardial infarction at 52 years of age, her mother is still alive but frail.

Mrs Ramnath is transferred to the cardiac care unit eight days after her original admission to the hospital as her condition has deteriorated. A full nursing assessment is carried out by the nursing staff admitting her. She has developed a grade 3 pressure sore. An investigation is undertaken as to how she developed the pressure sore.

On assessment upon admission Mrs Ramnath was considered to be high risk for the development of a pressure sore and a request for a pressure-relieving mattress was made. During her stay she was transferred three times from ward to ward within her first week. Initial assessment and her subsequent plan of care identified her need for a pressure-relieving mattress, however this never arrived. During her time on the various wards her skin had started to break down. A request was made again for a pressure-relieving mattress, but again due the numerous moves and poor communication between the teams this never arrived and there was a delay in the patient receiving the equipment.

As a result of the above the hospital has instigated a system whereby transferring of patients between wards and departments (regardless of length of stay) will necessitate a full nursing assessment of needs with detailed and appropriate information being given to the receiving nurse from the transferring ward. The movement of high-risk patients from ward to ward has now been reviewed and revised. There is now provision for ward staff to request and receive emergency equipment outside of normal hours as opposed to having to wait for the equipment to arrive.

Many of the types of abuse listed in Table 2.1 may be the result of deliberate intent, negligence or ignorance. There are a number of forms of abuse that could constitute a criminal offence and in this case this should involve the police: vulnerable people are entitled to the same protection of the law as another person. Examples of abuse that may constitute a criminal offence according to the Department of Health and Home Office (2000) will include:

- Assault (physical or psychological)
- Sexual assault or rape
- Theft
- Fraud or other forms of financial exploitation
- Discrimination based on gender, race, age.

It can be seen that there are a wide range of actions that can be considered as abuse. The same is also true of those who may abuse.

Who are the abusers?

Family members, relatives, professional staff, paid care workers, other service users, neighbours, friends, strangers, a teacher, a member of the clergy and those who deliberately exploit vulnerable people may abuse. Abusers can be male or female. Those in positions of power or authority who use their status to the detriment of the health, safety, welfare and general well-being of people in their care are also in a position to perpetrate abuse (see Case study 2.1).

Abuse can take place anywhere:

- in public places;
- in a prison;
- in the person's own home;
- at work;
- in hospital;
- in places of worship;
- in care homes;
- at day care.

What justifies intervention?

The seriousness or extent of abuse is not always clear, therefore it is essential that consideration be given to the appropriateness of intervention and that a comprehensive assessment is undertaken. The Department of Health and Home Office (2000) assessment of seriousness will take into consideration the following:

- the vulnerability of the individual;
- the nature and extent of the abuse;
- the length of time it has been occurring;
- the impact on the individual;
- the risk of repeated or increasingly serious acts involving this or other vulnerable adults.

Taking action and raising concerns

You must act within legal frameworks and also according to local policies in relation to safeguarding those who may be in vulnerable situations. Situations may arise that will necessitate that you work with others to implement and monitor any strategies within your work place to safeguard and protect others. Any information that is gained is shared appropriately with other appropriate colleagues and that advice (you may receive this from a number of sources) is sought if you have any concerns. Information sharing can be within your sphere of practice or it can include the sharing of information across agency boundaries with the prime aim of safeguarding and protecting the individual and the public. You might also need to make referrals to others, for example, to social workers or the police, and it is important that you remember that the people you care for have a right to confidentiality and you have a duty to ensure that any information you disclose corresponds to local policy and guidance and that the person you are caring for has given their consent. There may be some exceptional circumstances whereby disclosure of information can be made without consent, but these are usually complex and as such you must seek advice prior to disclosing any information. You must also ensure that you have support systems in place that will help you to manage and deal with any emotions that may arise out of the situation (Peate and Potterton 2010).

Immediate concerns associated with abuse must be dealt with in the first instance under local safeguarding policies and procedures. The National Patient Safety Organisation (2009) has produced information that can help you if you are concerned about patient safety incidents.

When raising concerns this has to be done in an appropriate manner and this includes using local policies, clinical governance and risk-management procedures. Go back to the first case study presented in this chapter and think about how Javelle may have felt when she had to raise concerns about a senior member of the ward team. It may not always be easy to report concerns; you may not know how to do this, you might be afraid of reprisals, you could even feel you are being disloyal. This can appear even more complex and frightening if you are working alone or if you work in remote, small communities. Always keep in mind that the person you care for is your primary concern. Remember that raising issues early has the potential to prevent their becoming more serious and in effect causing more harm to those you care for.

There are a number of sources of advice that you can access to seek assistance if you are unsure. These include your manager, your tutor or your mentor/facilitator, your trade union (for example, UNISON), your professional body (for example, the Royal College of Nursing) or the charity Public Concern at Work (this is an independent whistleblowing charity). These organisations can raise issues formally and sometimes can act for you or on your behalf; they may also be able to offer you personal support. Examples of concern may include (NMC 2010):

- issues related to health and safety violations where there may be risk to health and safety;
- unprofessional staff behaviour or attitudes;
- concerns about the standard of care being delivered;
- reservations about the environment in which care is being delivered;
- the health of a colleague and the impact this is having on their ability to practise safely;
- a shortage or lack of the availability of clinical equipment, this may also include a lack of adequate training;
- any criminal activity, fraud and financial mismanagement.

You have to report your concerns to the right person or authority immediately if you believe or see risk to the safety of those in your care. If there is immediate risk or harm, you should report this without delay.

Silence is not always golden. An everyday aspect of your work is to speak up for the people you care for: not to do anything and report concerns is unacceptable. Raising concerns and speaking up demonstrates your commitment to the people you care for.

More often than not you will raise your concern directly with the nurse in charge and for most of the time this will be dealt with and a satisfactory conclusion will emerge. However, if this fails there may be a need to take your concerns through a formal route, and at this stage you might wish to seek support and advice from a professional body, trade union, mentor, tutor or facilitator. Figure 2.2 outlines the stages for raising and escalating concerns.

Myths and facts

Many individuals have a number of misconceived ideas concerning the facts about the abuse and neglect of adults.

Mistaken beliefs that are not checked out may be detrimental to the health and well-being of the vulnerable or abused person. Below are some common myths and facts that are coupled with abuse and vulnerability:

Myth: Abuse and neglect of adults is rare.

Fact: It is difficult to determine an accurate percentage of the occurrences of abuse because many of those people who have been abused hide behind a sense of shame and embarrassment. For a variety of reasons some people can find it difficult speak out about their abuse, because of this the incidence of adult abuse is biased; this also makes it difficult to measure.

Myth: Most abuse of adults occurs in care or nursing homes.
Fact: Abuse can occur just as easily in a person's own home, a busy hospital ward or in day care.

Myth: Abuse in later life only happens to those people who are very frail.
Fact: Abuse can happen to anyone and comes in many forms including physical abuse, emotional abuse and financial abuse. Emotional abuse is just as harmful as physical abuse.

Myth: Adult abuse only occurs to older women, older people, those who are isolated or those with disabilities.

Fact: Anyone can be abused. Often the abuser is a loved one whom the person trusts. It is this bond of trust that can permit the abuser to destroy the person's self-confidence and also challenge their feeling and sense of self-worth.

Myth: Most abuse of adults concerns physical abuse.
Fact: Physical abuse is often the easiest type of abuse to notice as there is easily recognisable physical evidence that can include bruises, scratches, biting or scarring. When verbal, emotional or psychological abuse is present, external indicators can come in the form of behavioural modifications.

Ethical considerations

Ethical issues are apparent in all aspects of care and instinctively concluding that something is fair or unfair requires criteria to be called upon to make that judgement. Having an understanding of ethics will help the nurse when caring for patients in acute care settings and will help them make certain judgements that are based on protecting the public from harm. Whatever element of nursing intervention is being undertaken will have the potential to impact positively and also negatively on the patient's physical and psychological well-being. A continuous awareness

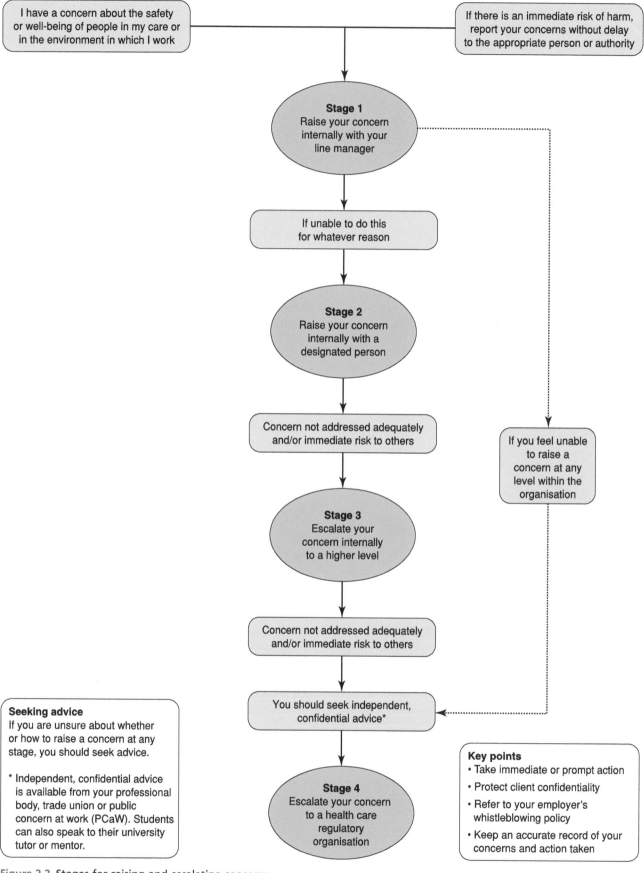

Figure 2.2 Stages for raising and escalating concerns

Source: Nursing and Midwifery Council (2010) *Raising and Escalating Concerns: Guidance for Nurses and Midwives*. London: Nursing and Midwifery Council, pp. 12–13. This flow chart should be read in conjunction with the full guidance available at www.nmc.uk.org/guidance.

of this, no matter how short-lived the interaction is with the patient, is required. Nurses are engaged with the ethical practice of nursing and are confronted with ethical issues, challenges and dilemmas almost every day.

Nurses are, at all times, accountable for their own practice (or omissions) regardless of the advice and directions given to the nurse by another health care professional, for example a doctor (NMC 2008). If a nurse carries out actions on the directions of another health care professional, this will not relieve the nurse of their personal and professional responsibility if the nurse is acting unethically or unlawfully. It is essential that the nurse is fully aware of the legal and ethical issues that surround patient care. Nurses must have skills in ethical reasoning as well as an understanding of the ethical theories that may inform practice.

The key element of the chapter is associated with ensuring that the patient's best interests and well-being are respected. A number of ethical perspectives have to be considered by the nurse when working with patients in any health and social care setting.

Ethical dilemmas can arise when there is or may be conflict between various interests and interested parties. Decisions need to be taken, care has to be prioritised and resources managed on a daily basis, and undertaking these tasks will unavoidably involve ethical considerations.

Each person is important and is entitled to be treated with respect. The Royal College of Nursing (RCN 2009) suggests that this value, respect, is upheld in law and must underpin all aspects of nursing practice. Ethical theories are complex theories that philosophers use to help consider moral beliefs and practices.

Advocacy

Another ill-defined concept is patient advocacy; it is subject to ambiguity of interpretation. Advocacy has been described in legal and ethical frameworks; nurses often associate this with ethical obligations to act as an advocate for the people they care for and in so doing treat people in a dignified way. Acting as an advocate means that the nurse has to promote the patient's rights to autonomy, free choice and self-determination (Terry 2007). One of the most important roles of the nurse is to act as patient advocate, to protect the interests of the people they care for when those people cannot because of illness or inadequate health knowledge. There are some patients, however, who may be unable to make independent decisions concerning their health and well-being (LeMone and Burke 2008). People who are, or may be, in vulnerable situations will need an advocate who will be required to help them assert their human rights. You might be this advocate; if this

is the case, then you must ensure you are up to date with current legislation and local policy. If you observe any activity that you consider does not safeguard those people in need of support then you have a responsibility to challenge this practice.

According to the Royal College of Nursing (RCN 2003) advocacy is defined as the act of speaking or acting on behalf of another: an advocate is somebody who expresses and defends the cause of another. Nursing interventions are concerned with helping and empowering people, assisting them to achieve, maintain or recover independence if this is needed. Promotion of a safe environment is also an essential element of advocacy (International Council of Nursing 2002).

The overall role of the advocate is to protect patients' rights (Kozier et al. 2008). There are a number of ways in which this role can be accomplished. The role of the nurse is multifaceted, nurses are patient educators and have a responsibility for explaining procedures and treatments to people they care for. Nurses teach patients and their families how to eat more healthily, take medicines, change dressings and use medical equipment. They also empower patients, directing people toward healthy behaviours and supporting them in times of need. If the patient is able the nurse encourages and teaches them how to be self-caring. Nurses intervene and provide care only when patients cannot do this for themselves.

Nurses provide dignity to individuals near the end of their lives by advocating for sufficient and appropriate pain medication and offering them choice, helping them make decisions concerning the way they wish to die.

Health care systems can be complex and often difficult to navigate; people who are acutely ill may find dealing with this complex system is too much for them, and the nurse is ideally placed to help people here. Kozier et al. (2008) suggest that there are three values basic to patient advocacy (see Table 2.2).

There are barriers that can affect or impact on the nurse's ability to act as advocate. These can include:

- **Apathy**
- **Disempowerment**
- Feelings of inadequacy, preparedness
- Lack of knowledge, education
- Lack of time.

The *Code* of professional conduct (NMC 2008) states that in order to make people your first concern, treating them as an individual and respecting their dignity may mean that you will have to act as their advocate. This can include helping them to access relevant health and social care, information and support. Rooted in the role of advocate are, according to Maude and Hawley (2007), two

Table 2.2 Values associated with patient advocacy

1 The patient is an holistic being who has the right to make choices and decisions.
2 Each patient has the right to expect a nurse–patient relationship that is based on shared respect, trust, collaboration solving problems related to health and health care along with consideration of their thoughts and feelings.
3 The nurse has a responsibility to ensure that the patient has access to health care services that meet their health needs.

Source: Adapted from Kozier *et al.* (2008).

moral concepts – fidelity (this is about being honest and truthful) and respect. Respect extends to dignity, privacy, self-determination and choice. When acting as advocate the nurse must be ready to intervene directly on the patient's behalf. This can usually be achieved by influencing others, using interpersonal skills, applying a sound knowledge base and having a desire to ensure that fairness and equity are paramount.

Caring with confidence

Providing care has become more complex than ever and this can be in the person's own home or in an acute care setting. Changes in health care have come about for a number of reasons, for example, the increase used of technology, the increased use of a number of specialist practitioners and the provision of more specialist care; this is also coupled with more complex patient needs. Regardless of this the more fundamental aspects of care remain the same; people expect to be safe, to be treated with kindness, courtesy and compassion. Providing these fundamental aspects of care can help the people you care for feel that they are being cared for in a competent way. These issues matter to patients.

Nursing is often described as an art and science. It is essential that nurses 'care for' and 'care about' in equal measures (DH 2008), providing care with kindness takes no more time. The following are cited as confidence creators – patients see these as core to care that is provided:

- a calm, clean, safe environment;
- a positive friendly culture;
- good teamwork and good relationships;
- well-managed care with efficient delivery;
- personalised care for and about every patient.

All of these carry equal importance; there is no one point that matters more than another. Considering them all them will demonstrate that they are all interrelated and

Table 2.3 Summary of what patients want from health care providers

• A healthcare provider who looks and acts professionally; is caring, kind, compassionate and knowledgeable. A care provider who offers individualised care that is personalised, holistic, timely, seamless and provides information.
• A champion who puts their interests first and protects them when they are vulnerable.
• A care provider who works with patients and relatives to plan care, offers constant feedback and reports, and assists them to navigate health and social care systems.
• A coordinator who is constant, accessible and accountable for communicating the plan and monitoring the delivery of care. Patients want to know that their care is being actively managed.

Source: Adapted from DH (2008).

require input from the whole health care team. Table 2.3 summarises what patients want from health care providers.

Conclusion

There is a growing literature relating to vulnerability and all health and social care providers in all settings should be aware of the developments in this sphere of health and social care. This chapter has defined key terms and has demonstrated that there are challenges present when trying to define terms such as abuse and vulnerability, there are also challenges when attempting to define who is vulnerable or at risk. Vulnerability is a dynamic and ever-changing concept relating to all entities that waxes and wanes.

People being cared for in a variety of care environments are potentially vulnerable. This is applicable to those people you may care for in the acute care setting. There are a number of rights all people have that help to ensure they are safe and free from risk, for example human rights.

Provision exists that provides guidance and support to practitioners to help them identify, protect and monitor those people who are at risk of abuse and who are vulnerable. Professional bodes such as the Nursing and Midwifery Council also provide support, advice and guidance for students, registered nurses and midwives, helping to ensure that the voice of the vulnerable person is heard and acted upon.

Acting as a patient's advocate requires a practitioner who is knowledgeable as well as one who understands ethical theories and how these apply to practice. Understanding ethical behaviour and acting ethically can have an impact on the quality of care.

Glossary

Apathy Lack of interest or concern.

Autonomy The right of patients to make decisions about their health care without the health care provider trying to influence the decision.

Clinical governance A framework through which organisations are accountable for continually improving the quality of services and safeguarding high standards of care.

Coercion Applying either physical or moral force to another.

Dignity Providing dignity in care focuses on three integral aspects: respect, compassion and sensitivity.

Discrimination This can be direct or indirect and is associated with treating a person or a group of people less favourably than others in the same situation.

Disempowerment Processes that lead to a reduction of the power which individuals have to make their own choices and shape their own lives as well making decisions about their own health care and health care needs.

Ethics A system of moral principles, rules of conduct.

Fraud A crime associated with deception deliberately practised in order to secure unfair or unlawful gain.

Harassment Any unwanted or uninvited behaviour which is offensive, embarrassing, intimidating or humiliating.

Health Service Ombudsman Exists to provide a service to the public by undertaking independent investigations into complaints about health services that have not acted properly or fairly or have provided a poor service.

Insomnia Inability to obtain an adequate amount or quality of sleep.

Malnutrition Any condition in which the body does not receive enough nutrients for effective function. Malnutrition may range from mild to severe and life threatening.

Neglect This is a type of abuse where a person has been remiss in their provision of care or treatment.

Paranoia Unfounded or exaggerated distrust of others.

Physiological needs Physiological needs are those required to sustain life, such as air, water, nourishment and sleep.

Racism Discrimination or prejudice based on race.

Respect To show regard or consideration for another person, respect a person's rights.

Self-esteem Central to a person's survival, the basis of our well-being, the degree of worth and competence one attributes to oneself.

Sensory depravation Deprivation of adequate and appropriate interpersonal or environmental experience and deprivation of usual external stimuli and the opportunity for development.

Sexism Discrimination or prejudice based on sex.

Statute A law enacted by a legislator.

Test yourself

1   What is the primary role and function of the Nursing and Midwifery Council?

2   Nurses are accountable to the NMC. True or false?

3   If you are concerned about the health and well-being of somebody you should:
   a. suspend judgement until you have definitive evidence
   b. report this immediately
   c. wait until you get back to university and report it to your lecturer
   d. say nothing as you are a student

4   The most vulnerable people in our society are children. True or false?

5   Which of the following may be signs of abuse:
   a. change in a person's behaviour
   b. unexplained burns in unusual locations
   c. unexplained fractures to any part of the body
   d. all of the above

6   How would you define whistleblowing?

7   An advocate can be defined as:
   a. a person who needs help and assistance
   b. another name for a midwife
   c. somebody who acts on behalf of another, somebody who expresses and defends the cause of another
   d. none of the above

8   Racism can mean:
   a. abuse of person because of their culture
   b. belief that one religion is superior to other
   c. disregarding a person's requests concerning their care
   d. belief in superiority of a particular race

9   True or false: abuse can be a criminal offence?

10 Which of the following might constitute deprivation of liberty:
   a. locking a person in their room as punishment for long periods of time
   b. excessively restraining a person for long periods of time
   c. sedating a patient because they are 'causing trouble'
   d. all of the above

References

Criminal Records Bureau (2011) *Definitions*. Available from http://www.crb.homeoffice.gov.uk/faqs/definitions.aspx, accessed February 2011.

De Chesnay, M. (2008) Vulnerable populations: Vulnerable people. In De Chesnay, M. and Anderson, B. A. (eds) *Caring for the Vulnerable: Perspectives in nursing theory and practice and research*, 2nd edn. Boston: MA: Jones and Bartlett, pp. 3–14.

Department of Health and Home Office (2000) *No Secrets: Guidance on developing and implementing multi-agency policies and procedures to protect vulnerable adults from abuse*. London: Department of Health.

DH (Department of Health) (2010) *Clinical Governance and Adult Safeguarding; An integrated process*. London: Department of Health.

DH (Department of Health) (2009) *Safeguarding Adults. Report on the consultation on the review of 'No Secrets'*. London: Department of Health.

DH (Department of Health) (2008) *Confidence in Caring – a framework for best practice*. London: Department of Health.

Equalities and Human Rights Commission (2010) *How Fair is Britain? Equality, human rights and good relations in 2010*. London: Equalities and Human Rights Commission.

Healthcare Commission (2009) *Investigation into Mid Staffordshire NHS Foundation Trust*. Available from http://www.cqc.org.uk/_db/_documents/Investigation_into_Mid_Staffordshire_NHS_Foundation_Trust.pdf, accessed March 2011.

International Council of Nursing (2002) *The ICN Definition of Nursing*. Geneva: ICM.

Kozier, B., Erb, G., Berman, A., Snyder, S., Lake, R. and Harvey, S. (2008) *Fundamentals of Nursing. Concepts, process and practice*. Harlow: Pearson.

LeMone, P. and Burke, K. (2008) *Medical-Surgical Nursing. Critical thinking in clinical care*. Old Tappan, NJ: Pearson.

Lord Chancellor's Department (1998) *Who Decides?: Making decisions on behalf of mentally incapacitated adults*. London: The Stationery Office.

Maslow, A. (1954) *Motivation and Personality*. New York: Harper & Row.

Maude, P. and Hawley, G. (2007) Clients' and patients' rights and protecting the vulnerable. In Hawley, G. (ed.) *Ethics in Clinical Practice: An interprofessional approach*. Harlow: Pearson, pp. 54–75.

Mencap (2007) *Death by Indifference*. London: Mencap.

Michael, J. and the Independent Inquiry into Access to Healthcare for People with Learning Disabilities (2008) *Healthcare for All: Report of the independent inquiry into access to healthcare for people with learning disabilities*. Available from http://www.dh.gov.uk/prod_consum_dh/groups/dh_digitalassets/@dh/@en/documents/digitalasset/dh_106126.pdf, accessed March 2011.

Michaels, C. and Moffett, C. (2008) Rethinking vulnerability. In De Chesnay, M. and Anderson, B. A. (eds) *Caring for the Vulnerable: Perspectives in nursing theory and practice and research*, 2nd edn. Boston: MA: Jones and Bartlett, pp. 15–24.

National Assembly for Wales (2000) *In Safe Hards: Implementing adult protection procedures in Wales*. Guidance Issued by the National Assembly for Wales under s7 of the Local Authority Social Services Act 1970. Cardiff: National Assembly for Wales.

National Patient Safety Organisation (2009) *Being Open: Communicating patient safety incidents with patients, their families and carers*. Available from http://www.nrls.npsa.nhs.uk/resources/?entryid45=65077, accessed March 2011.

NMC (Nursing and Midwifery Council) (2010) *Raising and Escalating Concerns. Guidance for nurses and midwives*. London: NMC.

NMC (Nursing and Midwifery Council) (2009) *Guidance for the Care of Older People*. London: NMC.

NMC (Nursing and Midwifery Council) (2008) *The Code. Standards of conduct, performance and ethics for nurses and midwives*. London: NMC.

Parliamentary and Health Service Ombudsman (2011) *Care and Compassion? Report of the Health Service Ombudsman on ten investigations into the NHS care of older people*. London: The Stationery Office.

Peate, I. and Potterton, J. (2010) The vulnerable adult. *British Journal of Health Care Assistants* 5 (1), 8–11.

Penhale, B. and Parker, J. (2008) *Working with Vulnerable Adults*. London: Routledge.

RCN (Royal College of Nursing) (2009) *Research Ethics. RCN guidance for nurses*. London: RCN.

RCN (Royal College of Nursing) (2003) *Defining Nursing*. London: RCN.

Terry, L. M. (2007) Complex care: Ethical problems in the emergency department, perioperative, intensive and coronary care units. In Hawley, G. (ed.) *Ethics in Clinical Practice: An interprofessional approach*. Harlow: Pearson, pp. 276–99.

Further reading

Dartington, T. (2011) *Managing Vulnerability: The underlying dynamics of systems of care*. London: Karnac Books.

Francis, R. (2010) *Independent Inquiry into Care Provided by Mid Staffordshire NHS Foundation Trust January 2005–March 2009*. London: The Stationery Office.

Mandelstam, M. (2011) *How we Treat the Sick. Neglect and abuse in our health services*. London: Jessica Kingsley.

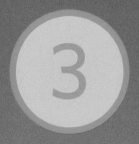

3

The cell and tissues

John Mears

Aims

The aim of this chapter is to provide you with an introduction to the structure and function of cells, along with the composition of the main tissue types, functions, tissue repair and the inflammatory process.

Objectives

After reading this chapter you will be able to:

→ Identify the component parts of a human cell and discuss their function

→ Explain the role of the plasma membrane and mitotic cell division

→ Explain transmembranal and intracellular transport mechanisms

→ Outline the pathway for the production of adenosine triphosphate (ATP)

→ Describe the structure and function of the main types of tissue

→ Describe inflammation and the process of healing and tissue repair

→ Discuss the consequences of disruption of normal cellular function, particularly the consequences of disrupted ATP production

Introduction

Understanding how to care for people safely and effectively requires the nurse to appreciate the microscopic and macroscopic aspects of the human. Studying the human from a cellular level as described in this chapter will help you recognise factors that impact on health and a person's vulnerability to illness. Observing the person from a cellular level is only one aspect of a wider understanding, this chapter sets the scene for the following chapters, providing a fundamental basis concerning the chemical foundations of life and how the body's cells are built and operate. The chapter then explores the how the body's tissues function allowing you to appreciate what occurs when cells, tissues and organ systems fail.

The cell and its environment

Before considering the basic structure of the cell it is important to consider the physiological environment of the cell. All human cells contain an aqueous fluid (intracellular fluid) identified as cytosol. Apart from the organelles, this fluid contains substances such as protein, other nutrient molecules, metabolic products and also a range of chemicals known as electrolytes. Outside the cells there is the extracellular fluid, which is composed of the interstitial fluid just mentioned and the circulating fluid; this is composed of blood in the vascular system and the lymph found in the lymphatic vessels. The extracellular fluid has a similar composition to the intracellular fluid. However, there are important differences in the composition of these fluids, particularly in the type and quantity of electrolytes and in the distribution of protein molecules.

The intracellular and extracellular environments are separated by the cell membrane, which is selectively permeable; it is able to control the movement of electrolytes and other molecules across it. This is discussed later in the chapter. The correct balance and movement of these chemicals between the intracellular and extracellular environments is vital to the maintenance of normal function and therefore health. A disruption of this balance is one of the factors that can cause homeostatic imbalance and potentially lead to a medical emergency.

Electrolytes

Electrolytes are charged atoms or molecules in solution which can conduct electricity. They may be cations, which have lost an electron and therefore carry a positive charge,

Table 3.1 Common cations and anions

	Normal values and location
Cations	
Sodium (Na^+)	135–145mmol/L main extracellular fluid cation
Potassium (K^+)	3.5–5.0mmol/L main intracellular fluid cation
Calcium (Ca^{2+})	Found in both fluid compartments
Magnesium (Mg^{2+})	Found in both fluid compartments
Hydrogen (H^+)	Found in both fluid compartments
Anions	
Chloride (Cl^-)	95–108mmol/L main anion in extracellular fluid
Phosphorus (P^-)	2.5–4.5mmol/L main anion in intracellular fluid
Bicarbonate (HCO_3^-)	22–28mmol/L found in both fluid compartments

or anions which have gained an electron and therefore have a negative charge. An example of this is common salt which is composed of sodium (Na) and chlorine (Cl) and is crystalline in structure. When the salt is dissolved in water the sodium and chlorine dissociate and become sodium cations (Na^+) and chloride anions (note the change of nomenclature) (Cl^-). In so doing the sodium loses an electron and the chloride gains an electron.

Electrolytes are not evenly distributed through the body. The concentrations of electrolytes (cations and anions) inside and outside the cells are different (see Table 3.1).

The key electrolyte differences are that potassium (K^+) is the main cation inside the cell and sodium (Na^+) is the main extracellular cation. Phosphorus (P^-) is the main intracellular anion and chloride (Cl^-) is the main extracellular anion. Other electrolytes of significance such as calcium (Ca^+), magnesium (Mg^{2+}) hydrogen ion (H^+) and bicarbonate (HCO_3^-) are distributed more evenly but concentrations will vary depending on the actual function of the cell concerned. Changes in the distribution of electrolytes and the ability of the cell to control their concentrations are very significant in disease processes.

Changes in the balance of electrolytes can have a dramatic effect on the functioning of the body. When the myocardial muscle is damaged by myocardial infarction, the damaged cells release potassium which increases the amount of this electrolyte in the interstitial fluid and circulation. This change alters the electrical potential across cells, especially the muscle cells of the heart, and may cause the electrical stimulation to become irregular leading to arrhythmias. These arrhythmias may affect the ability of the heart to pump effectively and therefore lead to a decrease in the oxygen supply to the body's cells, which, in turn, will lead to malfunction.

Acidity, alkalinity and pH balance

All physiological processes in cells are dependent on the correct pH. The pH is a measure of the hydrogen ion (H^+) concentration or acidity/alkalinity of the environment and is represented by a number between 0 and 14 where 0 is the most acidic, 14 is the most alkaline and 7 is neutral. The normal pH of blood, for example, is between 7.35 and 7.45. The pH of the blood and therefore the pH of the body is regulated by the lungs and kidneys. This balance is represented by the equation

$$CO_2 + H_2O \rightleftharpoons H_2CO_3 \rightleftharpoons H^+ + HCO_3^-$$

(carbon dioxide + water $\rightleftharpoons$ carbonic acid $\rightleftharpoons$ hydrogen ion + bicarbonate ion)

Alteration of this balance leads to malfunction of cells. If the CO_2 increases in the body because of poor respiration then the equation will be driven to the left, increasing the amount of H^+ ions and therefore an increase in acidity and vice versa. If the kidneys are not able to function properly then removal of bicarbonate ion will decrease and there will be an increase in alkalinity. The overall process is much more complex than this but these examples are given as an example of the control of the cellular environment.

Basic structure of cells

All cells have the same basic structure with a plasma membrane, a nucleus and cytoplasm. The cytoplasm consists of a water-based fluid, referred to as cytosol, which contains a range of organelles, inclusions and electrolytes (see Figure 3.1).

Exceptions to this are erythrocytes (red blood cells) and corneocytes (the cells on the surface of the epidermis of the skin), which do not contain nuclei. A third variation is found in cells of skeletal muscle which are multinucleate, i.e. each muscle cell has more than one nucleus. There are significant differences in shape and size of cells depending on the particular tissue type and their function. Some neurons (nerve cells) have axons that are over a metre long whilst red blood cells are only 7 microns in diameter and 2 microns deep. Some types of cell have more of one type of organelle, e.g. muscle cells have many mitochondria as they need to produce large quantities of energy.

Plasma membrane

All cells and their organelles are surrounded by plasma membranes (see Figure 3.2). This is a lipid bilayer that also contains a range of proteins and other molecules and

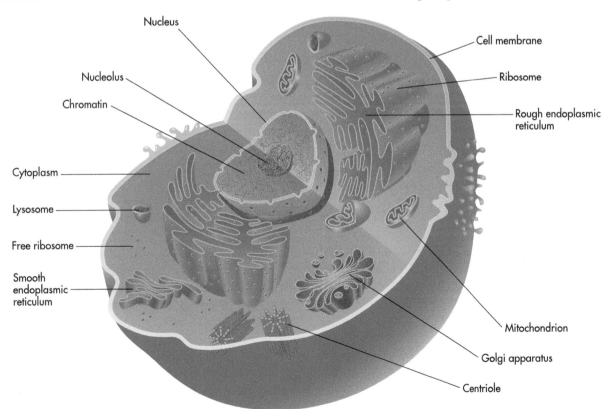

Figure 3.1 Cellular components

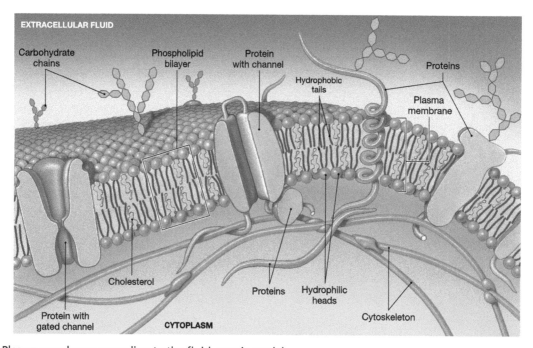

Figure 3.2 Plasma membrane according to the fluid mosaic model

Source: Martini, F. H. and Bartholomew, E. F. (2009) *Essentials of Anatomy & Physiology*, 5th edn, San Francisco: Pearson Benjamin Cummings, Fig. 3.3, p. 63.

is only 5–7 nanometres thick. Some of the proteins in the cell membrane cross the full thickness of the membrane (transmembranal) whilst others only penetrate partway into the membrane or are on the surface, effectively floating in the lipid layer. There are a range of glycoproteins that are attached to the outer surface of the cell membrane, mainly on the transmembranal proteins. The phospholipids and proteins of the membranes are not physically connected to each other but are held in place by molecular and atomic attractions. This means that sections of plasma membrane can move into and out of the outer membrane of the cell (see exocytosis and endocytosis in this section).

The molecules that make up the lipid bilayer are phospholipids. Phospholipids are neutral fats that have had one of the three fatty acids replaced by a phosphate molecule (PO_4^-) which is anionic and therefore is compatible with water. The consequence of this is that the molecules have a hydrophilic (water-attracting phosphate) end and a hydrophobic (water-repelling fatty acid) end. On both layers; the hydrophilic end is on the outer face with the fatty acid, hydrophobic end on the inside of the layer. This means that the outside of the membrane is compatible with the aqueous medium both inside and outside the cell but because of the hydrophobic nature of the interior of the bilayer water and electrolytes cannot cross the lipid sections of the membrane. The movement of electrolytes is facilitated by protein channels.

The structure of the membrane is also the reason why most drugs are fat soluble: this facilitates their transport into the cell in which they will have their action. The hydrophobic barrier is one of the ways in which the differences in concentrations of electrolytes inside and outside the cell are maintained. The membrane also acts as a selectively permeable membrane to help control the movement of water into and out of the cell.

The cell membrane is stabilised by molecules such as cholesterol and vitamin E. Without these stabilising molecules the cell membrane would not be able to maintain its integrity.

As identified earlier, some of the proteins in the plasma membrane cross the full width of the membrane whilst others penetrate only part way through. Some of the membrane proteins form channels through the cell membrane that under the right conditions allow the movement or transport of electrolytes and other lipid-insoluble substances into and out of the cell (see Figure 3.3).

Some channels allow passive movement of electrolytes but most of this movement is dependent on energy supplied by ATP and also on other transport proteins. In this way, the cell is able to control the movement of electrolytes and other molecules into and out of the cell. There are exceptions to this mechanism. One is normal and involves the pacemaker cells of the heart where sodium is able to passively move into the cells, through ion channels, altering the membrane potential. The second is an abnormal situation found in damaged nerves where the normal stable ion channels are replaced by unstable channels that allow the movement of sodium and therefore set off action potentials that lead to neuropathic pain.

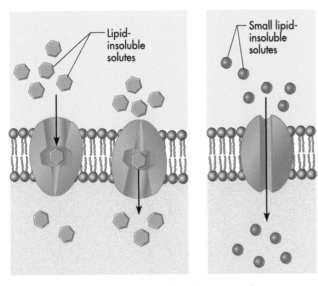

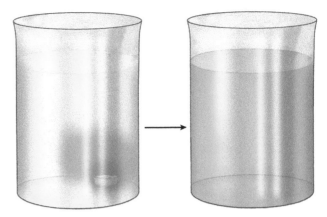

Figure 3.4 Diffusion of a substance from an area of high concentration to an area of lower concentration until the concentration of the substance is uniform throughout the solution

Figure 3.3 Protein channels in the plasma membrane

Source: Marieb, E. N. and Hoehn, K. (2010) *Human Anatomy and Physiology*, 8th edn. Uppser Saddle River, NJ: Pearson, p. 69, Fig 3.7. Copyright © 2010. Reproduced by permission of Pearson Education, Inc.

Attached to the outside of the plasma membrane, particularly to the protein molecules, there are a range of carbohydrates and glycoproteins that have a wide range of functions. Some are signalling molecules while others are used for attachment to other cells and for attracting and attaching other cells such as neutrophils, yet others are part of the immune system, including antibodies.

Each cell in the body, except sperm, have marker molecules on the cell surface that identify them as belonging to that individual. This is part of the histocompatability system of the body and one of the main reasons why individuals undergoing organ transplant need to be immunosuppressed following transplantation. As the donor cells do not carry the correct marker molecules they are attacked by the host's immune system.

Transmembranal transport

There are two broad types of transport across plasma membranes. The first is passive transport, which by its very nature does not require any energy input. Passive transport can be subdivided into four categories; diffusion, facilitated diffusion, osmosis and filtration.

The second is active transport and this requires energy input, usually in the form of ATP. This type of transport is energy dependent and requires the continual production of ATP for the mechanisms to work. As the body only has enough ATP available at any time to last a few seconds if the supply ceases then not only is active transport of electrolytes and other chemicals into and out of the cell compromised but the normal functioning of the cell is also potentially seriously affected.

Passive transport

Diffusion is the movement of a substance from an area of higher concentration to an area of lower concentration. Figure 3.4 illustrates this principle. If dye is added to a beaker of liquid the molecules will gradually spread throughout the liquid (a). This happens because the molecules of dye move into the solution and are constantly moving and bumping into each other. The consequence of this is that they gradually spread until they are evenly distributed throughout the solution (b).

The difference is called the concentration gradient. The concentration may simply refer to the number of atoms or molecules in a given volume or may refer to the electrical concentration. Examples of diffusion would be the movement of dissolved oxygen from the alveoli of the lungs to the blood in the capillaries surrounding the alveoli. The movement of carbon dioxide in the opposite direction is also achieved by diffusion. The diffusion across the alveoli is dependent on the distance (the diffusion pathway). If this is extended for any reason, e.g. if there is inflammation or scarring from previous episodes of healing, then the distance across the diffusion pathway is extended which can seriously affect the supply of oxygen and the removal of carbon dioxide.

Facilitated diffusion is a process in which molecules are assisted in moving down their concentration gradient across the plasma membrane. A good example of this facilitation is the movement of glucose molecules into the cell. There are receptor molecules on the surface of the cell membrane which are activated by the attachment of insulin. Once the receptor is activated it in turn activates the carrier molecules in the plasma membrane. The carrier molecules are specifically designed to interact with the

Capillary   **Interstitium**   **Cell**

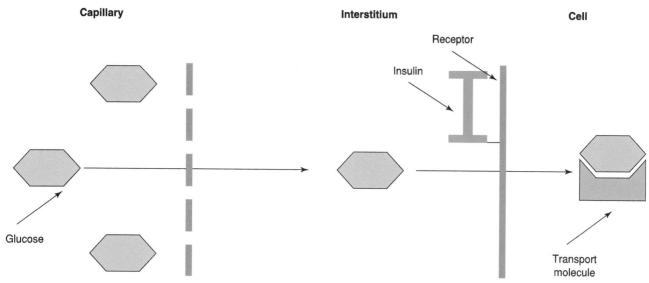

Figure 3.5 The movement of glucose from capillary to cell
Source: © Mears Associates 2011.

glucose molecules. No extra energy is required because the carrier molecules are designed to move into the cell when they connect with the glucose molecule. There are in fact two types of carrier that operate like taxis. Some are waiting in the cell membrane (taxi rank) and others are cruising waiting to pick up free glucose molecules. If these transport molecules are missing or if they malfunction glucose transport into the cells is reduced. The transport of glucose is also critically dependent on insulin being attached to the cell plasma membrane to enable the glucose transport to take place (see Figure 3.5).

Osmosis is the term used for the movement of water across a selectively permeable membrane (a cell plasma membrane for example) from an area of lower solute concentration to an area of higher solute concentration to equalise the concentrations on either side of the membrane (see Figure 3.6).

It should be remembered that, in effect, this is water moving along its own concentration gradient. An example of this in action would be if a person were dehydrated. When we dehydrate, e.g. when we are unwell and sweating or not drinking sufficient fluid, we lose water from the spaces around the cells (interstitial space). This makes the remaining interstitial fluid more concentrated so water moves from inside the cells (intracellular space) into the interstitial space. Unfortunately, this makes the cytosol in the cells more concentrated and affects their ability to function properly. In the central nervous system this may lead to confusion or loss of consciousness.

Filtration

Filtration is the movement of a fluid under pressure from one space to another through the plasma membrane. An

extremely important example of this is the movement of plasma across the arteriolar wall in the systemic circulation and particularly in the glomerulus of the nephron in the kidney. Under normal circumstances approximately 125mL of plasma a minute are filtered in the kidney. If the blood pressure drops drastically this filtration ceases and the individual develops acute renal failure.

In the systemic circulation, between three and four litres of fluid are filtered out of the arterioles into the interstitial spaces every day. In healthy individuals, this is returned to the circulation through the vennules or is cleared by the lymphatic system. In some situations, this process is interrupted, e.g. if the venous pressure is high, as in cardiac failure, less of the fluid is returned to the circulation. The excess fluid that remains in the interstitial

Both solutions have identical osmolarity, but volume of the solution on the right is greater because only water is free to move

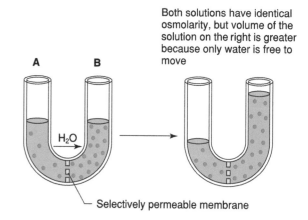

The membrance is selectively impermeable: it allows the movement of water across it from A to B but not solute. Water moves from the area of low solute concentration until the conventration of solute is the same on both sides of the membrane (isotonic)

Figure 3.6 Osmosis

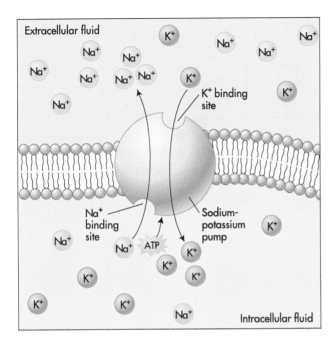

(a)

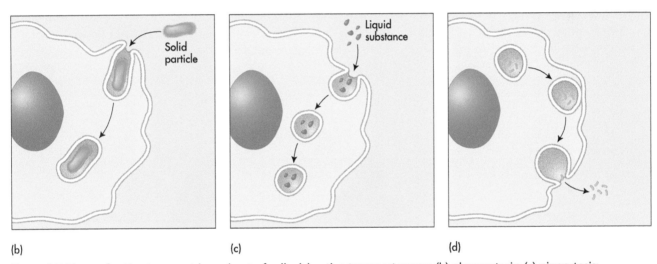

(b)   (c)   (d)

Figure 3.7 Types of active transport in and out of cells: (a) active transport pump; (b) phagocytosis; (c) pinocytosis; (d) exocytosis

spaces is called oedema. This oedema can have a significant effect on the diffusion pathway, creating a similar problem to that in the lungs identified earlier in the chapter.

Active transport

Active transport pumps require energy input in order to function (see Figure 3.7).

This energy is supplied by ATP which loses a phosphate group to become adenosine diphosphate (ADP) with the release of energy. This type of transport is involved in moving electrolytes against their concentration gradients, e.g. returning potassium to the cell and removing sodium

from the cell to the interstitial fluid. This process is known as primary active transport.

Endocytosis and exocytosis

The two processes involve the formation of a vesicle by pinching off sections of plasma membrane containing particles or fluid (see Figure 3.7).

In endocytosis water, large food particles that are too large to cross the plasma membrane or microorganisms such as bacteria are transported from outside the cell to the inside. If water is being transported the process is called pinocytosis. The same principle is used in phagocytosis to engulf bacteria and cell debris (see Figure 3.7).

Exocytosis is the reverse process. Vesicles created by budding from the endoplasmic reticulum and Golgi apparatus move to the surface of the cell and the vesicle membrane joins the cell membrane and expels its contents into the interstitial space. Always remember that the molecules of the plasma membrane are not physically linked so this kind of manoeuvre is easily and effectively accomplished.

Cytoplasm

Cytoplasm is the name given to the contents of the cell within the plasma membrane and outside the nucleus. It is composed of an aqueous fluid (cytosol) in which are dissolved or suspended proteins, salts (electrolytes), sugars and other molecules necessary for the function of the cell as well as metabolic by-products and organelles and inclusions required for the normal function of the cell (see Figure 3.8).

The inclusions will vary from cell to cell but may be glycogen granules in liver and muscle cells, fat globules in fat cells or melanin in epidermal melanocytes.

Mitochondria

Mitochondria are small double-walled sausage-shaped structures in which most of the energy required for metabolism and cellular function is produced. It is within these structures that oxygen is utilised to produce adenosine triphosphate.

The number of mitochondria within specific types of cells is dependent on the activity of those cells. In liver and muscle cells, there are many mitochondria because these cells are very metabolically active. Bone cells (osteocytes) have few as they are not very metabolically active.

Ribosomes

These small organelles are found attached to the endoplasmic reticulum and floating freely in the cytosol. They are composed of ribosomal ribonucleic acid and proteins and are manufactured in the nucleolus of the nucleus and then transported into the cytosol. Their function is to act as centres for the production of proteins, which include enzymes. The proteins produced are used for metabolism, repair and replication within cells and for transport into the extracellular matrix.

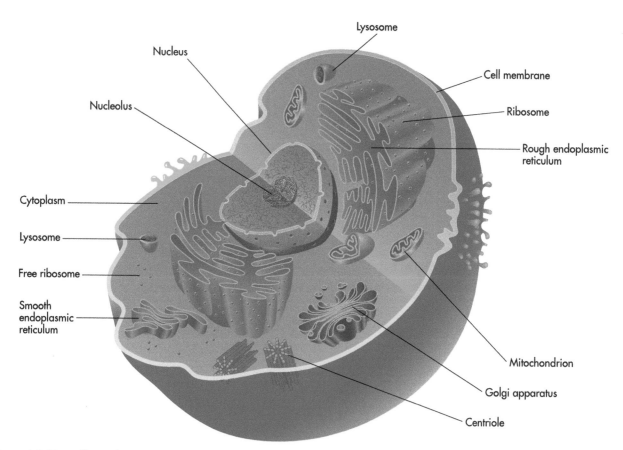

Figure 3.8 The cell membrane, cytoplasm, nucleus, ribosomes, centrosomes, mitochondria, endoplasmic reticulum, Golgi apparatus and lysosomes

Endoplasmic reticulum

The endoplasmic reticulum is a series of tubes and flattened fluid-filled cavities (cisternae) that are continuous with the nuclear membrane. Like all the membranes in the cell they are lipid bilayers.

There are two distinct types of endoplasmic reticulum; some of it has ribosomes attached and is known as rough endoplasmic reticulum; this is found in all cells. The other is known as smooth endoplasmic reticulum as it has no ribosomes attached. It is found in a limited number of cells. The two types of endoplasmic reticulum have different roles.

The ribosomes on the rough endoplasmic reticulum produce all the proteins that are secreted from the cells. The various molecules necessary for the production and maintenance of the cell are also produced by this type endoplasmic reticulum.

Smooth endoplasmic reticulum is composed mainly of loops and is not involved in protein synthesis. Rather the integral proteins of the membrane have specialist catalytic roles, e.g. cholesterol synthesis in the liver, steroid-based hormone production in the cells of the testes, detoxification of some drugs and pesticides in the liver and kidney.

Golgi apparatus

The Golgi apparatus is an assembly of flattened, stacked plasma membranes. This structure is the finishing shop and transport centre for molecules produced in the cell. The Golgi apparatus receives the molecules produced by the endoplasmic reticulum, makes adjustments to the chemical structure and then transports the finished items in vesicles. Some of the products are for use within the cell and its membranes and others are exported. Most of the chemicals produced are transported in vesicles composed of pinched-off plasma membrane. Export from the cell is achieved by exocytosis.

Lysosomes

Lysosomes are small spherical organelles surround by plasma membrane. They contain enzymes that are capable of degrading and breaking down all sorts of material from bacteria and toxins to worn out organelles. They are therefore abundant in phagocytic cells (cells that engulf and destroy bacteria and cell debris in the inflammatory process) such as macrophages and neutrophils. These small structures create a safe area for the destruction of unwanted material within cells. The digestive environment is very acidic and requires energy in the form of ATP to pump hydrogen ions into these organelles. If the pump fails because of lack of ATP associated with poor oxygen supply then the lysosomes do not function properly and the degradation process is inhibited leading to a breakdown in cellular function.

Peroxisomes

Peroxisomes are membranous sacs that are similar to lysosomes but are self-replicating and are not produced by the usual endoplasmic reticulum and Golgi apparatus route. They contain a number of enzymes including oxidases that are important in the detoxification of substances such as alcohol but just as importantly they are involved in the neutralising of free radicals. These organelles are found in large numbers in kidney and liver cells which are metabolically very active and are primary sites for detoxification.

Cytoskeleton

Each cell has a collection of microtubules and filaments that are associated with the cytoplasmic side of the plasma membrane and also form a network throughout the cell. They are composed of proteins, some of which are similar to those found in muscle cells. They help to give the cell shape, attachment for organelles and enable cell movement. The movement is particularly important in white cells such as monocytes, macrophages and neutrophils that have to change shape to pass through capillaries and to be able to move through the pores in capillary walls to reach areas of inflammation and infection.

The cytoskeleton is significant in maintaining cell shape and as a consequence ensuring that the cell has sufficient volume to remain adequately hydrated. As humans age connective tissue protein production decreases, reducing the volume of the cell. This can be extremely significant in situations where patients are sitting or lying in one position for a period of time as the cell can be more easily damaged which can lead to the production of pressure ulcers. This is a particular problem in the very ill and malnourished and those with reduced mobility.

Centrosome and centrioles

The centrosome is an area near the nucleus that contains a pair of rod-like structures called the centrioles. This area and the centrioles are associated with the process of cell division. They produce the mitotic spindle in dividing cells.

The centrioles also form the basis of cilia and flagellae. Cilia are typically found on the columnar epithelium of the lining of the respiratory tract. They are involved in the movement of dust particles up the respiratory tract. The only example of a flagellum found in humans is in sperm.

Nucleus

The nucleus is a structure found in all human cells except those identified earlier in the chapter. It is protected by a double nuclear envelope, the outer layer of which is continuous with the endoplasmic reticulum. The envelope has gaps in it called pores that allow the movement of specified molecules into and out of it. Protein molecules enter and ribosomes and messenger ribonucleic acid (mRNA) exit. Signalling chemicals that can stimulate the DNA transcription can also enter through these pores.

Within the nucleus there is an area called the nucleolus. The nucleolus is primarily responsible for the production of ribosomal RNA (rRNA) which combines with proteins imported from the cytoplasm to make the ribosomes, which then leave the nucleus and enter the cytoplasm to attach to endoplasmic reticulum or to attach to the cytoskeleton as individual units.

The nucleus of the cell is where the DNA is stored. The DNA is normally shared out amongst the 46 chromosomes that are the typical karyotype of humans. This number can vary between 45 and 49 depending on events that take place during the production of ova and sperm. In cells that are not undergoing division the DNA combined with special proteins called histones is unravelled and takes the form of long filaments called chromatin. It is only as the cell begins the process of division that the DNA coils up to produce the familiar shapes that we recognise as chromosomes.

DNA is a double helix that carries our genes which in turn determine what we look like and how we function. DNA carries the code for nearly all the proteins that are produced in the cell by ribosomes. These proteins can be enzymes, surface markers and antibodies. They can also be structural proteins or command molecules that regulate the production of the other molecules produced in the cell.

Cell cycle and cell division

Cells, like the organism they form, are mortal, but they are able to postpone their death by asexual reproduction or simply dividing in two. They can do this only a certain number of times before they lose the ability and die. This process is called mitosis. Mitosis or the mitotic phase takes up a small part of the overall life of a cell. Only a proportion of cells are dividing at any time so most of the cells are not involved in producing new cells but are involved in the normal day-to-day cellular function. This non-dividing phase is called interphase. During interphase the

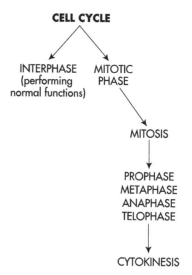

Figure 3.9 Flow chart of the cell cycle

cells also grow and replicate (double by making exact copies) their DNA and organelles ready for the next mitotic phase. The combination of interphase and the mitotic phase is known as the cell cycle (see Figure 3.9).

Mitosis is asexual reproduction, as there is only one cell involved. The process of mitosis is complex and is divided into four phases with the last phase being combined with cytokinesis, which describes the process of the non-nuclear part of the cell dividing in half. The four phases are prophase, metaphase, anaphase and telophase (see Figure 3.10). These phases are not discrete but are part of a continuous process and indicate the significant stages that can be identified in the overall process.

Prophase

In prophase the nuclear membrane breaks down, the nucleus disappears and the long strands of chromatin condense (become densely coiled) to form the familiar chromosome shapes (remember that the cell has already made duplicate copies of its DNA ready for the two daughter cells). The centrioles discussed earlier produce guiding filaments that create a cage-like structure called the spindle. The chromosomes begin to migrate towards the middle of the cell.

Metaphase

Metaphase sees the chromosomes, or chromatids as they are more correctly known at this stage, finishing their migration to the middle of the cell and lining up across the middle of the cell. This arrangement is known as the metaphase plate.

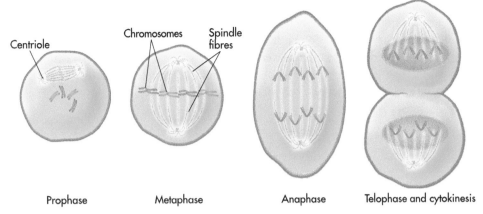

Figure 3.10 Phases of mitosis

Anaphase

Anaphase is the stage in which the duplicate pairs of chromatids become separated and the spindle retracts, pulling and separating the pairs of chromatids and moving them towards each end of the cell.

Telophase

In telophase the chromatids complete the journey to each end of the cell, the spindle disappears and the nuclear membranes form.

Cytokinesis

The division is then completed by the mother cell dividing in two along the midline to create to identical daughter cells.

Energy production in the cell

Normal metabolic function is dependent on the production of energy to drive the reactions and processes necessary to maintain homeostasis. The main energy source for cellular activity is ATP. This molecule is key to continued normal function of the cell and therefore its production needs to be continuous in order to provide the necessary energy.

ATP is required to fuel:

- Energy production itself. It is necessary to initiate glycolysis and fatty acid oxidation.
- Active transport of electrolytes across the plasma membrane, e.g. the Na^+/K^+ pump that restores the resting potential of the heart's pacemaker cells.

- The amplification of second messenger systems in cells. This process involves small amounts of signalling molecules attaching to the surface of the cell and initiating a process involving a number of membrane and intracellular proteins that amplify the message to ensure that there is a sufficient response within the cell. This means that a relatively weak signal can produce a significant cellular action. The amino acid endocrines such as antidiuretic hormone function in this way.
- Contraction of skeletal, cardiac and smooth muscle cells.
- Phosphorylation of molecules to enable and enhance reactions in the cell.

Any interruption in the production of ATP will have a devastating effect on cell function.

ATP can be produced from a number of nutrients including glucose, glycerol and fatty acids, which are the component parts of triacylglycerols (also known as triglycerides or neutral fats) and some amino acids. At rest many cells use glycerol and fatty acids but this process is relatively slow and only yields 50% of the ATP yielded by glucose under ideal conditions. Therefore even moderate activity requires the use of glucose. Glucose is found free in the blood or stored as glycogen in the liver and skeletal muscle. If glucose is in short supply the other molecules including amino acids are used for the production of glucose. This is a process known as gluconeogenesis.

In order to produce sufficient ATP it is necessary to have an adequate supply of oxygen through the lungs and effective delivery of oxygen into the cells. This means that any acute or chronic respiratory problem could affect the availability of oxygen for distribution to the cells. Similarly many cardiovascular problems, such as myocardial infarction, heart failure, peripheral vascular disease or a significant reduction in systemic arterial blood pressure as in shock could also lead to a situation of insufficient oxygen delivery. Where there has been injury followed by inflammation or scarring following injury the diffusion pathway can be compromised, potentially reducing oxygen delivery. All of these situations will also affect the removal and disposal of carbon dioxide and other metabolic products that could alter pH or prove toxic to the cells, further compromising their ability to function effectively.

As identified earlier in the chapter, ATP can be produced from a variety of substrates. The processes are extremely complex, but the pathway is quite straightforward (see Figure 3.11).

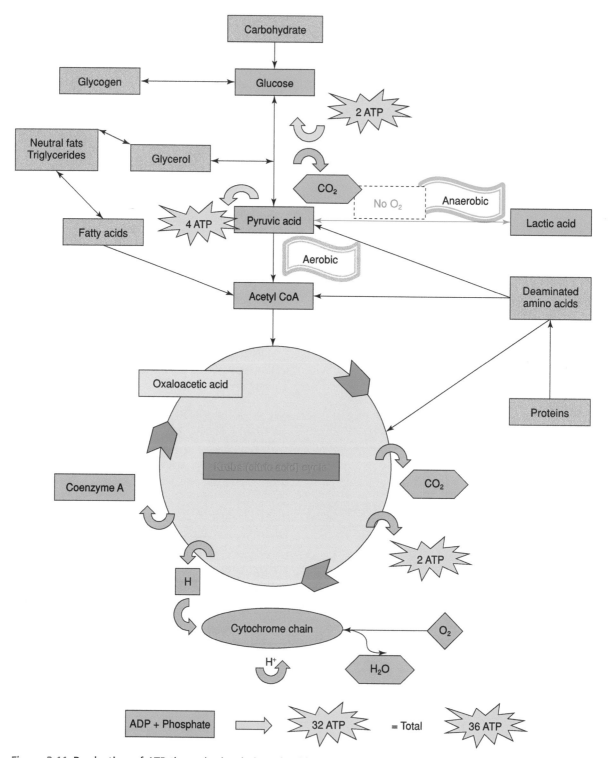

Figure 3.11 Production of ATP through glycolysis and oxidative phosphorylation showing the aerobic and anaerobic pathways and relation to macronutrients

Source: © Mears Associates 2011.

The process can be summarised by the following equation:

$$C_6H_{12}O_6 + 6O_2 \rightarrow 6H_2O + 6CO_2 + \text{energy}$$
$$(36 \text{ molecules of ATP})$$

glucose   oxygen   water   carbon dioxide

Within the cytosol each molecule of glucose is converted to two pyruvic acid molecules through a number of stages. The process is termed glycolysis. This yields a total of two ATP molecules. There are actually four molecules produced but two molecules are required to initiate the process. The pyruvic acid therefore retains much of the chemical energy of the original glucose. The fate of the pyruvic acid molecules is dependent on the availability of oxygen.

Aerobic pathway (oxygen present)

In the presence of oxygen the pyruvic acid moves into the mitochondria and is converted into acetyl coenzyme A (acetyl CoA) and enters the Krebs or citric acid cycle. This part produces the hydrogen ions that will combine with oxygen in the next phase of the process. It is during the Krebs cycle that the carbon dioxide is produced. During the cycle the coenzyme A is released and the pick-up molecule oxaloacetic acid is regenerated ready for the next cycle. During the cycle molecules that are the building blocks for non-essential amino acids and fatty acids are produced. It can therefore be seen that this is a very efficient energy production system.

The final phase of ATP production involves a complex system called the cytochrome chain which facilitates the production of water from hydrogen ions and molecular oxygen (see Figure 3.11). It is the energy released from this reaction that is used to produce ATP from ADP and phosphate molecules. The vast majority of the 36 molecules of ATP are produced at this stage. The total output is 38 but we must remember the two molecules needed to initiate the process. The water produced is frequently referred to as the water of metabolism. Approximately 250–500mL are produced daily.

To give an illustration of how dependent we are on the process of ATP production we can turn to the well-known poison, cyanide. Its mode of action is to inhibit the action of one of the proteins (cytochrome A_3) in the cytochrome chain. If given in a large enough dose, death is almost instantaneous, so dependent are we on ATP production.

Anaerobic pathway (oxygen not present)

In the absence of oxygen, the pyruvic acid undergoes a very different fate. It remains in the cytosol and is converted to lactic acid. The total yield is only two molecules of ATP for each molecule of glucose. Initially, the process is faster than the aerobic route but this is only short-lived. The cells of the brain, for example, will suffer almost instant failure. A build-up of lactic acid will contribute to acidosis, which will affect the ability of cells to function. This can happen in acute medical emergencies.

Additional pathways

Both glycerol and fatty acids, the breakdown products of fats, are used as fuel for ATP production under normal circumstances. In fact, the liver and resting skeletal muscle will use them out of preference. The glycerol joins the pathway during glycolysis and contributes to the production of pyruvic acid. Fatty acids undergo a process leading to the production of acetyl coenzyme A.

This process is only effective if there is a sufficient supply of glucose. If there is a deficiency of glucose cells sequester oxaloacetic acid (the pick-up molecule in the Krebs cycle) for conversion into glucose. This means that acetyl CoA cannot be used. The acetyl CoA is then converted into ketone bodies, which are acidic and contribute to acidosis. This is the situation that arises in uncontrolled diabetes mellitus.

Amino acids can be converted to a variety of molecules that can be used for energy production. They are essentially converted to pyruvic acid or to other intermediates in the Krebs cycle. Under normal conditions excess amino acids are converted. Where there is a lack of carbohydrate there may be breakdown of protein to provide amino acids for ATP production.

Tissues

Cells are the basic building blocks of organisms. At the very simplest level the cell is actually an organism such as a bacterium and amoeba. Humans are much more complex than this and are composed of many, many cells which have different sizes, shapes and functions.

Similarly tissues are very different and within each tissue type there are wide variations in cellular morphology and function. The key is that the tissue types are generally composed of similar cells and carry out related functions, e.g. the epidermis of the face and the lining of the mouth (buccal mucosa) are the same tissue type with related functions, although their appearance is very different to the naked eye. Blood and bone look very different but both are classified in the same tissue type. At first it is a difficult to reason this out, but after some consideration we can see that they both have a support function that involves the whole body.

Four main tissue types are identified:

1 Epithelial
2 Connective
3 Nervous
4 Muscle.

Within these broad classifications, there are many subdivisions.

Epithelial tissue

Epithelial tissue is composed of layers of cells that cover the body surfaces especially those that are exposed directly to the atmosphere, such as the skin and respiratory tract, or those surfaces that have contact with foreign objects, such as the lining of the gastrointestinal system (the gastrointestinal tract runs from the mouth to the anus). The gastrointestinal tract is effectively a tube that runs *through* the body rather than being *of* the body. Other areas that are protected by epithelial tissue are the vessels of the cardiovascular system, secretory glands and the hollow structures in the liver and genito-urinary tract (see Figure 3.12).

All epithelial tissues are composed of cells held tightly together and adhered to a basal membrane composed mainly of connective tissue. Some form single layers of cells (simple epithelium) whilst others have multiple layers of cells (stratified epithelium). Epithelial tissues are classified as follows.

Simple squamous epithelium

This is a single layer of flattened cells that typically lines the vessels of the cardiovascular system and the alveoli of the lungs. These cells are narrow enough to allow the diffusion of gases and many nutrients. In the small arterioles, capillaries and vennules of the cardiovascular system they also have adjustable pores between the cells that can be dilated in response to injury thereby facilitate the inflammatory process.

Stratified squamous epithelium

This is a protective epithelium. Unlike squamous epithelium it has multiple layers designed to withstand physical trauma. Examples are to be found in the mouth, oesophagus

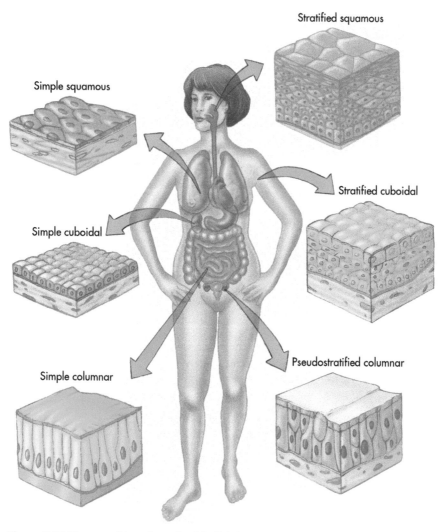

Figure 3.12 Types and location of epithelial tissue

and vagina. The epidermis is a special type of stratified epithelium in that it has a protein called keratin that holds the cells in very close proximity to each other, forming a highly effective barrier.

Simple cuboidal epithelium

Cuboidal cells are found in the tubules of the kidney and have an important role in controlling water and electrolyte levels in the body. They are also found in secretory tissues. Because of their shape they are able to control diffusion in and out of each side of the cell more readily than the flat squamous epithelium.

Stratified cuboidal epithelium

The human body contains little of this type of epithelium. It is found in mammary glands and sweat glands.

Simple columnar epithelium

Unciliated versions of this type of epithelium are found in the lining of the gastrointestinal tract. Ciliated versions are found in the small bronchi of the lungs and the reproductive tract. They are frequently secretory. In the bronchi, for example, they secrete the mucus that helps to trap dust particles.

Pseudostratified columnar epithelium

This particular epithelium looks like stratified epithelium but is, in fact, composed of cells of different sizes. These cells are typically found in the respiratory tract and some are known as goblet cells that produce mucus.

Transitional epithelium

This special epithelium is found in the urinary system. The cells change shape as the bladder fills and empties. In this way, the integrity of the wall is maintained at all times, whether contracted or distended.

Connective tissue

Connective tissue is extremely varied but is all derived from the same embryonic tissue (see Figure 3.13).

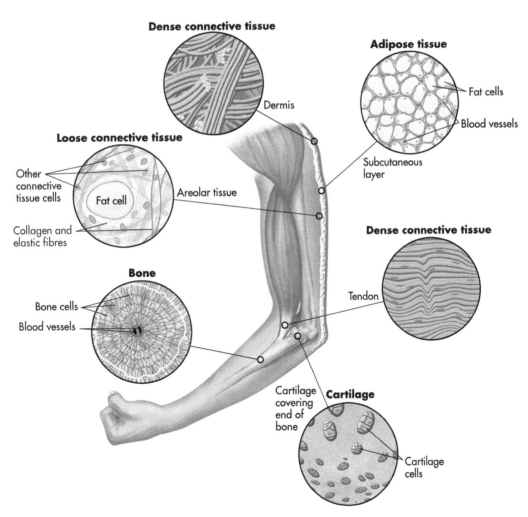

Figure 3.13 Types and location of connective tissue

This is the commonest type of tissue, found throughout the body, and is intimately connected to the other tissue types. Whereas the other three types of tissue are mainly composed of cells, connective tissue is made up of significant quantities of non-cellular material. It forms the basal membrane that supports epithelial tissue. All blood vessels have an outer support layer of connective tissue that is predominantly made up of filamentous proteins. Ligaments and tendons are structured to provide support for joints and attachment for muscles. Bones provide support for muscles and protection for the more delicate organs.

As with other tissues connective tissue is constantly being broken down and remade. If there is an imbalance in this process problems can arise, e.g. if there is an imbalance in the production and degradation of the connective tissue proteins that surround and protect blood vessels so that there is excess degradation then there is the possibility of developing aneurysms in arteries and varicosities in veins.

Nervous tissue

Nervous tissue is composed of two main types of cell (see Figure 3.14). Neurons are the cells that conduct signals very rapidly to and from the central nervous system. They are primarily composed of a cell body and long extensions called axons. Either at one end of the axon or on the cell body are a number of other projections called dendrites. Neurons conduct impulses in one direction only. The impulses arrive at the dendrites and are then passed along the axon, never the other way round. Unlike many other tissues the neurons do not touch each other: there is always a small gap known as a synapse between them. The electrical impulse that passes along the axon stimulates the release of chemicals that pass across the synapse to stimulate an electrical impulse in the next neuron. This works as a safety and control mechanism. If the neurons were actually in contact with each other the whole nervous system could be affected every time one neuron were stimulated.

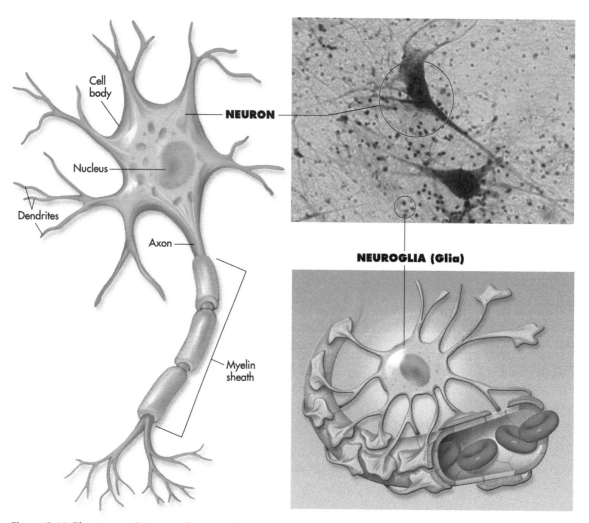

Figure 3.14 The two main types of nerve cell

Neuroglial cells act as the support system that ensures that the neurons receive nutrients and that they are protected and insulated. The neuroglial cells are non-conducting. The majority of the nervous tissue is found in the central nervous system: the brain and the spinal cord. Outside the nervous system there are neurons and ganglia (collections of nerve cell bodies and synapses) that make up the peripheral nervous system.

Muscle tissue

Muscle tissue is the tissue that is involved with movement of and within the body. Every time we move, our heart beats, we ingest food or pass urine muscle is involved. Three types of muscle are found in the human body (see Figure 3.15).

Skeletal muscle

We are all familiar with skeletal muscle (often referred to as striated muscle because of the patterns that are seen when the muscle is examined under a microscope). This type of muscle is also known as voluntary muscle because we are able to control its activity. The cells of skeletal muscle are long and thin with multiple nuclei. They are gathered into bundles that are then bundled together similar to multicore electrical cables. The muscle fibres, however, are able to contract and extend. You can easily demonstrate this by looking at the biceps muscle of the upper arm. As you flex your elbow the biceps muscle on the upper arm bulges up and as you straighten your arm the muscle flattens again. This process is complex and involves a number of elastic proteins and a very precise balance and exchange of electrolytes, especially calcium and magnesium.

Cardiac muscle

This, as its name implies, is found only in the heart. Indeed, apart from the epithelial lining of the chambers and the connective tissue outer coat, the heart is made entirely of cardiac muscle. It is similar to skeletal muscle but the muscle fibres interlock with each other. This ensures that when the muscle is stimulated all the stimulated fibres contract together and in a programmed sequential manner. Both atria contract at the same time to force blood through atrioventricular valves into the ventricles. Similarly the ventricles contract together, starting at the apex, in order to force blood into the aorta and pulmonary artery.

The muscle of the heart is stimulated by impulses from a specialised collection of cells known as the sino-atrial node (pacemaker) and is therefore not under voluntary control. The frequency and strength of the contraction of

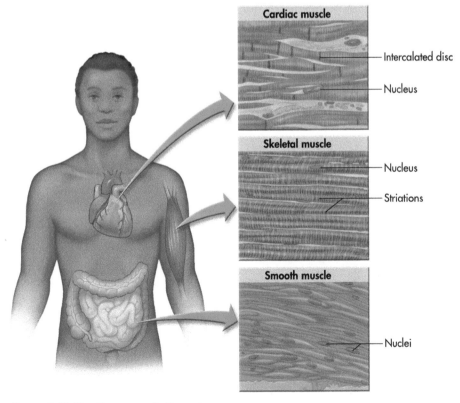

Figure 3.15 The three muscle tissue types

cardiac muscle is controlled by the nervous system but is also influenced by hormones (endocrines) and a variety of other chemicals, e.g. caffeine.

Smooth muscle

This type of muscle is quite different from the other two types. It is composed of narrow leaf-like mononucleate cells that are held together by connective tissue and have bands of elastic protein wrapped around them. It is the contraction and extension of this protein that lengthens and shortens the muscle.

Smooth muscle is found in the walls of all the hollow structures and vessels of the body, e.g. the blood vessels, bronchioles, ureters, bladder, urethra, uterus and the gastrointestinal tract. It is termed involuntary because we have no conscious control over its function, although we can influence some of its activity by lifestyle changes. Preventing uterine contraction, however, is simply not possible.

Hypertension, which is a permanent upward adjustment of blood pressure and a major factor in the development of atherosclerosis and consequently acute myocardial emergencies, is related to factors that cause continued stimulation and contraction of the smooth muscle of the blood vessels leading to an increase in total peripheral resistance.

The sudden narrowing of bronchioles in an acute asthma attack is a result of the stimulation of the bronchiolar smooth muscle by inflammatory chemicals causing extreme and prolonged contraction and sensitisation of the muscle.

Tissue injury

Tissue injury is caused by a range of factors. Some examples are:

- *Mechanical* – blunt force trauma, gunshot, surgery;
- *Chemical* – acids and alkalis, poisons, drugs, alcohol;
- *Heat* – sunburn, sunstroke, flame, hot liquids and gases;
- *Allergens* – pollen, bee sting venom, medications;
- *Pathophysiological* – dehydration, hypoxia, hypercapnia;
- *Microbial* – bacteria and/or their toxins, protozoa, viruses.

When we talk about tissue damage what we are really talking about is damage to cells. In any tissue injury, it is likely that there will be cells that are damaged beyond repair, others that are injured but are repairable and around the damaged area there will be cells that are fully functional. Cells and non-cellular material (mainly connective tissue)

that are damaged beyond repair and die are termed necrotic.

The process of necrosis is uncontrolled. In extreme conditions under the influence of bacterial toxins, this situation can progress from the original site of infection at an alarming rate, as in the case of necrotising fasciitis. Necrotic tissue is non-viable, can act as a focus for bacterial growth and inhibits tissue repair. If the necrotic material is not removed it can spread out from the original site of injury, causing damage elsewhere.

The dead and dying cells, as well as those that are injured but survive, release and produce a range of chemicals that are designed to try to counteract the insult and also to initiate the repair cycle. These will be discussed in more detail in the section on tissue repair.

There is however a more controlled form of cell death that is called apoptosis. In this process, the cell shrinks and wraps important chemicals and structures in plasma membranes and signals phagocytic cells to dispose of them. It is usually associated with development. The webs between our toes and fingers, found in the embryo, are removed in this way. More significantly it happens in severely hypoxic cells, particularly in relation to myocardial infarction and stroke (Marieb and Hoehn 2010). This is one of the reasons why patients are very carefully monitored if any hypoxia is suspected.

Tissue repair

There are two possible pathways for healing when tissue is damaged.

Regeneration

There are only a limited number of cell types that can regenerate: some liver cells, neurons and epidermis (although the range of cell types is limited, e.g. melanocytes are not produced, hence the pale colour of mature scar tissue).

Repair

This includes all other cells and non-cellular material. The damaged area is filled with scar tissue which is essentially a type of collagen. Collagen is a filamentous protein which in scar tissue is crosslinked with carbohydrate-based molecules to give strength and structure.

The repair process follows a well-identified pathway to healing provided that there are no obstructing factors such as necrotic tissue, foreign matter or infection. It is also important that the individual has an acceptable pO_2, an effective circulation and is well nourished. The healing pathway is as follows.

Vasoconstriction

Thromboxane and endothelin are two vasoconstrictor chemicals that are very rapidly released by damaged tissue, particularly the vascular endothelium. They cause vasoconstriction that helps to minimise bleeding at the site of the injury. This response is variable from individual to individual.

Haemostasis

Tissue injury leads to the activation of the intrinsic and extrinsic clotting pathways. These clotting mechanisms reduce blood loss where there is vascular damage. The intrinsic mechanism is activated from within the blood itself. The extrinsic pathway is activated by chemicals released when tissue is damaged.

Inflammation

The inflammatory response is a universal reaction to tissue damage and is characterised by four signs:

1 Rubor – redness
2 Tumor – swelling
3 Calor – heat
4 Dolor – pain.

A fifth, loss of function, was later added to the original four.

When cells are damaged there are a number of events that happen almost immediately:

1 Vasodilation
2 Release of messenger molecules
3 Activation of complement
4 Extravasation of vascular components
5 Phagocytosis
6 Pain.

Vasodilation
There is a rapid vasodilatation of the blood vessels around the site of injury or infection. This causes slowing and pooling of the blood in and around the damaged area and is responsible for the redness that is associated with inflammation.

Vasodilatation is produced by four main mechanisms:

- First, the kinin system in the cell produces bradykinin which is a vasodilator. It also stimulates the production of pain.

- Second, the damaged plasma membranes release a fatty acid called arachidonic acid which is a precursor to prostaglandins. The prostaglandins are vasodilators. They also lower the threshold of the pain receptors which are then stimulated by bradykinin. The prostaglandins are hyperalgesic (increase pain).

- Third, mast cells (one of the family of white cells) degranulate releasing histamine. The histamine has the added effect of increasing the pore size between the cells of the capillaries which allows the movement of macromolecules (mainly proteins) into the interstitial spaces. The abnormal release of histamine in response to allergens and immunoglobulin E causes the massive vasodilatation associated with anaphylactic shock.

- Fourth, nitric oxide (NO) is released from vascular epithelial cells. This molecule, which has a lifespan of fractions of a second, is a powerful vasodilator. Macrophages can also release large quantities of NO. However, they generally do not arrive at the site of injury until about 24 hours after injury.

Release of messenger molecules
The key molecule released is interleukin 1, which attracts neutrophils and macrophages to the site of injury. These are the phagocytic cells that will clear the debris from the injured area.

Chemical messengers that attract and activate lymphocytes are also released and thereby initiate the production and release the antibodies of the immune system.

Activation of complement
Complement is an intriguing group of proteins that come together to help activate the immune system. It is also responsible for labelling invading microorganisms to facilitate their destruction by the phagocytic neutrophils and macrophages.

Extravasation of vascular components
Fluid from the vascular system along with proteins such as thrombin and fibrinogen move into the interstitial space around the injury. These are rapidly followed by neutrophils. This movement of fluid creates the swelling that we associate with inflammation.

The proteins that transfer are involved in the clotting mechanism. When there is a bacterial presence they are also involved in 'walling-off' the area and again classically creating an abscess.

Phagocytosis
The neutrophils arrive at the site of injury quickly and begin the process of removing cell debris and microorganisms. Macrophages arrive about 24 hours later. Macrophages are monocytes that transformed as they left

the vascular system. Phagocytosis is a very metabolically intense activity and accounts for a great deal of the heat produced during inflammation.

Pain

Pain is generated by the action and interaction of bradykinin and prostaglandins. The prostaglandins reduce the threshold of the pain receptors, therefore increasing the sensation of pain in inflammation. There are a number of other chemicals that can be involved in stimulating pain following injury. Lactic acid, which is produced through anaerobic cellular respiration, is an example. Hydrogen ions and potassium released from damaged cells also stimulate the pain receptors.

Proliferation

During the process of inflammation the next stage of healing begins. Fibroblasts are attracted to the site of injury and begin producing the collagen and crosslinking chemicals that make up the bulk of scar tissue. Where there is significant tissue loss angiogenesis (the production of new blood vessels) also takes place so that the active cells can be supplied with oxygen and nutrients. During this proliferation phase the swelling decreases as the exuded fluid is reabsorbed.

Maturation

Finally, there is a prolonged period of maturation that may take weeks. During this time the collagen bundles thicken and align and the new blood vessels, if they were produced, atrophy. Metabolic activity decreases, the damaged area cools and lightens if on the surface of the body.

Conclusion

This chapter has introduced the cell and the tissues that are formed from combinations of cells. The structure and function of the cell membrane, the cytosol and the organelles found in the cell have been examined. Transport across the cell membrane has been discussed and the importance of the mechanisms involved has been stressed. The significance of the environment of the cell has been considered with the introduction of the concept of electrolytes and pH. Some emphasis has been placed on the production of ATP and the consequences of an interruption of production in the rapid deterioration that can take place in acute illness.

The cell cycle was discussed with an emphasis on mitosis or asexual cell division.

The structure of different tissues has been outlined, demonstrating the combination of a variety of cells to form these structures. The combination of different tissue types to form organs and systems was introduced.

There has been a brief examination of the inflammatory process and tissue regeneration and repair. The significance of inflammation on the ability of cells continue normal function was identified. There was emphasis on cell function and ATP production by changes in electrolyte balance, pH changes and interruption of oxygen supply.

Finally, the chapter has identified the importance and significance of the cell and its function on the health of tissues, organs and the organism itself. If normal function, particularly ATP production, cannot be maintained then the cell will malfunction and may even die.

Glossary

Active transport Any movement of substances across a membrane that requires the input of energy.

Adenosine triphosphate Usually abbreviated to ATP, this is a molecule that stores and provides energy for the metabolic activity of cells.

Anion A negatively charged electrolyte.

Aqueous Pertaining to water or water-based environments.

Arrhythmia Any electrical activity in the heart that differs from the normal.

Cation A positively charged electrolyte.

Cell The basic structural unit of living organisms.

Centriole Rod-like structures in the centrosome that are responsible for the production of the mitotic spindle.

Centrosome An area near the nucleus that contains the centrioles and is involved in mitosis.

Corneocytes The outer cells of the epidermis that are flattened and contain no nucleus. These are the cells that are shed from the surface of the skin.

Cytoplasm The contents of a cell inside the plasma membrane excluding the nucleus.

Cytoskeleton An array of connective tissue within the cell which helps to give the cell shape and to act as an attachment for organelles and inclusions.

Cytosol The viscous liquid component of the cytoplasm of cells in which organelles and inclusions are suspended.

Electrolytes Atoms or molecules in an aqueous solution that have an electrical charge produced by the gaining or losing of an electron and can therefore conduct electricity.

Endocytosis A process whereby molecules too large to pass across the cell membrane can enter the cell. This is achieved by pinching off of a small section of the plasma membrane and forming a vesicle that can then pass into the cell. Water can be transported this way (pinocytosis) as can cell debris and microorganisms (phagocytosis).

Endoplasmic reticulum The array of tubes and discs in the cell that is responsible for production and processing of a variety of molecules in the cell. It has two forms: rough, which has ribosomes attached, and smooth which does not.

Exocytosis This is the reverse of endocytosis and involves a vesicle formed in the interior of the cell joining the cell membrane and expelling its contents into the interstitial space.

Extracellular Relating to the internal areas of the body that are not cellular. The extracellular space is usually divided into interstitial and vascular space.

Extracellular matrix The fluid and connective tissue that fills the space between cells in the body.

Filtration The movement of dissolved substances across a membrane. The term implies that some molecules, protein and other insoluble substances will not be filtered.

Glomerulus The part of the nephron where the blood is filtered as the first step of urine production.

Glycoproteins Molecules that are composed of elements of carbohydrates and proteins.

Golgi apparatus A series of flattened discs that are involved in finishing molecular production in the cell.

Histocompatability This is the term used to describe the body's identification system and is usually based on molecules attached to the surface of cells identifying that the cell belongs to the particular person.

Hydrophillic Any substance that interacts with water.

Hydrophobic Any substance that does not interact with water.

Inclusions These are found in cells and are large unspecified molecules, food particles or cell debris.

Inflammation One of the body's non-specific responses to trauma or infection involving dilatation of blood vessels and movement of blood components into the interstitial space.

Interstitial This refers to the space around cells that contains fluid (interstitial fluid) or connective tissue.

Intracellular The contents of, or any activity that takes place inside, the cell.

Lymphatic system A collection of capillaries, nodes and ducts that removes excess fluid and cell debris from the interstitial spaces and returns it to the vascular system via the subclavian veins.

Lysosome Intracellular organelle that is involved in processing microorganisms and cell debris entering the cell through phagocytosis.

Membrane potential This is the voltage across the cell membrane created by the distribution of electrolytes. Changes in voltage across the cell membrane are important for stimulating electrical potential in nerves and muscles and also for ion pumps.

Metabolism The term that describes all the chemical reactions that take place in the body.

Mitochondrion An intracellular organelle in which oxidative phosphorylation takes place.

Mitosis Asexual cell division involving the production of two daughter cells that are copies of the parent cell. Also known as mitotic cell division.

Mitotic cell division See Mitosis.

Multinucleate Cells that contain more than one nucleus.

Myocardial infarction Death of cardiac muscle usually caused by acute lack of blood supply following blockage of coronary arteries.

Nephron The functional unit of the kidney, where blood is filtered and urine is produced.

Neuropathic pain Pain that is generated by damaged nerves or central nervous system structures rather than in response to inflammation through pain receptors.

Oedema Excess fluid, above the normal, found in the interstitial spaces that is not rapidly removed.

Organ A combination of two or more tissues adapted to carry out a specific function.

Organelles Structures within the cytosol that are the sites of specific cellular activity.

Osmosis The movement of water from an area of high solute concentration to one of lower concentration.

Peroxisomes Membranous sacs that are involved in intracellular detoxification.

pH A logarithmic scale representing H^+ concentration where '0' is the highest acidity and '14' is the lowest.

Phagocytosis See Endocytosis.

Phospholipid A triacylglycerol (triglyceride) fat that has one of the three fatty acid components replaced by a phosphate molecule.

Pinocytosis See Endocytosis.

Plasma membrane A membrane composed of phospholipids, proteins and cholesterol that surrounds cells and intracellular organelles.

Ribosome An intracellular organelle composed of protein and ribonucleic acid which is responsible for protein production in the cell.

Selectively permeable A membrane that is able to control molecules that can cross it. It is usually referred to in connection with the movement of water from an area of high solute concentration to one of lower concentration. This is also known as osmosis.

Tissue Combination of similar cells and extracellular substances that perform a specific function.

Transport molecules These are molecules attached to the surface of the cell or free-moving inside the cell that act as transport or carrier molecules for other molecules being brought into the cell or transferred from one organelle to another.

Triacylglycerol Known as triglycerides or neutral fats. These molecules are composed of a glycerol molecule joined to three fatty acid molecules.

Vennule Small vessel connecting the capillary bed and vein.

Vesicle A small fluid-filled sac. In cellular terms it is surrounded by plasma membrane and may also contain particulate matter and a variety of metabolic intermediates and products.

Test yourself

1 Cells that contain a nucleus are termed:

   a. edentate
   b. prokaryotic
   c. akinetic
   d. eukaryotic

2 Cells join together to form which of the following?

   a. organs
   b. tissues
   c. systems
   d. colonies

3 Which of the following cells is multinucleate?

   a. skeletal muscle
   b. motor neuron
   c. smooth muscle
   d. squamous epithelium

4 Which of the following is involved in protein synthesis in the cell?

   a. peroxisome
   b. centriole
   c. ribosome
   d. lysosome

5 What is the main component of the cell membrane?

   a. protein
   b. phospholipid
   c. cholesterol
   d. vitamin E

6 How many types of muscle tissue are there?

   a. 3
   b. 1
   c. 4
   d. 2

7 Which of the following is the main intracellular cation?

   a. Mg^{2+}
   b. Ca^{2+}
   c. K^+
   d. Na^+

8 Which of the following are exclusively involved in glycolysis?

   a. fatty acids and glucose
   b. glucose and amino acids
   c. fatty acids and amino acids
   d. glycerol and glucose

9 Which of the following are vasoconstrictors?

   a. endothelin and nitric oxide
   b. nitric oxide and bradykinin
   c. bradykinin and thromboxane A_2
   d. endothelin and thromboxane A_2

10 Which organic acid is produced in anaerobic cellular respiration?

   a. pyruvic
   b. lactic
   c. acetic
   d. succinic

Reference

Marieb, E. and Hoehn, K. (2010) *Human Anatomy and Physiology*. San Francisco: Benjamin Cummings.

Further reading

Alberts, B. (2004) *Essential Cell Biology*, 2nd edn. New York: Garland.

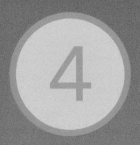

4

Body fluids and electrolytes

Liz Allibone

Aims

The aims of this chapter are to improve your understanding of the underlying pathophysiology and factors compromising fluid and electrolyte balance, as well as the essential nursing assessment and management required to prevent further deterioration and a medical emergency.

Objectives

After reading this chapter you will be able to:

→ Describe the fluid compartments of the body

→ Outline the transport mechanisms of water and solutes which allow them to move between compartments

→ Describe the mechanisms which help to regulate body fluid balance

→ Explain four acute disorders of body fluid balance and the underlying pathophysiology

→ Describe the nursing assessment of the patient with an acute fluid and/or electrolyte imbalance using an ABCDE approach

→ Describe the nursing management and treatment of a patient with a fluid and/or electrolyte imbalance

Introduction

Blood is a life-maintaining fluid and is the only liquid connective tissue. It comprises 8% of total body weight (5 litres in a normal adult) and consists of red blood cells (erythrocytes), plasma, white blood cells (leukocytes) and platelets (thrombocytes). The blood helps transport gases, nutrients and waste products, defends against infections and injury, aids in the immune process and helps regulate temperature, acid-base balance and fluid exchange.

Cell function depends on both a stable supply of nutrients and removal of waste products, as well as on homeostasis of the surrounding fluids. Fluctuations in fluids affect blood volume and cellular function, and a disturbance in cellular function can be life threatening. Fluid or electrolyte loss, retention or redistribution are common clinical problems in many areas of clinical practice.

Physiology of fluid and electrolyte balance

Distribution of body fluids and electrolytes

Water

Water is the universal solvent and is essential for life, and body fluids are dilute solutions of water and electrolytes. Water accounts for approximately 50% body mass and total body water depends on a number of factors including sex, weight, age and relative amount of body fat. Total water content declines throughout life and accounts for only about 45% of body weight, so the risk of suffering from a fluid imbalance increases with age. Whilst a healthy young man is around 60% water a healthy young woman is about 50% water. This male/female difference is because women have a relatively larger amount of body fat and a smaller amount of skeletal muscle. Skeletal muscle is around 65% water, whilst adipose tissue is only around 20% water (Marieb and Hoehn 2010). People with greater muscle mass have proportionately more body water whilst an obese person may have a relative water content level as low as 45%.

Body fluids are distributed within two major biochemically distinct fluid compartments in the body; inside the cells (intracellular) and outside the cells (extracellular). In adults approximately two-thirds of the body's fluid is intracellular (ICF) and is contained within the body's more than 100 trillion cells, which amounts to approximately 28 litres in the average 70kg male. As this huge number of cells is not united physically the intracellular

fluid compartment is actually a virtual compartment. However, these discontinuous small collections of fluid have similar behaviour, composition and location so it is physiologically appropriate to discuss intracellular fluid as if it were one single compartment.

The extracellular fluid (ECF) consists of fluid outside the cells, decreases with advancing age and is more readily lost from the body than intracellular fluid. This fluid is commonly subdivided into smaller compartments; the intravascular and the interstitial compartments or spaces. The intravascular compartment consists of fluid within the blood vessels (i.e. the plasma volume). The average adult blood volume is approximately 5–6 litres, of which about 3 litres is plasma (Edwards 2001, Marieb and Hoehn 2010). The interstitial fluid is water in the 'gaps' between the cells and outside the blood vessels and also includes lymph fluid (sometimes called the 'third space'). Transcellular fluid is contained within specialised cavities of the body, e.g. pleural, synovial, pericardial fluids and digestive secretions which are separated from the interstitial compartment by a layer of epithelium. This fluid is similar to interstitial fluid and is often considered as part of interstitial volume (Edwards 2001). At any given time transcellular fluid is approximately 1 litre (Heitz and Horne 2004). Figure 4.1 shows how the fluids are distributed in the body.

The intracellular and extracellular compartments are divided by the plasma membrane, whilst the interstitial and transcellular compartments are divided by specialised cell layers. The capillary wall separates the blood from the interstitial fluid. The capillary wall is a semipermeable membrane, which is permeable to most molecules in the plasma except plasma proteins and red blood cells which are too large to move through the capillary wall. This selective permeability helps to maintain the unique composition of each compartment while allowing for movement of nutrients from the plasma to the cells, and

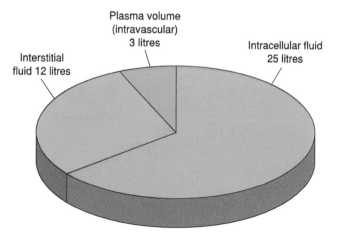

Figure 4.1 Fluid compartments

movement of waste products out of the cells and into the plasma.

Solutes

In addition to water, body fluids contain two types of dissolved substance (solutes): electrolytes and non-electrolytes.

Electrolytes

An electrolyte is a substance which develops an electrical charge when dissolved in water. Electrolytes which develop a positive charge in solution are called cations. The primary extracellular cation is sodium (Na^+) whereas the primary intracellular cation is potassium (K^+). Electrolytes which develop a negative charge in solution are called anions; the primary extracellular anions are chloride (Cl^-) and bicarbonate (HCO_3^-) whereas the primary intracellular anion is phosphate ion (PO_4^{3-}). The number of cations and anions in body fluids, as measured in milliequivalents, is always equal because positive and negative charges must be equal. All solutions are electrically neutral and this balance is called electroneutrality.

Non-electrolytes

The non-electrolytes have bonds which prevent them from dissociating in solution so they have no electrical charge. Most non-electrolytes are organic molecules: glucose, lipids, creatinine and urea.

The electrolyte content of the plasma and interstitial fluid is not routinely measured in clinical situations, as it is essentially the same, so plasma electrolyte values reflect the composition of the extracellular fluid. However, plasma electrolyte values do not necessarily reflect the electrolyte composition of the intracellular fluid. In situations such as tissue trauma or acid-base imbalances electrolytes might be released from or move into or out of the cells, and this will significantly alter plasma electrolyte values.

Transport processes of solutes and water

Fluids

Body fluids, nutrients and waste products are in constant motion within the body's compartments maintaining healthy living conditions for body cells. The ECF is modified by external factors whilst the ICF remains stable. A change in one compartment can affect all of the others, and the continuous shifting of fluid can have important implications for patient care.

Normal movement of fluids through the capillary wall from the vascular system (capillary filtration) into the tissues depends on two forces – like a 'push and pull' mechanism – and it is a delicate balance. Hydrostatic pressure (a pushing force) is created by the pumping action of the heart and also the effects of gravity on the blood within the blood vessels. Hydrostatic pressure is the same as capillary blood pressure and it is higher at the arterial end than at the venous end of the capillary bed. When the hydrostatic pressure inside a capillary is greater than the pressure in the surrounding interstitial space, fluids and solutes inside the capillary are forced out into the interstitial space. When the pressure inside the capillary is less than the pressure outside of it, fluids and solutes move back into the capillary. The hydrostatic pressure in the interstitial space ranges from about +2mmHg and −2mmHg, whilst by the time the blood has crossed the capillary bed the pressures have fallen to about 15mmHg (Casey 2004, Marieb and Hoehn 2010). There is therefore a pressure gradient that tends to force water from the capillaries to the interstitial space. Figure 4.2 demonstrates the direction of push and pull forces, and Table 4.1 summarises the push and pull forces at the capillary bed.

Osmotic pressure (the 'pull') is generated by molecules in solution. Osmotic pressure generated by protein molecules (predominantly albumin) is called colloid oncotic pressure; osmotic pressure created by electrolytes is called crystalloid osmotic pressure. Albumin is a large protein molecule and works like a magnet, attracting water and holding onto it inside the blood vessel. Blood contains more protein than interstitial fluid so the colloid oncotic

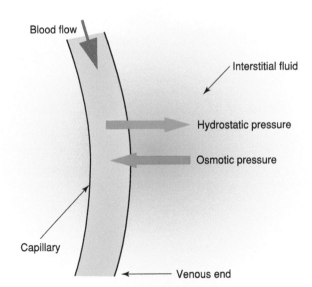

Figure 4.2 Osmotic versus hydrostatic pressure in the capillaries

Table 4.1 Summary of 'push and pull' forces at capillary bed

Push	Pull
• Hydrostatic pressure, generated by blood pressure	• Colloidal osmotic pressure, generated by pressure of plasma proteins
• Forces fluid and solutes through the capillary wall into the interstitial fluid	• Pulls fluid back from the interstitial space into the capillary circulation

pressure of blood is greater than the colloid oncotic pressure of interstitial fluid. The crystalloid osmotic pressure between the two compartments is similar.

In health, the colloid oncotic pressure generated by the high protein level of the blood draws water out of the interstitial space and into the blood by osmosis and prevents the formation of tissue oedema because the amount of fluid moving out of a vessel equals the amount moving in. If patients are albumin depleted, e.g. owing to sepsis, nephrotic syndrome or injury such as burns, they can develop generalised oedema. In a healthy person, there are virtually no plasma proteins in the interstitial fluid (Casey 2004).

Plasma colloid oncotic pressure opposes hydrostatic pressure with a constant pressure of around 25mmHg (Marieb and Hoehn 2010). The balance between the two opposing push and pull pressures leads to a net outward flow of water at the arterial end of the capillaries and inward flow of the venules; a process of reabsorption. If extra fluid or plasma proteins filter out of the capillary the excess fluid shifts into the lymphatic vessels which return

it to the heart for recirculation. However, if the lymphatic system is unable to remove any escaped plasma proteins localised oedema can occur, e.g. following surgical removal of lymph nodes or a tumour causing obstruction.

Adequate venous return is also aided by the action of the skeletal muscle pump. This requires the muscles (especially in the legs), to compress the vein and push blood back towards the heart. Good respiratory function is also important; the thoracic cavity generates pressure on inspiration and pulls blood back up to the heart. Venous valves help prevent backflow. Obstructions such as a tumour either inside or outside of the veins can lead to venous hypertension and valve failure. This increases hydrostatic pressure in the capillaries and separates the cells in the capillary wall, which causes fluid and proteins to shift into the tissues.

Solutes

There are also several factors which help to maintain the difference in solute composition between the ECF and ICF. Some solutes move freely across the plasma membrane but most require some form of assistance.

Diffusion is the random movement of particles in all directions through a solution or gas. Particles move from an area of high concentration to an area of low concentration along a concentration gradient which eventually results in an equal distribution of solutes within the two areas. The energy for diffusion is produced by thermal energy. Factors which increase diffusion include increased temperature, increased concentration of the particle, increased surface area available for diffusion and decreased size or molecular weight of the particle. See Figure 4.3.

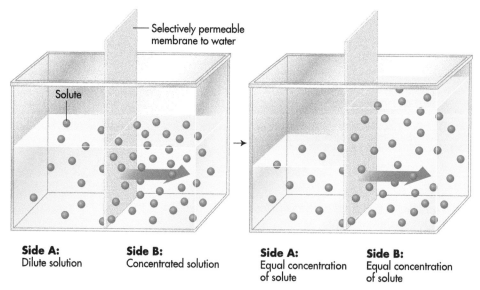

Figure 4.3 Osmosis moves water from an area of low concentration to an area of high concentration

Table 4.2 Regulation of body fluid and solutes

Osmosis	The passive movement of water through a semipermeable membrane from an area with a low concentration of solutes to an area with a high concentration of solutes
Diffusion	Gas or solutes moving from an area of high concentration of solute to an area of low concentration of solute
Filtration	Movement of a gas or solute through a material that prevents the passage of certain molecules
Active transport	Movement of gas or solute particularly into and out of cells and across epithelial layers resulting directly from expenditure of metabolic energy

Facilitated diffusion is the passive movement of specific molecules, e.g. sodium ions, glucose and amino acids, down a concentration gradient (high to low concentration) passing through the membrane requiring the assistance of a specific carrier protein. So, rather like enzymes, each carrier has its own shape and only allows one molecule (or one group of closely related molecules) to pass through.

Active transport facilitates particle movement from an area of lower concentration to an area of higher concentration, but this process requires energy to make it happen. The energy required for active transport comes from adenosine triphosphate (ATP), a molecule stored in all cells. Many important solutes are transported actively across cell membranes including sodium, potassium (the sodium potassium pump), hydrogen and glucose. Active transport is vital for maintaining the unique composition of both the ICF and ECF.

Osmosis is the passive movement of water across a semipermeable membrane from an area of lower solute concentration to an area of higher solute concentration. The membrane is permeable to water but selectively permeable to solutes. Osmosis ceases when there has been enough fluid movement to equalise the solute concentration. In clinical practice, you may hear the expression 'water follows salt'.

Osmolality: changes in the concentration of body fluids affect the movement of water among fluid compartments by osmosis. The measure of a solution's ability to create osmotic pressure and affect the movement of water is called osmolality. The term osmolarity refers to the concentration of particles in a solution and these terms are sometimes used interchangeably. An increase in extracellular osmolality increases movement from the intracellular space to the extracellular space. Decreased extracellular fluid osmolality moves the water to the cells from the intravascular space.

Filtration is the movement of water and solutes from a region of high hydrostatic pressure to an area of low hydrostatic pressure through a semipermeable membrane. The pressure is created by the weight of the fluid, and enables the glomerulus in the kidneys to filter blood.

A summary of the movement of molecules is given in Table 4.2.

Mechanisms which regulate body fluid balance

Most of the body's major organs work together to maintain body fluid balance. The amount of fluid and electrolytes gained throughout the day must equal the amount lost. Some of the fluid can be seen or measured, such as urine, but fluid loss from the skin through perspiration and lungs through water vapour is referred to as 'insensible loss' and is at least 800ml per day, although a number of factors can increase this. When fluid balance is critical all routes of loss must be taken into consideration, e.g. the loss can be much greater with increased respiratory rate or if the patient is pyrexial.

There are a number of organs and systems that regulate body fluid and electrolyte balance including kidneys, the renin–angiotensin–aldosterone system and hormones such as antidiuretic hormone play a vital role in fluid balance and these are discussed in more detail in Chapters 8 and 11.

However, there are also other homeostatic mechanisms.

ANP and BNP

Two cardiac hormones, atrial-natriutetic peptide (ANP) and B-type natriuretic peptide (BNP), also provide short-term assistance to maintain balance.

ANP is stored in the cardiocytes in the right atrium and is released when atrial 'stretch' is sensed. It opposes the effect of the renin–angiotensin–aldosterone system and causes vasodilation, increases glomerular filtration and decreases ADH release from the pituitary gland.

BNP or brain-type or B-type natriuretic peptide is secreted by the cardiac ventricles in response to 'stretch'. Its actions are similar to ANP but with a longer half-life. BNP is an indicator for heart failure because it is raised in the serum of patients who have enlarged hearts.

Thirst

The thirst mechanism is the simplest mechanism for maintaining extracellular fluid concentration and is experienced when water loss equals 2% of body weight (approximately 700ml) or when there is increased osmolality (Marieb and Hoehn 2010). Volume depletion, increased plasma osmolarity, dry mucous membranes and hypotension stimulate the osmoreceptors (thirst centre) in the hypothalamus (Edwards 2001). Nurses must be aware that in older patients or people unable to ask for water the thirst mechanism is less effective which makes them more prone to symptomatic hyperosmolarity, i.e. thirst and dehydration.

Gastrointestinal (GI) system

The GI system also works to absorb and excrete fluids and electrolytes. Sodium, potassium and chloride are lost from the GI tract and this can increase as a result of vomiting, diarrhoea or fistulae. If more water than sodium is lost from the GI tract, this can lead to hypernatraemia – especially in infants and babies.

Acute disorders of fluid and electrolyte balance

In health, there is a steady balance between the fluids and electrolytes gained and lost by the body. However, normal fluid and electrolyte balance can be disrupted by illness and there are situations when the body is unable to cope with fluid deficits or excesses that may be seen in acute care. These common acute problems will now be explored, with a more detailed nursing assessment, action and management principles later in this chapter.

Acute fluid imbalances

Dehydration
Loss of body fluids increases the osmolality of the blood. This causes water molecules to shift out of the intracellular space into the more concentrated intravascular compartment. If this is balanced by increasing the water intake and reducing urine output the body's fluid volume can be restored. However, if there is an inadequate supply or water, or if the kidneys are unable to retain water, the fluid from the cells continues to shift to the intravascular space causing cell shrinkage and reduced cellular function.

Patients often rely on health professionals to ensure that they have an adequate supply of food and drink. They may also be confused or unable to express feelings of thirst, they may be tired, frail or unconscious preventing a normal oral intake, and mental health problems may cause personal neglect. Infants also are unable to drink

fluid on their own, and they have immature kidneys, unable to efficiently concentrate urine. Co-existing illnesses may also exacerbate fluid loss, e.g. diarrhoea causing excessive GI loss, pyrexia causing excessive perspiration. Hyperglycaemia has an osmotic diuretic effect as glucose spills into the urine and takes water and electrolytes with it leading to polyuria and in turn dehydration.

> Patients are often unable to drink when they feel thirsty because they have less control over their environment and they rely on health professionals to provide adequate fluids.

Patient presentation may show changes in mental status as dehydration progresses. The person may complain of weakness, dizziness or excess thirst. They may be pyrexial, with dry skin or dry mucous membranes. They may be tachycardic and hypotensive. In severe cases, seizures and coma may result. The patient's urine may be more concentrated unless they have diabetes insipidus – when it will be in large volumes and very pale in colour. Blood results may show an elevated serum sodium, elevated serum osmolarity and elevated haematocrit.

Hypovolaemia
Depletion of extracellular fluid or isotonic fluid loss is termed as hypovolaemia. Older people and children are particularly vulnerable to hypovolaemia. It can occur because of abnormal renal, GI or skin losses, bleeding, decreased intake, or fluid movement into the interstitial space, e.g. pleural effusion, peritonitis or burns as a result of increased permeability of the capillary membrane, or decreased plasma colloid osmotic pressure. Untreated, hypovolaemia (less than 40% of intravascular volume loss) can progress to hypovolaemic shock and acute renal failure (Heitz and Horne 2004, Metheny 2010).

Hypovolaemic shock is a medical emergency where cardiac output falls and mental status can deteriorate to unconsciousness. The patient will present with supine hypotension, rapid, thready pulse, flat jugular veins and decreased central venous pressure with cool and clammy skin.

Third spacing of body fluids is a unique situation (which may lead to hypovolaemia) referring to a shift of fluid from the intravascular compartment to an interstitial space as a result of an alteration in capillary permeability secondary to inflammation, injury or ischaemia. Whilst this fluid is still technically within the body it is biologically unavailable for functional use as it is outside of the extracellular compartment. A patient with significant third space loss may appear hypervolaemic (with weight gain and oedema) but they are clinically hypovolaemic.

Table 4.3 Common causes of hypovolaemia

• Vomiting and diarrhoea	• Excessive sweating
• Excessive laxative use	• Renal impairment with excessive urination
• Fistulae	• Nasogastric suction
• Abdominal surgery	• Excessive diuretic use
• Haemorrhage	• Decreased intake, e.g. anorexia, nausea, inability to access fluids, depression
• Diabetes mellitus (with polyuria)	
• Pyrexia	

Table 4.4 Common causes of third space fluid shifts

• Acute intestinal obstruction	• Pancreatitis
• Acute peritonitis	• Heart failure
• Burns (first 24 hours but greatest movement in first 8–12 hours)	• Liver failure
	• Hypoalbuminaemia
• Sepsis	• Pleural effusion

Table 4.5 Common causes of hypervolaemia

• Excessive IV administration of normal isotonic 0.9% saline solution or hypertonic fluids such as mannitol or hypertonic saline
• Blood or plasma replacement
• High intake of dietary sodium
• Compromised regulatory systems, e.g. heart failure, cirrhosis of the liver, nephrotic syndrome
• Corticosteroid therapy
• Hyperaldosteronism

Tables 4.3 and 4.4 outline common causes of hypovolaemia and hyovolaemia due to third spacing of fluid.

Hypervolaemia

Excessive isotonic fluid gain in the extracellular compartment is termed hypervolaemia. The volume can increase in either the intravascular and interstitial fluid compartments and can lead to heart failure and pulmonary oedema. Fluid is forced out of the blood vessels and shifts into the interstitial spaces, causing tissue oedema. It is caused by excessive sodium or fluid intake, fluid or sodium retention or a shift from the interstitial space to the intravascular space. It may be a result of renal failure. The body will try to compensate by releasing ANP and decreasing the release of ADH and aldosterone.

A person with acute hypervolaemia may present with shortness of breath, cough and orthopnoea, with an elevated blood pressure, tachycardia and bounding pulse. Wheezes may be audible and chest auscultation may reveal crackles. The neck veins may be distended and the skin moist. If the patient is being haemodynamically monitored their CVP will be elevated. For causes of hypervolaemia see Table 4.5. If left untreated hypervolaemia can progress to acute pulmonary oedema, which is a medical emergency (see Chapter 6 for more information).

Water intoxication

Water intoxication occurs when excess fluid moves from the extracellular space to the intracellular compartment. The fluid shift happens when there is excess fluid low in sodium in the intravascular space, so it becomes hypotonic to the cells whilst the cells are hypertonic to the fluid. As a result the fluid moves by osmosis to the cells, which have comparatively more solutes and less water.

Water intoxication can also occur with rapid infusions of hypotonic solutions or if a person continues to drink water or other fluids in large amounts. This can be a result of mental health problems or in situations where the person is perspiring excessively as well as consuming large volumes of fluid, e.g. athletes, after consumption of amphetamine-type substances such as ecstasy. This can be a life-threatening situation.

Causes of water intoxication can be syndrome of inappropriate antidiuretic hormone secretion (SIADH), which causes the kidneys to retain water, leading to dilutional hyponatraemia.

Signs and symptoms may include headache and confusion owing to increased intracranial pressure as the cells in the brain expand. Nausea, vomiting, cramps, muscle weakness and thirst may also be experienced. Later signs may include seizure and coma, bradycardia and widening pulse pressure.

Causes of syndrome of inappropriate antidiuretic hormone secretion

- Neurological injury.
- Central nervous system disorders.
- Malignancy, e.g. small-cell lung cancer, pancreatic cancer.
- Pulmonary disorders, e.g. asthma, chronic obstructive pulmonary disease.
- Certain medications, e.g. some cytotoxic drugs, diuretics, barbiturates, oral diabetic therapy.

Oedema

Oedema is as a result of interstitial compartment expansion, i.e. an excess of fluid in the tissues, and can be caused by changes in the fluid pushing pressure or insufficient pulling pressure causing either excess fluid formation or too little removal.

Localised oedema can occur where there is obstruction or reduced venous flow in part of the venous system raising the hydrostatic pressure at the venular end of the capillary. Causes include thrombus, tumour, advanced pregnancy, or reduced activity of the skeletal muscle pump.

Generalised oedema is widespread and may be caused by sodium retention or decreased plasma proteins. A major consequence of untreated generalised oedema is circulatory overload and pulmonary oedema, which is covered in more detail in Chapter 6.

Acute electrolyte imbalances

Sodium

Sodium is the major extracellular cation accounting for 90% of extracellular fluid cations and exerts significant osmotic pressure. It attracts fluid, and in turn plays a vital role in determining the volume and osmolality of the extracellular fluid and regulates body water. It also helps transmit impulses in nerve and muscle fibres by participating in the sodium potassium pump. Sodium influences the level of potassium and chloride by exchanging for potassium and attracting to chloride: it also combines with bicarbonate and chloride and assists in acid-base balance (Marieb and Hoehn 2010, Metheny 2010).

The normal serum range is 135–145mmol/L. The amount of sodium inside a cell is approximately 10mmol/L. Whilst sodium requirements vary depending on the size and age of the person, and the average daily intake of sodium far exceeds the body's normal daily requirements, renal and endocrine mechanisms help regulate sodium balance, keeping the levels fairly constant.

Sodium plays a major role in maintaining fluid balance; where sodium goes, water will follow.

Sodium is lost through the skin, GI tract and genitourinary tract and when the concentration of sodium changes, water in the extracellular compartment also changes accordingly. For example, if the serum sodium rises because of dehydration (i.e. a water deficit), serum osmolality rises causing the thirst mechanism to be activated and ADH will also be released decreasing renal water excretion, which increases extracellular water to normalise the serum osmolality of sodium. Therefore changes in the serum sodium levels typically reflect changes in the water balance.

Drugs associated with hyponatraemia
- Diuretics (especially loop and thiazide diuretics)
- Anticoagulants (heparin)
- Anticonvulsants (carbamazepine)
- Desmopressin acetate (DDAVP)
- Recreational (MDMA, ecstasy)
- Antidepressants and antipsychotics (fluoxetine sertraline, SSRIs)
- Antineoplastics (cyclophosphamide and vincristine).

Hyponatraemia

Hyponatraemia is the most common electrolyte imbalance in hospitalised patients and refers to a serum sodium of below 135mmol/L (Beckett et al. 2010, GAIN 2010, Metheny 2010). Clinical indicators and treatment depend on the rapidity of onset and cause of hyponatraemia and whether it is associated with a normal, decreased or increased ECF volume. Severe hyponatraemia can lead to seizures, coma and permanent neurological damage. Even mild hyponatraemia (126–134mmol/L) can have significant effects on gait stability and inpatient mortality (Sterns et al. 2010). Increasingly patients are on multiple medications and sodium loss can be caused by a number of different drugs. The nurse should be familiar with possible side effects of common medications.

Hyponatraemia can develop because of a loss of sodium, net gain in water, or inadequate intake of sodium. Table 4.6 identifies common causes of hyponatraemia. As sodium levels decrease, fluid shifts can occur. The most feared complication of hyponatraemia is cerebral oedema (Sterns et al. 2010) due to the shift of water into the intracellular fluid compartment by osmosis because the blood

Table 4.6 Common causes of hyponatraemia

Causes	Outcomes
Hypovolaemic hyponatraemia (both extracellular fluid and sodium are depleted, but the sodium deficit is greater)	• Loss of GI fluids, diuretic abuse, cystic fibrosis, burns, adrenal insufficiency, osmotic diuresis, salt-losing nephritis
Isovolaemic hyponatraemia (low serum sodium with no evidence of hypovolaemia or oedema)	• SIADH, glucocorticoid therapy, renal impairment
Hypervolaemic hyponatraemia (both extracellular water and serum sodium levels are increased but water gain is increased to a greater extent)	• Heart failure, liver failure nephrotic syndrome, hyperaldosteronism, excessive administration of hypotonic IV solutions

vessels contain more water and less sodium than the intracellular compartment.

An acute sodium decrease will produce significant neurological changes, whilst chronic hyponatraemia is associated with less symptoms because the brain is able to adapt over time to by reducing intracellular solutes, which in turn limits the shift of water into the brain cells.

Neurological signs do not usually occur until the serum sodium level falls below 120–125mmol/L, when the patient may complain of nausea and a headache. As the sodium level drops further irritability, muscle tremors and twitching may develop or the patient may become disorientated. If the levels fall to 110mmol/L and below symptoms may progress to stupor, delirium, psychosis, seizures and possibly coma and permanent neurological damage or even death.

Hypernatraemia

Hypernatraemia is defined as serum sodium greater than 145mmol/L. It is much less common than hyponatraemia and is found in approximately 1–3% of hospitalised patients (Metheny 2010). This is caused by an acute gain in sodium or a loss of water. It is always associated with hyperosmolarity. As with hyponatraemia, severe hypernatamia can lead to seizures, coma and permanent neurological damage or even death. The mortality is around 40–70%, depending on the severity of the underlying diseases (Metheny 2010).

Hypernatraemia usually occurs in people who have lowered osmotic stimulation of thirst and restricted access to water, e.g. confused or elderly people, infants and immobile or unconscious patients. Normally the body protects itself against the development of hypernatraemia by releasing ADH and stimulating the thirst mechanism, but if there is failure in these responses hypernatraemia can develop.

As the hypernatraemia develops the cells shrink as fluid is pulled away from them by osmosis to the hypotonic ECF. As the cells in the brain become dehydrated the brain can contract on delicate cerebral vessels and lead to vascular trauma and bleeding. As with hyponatraemia, acute, fast-developing hypernatraemia over a period of 24 hours or less is often fatal, whereas slow-developing high serum sodium levels enable the brain to adapt by raising the amount of intracellular solutes and in turn reduce the water loss.

> **Hypernatraemia** is almost never seen in an alert patient with a normal thirst mechanism and access to water.
>
> **Severe hypernatraemia** can lead to seizures, coma and permanent neurological damage.

Signs and symptoms of hypernatraemia include thirst, elevated body temperature, dry mucous membranes, disorientation and confusion, lethargy, muscle irritability and convulsions.

Potassium

Potassium is a major intracellular cation (98% of the body's potassium is inside the cells) and plays an important role in many metabolic cell functions. The remaining 2% in the extracellular fluid is important for nerve impulse transmission. The sodium–potassium pump is critical in maintaining the balance between intracellular and extracellular potassium and even slight changes in potassium concentration can have significant effects on neurons and muscle fibres. Potassium also helps maintain cells' electrical neutrality and osmolality, and assists with skeletal and cardiac muscle contraction and electrical conductivity.

> Normal serum potassium level ranges from 3.5–5mmol/L.

Distribution of potassium between the extracellular and intracellular fluid is affected by extracellular pH and insulin levels. Alterations in the acid-base balance and the shifting of hydrogen ions can have a significant effect on potassium distribution. Potassium ions move into the cells during alkalosis (as hydrogen ions move out) and out of the cells during acidosis (as hydrogen ions move in). Severe cell damage or cell death can also cause potassium to move out of the cells.

> Insulin and alkalosis decrease serum K^+.
> Acidosis increases serum K^+.

The kidneys are the primary regulators of potassium balance. About 80% of the potassium excreted daily from the body is via the kidneys. The remaining 20% is lost through faeces and sweat (Marieb and Hoehn 2010). As the serum potassium rises after a potassium load so does the level in the renal tubular cell. This increases the concentration gradient which promotes the movement of potassium into the renal tubule to be excreted in the urine. Aldosterone also increases the urinary excretion of potassium. However, the kidneys are not able to conserve potassium and may continue to excrete it even when the serum potassium level is low.

> The body is unable to conserve potassium and the kidneys may continue to excrete it even when the serum levels of potassium are low.

Disturbances in potassium balance are common because they are associated with a number of diseases, injuries and therapies.

Hypokalaemia

Hypokalaemia refers to a below normal serum potassium concentration. Mild hypokalaemia (between 3.0mmol/L and 3.5mmol/L) is usually asymptomatic in the absence of disease. Moderate hypokalaemia ranges from 2.5mmol/L to 3.0mmol/L, whereas severe hypokalaemia is usually defined as below 2.5mmol/L.

Hyperaldosteronism

- Excessive levels of aldosterone act at the distal tubule, promoting sodium retention, leading to water retention and volume expansion. Hypertension then follows.
- Potassium excretion is increased resulting in hypokalaemia.

Hypokalaemia occurs if there is inadequate intake of potassium, a loss of potassium from the body or a movement of potassium into the cells. It is also possible to obtain a false low result owing to a blood sample collection from a vein site or an intravenous infusion where the fluid is low in potassium. However, it is rarely the result of inadequate intake alone, and frequently a combination of factors lead to hypokalaemia.

The most common causes of hypokalaemia are diuretic treatment and hyperaldosteronism. Abnormal GI loss, e.g. vomiting and diarrhoea, laxative abuse, ileostomies and nasogastric aspiration are also causes. Potassium depletion can also occur when insulin treatment is initiated because insulin promotes the movement of potassium into the cells.

Hypokalaemia danger signs!

- Arrhythmias
- Paralytic ileus
- Muscle paralysis
- Respiratory and cardiac arrest.

If your patient is taking **digoxin** check serum for digoxin levels for toxicity. Hypokalaemia enhances the efficiency of the drug.

Severe hypokalaemia can lead to death from cardiac or respiratory arrest. Clinical signs are usually not present until the potassium level falls below 3.0mmol/L but patients with liver or cardiac failure are sensitive to hypokalaemia.

Skeletal muscle weakness and leg cramps are a sign of moderate potassium loss, which can then progress to paraesthesia. The patient may also complain of constipation and may present with a paralytic ileus. However, the major cardiac effect of hypokalaemia is atrial and ventricular arrhythmias (also discussed in Chapter 6).

Hyperkalaemia

Hyperkalaemia can be a serious, life-threatening medical condition. It occurs when the serum potassium level rises above 5.5mmol/L (GAIN 2008) and seldom occurs in patients with a normal renal function. An increased intake of potassium, a decreased urinary excretion of potassium or movement of potassium out of the cells may result in hyperkalaemia. When cells die or are damaged, e.g. after burns, crush injuries, chemotherapy or severe infections they can release potassium into the extracellular space. Therefore alterations in serum potassium levels reflect changes in the ECF potassium, not necessarily changes in the total body levels. See Table 4.7 for common causes of hyperkalaemia.

Cardiac arrest is more frequently associated with **hyperkalaemia** than hypokaleamia.

Digoxin toxicity can cause hyperkalaemia.

'Pseudohyperkalaemia' can also occur and the nurse must always be on guard to be sure that the serum potassium results are true. Causes of false readings include haemolysis of blood samples, or if the tourniquet is too tight or if the sample was taken from a site close to an intravenous infusion containing potassium (Beckett *et al.* 2010, Metheny 2010). False high reading of potassium should be suspected if there is no apparent cause for hyperkalaemia, and there are no changes in the ECG reading or muscle strength.

Excessive use of salt substitutes may cause hyperkalaemia because most use potassium as a substitute for sodium.

Most of the signs and symptoms of hyperkalaemia are related to its effect on cellular membrane potential, and in turn its neuromuscular and cardiac functions in the body.

Table 4.7 Common causes of hyperkalaemia

- Decreased renal excretion; untreated renal failure or renal damage
- Addison's disease
- Potassium-sparing diuretics
- ACE inhibitors
- Non-steroidal anti-inflammatory drugs
- Acid-base imbalances
- Cell injury and cell death e.g. from infection, crush injury, chemotherapy
- Donated blood (if close to expiry date)
- High potassium intake e.g. diet or supplements

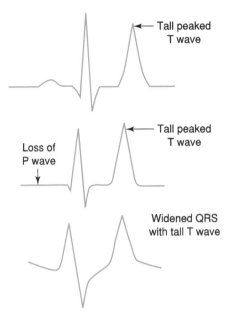

Figure 4.4 ECG trace showing changes with progressive hyperkalaemia

By far the most prominent effect of hyperkalaemia is on cardiac conduction and the myocardium. The earliest changes are a peaked, narrow T wave and a shortened QT interval on the ECG trace. As the serum level rises further, the P wave will flatten with a prolonged PR interval and the QRS will widen. Heart block, ventricular arrhythmias and cardiac arrest may occur at any point in this progression. In severe hyperkalaemia the heart may become dilated and flaccid and the strength of myocardial contraction will be decreased (see Figure 4.4).

Hyperkalaemia may also cause skeletal muscle weakness and paralysis related to a depolarisation block of the muscle, although this often does not occur until the serum potassium level is greater than 8mmol/L. The muscle weakness can spread from the large muscles in the lower extremities to the trunk and then arms and respiratory muscles. The patient may also complain of abdominal cramps, nausea and diarrhoea.

Magnesium

Magnesium is the body's fourth most abundant cation and, after potassium, the most abundant cation in intracellular fluid. About 50% of the body's magnesium is located in the bone and one-third is in the intracellular fluid. The extracellular fluid only contains about 1% of the body's magnesium (Heitz and Horne 2004).

Normal serum level of magnesium is 0.75–1.1mmol/L.

Magnesium affects a number of important functions in the body and cells. It plays a vital part in helping the body produce and use adenosine triphosphate (ATP) for energy and is implicated in neuromuscular transmission, hormone receptor binding and cardiovascular tone (myocardial contractility). Magnesium also promotes the production of parathyroid hormone and triggers the sodium potassium pump, so it is closely related to potassium levels inside and outside the cells. Magnesium also influences the body's calcium levels through its effect on the parathyroid hormone, so excretion of magnesium is decreased with increased PTH or decreased excretion of sodium or calcium.

The body will try to balance the magnesium level. The kidneys are the main route of magnesium excretion, but (unlike potassium) they are also able to conserve magnesium when required. The GI system (mainly the jejunum and ileum) absorbs dietary magnesium.

Approximately 25–30% of serum magnesium is bound to protein, a small portion is combined with other substances and the rest is free (ionised). While it is the free portion which is physiologically important, it cannot be measured alone. Therefore the serum magnesium level reflects the total amount of circulating magnesium, and the serum albumin levels need to be measured with serum magnesium levels and a low serum albumin will decrease the total magnesium level, whilst the amount of free magnesium may be unchanged (Metheny 2010).

Magnesium levels should be reviewed in line with serum albumin levels because 25–30% of the body's magnesium is bound to protein.

Hypomagnesaemia

Hypomagnesaemia occurs when the serum magnesium falls below 0.75mmol/L. This condition is very common among critically ill patients, and if left untreated, can lead to cardiac arrhythmias, respiratory muscle weakness and seizures. It can occur owing to a shift to the intracellular space, decreased GI absorption (e.g. malabsorption syndromes, fistulae, Crohn's disease, bowel resection, cancer) or decreased intake or increased urinary loss (e.g. diabetic ketoacidosis, hyperparathyroidism, loop diuretics). Whilst a healthy balanced diet provides sufficient magnesium, patients who eat a poor diet, e.g. chronic alcoholics and critical care patients are at risk of hypomagnesaemia.

Hypomagnesaemia is most common in critically ill patients, even those with normal renal function.

Hypomagnesaemia is often associated with hypercalcaemia and hypokalaemia.

Signs and symptoms of hypomagnesaemia are similar to potassium and calcium imbalance, however some patients may not show any clinical manifestations even if the level is well below 0.75mmol/L. The symptomatic patient may have an altered level of consciousness, psychosis, vertigo or develop seizures, they may complain of leg cramps, muscle weakness or tremors. Deep tendon reflexes might be hyperactive, with also a positive Chvostek's and Trousseau's sign (this is explained more detail later). Magnesium deficiency is also associated with a high frequency of cardiac arrhythmias (atrial and ventricular) and sudden death. Respiratory muscles may also be affected leading to laryngeal stridor. There is also a link between hypomagnesaemia and hypertension.

Hypermagnesaemia

Hypermagnesaemia is less common than hypomagnesaemia and occurs when the serum magnesium is greater than 1.1mmol/L. It is caused by impaired renal excretion and excessive magnesium intake.

Whereas decreased serum magnesium over-stimulates the neuromuscular system, an increase level diminishes or suppresses it. Therefore the patient may develop bradycardia, heart block and progress to asystole. Vasodilation may also occur leading to hypotension and the patient may appear flushed. Deep tendon reflexes may be hypoactive and the patient may have generalised weakness. As the serum level increases the patient's level of consciousness may deteriorate from drowsiness to a coma and finally (with a level at 10mmol/L) cardiorespiratory arrest.

Calcium

Calcium is the most abundant mineral in the body and is primarily bound with phosphorus to form the mineral salts of the bones and teeth. It also has important intracellular functions, such as the development of the cardiac action potential and muscle contraction and relaxation. Less than 1% of the body's calcium is contained within extracellular fluid and this is regulated carefully by the parathyroid hormone, vitamin D and calcitonin (Heitz and Horne 2004, Beckett et al. 2010).

Calcium is present in three different forms in the plasma; ionised calcium, protein bound calcium and complex calcium. Almost half of the calcium is free, ionised calcium. Around 40% of calcium is bound to protein, primarily to albumin. The remaining calcium is combined with non-protein anions such as phosphate, carbonate and citrate. Only the ionised calcium is physiologically important and plasma calcium (Ca^{2+}) refers solely to the concentration of ionised calcium (Heitz and Horne 2004, Metheny 2010).

Serum calcium
- Normal serum levels of total serum calcium in an adult range from 2.1–2.6mmol/L.
- Normal serum levels of serum ionised calcium is 1.1–1.3mmol/L.

The percentage of calcium which is ionised is affected by plasma pH, phosphorus and albumin levels, so if a patient develops alkalosis causing an increase in arterial blood pH, more calcium becomes bound to protein (Malster 2008). This means that the total serum calcium remains unchanged, but the ionised portion decreases.

Changes in the plasma albumin level affect the total serum calcium level without changing the level of free calcium, so in cases of hypoalbuminaemia, less protein is able to bind with calcium, and the total calcium level drops but the level of ionised calcium is unchanged. Therefore when evaluating total calcium levels these factors must be taken into consideration as must acid-base balance.

Hypocalcaemia

Left untreated or poorly managed hypocalcaemia emergencies can lead to significant morbidity or (more rarely) death.

Hypocalcaemia can be asymptomatic and symptomatic. Asymptomatic hypocalcaemia is often caused by hypoalbuminaemia which is sometimes described as 'pseudohypocalcaemia' because there is a reduced total serum calcium concentration but the ionised calcium remains normal

Symptomatic hypocalcaemia occurs when there is a decrease in the percentage of calcium which is ionised (although the total serum calcium level is normal). Common causes are listed in Table 4.8.

Table 4.8 Common causes of symptomatic hypocalcaemia (decrease in percentage of ionised calcium)

- Increased calcium loss e.g. loop diuretics
- Reduced intake e.g. inadequate vitamin D consumption or exposure
- Decreased regulation e.g. hypoparathyroidism
- Decreased intestinal absorption
- Post-partial parathyroidectomy or thyroidectomy
- Chronic alcoholism
- Acute pancreatitis

Clinical manifestations of hypocalcaemia include enhanced neuromuscular irritability and tetany (involuntary muscle contractions), tingling of the fingers, muscle cramps, numbness and convulsions. Alterations in mental status might include anxiety or depression. Sudden drops in plasma calcium levels can lead to decreased myocardial contractility, hypotension and heart failure. Other cardiovascular manifestations may include arrhythmias and bradycardia.

Hypercalcaemia

Hypercalcaemia is a common metabolic emergency which occurs when the serum level of calcium rises above 2.6mmol/L, or if ionised serum calcium level rises above 1.3mmol/L or if more calcium enters extracellular fluid than the rate of renal excretion of calcium. It has been suggested that the prevalence of hypercalcaemia in the hospital inpatient population ranges from 0.6–3.6%.

Any situation which increases the level of total serum or ionised calcium may cause hypercalcaemia. Hyperparathyroidism and malignancy are the two main causes. Cancer (commonly breast and lung cancers and lymphoma) which invades and destroys the bones may cause more calcium to be released into the bloodstream. Immobility can result in loss of bone mineral leading to an increase in total calcium in the bloodstream.

Hypercalcaemia danger signs!
- Arrhythmias
- Bradycardia
- Heart block
- Cardiac arrest
- Coma
- Stupor
- Paralytic ileus.

If the patient develops acute hypercalcaemia the signs and symptoms are more severe. The patient may complain of fatigue and lethargy or exhibit confusion. Muscle weakness, hyporeflexia and decreased muscle tone may occur. Hypercalcaemia can also alter myocardial muscle function, causing rhythm disturbances such as bradycardia, heart block and a shortened QT interval. Severe hypercalcaemia can lead to ventricular arrhythmias and cardiac arrest.

Nursing assessment of fluid and electrolyte status in the patient

Nurses are directly responsible for monitoring patients for actual or potential fluid and/or electrolyte disturbances and the NMC (2010) requires nurses to be able to carry out accurate assessment of people of all ages using appropriate diagnostic and decision-making skills. While nurses often keep fluid balance charts and perform vital signs as part of daily practice it is also important to have a good understanding of normal physiological mechanisms as well as the signs and symptoms of fluid and electrolyte problems. The nurse is responsible for reviewing the patient's history and laboratory data as well as close clinical observation and assessment, and analysis of the effectiveness of interventions. The nurse should also recognise when specialist knowledge and expertise is required and seek advice accordingly.

Airway

The look, listen and feel approach is the best way to assess the airway for obstruction or use of accessory muscles. A patient with fluid volume overload may have wheezing or excess secretions. (See Chapter 5 for a broader explanation.) If the patent is in shock the airway must be secured for tissue oxygen delivery, and in severe situations endotracheal intubation may be required.

Breathing

Deep, rapid respirations may indicate a change in the acid-base balance, e.g. a compensatory mechanism if the patient is in metabolic acidosis (the lungs attempt to 'blow off' excess carbon dioxide). Slow shallow breathing may be a compensatory mechanism for metabolic alkalosis (the lungs try to retain carbon dioxide). In situations such as severe hypokalaemia or hyperkalaemia there may be weakness or paralysis of the respiratory muscles. Crackles or wheezing may be audible or present on auscultation which may indicate fluid volume overload and pulmonary oedema. The patient might expectorate pink, frothy sputum and they might be using their accessory muscles. Pulse oximetry may also decrease if the patient is developing pulmonary oedema or is hypovolaemic.

Circulation and fluid balance

The look, listen and feel approach is also an important part of assessing your patient's circulatory status. Blood pressure is a sensitive method for assessing fluid depletion. Hypotension may occur as a reduction of stroke volume. Electrolyte disturbances which can cause arrhythmias may also then lead to hypotension if heart rate or stroke volume is affected. Lying and standing blood pressures and pulse rate might be recorded to assess for hypovolaemia. Standing from a supine position causes an abrupt drop in venous return for which the body usually compensates through increasing peripheral resistance and a slight increase in heart rate. However, a fall in systolic pressure greater than 15mmHg or more and an increase in heart rate greater than 15 beats per minute may suggest fluid volume deficit. Orthostatic changes may also occur with autonomic neuropathy, e.g. diabetes mellitus, as well as some antihypertensive medications.

The jugular veins often follow the changes in central venous pressure (CVP), which may help assess fluid status. Normal CVP ranges from 2–8mmHg. Central venous pressure measures the pressure in the right atrium or vena cava and helps to monitor the effectiveness of the heart's pumping mechanism and vascular tone. Flat neck veins in the supine position may indicate decreased plasma volume and a low CVP, whereas distended neck veins and an elevated CVP may be seen in hypervolaemia.

Elevated blood pressure and a bounding pulse may be present in hypervolaemia as stroke volume increases. The pulse should be palpated manually and an ECG may show conduction disturbances, e.g. a long or short QT interval, arrhythmias or ectopics. Tachycardia or arrhythmias are usually the earliest sign of hypovolaemia but may also be associated with electrolyte disturbances such as hypokalaemia. Bradyarrhythmias may be present with hypercalcaemia. A bounding pulse may be felt in hypervolaemia as the strength of the contraction of the left ventricle and the amount of blood it ejects increases, whilst a thready, weak pulse may indicate fluid volume deficit because of a reduced circulating blood volume. At the same time the patient's skin temperature should be assessed, e.g. is it cold and clammy, or hot and sweaty? The more dehydrated the patient is the further up the limb the coolness will extend owing to compensatory vasoconstriction.

> Palpating the pulse manually can give you vital information about a patient's fluid and/or electrolyte status.

Disability

The AVPU approach should be used to assess the patient's level of consciousness as a change in serum osmolality, acid-base balance or electrolyte balance may affect the patient's level of consciousness, personality, behaviour and neurological function. The patient may be restless or anxious or complain of dizziness if they are dehydrated or water intoxicated. In severe cases, seizures and coma may result. In situations of water intoxication, the patient may develop raised intracranial pressure and may complain of a headache as an early symptom. Later they may become lethargic and irritable. Late signs of raised intracranial pressure include pupillary changes and a widening pulse pressure.

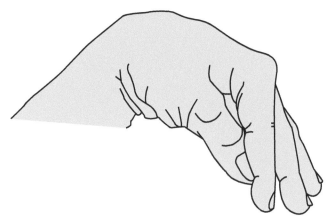

Figure 4.5 Trousseau's sign for hypocalaemic tetany

Patients should also be assessed for neuromuscular irritability if calcium or magnesium imbalances are suspected, by checking for Chvostek's sign (tapping over the facial nerve causes facial muscles to twitch) and Trousseau's sign, a spasm presenting with adduction of the thumb, flexed wrist and extended fingers two and four after inflating a blood pressure cuff on the upper arm (see Figure 4.5), as well as deep tendon reflexes which may be hypoactive or hyperactive when imbalances in electrolytes are suspected. Deep tendon reflexes may be altered with some electrolyte disturbances, but should be evaluated in light of other clinical signs and laboratory data such as sensation, neurological status and fatigue level.

The patient may also be complaining of thirst or nausea. They may have absent or reduced bowel sounds as for example in hypokalaemia, or experience diarrhoea. Thirst can be affected by fluid volume and electrolyte changes such as hypernatraemia, hypercalcaemia and hyperglycaemia. However, patients with altered levels of consciousness who are debilitated or who have altered mental status may not be able to respond to thirst.

Exposure and investigations

Oedema formation may be localised, often as a result of inflammation (e.g. thrombophlebitis), or generalised (as a result of water or salt retention), so the nurse may need to examine the whole body. Dependent oedema is when fluid accumulates mostly in the lower extremities (or in the sacral region when the patient is lying down) whilst generalised oedema is spread throughout the body and may accumulate in periorbital and scrotal regions because of the relatively lower tissue hydrostatic pressure in these areas of the body. Pitting oedema can be evaluated by pressing a fingertip into the skin over a bony surface for a few seconds. After the pressure is removed, the indentation can be assessed (see Figure 4.6). Commonly the amount of pitting oedema is assessed using plus signs although it is a subjective process. A slight imprint can be charted as +1 while a deep, persistent imprint with the skin slow to return to its original contour may be documented as +4 (Heitz and Horne 2004, Metheny 2010).

Skin turgor can be assessed by gently pinching the skin over the forearm, sternum or dorsum of the hand (see Figure 4.6). If the patient is adequately hydrated the skin will return to its original position when released. In hypovolaemia, the pinched skin may remain elevated for several seconds. However, an older patients' skin may lose elasticity so this can be an unreliable measure of dehydration.

A dry mouth and flushed dry skin may also signal dehydration. The tongue may have increased furrowing if the patient is dehydrated. Hypernatraemia may cause the tongue to become red and swollen. As the tongue turgor is not affected by age it is considered to be a more reliable physical sign of dehydration than skin turgor.

Acute weight changes may also be indicative of acute fluid imbalances. Each kilogram lost or gained suggests one litre of fluid lost or gained. The weight gain may be as a result of an increase in total body water which could be in any of the compartments. Ideally the patient should be weighed daily at the same time in the morning before breakfast using the same scales, wearing similar clothes and after voiding.

Urine is usually straw coloured, but if the patient is dehydrated the volume of urine will be reduced and it will darken in colour. However, there are a number of factors

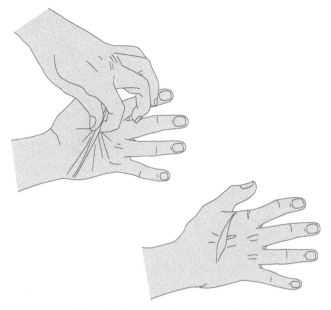

Figure 4.6 Skin with decreased tugor remains elevated after being gently pinched and released

which can alter urinary volume including fluid intake, blood volume, renal concentrating ability and insensible loss. Some drugs, for example tuberculosis medication, can alter the colour of urine. In cases of hypervolaemia, the urine will become pale and dilute as the kidneys excrete water to normalise the fluid balance. The patient's urine may be assessed for specific gravity, glucose and protein and serum blood sugars may also be assessed if hyperglycaemia is suspected.

CASE STUDY 4.1 Faith, a patient with electrolyte imbalance – Part 1

SITUATION AND BACKGROUND

Faith is an 81-year-old lady who was admitted onto the medical ward 36 hours ago with pneumonia, dehydration and generalised weakness. Faith lives alone and often prefers not to drink too much fluid because she does not 'want to keep going to the toilet'. She is being treated with intravenous antibiotics and, because of her dehydration and lethargy, intravenous fluids of 5% dextrose (3 litres per day) were commenced shortly after admission. She has also been encouraged to drink clear fluids. Faith has had an uneventful past medical history.

When Faith was admitted she was pyrexial with a temperature of 38.7° centigrade but since the administration of antibiotics she now has a temperature of 37.5°. However, Faith has recently developed nausea and diarrhoea which the doctor suggests might be a side effect of the antibiotics.

This morning when you come on duty Faith appears very weak and lethargic, disorientated and she is refusing to drink because she says she feels 'sick and ill'. She has also had two occasions of being incontinent with loose, watery stools.

You introduce yourself and explain that you would like to take Faith's vital signs and assess her to see how she is doing and try to find out why she is feeling unwell today. You apply hand gel.

ABCDE ASSESSMENT

Airway

Faith's airway is patent and she is able to talk. She does not appear to be using her accessory muscles and there are no signs of cyanosis. Faith does have some lower airway secretions and she had been able to cough and expectorate with encouragement, but today she is rather disorientated

---

CASE STUDY 4.1 Faith, a patient with electrolyte imbalance – Part 1 (*continued*)

and too weak to follow instructions. However, at this stage Faith does not appear to have a high risk of aspiration.

Breathing

Faith has a few crackles in the bases and upper airways on auscultation secondary to retained secretions. Her respirations are 28 per minute this morning which are consistent with previous observations and her breathing does not appear laboured. Faith's pulse oximetry is 98% on 2 litres of oxygen via nasal cannula which was prescribed and commenced on admission, however she occasionally tries to remove her nasal cannula saying that it makes her 'head hurt'. As Faith's saturations are within the target as set by the British Thoracic Society Guidelines (O'Driscoll *et al.* 2008) you do not increase the oxygen flow and at this stage a mask is not required. You note equal lung expansion on palpation and the trachea is midline.

Circulation

Faith is currently having an intravenous infusion of 5% dextrose at a rate of 125ml per hour as prescribed and it is running via an infusion pump. Faith appears pale but there are no obvious signs of blood loss. Her peripherals are cool to touch but her capillary refill is 2 seconds. Her heart rate is currently 100 beats per minute and is regular. Her pulse neither feels weak nor bounding to touch. Previous recordings have shown a heart rate of 80–90 beats per minute. Her blood pressure is 140/85 which is within her usual parameters. Her neck veins do not appear distended. Skin turgor is not an accurate assessment measure as Faith's skin has decreased elasticity. There are no signs of pitting oedema. Faith has been doubly incontinent this morning with two episodes of watery, light-brown stools so it is difficult to maintain an accurate fluid balance or test her urine. Faith's mouth appears dry and her tongue is a little furry.

Disability

Faith's Glasgow Coma Scale score is 14/15 (E4, V4, M6) which shows a new deterioration in neurological status. Faith is alert but disoriented, restless and forgetful and keeps assuming that she is at home. She is also now weak and unable to cough effectively. Her face twitches when she is still. When asked how she is feeling she says her 'legs and head hurt'. Blood sugar is 5.9mmol/L. Her pupils are equal and reactive to light.

Exposure

Faith has a peripheral intravenous catheter in her left arm through which she is receiving an intravenous infusion of 5% dextrose. You assess her IV site using the Visual Infusion Phlebitis Score (Jackson 1998) and her IV site appears patent with no signs of phlebitis. Her skin does not show any rashes. Faith has been doubly incontinent of watery, loose stools but her urine has appeared light straw coloured. Her tongue and oral mucosa is dry but this may be due to the fact that she is declining to clean her teeth.

EWS

Using an early warning score, you notice that Faith's heart rate and her deteriorating neurological status triggers a call to the doctor. She passes more loose stools with increasing frequency, and is complaining of a headache and pains in her legs. You are concerned that Faith is at risk of a worsening of her neurological status as well as a fall and dehydration. The two triggers generate a medium score on the EWS, which means that her doctor must be informed and attend to review her within 30 minutes.

You check that she has all the information she needs, and use SBAR to structure her conversation with the doctor, as hospital policy dictates. The doctor says he will assess Faith within 30 minutes.

Maximising fluid and electrolyte balance

The events which lead to fluid volume disturbances often also lead to electrolyte problems. The nurse needs to be alert to the risk of medical care itself precipitating disturbances in fluid or electrolyte balance, particularly in frail elderly or critically ill patents. Therefore the nurse has an important clinical and professional role to play in the assessment, management and treatment and for monitoring effectiveness. In most situations, the underlying problems must be resolved alongside correcting the fluid or electrolyte imbalance. Fluid, sodium and potassium imbalances are particularly common metabolic abnormalities caused by a wide variety of conditions, but if left untreated, they can rapidly become life threatening.

Fluid balance charts are an important part of hydration monitoring. The nurse completing the chart should be aware of the target fluid balance and patient specific parameters and report any issues to members of the multidisciplinary team. However, fluid balance charts are often poorly maintained and inaccurate. This may be due to lack of training or time or poor handover between shifts or staff.

Nurses have a professional responsibility to ensure that their patients have an accurate and adequate fluid balance but there have been reports of failures to recognise, report and act on observations when a patient has been deteriorating (NPSA 2007). The NMC (2009) *Record Keeping: Guidance for nurses and midwives* and the NMC (2010) competencies for entry to the professional register also require nurses to maintain clear, accurate and complete records. The NMC (2008) code of conduct goes on to emphasise the importance of the personal accountability of the registered nurse in ensuring complete and accurate documentation, and suggests that good record keeping helps to identify risk and early detection of complications. The Department of Health (2010) *Essence of Care* guidance includes benchmarks in food and nutrition and record keeping so that health professionals can share and compare practice, and develop action plans to remedy poor practice. The NPSA and RCN (2007) developed a toolkit to protect the safety and well being of hospitalised patients by encouraging hydration best practice. For further information see http://www.rcn.org.uk/news-events/campaigns/nutritionnow/tools_and_resources/hydration.

Fluid replacement for hypovolaemia

The type of fluid replacement depends on the type of fluid lost and the severity of the deficit. Acid-base status, serum electrolyte levels and serum osmolality must be taken into consideration.

If oral replacement is not sufficient or if the situation is severe, intravenous therapy solutions are used to replace and restore the circulating blood volume. As the body needs more than water for maintenance, electrolytes are also required. The fluids should be administered at a rate rapid enough and in sufficient quantity to maintain adequate tissue perfusion, taking the patient's cardiac and renal functions into consideration. The patient might require a fluid challenge when specific volumes are administered at a specific rate and interval whilst monitoring the patient's haemodynamic status and response.

Intravenous solutions are classified as crystalloids and colloids. Crystalloids are electrolyte solutions and can be described as hypotonic, isotonic or hypertonic depending on their contents, for example their osmolality.

Crystalloids

Water and electrolyte solutions may be given to hydrate, correct electrolyte disturbances, or to expand the intracellular and intravascular volume.

Hypotonic solutions, e.g. 0.45% sodium chloride or 0.18% sodium chloride, provide a basic fluid for maintenance needs and a small amount of sodium chloride and are suitable for patients who are hypovolaemic with hypernatraemia. However, excessive use may cause a shift of water into the hypertonic intracellular space to balance the osmolality of the compartments.

Isotonic fluids such as 0.9% sodium chloride ('normal saline'), 5% dextrose, Hartmann's and Ringer's lactate remain in the intravascular space and help expand the plasma volume when infused, making the solution suitable for restoring fluid volume. However, owing to the amount of chloride and sodium content caution should be exercised if the patient has hypernatraemia or renal failure.

Hypertonic solutions such as 3% sodium chloride or 10% dextrose are used to treat severe deficits in serum sodium or dextrose. Small volumes must be infused slowly and usually in a clinical area where the patient is closely monitored because of the osmotic 'pull' of the solution, which can lead to a shift of fluid into the intravascular space causing fluid overload.

Colloids

Increase the osmotic pressure of plasma and increase blood volume. They may be used to help pull fluid from the interstitial to the intravascular space e.g. in oedematous hypovolaemic patients and/or those with third space fluid shifts.

Colloid solutions, e.g. gelofusine and albumin, contain substances of high molecular weight which do not readily migrate across the capillary walls. They increase the osmotic pressure of the plasma and pull fluid from the other compartments into the intravascular space to increase the volume, and are indicated when there is depletion of circulating plasma proteins or if there has been a movement or loss of fluid into the interstitial space, e.g. septic shock, anaphylaxis, extensive burns.

Hypervolaemia

Reversal of the primary problem is the initial goal of treatment. Alongside this restriction of sodium and fluids may be required as well the administration of diuretics (however the patient should be monitored for hypokalaemia if loop diuretics are prescribed). Renal dialysis may be required if the underlying cause is renal failure.

For more information, advice and guidance on intravenous therapy best practice in the UK, please see the RCN (2010) *Standards for Infusion Therapy*.

Sodium imbalances

Sodium imbalances can cause significant neurological complications. The patient should be nursed in an observable area and a safe environment must be maintained. The person may be confused or agitated and at risk of seizures, or even coma and death.

Hyponatraemia

Treatment depends on fluid volume status and the severity of the condition. In situations of mild hyponatraemia with hypervolaemia or isovolaemia water intake is usually restricted to allow the sodium and water to balance naturally. If the patient is hyponatraemic they may require isotonic IV fluids, e.g. normal saline. Hypertonic saline (3% sodium chloride) may be administered but this must be with extreme caution because it 'pulls' water from the intracellular to the intravascular compartment owing to the osmotic pull of this highly concentrated solution, and this causes cell shrinkage. In these situations, patients may be moved to high dependency or intensive care environments. If the shift of water happens too quickly it

can cause the brain cells to contract and bleed, and the intravascular volume to be overloaded leading to heart failure. As the patient can develop neurological changes they must be nursed in an observable position to prevent risk and for any signs of deterioration to be reported immediately.

Hypernatraemia

Sometimes, inappropriate treatment itself may cause serious consequences – for example, over-rapid rehydration risks cerebral oedema. Therefore management will depend on the cause and the speed of onset. If it has developed quickly over a few hours the patient may be given 5% dextrose and this may be given quickly because in these situations rapid correction improves prognosis without the risk of cerebral oedema. If it is of longer or unknown duration the patient may be prescribed hypotonic saline and hypotonic oral fluids. This will need to be administered with caution as there is a risk of fluid movement to the intracellular space as the body tries to normalise fluid balance. Where there is concurrent renal failure haemodialysis or filtration may be required.

CASE STUDY 4.2 Faith, a patient with electrolyte imbalance – Part 2

Faith has been admitted with pneumonia, dehydration and generalised weakness. She has received antibiotics and 5% dextrose as rehydration, but is now disorientated and has developed watery diarrhoea and nausea. As she has triggered in the medium score on the EWS, the doctor has been called to review her.

Medical assessment

The doctor assesses Faith's vital signs, fluid balance and neurological status. He notes that Faith was alert and oriented on admission. He reviews Faith's drug chart and prescribed treatment. He assesses Faith's pulse oximetry on air and notes it to be 94%. He takes a blood gas and it shows a PaO_2 of 10kPa, $PaCO_2$ of 5kPa, pH of 7.43, HCO_3^- of 24 and notes this to be a normal blood gas on air with normal acid-base balance. Therefore Faith is not hypoxaemic neither does she currently have signs of a metabolic or respiratory-related acid-base disturbance, e.g. hypercapnia, dehydration, acidosis.

He then reviews the morning's blood results and notes that Faith's sodium is now 120mmol/L while the other electrolytes levels are within normal limits. Faith's previous sodium was 134mmol/L.

Diagnosis

The doctor diagnoses that Faith has acute onset hyponatraemia most likely to have been cased by excessive

intravenous administration of 5% dextrose (i.e. water overload) because she appears normovolaemic, her blood pressure is normal and heart rate has not significantly increased. It is likely that the recent pyrexia (and sweating) and loss of fluid from the watery diarrhoea, while also contributing to sodium loss, may also have reduced the risk of fluid volume overload.

Faith is in danger of further neurological deterioration and even permanent neurological injury if her sodium levels drop further because of possible cerebral oedema caused by the shift of water from the extracellular to the intracellular compartment. The doctor suggests that Faith's headache may be due to movement of water into the cerebral cells and her leg pains are being caused by cramps due to the reduced sodium available for conduction of muscle and nerve tissue.

Intervention

Acute hyponatraemia can cause more symptoms than if the level drops slowly and treatment will usually be based on the presence or absence of symptoms, the rate of onset and the person's volume status.

The goal of treatment is to identify the underlying pathology, correct acute symptoms and gradually return Faith's sodium to a normal level. As Faith appears to have a normal extracellular fluid volume but has a deteriorating neurological status the doctor orders Faith's intravenous

CASE STUDY 4.2 Faith, a patient with electrolyte imbalance – Part 2 (continued)

infusion of 5% dextrose to be immediately discontinued, fluid intake to be restricted to 500ml per day and to immediately be administered 40mg furosemide intravenously. The doctor considers the treatment option of administration of hypertonic 3% sodium chloride intravenously but as this must be administered with caution and ideally in a high-dependency or intensive care environment the doctor decides to review Faith's serum sodium in 2 hours. If the fluid restriction and furosemide has not increased her serum sodium levels, or if her neurological symptoms have not improved, 3% sodium chloride may be required

The doctor is aware that the rate of correction of serum sodium concentration in hyponatraemia is still under debate. In Faith's case, he sets a target of raising the serum sodium by 0.5–1mmol/L per hour as she is not in a life-threatening situation, but she should be monitored closely. This is because a more rapid correction of serum sodium concentration may cause central pontine myelinolysis (or osmotic demyelination). This is a condition when the brain cells shrink owing to water moving too quickly out of the cerebral cells, causing irreversible brain damage (usually a few days after the serum sodium concentration is corrected).

The doctor asks the nurse to move Faith's bed into a position in which she can be closely observed, with suction and artificial airway equipment available. She is at risk of

seizures or a coma if her hyponatraemia worsens. The nurse is asked to record half-hourly neurological observations and to immediately report any worsening in Faith's condition. A urinary catheter is inserted and an accurate fluid balance chart is maintained. Faith is allowed sips of water and mouth care to keep her mouth comfortable. The outreach team is notified as well as the nurse in charge in case Faith needs to be moved into high-dependency or intensive care.

After the prescribed treatment Faith's urine output has been 750mL over the past 2 hours and her serum sodium rises to 122mmol/L. Her neurological observations have not deteriorated, and her heart rate and blood pressure are within her normal limits. The doctor prescribes a course of oral sodium supplements to be commenced later in the day when Faith is oriented and able to swallow and obey commands. Should Faiths' diarrhoea continue, he will prescribe isotonic (0.9% sodium chloride) intravenously.

The doctor reassesses Faith's serum sodium levels 6 hours after prescribed therapy and her sodium level continues to rise to 125mmol/L. She is more oriented and no longer complaining of a headache. Her vital signs are stable, and her Glasgow Coma Scale is 15/15. She has not had any more episodes of diarrhoea. Sodium supplements have been commenced and the doctor will recheck her serum sodium before he goes off duty in the evening.

Hypokalaemia

The management of hypokalaemia is usually by potassium replacement and the urgency of replacement depends on the severity and any underlying problems. The amount of supplementation required depends on the severity of the imbalance. Potassium may be replaced orally or intravenously. Oral replacement is generally preferable to supplementation for mild and low-risk hypokalaemia.

National Patient Safety Agency (NPSA) potassium patient safety alert

In 2002 the first safety alert from the NPSA was released in response to research from the UK and worldwide which highlighted risks to patients from errors occurring during intravenous administration of potassium solutions.

As a result all NHS trusts and primary care trusts have been required to store, prepare, check and prescribe intravenous potassium in accordance with specific NPSA guidelines to reduce potential harm to patients.

In high-risk patients or severe hypokalaemia, the patient will require being nursed in a hospital setting for intravenous replacement via an infusion. Intravenous potassium should never be given as a bolus dose as it can cause fatal arrhythmias, and it should never be given undiluted as it can cause extravasation (burning of the vein and surrounding tissues) so where possible it should be administered via a central line, but if given peripherally it should be adequately diluted in line with local guidelines (see Table 4.9). The recommended maximum dose of intravenous potassium is 20mmol/L per hour to prevent toxic effects.

If the patient is taking non-potassium-sparing diuretics, supplements may be prescribed as a preventative measure.

Hyperkalaemia

Treatment will depend on the underlying cause and severity of the situation. Restriction of dietary potassium and/or discontinuation of medications or factors increasing the serum level may resolve the condition. In acute or emergency situations intravenous administration of agents

Table 4.9 Intravenous potassium administration

- Do not administer more than 20mmol/L per hour
- Never give potassium as a bolus
- Use premixed potassium solutions where possible for all intravenous routes
- Use an intravenous infusion device to control flow rate
  - ideally administer via a central line (level 2 and level 3 care)
  - if administering via a peripheral line the total intravenous solution must be at least 50 times the volume of the potassium. For example if 20mmol/L of potassium is in 10ml, it must be infused in at least 500ml solution
  - make sure the peripheral line is patent before administration
- Monitor your patient's cardiac status throughout the infusion and report any changes
- Monitor IV site closely for signs of local irritation and infiltration
- Monitor serum potassium every 1–3 hours and monitor for signs of toxic reaction, e.g. paralysis or weakness
- Monitor urine output and report of less than 0.5ml/kg/hr
- Potassium can layer in the solution:
  - avoid adding to hanging containers, use premixed solutions where possible
  - if necessary to add, invert the container before and after adding the potassium and mix well

Sources: Adapted from NPSA (2002), Metheny (2010) and Datapharm communications (2011).

to antagonise the effects of hyperkalaemia or shift the potassium into the cells or even dialysis may be required. This is discussed further in Chapter 8.

Calcium imbalances

As with sodium and potassium imbalances, treatment depends on the duration or onset and the severity and the underlying condition. In acute hypocalcaemia the symptomatic or high-risk patient should be treated with intravenous calcium gluconate as well as oral calcium preparations. Vitamin D tablets may also be prescribed if hypovolaemic. If the hypocalcaemia is persistent the patient may be prescribed oral calcium replacement as well as vitamin D tablets, but once the serum calcium has stabilised the calcium supplement may be discontinued.

Hypercalcaemia usually requires the patient to be nursed in hospital under specialist advice. A patient with chronic hypercalcaemia is prone to pathological fractures and may need assistance to reposition if bedridden. The patient may require intravenous fluids to increase the urinary output of calcium as well as the administration of drugs to inhibit bone reabsorption. Haemodialysis may be required if the condition is secondary to renal failure. Surgery to remove part of the parathyroid gland may also be considered.

Conclusion

Maximising fluid and electrolyte balance is a crucial aspect of nursing knowledge and practice. Nurses should have a thorough understanding of the normal mechanisms which control fluid and electrolyte balance in order to be able to perform a comprehensive assessment of a patient's fluid and electrolyte status to identify patients at risk of deterioration, and monitor patients appropriately to prevent further complications. Nurses also have a professional requirement to maintain accurate fluid balance records and formulate plans to resolve fluid or electrolyte imbalances.

Glossary

Amino acid The building blocks of proteins.

Capillary The smallest of the body's blood vessels.

Delirium Acute confusional state.

Diuretic A drug that elevates the rate of urine production.

Effusion Excess accumulation of fluid in a space.

Enzyme Proteins causing chemical reactions.

Fistulae An abnormal connection or passageway between two epithelium-lined organs or vessels that do not usually connect.

Hypertension High blood pressure.

Ileum The final section of the small intestine.

Ischaemia A restriction of blood supply.

Jejunum The middle aspect of the small intestine.

Neuropathy Damage to nerves.

Node Localised swelling.

Orthopnoea Shortness of breath when lying flat.

Pancreatitis Inflammation of the pancreas.

Peritonitis Inflammation of the peritoneum.

Polyuria The passage of large amounts of urine.

Sepsis A life-threatening illness caused by the body overreacting to an infection.

Stridor A high-pitched wheezing sound.

Tumour A lump or growth of tissue made up from abnormal cells.

Venule A small blood vessel in the microcirculation.

Test yourself

1 Which are the correct terms for the fluid compartments of the body?

   a. intracellular, intrastitial, extracellular
   b. intracellular, extracellular, extravasular
   c. intracellular, interstitial, intravascular
   d. intercellular, interstitial, intervascular

2 Hydrostatic pressure

   a. pushes fluid and solutes out of the capillaries
   b. has a pulling power of albumin to reabsorb water
   c. is generated by blood flowing from the heart through the venous system
   d. does not change with blood pressure

3 Osmosis is the passive movement of solutes through a semipermeable membrane from a region of high osmolality to low osmolality. True or false?

4 Which is not a common cause of hypovolaemia?

   a. haemorrhage
   b. vomiting and diarrhoea
   c. heart failure
   d. excessive diuretic therapy

5 One sign of hypervolaemia is:

   a. acute weight loss
   b. distended neck veins
   c. extreme thirst
   d. weak and thready pulse

6 Signs and symptoms of hyponatraemia include:

   a. flushed skin, thirst, restlessness
   b. abdominal cramping, arrhythmias, muscle weakness
   c. skeletal muscle weakness, constipation, irregular and weak pulse
   d. changes in level of consciousness, muscle twitching, nausea and vomiting

7 Signs and symptoms of hypokalaemia include:

   a. skeletal muscle weakness, tachycardia, arrhythmias
   b. changes in level of consciousness, muscle twitching, nausea and vomiting
   c. chest pain, shortness of breath, cough
   d. Tetany, anxiety, confusion

8 Blood pressure and pulse are sensitive measures for detecting hypovolaemia. True or false?

9 Intravenous potassium can cause vein irritation and extravasation if it leaks into the tissues. True or false?

10 Colloids are water and electrolyte solutions given to hydrate or correct electrolyte disturbances. True or false?

References

Beckett, G., Walker, S. W., Rae, P., Ashby, P. (2010) *Lectures Notes; Clinical biochemistry*, 8th edn. Oxford: Wiley-Blackwell.

Casey, G. (2004) Oedema: Causes, physiology and nursing management. *Nursing Standard* 18 (51), 45–51.

Datapharm Communications (2011) *Electronic Medicines Compendium*. Available from http://www.medicines.org.uk/emc/medicine/20910/SPC/, accessed 14 October 2011.

Department of Health (2010) *Essence of Care*. London: The Stationery Office.

Edwards, S. (2001) Regulation of water, sodium, and potassium: Implications for practice. *Nursing Standard* 15 (22), 36–44.

GAIN (Guidelines and Audit Implementation Network) (2010) *Hyponatraemia in Adults (On or After 16th Birthday)*. Belfast: GAIN.

GAIN (Guidelines and Audit Implementation Network) (2008) *Guidelines for the Treatment of Hyperkalaemia in Adults*. Belfast: GAIN.

Heitz, U. E. and Horne, M. M. (2004) *Pocket Guide to Fluid, Electrolytes and Acid-base Balance*, 5th edn. St Louis, MO: Mosby.

Jackson, A. (1998) Infection control: A battle in vein infusion phlebitis. *Nursing Times* 94 (4), 68–71.

Malster, M. (2008) Fluid and electrolye balance. In Dougherty, L. and Lamb, J. (eds) *Intravenous Therapy in Nursing Practice*, 2nd edn. Oxford: Wiley-Blackwell, pp. 49–86.

Marieb, E. and Hoehn, K. (2010) *Human Anatomy and Physiology*. San Francisco: Benjamin Cummings.

Metheny, N. M. (2010) *Fluid and Electrolyte Balance: Nursing considerations*, 5th edn. London: Jones and Bartlett.

NMC (Nursing and Midwifery Council) (2010) *Standards for Pre-registration Nursing Education*. London: NMC. Available from http://standards.nmc-uk.org/PublishedDocuments/Standards%20for%20pre-registration%20nursing%20education%2016082010.pdf.

NMC (Nursing and Midwifery Council) (2009) *Record Keeping: Guidance for nurses and midwives*. London: NMC.

NMC (Nursing and Midwifery Council) (2008) *The Code: Standards of conduct, performance and ethics for nurses and midwives*. London: NMC.

NPSA (National Patient Safety Agency) (2007) *Safer Care for the Acutely Ill Patients: Learning from incidents*. London: NPSA.

NPSA (National Patient Safety Agency) (2002) *Potassium Chloride Concentrate Solution – Patient Safety Alert 01*. London: National Patient Safety Agency Safety.

O'Driscoll, B. R., Howard, L. S. and Davison, A. G. (2008) British Thoracic Society guideline for emergency oxygen use in adult patients. *Thorax* 63 (supp 6), v1–v169.

Royal College of Nursing IV Therapy Forum (2010) *Standards for Infusion Therapy*, 3rd edn. London: Royal College of Nursing.

Sterns, R. H., Hix, J. K. and Silver, S. (2010) Safely treating hypokalaemia in high-dependency cardiac surgical patients. *Nursing in Critical Care* 11 (6), 267–72.

Further reading

Adam, S., Odell, M. and Welsh, J. (2010) *Rapid Assessment of the Acutely Ill Patient*. Oxford: Wiley-Blackwell.

Benoit, R. and Svendsen, A. (2004) Hyponatremia and the nursing implications. *Canadian Journal of Cardiovascular Nursing* 14 (3), 4–7.

Cowen, M. D. (2009) Principles of fluid management. In Childs, L., Coles, L. and Marjoram, B. (eds) *Essentials Skills Clusters for Nurses: Theory and practice*. Oxford: Wiley-Blackwell, pp. 185–99.

Criddle, L. (2006) Pinch of salt: Dealing with hyponatraemic emergencies. *American Journal of Nursing, Critical Care Extra* 106 (10), 72CC–EE.

Docherty, B. and Coote, S. (2006) Fluid-balance monitoring as part of track and trigger. *Nursing Times* 102 (45), 28–9.

Elgart, H. N. (2004) Assessment of fluids and electrolytes. *AACN Clinical Issues* 15 (4), 607–21.

Finlay, T. (2004) *Intravenous Therapy: Essential clinical skills for nurses*. Oxford: Wiley-Blackwell.

Given, S. B. (2010) Action stat. hypernatremia. *Nursing* 40 (10), 72–73.

Hankins, J. (2006) Role of albumin in fluid and electrolyte balance. *Journal of Infusion Nursing* 29 (5), 260–265.

Higgins, C. (2007) *Understanding Laboratory Investigations; For nurses and allied health professionals*, 2nd edn. Oxford: Blackwell.

Holman, C., Roberts, S. and Nicol, M. (2005) Promoting adequate hydration in older people. *Nursing Older People* 17 (4), 31–2.

Humphreys, M. (2007) Potassium disturbances and associated electrocardiogram changes. *Emergency Nurse* 15 (5), 28–34.

Scales, K. and Pilsworth, J. (2008) The importance of fluid balance in clinical practice. *Nursing Standard* 22 (47), 50–57.

Sladdin, C. and Lee, G. (2006) Safely treating hypokalaemia in high dependency cardiac surgical patients. *Nursing In Critical Care* 11 (6), 267–72.

Sterns, R. H., Hix, J. K. and Silver, S. (2010) Treatment of hyponatraemia. *Current Opinion in Nephrology and Hypertension* 19, 493–8.

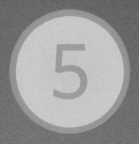

5

The patient with acute respiratory problems

Carl Margereson and Sarah Withey

Aims

This chapter aims to help you respond appropriately where a patient presents with an acute respiratory problem in the clinical environment.

Objectives

After reading this chapter you will be able to:

→ Describe the major structures of the respiratory system

→ Identify the determinants of external and internal respiration

→ Differentiate between oxygen delivery (DO_2) and oxygen consumption (VO_2)

→ Describe the functions of the respiratory epithelium including neurohormonal control of the airways

→ Describe how acute respiratory problems may compromise respiratory status

→ Describe the nurse's role in undertaking a respiratory assessment and delivering care to maximise respiratory status

Introduction

Patients who are acutely ill are in a stressed, hypermetabolic state where the body is attempting to cope with crisis and maintain homeostasis. This inevitably results in an increase in the amount of oxygen (O_2) required by the cells for aerobic metabolism. The nurse has a key role in ensuring that oxygenation is maximised both at pulmonary and cellular level. Where patient assessment is underpinned with a sound knowledge of respiratory and cardiac physiology then factors possibly compromising O_2 delivery (DO_2) can be detected early and prompt action taken to avoid further deterioration and a medical emergency.

Applied respiratory physiology

Internal respiration

For effective cellular function an adequate mitochondrial oxygen pressure is important and hypoxia is a cause of cell injury and death. The oxidation of glucose is crucial if energy-rich adenosine triphosphate (ATP) is to be released for effective cellular functioning. Although oxidation of glucose can take place in the cytoplasm of the cell (glycolysis) only two ATP molecules per glucose molecule are formed. Compare this with inside the mitochondria of the cell, where in the presence of O_2 one glucose molecule can liberate 38 molecules of ATP (a process called oxidative phosphorylation), thus facilitating aerobic metabolism.

> ATP stores energy in the cell and the aerobic production of ATP is very effective in extracting energy from food sources.

The mitochondria can produce ATP without using O_2 (anaerobic metabolism) but this is less efficient and while some cells can function relatively effectively (e.g. skeletal muscle) for short periods this is not possible in some organs (e.g. brain and heart). Prolonged anaerobic metabolism will result in disruption to cellular function, increased waste products such as lactic acid and possibly irreversible cell damage and death. As a consequence of insufficient oxygen to the cells (ischaemia) cellular hypoxia will result in cellular injury, causing destruction of the cell membrane and cell structure.

Oxygen delivery

Oxygen delivery to rapidly metabolising cells must be optimised if cellular demand (VO_2) is to be met. It is

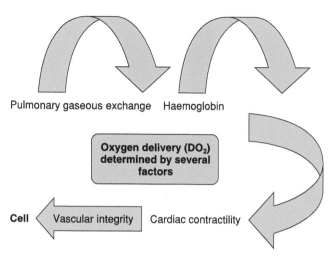

Figure 5.1 Determinants of oxygen delivery

useful to think of the steps facilitating O_2 delivery as connecting links in a chain (see Figure 5.1). The first link is at pulmonary level where external respiration with gaseous exchange takes place. Additional links include the haemoglobin which carries O_2 molecules, cardiac function which must maintain the systemic circulation and the integrity of the microcirculation which must facilitate gaseous exchange at cellular level. If any link is weak then O_2 delivery may well be reduced.

> **Factors determining oxygen delivery (DO_2):**
> - External respiration in lungs (including effective ventilation/perfusion)
> - Haemoglobin level
> - Cardiac output
> - Microcirculation.

The lungs and chest wall

The lungs are situated in the thoracic cavity with two lobes on the left and three lobes on the right (see Figure 5.2). The mediastinal cavity is found between the two lungs and accommodates the heart, great vessels, trachea, oesophagus, nerves and lymph nodes. The apices of the lungs extend just above the inner third of the clavicles, a fact that needs to be considered when a central line is being inserted! The bases of the lungs sit on the diaphragm. The anatomical and mechanical relationships of the lungs and chest wall facilitate effective ventilation. Each lung is surrounded by pleural membranes with the inner membrane (visceral pleura) attached to the lung surface and the outer membrane (parietal pleura) attached to the chest wall (also diaphragm). In the resting state there is inward recoil of the lungs (also visceral pleura) and outward movement of the chest wall (also parietal pleura). These two opposing forces on either side of the pleural membranes contribute to a negative pressure (less

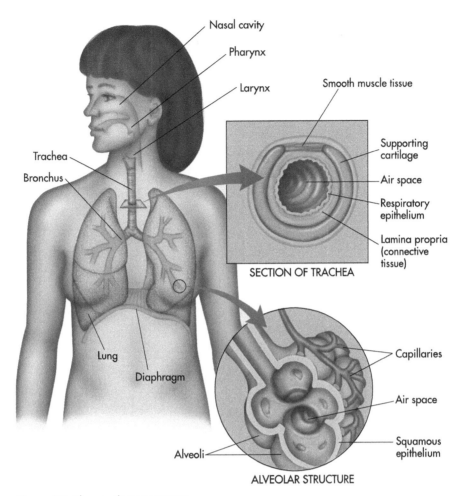

Figure 5.2 The respiratory system

than atmospheric pressure) in the pleural cavity which is important in keeping the lungs inflated. We will return to the significance of this later.

> Pressure difference between the alveoli and the pleural cavity is important in keeping lungs inflated.
> **Pleural cavity pressure:** negative (less than atmospheric).
> **Alveoli:** positive (atmospheric pressure).

The respiratory tract

The upper respiratory tract (URT) from the nose to the upper trachea has a large surface area and blood supply and for breathing is important in warming, moistening and filtering the air during inspiration. This is bypassed of course in patients who have a tracheostomy or endotracheal tube in place. The lower respiratory tract from the lower trachea to the respiratory bronchioles has evolved to conduct air efficiently into the lungs for gaseous exchange during inspiration and to remove air from the lungs during expiration.

The respiratory tract is described as a tree with different generations of branches (see Figure 5.3). The trachea is the trunk, referred to as generation zero. At the carina the trachea divides into the right and left major bronchi, referred to as first generation branches. These in turn branch again with each successive branch becoming smaller. The walls of the respiratory tree are made of cartilage to prevent collapse, smooth involuntary muscle and an inner lining of mucous membrane. At generation 16 the bronchi become terminal bronchioles, the cartilage disappears and the diameter is only approximately one millimetre. The walls of these bronchioles are made of simple ciliated epithelial cells, secretory Clara cells and smooth muscle. Because there are many of these

Respiratory defence mechanisms:
- Nasal hairs filter air
- Cough/gag reflex
- Lymphoid tissue
- Mucociliary escalator
- Immunoglobulin A (antibody)
- Alveoli macrophages.

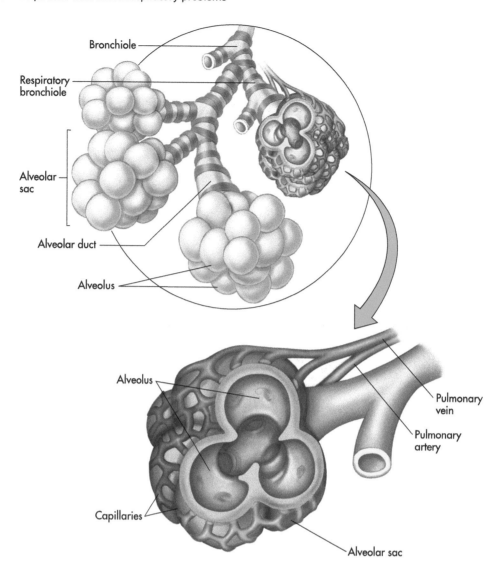

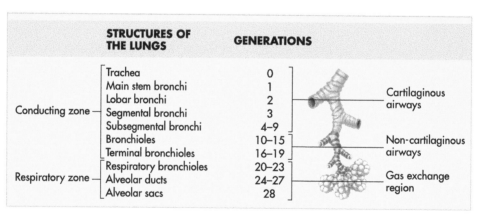

Figure 5.3 Conduction and gas exchange structures and functions

bronchioles the total resistance to flow is low but because they are so small in diameter the lumen can become further narrowed and obstructed by secretions and inflammation. Generations 20 onwards of the respiratory tree are the even smaller respiratory bronchioles which finally merge with the alveolar ducts and alveolar sacs.

The respiratory bronchioles together with the alveolar ducts and sacs are the site for gaseous exchange.

Clara cells are specialised non-epithelial cells in the airways and have both a protective and regenerative role.

Functions of the respiratory epithelium

It was once thought that the respiratory epithelial cells simply acted as a barrier to protect the inner layers of the respiratory tree. The respiratory epithelium does indeed have a huge role to play in protection. For most sections of the respiratory tree each epithelial cell has around 200 tiny hair-like projections called cilia. On top of the cilia sits a blanket of mucus which is constantly moved upwards by the cilia, all beating in the same direction (1000 beats per minute). Any debris in the air is thus trapped and moved upwards by the mucociliary escalator to be expectorated or swallowed. The creation of mucus (up to 100mls each day) is extremely complex but contributing are goblet cells which secrete mucus as well as submucosal glands found throughout the respiratory tract. Pathology, smoking, dehydration and dry gases (including O_2 therapy) can decrease the effectiveness of this protective mechanism. Additional defences include immunoglobulin A (IgA), an antibody produced by B lymphocytes and secreted onto the respiratory surface, irritant receptors and the cough reflex as well as lymphoid tissue and phagocytic macrophage cells in the alveolar wall.

Respiratory epithelial cells are also metabolically active and can produce a range of different substances including nitric oxide and cytokines. Nitric oxide (NO) is a potent bronchodilator but when produced in excessive amounts can contribute to inflammation. NO is also released by endothelial cells of blood vessels and is a vasodilator. Cytokines (e.g. interleukins) released by many different cells enable communication between cells and whilst most are important physiological regulators some may result in inflammation in a number of respiratory diseases.

> **Cytokines** are regulatory protein molecules released by a range of cells including lymphocytes. Examples:
> - Interleukins
> - Interferon
> - Tumour necrosis factor
> - Growth factor.
>
> Some cytokines are proinflammatory!

Neurohormonal control of the airways

Smooth muscle found in the lining of the respiratory tract enables the airway lumen to dilate and constrict. Each smooth muscle cell is supplied by branches of the sympathetic and parasympathetic nervous system. Parasympathetic nerves (also called cholinergic nerves) from the vagus nerve release acetylcholine and stimulate cholinergic receptors on the cell membrane resulting in contraction (the lumen becomes smaller). These nerves also supply glands and result in increased mucus secretion. Conversely, sympathetic nerves release noradrenaline (a neurotransmitter) which stimulate beta 2 receptors and result in relaxation of the muscle (the lumen dilates). The beta 2 receptors can also be stimulated by adrenaline (hormone) from the adrenal gland. Research has identified additional nerves in the respiratory system which result in bronchodilatation but the neurotransmitter released is nitric oxide. Although these nerves travel with the autonomic nerves they are described as non-adrenergic and non-cholinergic (NANC).

> Inflammatory cytokines and an increase in parasympathetic (cholinergic) activity narrow the airway lumen, thus increasing airway resistance.

Control of breathing

Fortunately, although breathing can be controlled voluntarily it becomes automatic and we do not need to think about it. In a rare congenital disorder (Ondine's curse) where autonomic control is lost then breathing stops during sleep. Air must be replenished in the lungs on a cyclical basis and inspiration and expiration facilitates this. It is carbon dioxide in arterial blood which stimulates the respiratory centre in the brainstem and so powerful is this that most of us can only hold our breath for a short period of time. As carbon dioxide (CO_2) increases in the blood it diffuses into the cerebrospinal fluid in the brain and hydrates with water to form weak carbonic acid. In turn, this then dissociates into hydrogen and bicarbonate ions, as can be seen in the following chemical equation, which is reversible:

$$CO_2 + H_2O \leftrightarrow H_2CO_3 \leftrightarrow H^+ + HCO_3^-$$

(carbon dioxide + water ↔ carbonic acid ↔ hydrogen + bicarbonate)

In fact, it is the liberated hydrogen (H^+) ions which stimulate special central chemoreceptors in the brainstem as a result of increased CO_2 levels. As a result of being stimulated nerve impulses in the medulla oblongata are generated and pass down the intercostal and phrenic nerves to the respiratory muscles. Peripheral chemoreceptors found in the carotid artery and aortic arch can also stimulate the respiratory centre but are sensitive to falling O_2 levels (hypoxaemia). As a result of contraction the external intercostal muscles raise the rib cage upwards and the diaphragm contracts, descending and pushing the abdominal contents out the way. This increases the dimensions of the thoracic cavity and as gas pressure is inversely proportional to volume, air is drawn into the lungs from the atmosphere.

In quiet inspiration, it is mainly the diaphragm followed by external intercostals which are used. Expiration in healthy individuals is passive: it simply involves muscle relaxation and no energy is needed. Energy expenditure for breathing accounts for only 3% of the body's O_2 consumption. This can increase dramatically in breathless patients where the use of accessory muscles for both inspiration and expiration can demand 30% of O_2 consumption.

> Muscles used during inspiration in health:
> - Diaphragm
> - External intercostals.
>
> Expiration does not require muscle contraction in health.

Lung volumes

At rest an adult takes in around 500 millilitres of air per breath and this is called tidal volume. Multiplying the tidal volume with the breathing rate per minute provides the ventilatory volume, referred to as pulmonary or minute volume, and with a ventilatory rate of 12 breaths per minute is 6 litres. Increasing tidal volume and rate, as for example during exercise, can increase the minute volume to 70 litres per minute. However, of the tidal volume, only 350ml reaches the respiratory bronchioles (generation 17–23) where gaseous exchange takes place. If 350ml is now multiplied by 12 breaths per minute this is referred to as alveolar volume (ventilation) which in adults is around 4.2 litres. The last portion of the tidal volume (150ml) remains in the larger airways (generations 0–16), and this is called the anatomical dead space.

> **Pulmonary or minute volume (MV):**
> $$MV = TV \times RR$$
> At rest:
> $$MV = 500 \times 12 = 6 \text{ litres}$$
> TV = tidal volume
> RR = respiratory rate

Given that it is alveolar volume which is available for gaseous exchange, this has real significance in clinical practice. There are a number of situations where patients may have reduced tidal volumes, e.g. pain and some respiratory disorders. With anatomical dead space fixed, there is always 150mL of the tidal volume not available for gaseous exchange. In this situation, then the dead space becomes a larger proportion of the total tidal volume. The body may attempt to maintain effective alveolar volumes by breathing at higher ventilatory rates. However, if this continues for long periods the patient will utilise a great

deal of energy for breathing and the respiratory muscles may fatigue very quickly.

> **Alveolar ventilation or volume (AV):**
> $$AV = (TV - DS) \times RR$$
> At rest:
> $$AV = (500 - 150) \times 12 = 4 \text{ litres}$$
> DS = anatomical dead space
> (approximately 2mL per kg body weight)

Another important lung volume is the functional residual capacity (FRC). This is the volume of air in the lungs at the end of expiration and consists of expiratory reserve volume (ERV) and residual volume (RV) (see Figure 5.4). An important aim in clinical practice, particularly where pulmonary status is compromised, is to maintain FRC so that alveolar volume does not fall further. Poor positioning, where patients are nursed flat or not well supported with pillows, can reduce FRC by up to 30% and may precipitate closure of alveoli (atelectasis) resulting in reduced oxygenation.

> Poor positioning, particularly in older people, will reduce the functional residual capacity and increase the risk of alveoli closure. Where possible position:
> - Sitting upright
> - High side-lying
> - Sitting in chair.

Fortunately, for most people with good lung function breathing takes very little effort. Nevertheless, breathing involves work as muscles must contract to move the lungs and chest wall out (compliance work) as well as move air through the airways (resistance work). Where there are

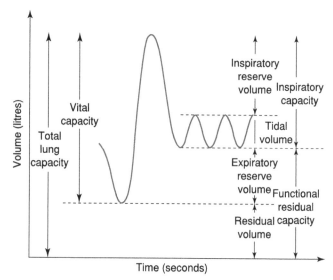

Figure 5.4 Lung volumes

respiratory problems which make the lungs stiffer (e.g. pneumonia/pneumothorax) then compliance is reduced and the patient becomes conscious of the increased effort needed to move the chest wall and lungs during inspiration. Similarly, where the lumen of the airways is narrowed then resistance is increased and once again there is much greater effort required to move air through the airways (e.g. asthma). Try breathing through a drinking straw! Where there is increased work of breathing then the cause should be established with management aimed at increasing compliance where possible, reducing airway resistance – or both.

Gaseous exchange

Following inspiration air is available in the respiratory bronchioles, alveolar ducts and sacs for gaseous exchange (alveolar volume) and there is a huge surface area available for this. Atmospheric air comprises a number of gases and each of these gases exerts a pressure independent of the others (i.e. each gas has its own partial pressure). Combining the partial pressures of all the gases present gives the atmospheric or barometric pressure, which at sea level is 101kPa (at higher altitudes pressures decrease). The proportion of O_2 in the air is around 21% and its partial pressure is approximately 21kPa. However, in alveolar air the proportion of O_2 is only 14% and because water vapour also exerts a partial pressure (6kPa), the partial pressure of alveolar O_2 is lower at 13.5kPa.

Alveoli are supplied with a vast network of pulmonary capillaries with each alveolus having a single capillary so

that alveolar air and pulmonary capillary blood is in close contact. The alveolar wall is extremely thin and is made up of pneumocyte cells and macrophage cells. Type I pneumocytes are flat squamous cells whilst type II are larger cells which release surfactant. The alveolar lining consists of an interface of water and gas molecules which increases the surface tension of each alveolus, creating instability and potential alveolar collapse. Surfactant is a detergent-like substance which reduces this surface tension thereby increasing compliance and reducing the work of breathing.

Pulmonary capillary blood returning from the tissues via the pulmonary arteries is deoxygenated with O_2 exerting a partial pressure of only 5.3kPa. With alveolar O_2 partial pressure at 13.5kPa and pulmonary capillary O_2 partial pressure at 5.3kPa a pressure gradient exists across the alveolar capillary membrane. O_2 molecules therefore diffuse across the membrane into the pulmonary capillary blood until equilibrium is achieved. Similarly, CO_2 moves down a pressure gradient diffusing from the blood into the alveolar air to be exhaled. Oxygenated blood returns to the left atrium via the pulmonary veins. Diffusion of gases across the alveolar capillary membrane is proportional to pressure gradient, surface area and gas solubility (O_2 is less soluble than CO_2) and is inversely proportional to membrane thickness and molecular weight of the gas (molecular weight of O_2 is less than CO_2).

For effective oxygenation, the relationship between ventilation (V) and perfusion (Q) is crucial. $\dot{V}$ is the abbreviation for 'volume per unit time' and in this context refers to alveolar ventilation, the air available for gaseous exchange per minute (4200mL). $\dot{Q}$ is the abbreviation for 'flow per unit time' and refers to perfusion of blood through the lungs, which is dependent on cardiac output (5L per minute). Overall perfusion is slightly greater than ventilation but in health gravitational forces result in varying $\dot{V}/\dot{Q}$ relationships in different areas of the lung. For example, at rest and before inspiration, ventilation is greater than perfusion in the apices of the lung, whereas at the base perfusion is greater. Pathology can result in abnormal $\dot{V}\dot{Q}$ relationships and this is a common cause of falling oxygen pressures. Where significant numbers of alveoli are not ventilated (low $\dot{V}/\dot{Q}$), as in pneumonia or alveolar collapse, then the blood perfusing these airless units will remain desaturated and result in a right to left

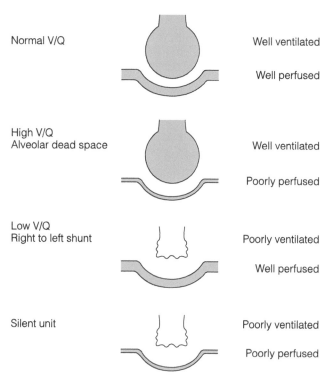

Normal V/Q — Well ventilated / Well perfused

High V/Q
Alveolar dead space — Well ventilated / Poorly perfused

Low V/Q
Right to left shunt — Poorly ventilated / Well perfused

Silent unit — Poorly ventilated / Poorly perfused

Figure 5.5 Ventilation and perfusion relationships in the lung

shunt. It is as if the blood from the right side of the heart has been shunted to the the left side of the heart bypassing the lungs completely. Figure 5.5 shows the different VQ relationships that can exist.

Transport of gases

Once O_2 has diffused across the alveolar capillary membrane into the pulmonary capillary blood it is transported in two ways. Most (97%) is attached to haemoglobin in the red cells and is transported as oxyhaemoglobin, whilst a small amount of O_2 (3%) is dissolved in plasma. Each molecule of haemoglobin is able to carry four molecules of O_2 and when this is so the haemoglobin is fully saturated (100%). In clinical practice, this is easily measured by a pulse oximeter using a finger probe with values of 96–100% in health. Where the inspired partial pressure of O_2 is too low or where there is a problem with gaseous exchange across the alveolar capillary membrane then the partial pressure of O_2 in arterial blood (PaO_2) will fall (hypoxaemia) and this will be reflected in falling saturations. Where there are increasing levels of reduced haemoglobin (without oxygen) then cyanosis may become evident where there is bluish discolouration of the skin and mucous membranes.

Normal PaO_2 range: 12–14kPa.
Normal $PaCO_2$ range: 4.6–6.0kPa.

When fully saturated each gram of haemoglobin is able to carry 1.39mL of O_2 and given a haemoglobin level of 15g/dL then a little over 20mL of O_2 can be carried in every 100mL of arterial blood: this is called O_2 capacity. Given a cardiac output of 5000mL then the amount of O_2 carried is approximately 1000mL and this is referred to as the O_2 delivery or DO_2. From this O_2 which is delivered to the cells each minute at rest, only 250mL is extracted by the cells (for oxidative phosphorylation) and this is called O_2 consumption or VO_2. This leaves a reserve of O_2 available in arterial blood which is required when VO_2 needs to increase during exercise or during illness to cope with cellular metabolic demand. The actual O_2 content of arterial blood (CaO_2) for each individual will depend on the saturation, amount of haemoglobin and cardiac output. All these parameters must be considered in ensuring that O_2 delivery (DO_2) is able to keep up with O_2 consumption (VO_2).

Anaemic patients with healthy lungs will have normal saturations but reduced oxygen content of arterial blood (CaO_2) may result in hypoxia!
Haemoglobin should be checked.

Just as O_2 moves down a pressure gradient from the lungs to the tissues, carbon dioxide (CO_2) moves down a pressure gradient from tissues to the lungs where it is exhaled (see Figure 5.6). CO_2 is more soluble than O_2 and there is more of it in the body and as CO_2 forms carbonic acid (H_2CO_3) in water it must be carried in an alternative form. Much of it is carried as bicarbonate (HCO_3) and some is carried attached to protein (e.g. haemoglobin) as carbamino compounds. The partial pressure of CO_2 in arterial blood ($PaCO_2$) can be measured through blood gas analysis which involves obtaining an arterial sample from the radial or femoral artery. Where ventilation is impaired and the lungs cannot remove CO_2 efficiently during expiration then its partial pressure in arterial blood ($PaCO_2$) will become elevated (hypercapnia) often accompanied by a fall in arterial O_2 (hypoxaemia).

Oxyhaemoglobin dissociation curve

The oxyhaemoglobin dissociation curve is described as S or sigmoid in shape (see Figure 5.7) and illustrates the relationship between PaO_2 (the horizontal axis) and haemoglobin saturation (the vertical axis). What is evident is that between a PaO_2 of 8 and 15kPa, the portion of the curve between these two points is relatively flat. That is, despite a fall in PaO_2 from 15kPa, saturations remain high. It is only when the PaO_2 falls to 8kPa (saturation

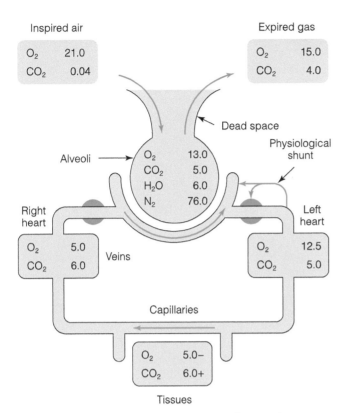

Figure 5.6 Diagram showing movement of gases down a pressure gradient (kPa)

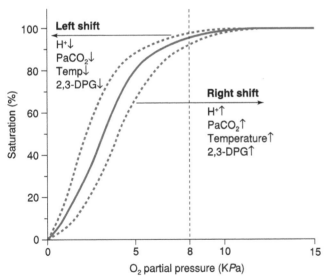

Figure 5.7 Oxyhaemoglobin dissociation curve. The unbroken curve is the normal position

- Temperature
- 2,3 diphosphoglycerate (2,3-DPG)
- Hydrogen ions or pH status
- PaCO$_2$.

Where the haemoglobin is affected by an increase in temperature (pyrexia), rising hydrogen ions (acidosis), and/or a rise in CO$_2$ then the bond is weakened and oxygen is readily off loaded to the tissues. An increase in 2,3 diphosphoglycerate (2,3-DPG) in the red cells during hypoxia can also facilitate oxygen release. During these times the oxyhaemoglobin dissociation curve shifts to the right. Conversely, where the haemoglobin is affected by a fall in temperature, a fall in hydrogen ions (alkalosis) or a fall in CO$_2$ then the bond is strengthened and less oxygen is released and the curve shifts to the left. These physiological changes in health ensure that when required oxygen is offloaded easily to metabolising tissues or conserved when metabolism is low (along with oxygen demand). There are clinical situations, however, in which abnormalities may shift the position of the curve and compromise the loading and offloading of oxygen at pulmonary and tissue level respectively.

Acute respiratory problems

There are many respiratory disorders but most fall into one of two groups – obstructive and restrictive disorders which may increase the work of breathing and result in breathlessness. Restrictive disorders develop when the compliance of the lungs and/or chest wall is reduced and the lungs become 'stiff'. Resistance disorders occur where there is an increase in airway resistance, often due to obstruction. Some patients may have mixed pathology with both restrictive and obstructive features. Breathlessness may be caused by disease affecting the airways, gaseous exchange units, chest wall/pleural membranes or the pulmonary circulation. Breathlessness can also be caused by cardiac problems as well as anaemia and non-cardiorespiratory causes such as anxiety states. Where there is acidosis the respiratory system will attempt to restore balance by increasing ventilation, thus removing carbon dioxide (therefore reducing carbonic acid) from the body.

This section will give a brief overview of common respiratory problems which may be seen in an acute care situation. Not only must nurses possess a broad knowledge of the structure and functions of the human body, they must have in-depth knowledge of common physical health problems (NMC 2010). Later sections will include assessment and general management principles.

90%) that the curve then falls steeply with low saturations. In practice, where PaO$_2$ falls below 8kPa respiratory failure is present and this has serious consequences for oxygen delivery. The nurse needs to be vigilant so that a trend in falling saturations is detected promptly and appropriate action taken.

The bond between haemoglobin and oxygen can be influenced by a number of factors:

Acute airway obstruction

Any part of the upper and lower respiratory tract may become obstructed. Obstruction around the laryngeal and tracheal area will result in high-pitched musical sounds (stridor) particularly on inspiration and the patient will be acutely distressed. Causes include inhaled foreign bodies, tumour invasion, infection/inflammation and severe allergic reactions such as anaphylaxis. Severe obstruction results in rapid desaturation with respiratory failure and possible cardiopulmonary arrest. Supportive management includes reassurance and positioning the conscious patient upright, well supported with pillows, and the administration of high-concentration oxygen through a high-flow device with a non re-breathing bag to correct hypoxaemia. A mixture of inhaled helium and oxygen (heliox) may be prescribed which reduces airway turbulence. It may be necessary for the doctor to perform tracheal intubation or tracheostomy with assisted ventilation, and where possible the cause of the obstruction should be identified and treated, possibly through fibre-optic bronchoscopy. Where allergy is the cause then this will necessitate the administration of drugs such as adrenaline, an antihistamine and hydrocortisone. If necessary then cardiopulmonary resuscitation should be performed. Current guidelines including treatment algorithms for anaphylaxis have been published by the Resuscitation Council UK (2008) and NICE (2010).

> Anaphylaxis is a type 1 hypersensitivity immune reaction (medical emergency!) where an allergen (e.g. foreign protein), immunoglobulin E (IgE) and mast cell complex results in a massive release of histamine from the mast cells.

Pneumothorax

The difference between subatmospheric pressure (negative) in the pleural cavity and atmospheric pressure (positive) in the lungs promotes lung inflation. A pneumothorax occurs when atmospheric air enters the pleural cavity and the pressure becomes positive, resulting in elastic recoil of the lung and either partial or total collapse. It may be spontaneous with no cause, as a complication in chronic lung disease, following trauma or inadvertently during hospital treatment (e.g. insertion of central line and mechanical ventilation). The visceral pleural membrane in the apices of either lung is usually involved as a result of gravitational forces and a small tear in the visceral pleura allows air to leak into the pleural space.

Presentation is usually sudden, often with sharp chest pain but that will depend on how large the pneumothorax is, with small volumes of air in the pleural cavity causing relatively few problems. With a larger pneumothorax perfusion of alveoli which remain non-ventilated may result in significant desaturation resulting in a greater proportion of the cardiac output leaving the left ventricle without oxygen. Apart from pain the patient will be breathless with increasing respiratory rate and tachycardia and will also be very anxious. There will be reduced chest expansion and breath sounds on the affected side. Cyanosis denoting reduced oxygenation may also be present. A pneumothorax may become a tension pneumothorax (a medical emergency) where air that has entered the pleural cavity cannot escape during expiration. The build up of air will compress the mediastinal space where the heart and great vessels are situated and this will result in cardiovascular collapse.

> In pneumothorax, high-concentration oxygen aids reabsorption of air (but not in patients with COPD!).

Depending on the degree of desaturation a high concentration of oxygen will be prescribed to restore saturations to within acceptable parameters, although this may be difficult to achieve if the pneumothorax is large. Although small volumes of air will be absorbed the doctor may decide to withdraw air using a needle and syringe, although for a large pneumothorax a chest drain attached to an underwater seal-drainage system will be necessary. This facilitates the removal of air during expiration but does not allow air to be drawn in during inspiration so that eventually all air is removed, with negative pressure restored in the pleural cavity and lung re-expansion.

A quick reference guideline is available on pleural disease (including pneumothorax) from the British Thoracic Society (2010).

> **Types of pneumothorax:**
> ● Primary spontaneous
> ● Secondary spontaneous
> ● Traumatic
> ● Iatrogenic
> ● Tension.

Bronchial asthma

Asthma is a chronic inflammatory disorder of the airways, commonly as a result of inhaled allergens leading to hypersensitivity. The inflammatory process is extremely complex and involves many different cells in the respiratory epithelium releasing mediators which are proinflammatory. Although there is widespread inflammation throughout the airways the sections that are particularly vulnerable to this inflammatory process are the terminal and respiratory bronchioles because there is no cartilage to maintain lumen patency. Swelling as result of inflammation, mucus plugging and smooth muscle contraction of these airways results in obstruction to airflow and wheezing. This airway obstruction in asthma is variable with symptoms often developing within a very short time frame. Symptom-free periods punctuated with acute episodes may occur in some individuals. Treatment in asthma is very successful and complete control of symptoms is possible in most cases with appropriate intervention including bronchodilators and steroids as well as patient education and the promotion of self-management.

The patient with acute asthma will be distressed and present with chest tightness, increased shortness of breath, wheezing and cough. The work of breathing is increased as a result of increased airway resistance due to narrowing. The patient must work much harder in order to drive air through these narrowed airways. This is evident by the position adopted to breathe, usually sitting upright and leaning forward, as well as the use of accessory muscles during inspiration and expiration. So much muscle contraction used for breathing will increase the need for oxygen at a time when air is unable to reach the alveoli and can lead to fatigue and serious compromise of cardiopulmonary status.

Asthma guidelines are available from the Scottish Intercollegiate Guidelines Network/British Thoracic Society (2011) and these are regularly updated. Features of acute severe asthma include the inability to complete sentences in one breath and a peak expiratory flow rate (PEFR) which is 33–50% of best or predicted. Known asthmatics will usually know their best PEFR value which should be recorded, otherwise the nurse will need to refer to a chart with predicted values. A respiratory rate greater than 25 breaths per minute (tachypnoea) and a tachycardia of more than 110 per minute are often present. High flow oxygen should be administered at 40–60% to those who are hypoxaemic to achieve saturations of 94–98% and the doctor will usually prescribe high-dose bronchodilators such as salbutamol or ipratropium nebulised with oxygen. Steroid medication is important and oral prednisolone and/or hydrocortisone intravenously are prescribed. Where there is no improvement the doctor may request additional doses of bronchodilators and occasionally these may be given intravenously. Where the desired level of bronchodilation has not been achieved additional agents such as magnesium sulphate and aminophylline may be prescribed.

Ongoing monitoring by the nurse is crucial. Where treatment is unsuccessful then deterioration may result in life-threatening asthma where the PEFR is less than 33% of best or predicted and the saturation (SpO_2) falls below 92% reflecting severe hypoxaemia. The patient may develop bradycardia, hypotension, cardiac arrhythmias and confusion. Arterial blood gas analysis may reveal respiratory failure where the PaO_2 is less than 8kPa. However, given the enormous ventilatory effort involved in breathing, exhaustion eventually ensues and the patient will be unable to ventilate sufficiently to remove CO_2. At this point blood gas analysis will reveal an elevated $PaCO_2$ (hypercapnia) as well as profound hypoxaemia (PaO_2 less than 8kPa). Given this scenario ventilatory support with positive pressure ventilation is necessary.

Where SpO_2 falls below 92% arterial blood gas analysis is required.

Increasing $PaCO_2$ in acute asthma reflects a near-fatal attack and is a medical emergency.

Exacerbation of chronic obstructive pulmonary disease

Chronic obstructive pulmonary disease (COPD) is also a chronic inflammatory disease of the airways but the cause and the inflammatory process is different to asthma, with the majority of cases due to the long-term effects of smoking. In fact, COPD is an umbrella term for chronic bronchitis and emphysema. In chronic bronchitis, irritation caused by smoking results in inflammation of airways and an increase in mucus-secreting glands as well as an increase in mucus-secreting goblet cells. There is increased production of sputum and the structural changes in the airways as a result of the inflammatory response leads to their narrowing. Emphysema, which often co-exists, affects the respiratory bronchioles, alveolar ducts and sacs where gaseous exchange takes place. There is distension and destruction of the tissue which may eventually affect gaseous exchange. This loss of elastic recoil of the respiratory bronchioles leads to early airway closure during expiration and air trapping.

As the disease progresses, particularly where smoking continues, the degree of airway obstruction which is irreversible will become worse. Increasing sputum production, breathlessness and disability, all more severe during winter, are usual. Initially, although there may be mild hypoxaemia, ventilatory drive is sufficient to remove CO_2. Indeed in some patients with severe emphysema the breathlessness can be profound but ventilatory effort keeps the CO_2 low. In time some patients may not be able to maintain this ventilatory drive and CO_2 excretion may be compromised so that chronic hypercapnia develops. Whilst rising levels of CO_2 will initially stimulate breathing as usual, eventually it is hypoxaemia which stimulates peripheral chemoreceptors in the carotid artery and aortic arch. This is referred to as hypoxic drive and is why caution is exercised when administering oxygen to patients with COPD.

It is during the winter months that patients with COPD may experience an exacerbation defined as 'rapid and sustained worsening of symptoms beyond normal day to day variations' (NICE 2010: 5). It is during these times that breathlessness and cough become worse with an increase in sputum which is purulent and indicative of infection. In addition there is often increased chest tightness, wheeze and fatigue with worsening hypoxaemia often resulting in confusion. With long-standing COPD low levels of O_2 in the lungs can result in narrowing of the pulmonary blood vessels, which can increase the work of the right ventricle of the heart, ultimately leading to cardiac failure. Cardiac failure which develops in this way following chronic lung disease is called cor pulmonale and the patient will have additional problems, including fluid retention with swollen ankles and possibly ascites (fluid in the peritoneal cavity).

It is often difficult making the decision as to whether the patient with acute exacerbation of COPD should be admitted to hospital or not. This will depend on what services are available locally. Where there is a community rapid response team or an intermediate care facility then escalation of treatment at home may avoid hospitalisation. Factors such as breathlessness, inability to cope, impaired level of consciousness and saturations below 90% would favour treatment in hospital. Treatment would necessitate the administration of inhaled bronchodilators (often nebulised with an air compressor) as well as corticosteroids (e.g. prednisolone) and antibiotics. Where there is fluid retention as a result of cardiac failure then diuretic therapy will also be necessary.

> Where a patient is known to have chronically elevated $PaCO_2$ levels (hypercapnic failure) then oxygen should be given at 24% initially to maintain SpO_2 at 88–92%.

During acute exacerbations the increased work of breathing with inevitable fatigue can result in poor ventilatory drive and the consequence of this is a falling PaO_2 and a rising CO_2. However, it is important to remember that a patient with long-standing COPD may have adjusted to living with chronic hypoxaemia and hypercapnia – this is the patient's 'normal' state. During acute episodes great skill is needed in reducing $PaCO_2$ levels without over-correction of PaO_2 oxygen levels and non-invasive ventilatory support and careful oxygen titration aims to achieve this, and is discussed later in this chapter.

Pneumonia

Pneumonia occurs when inflammatory material (exudate) accumulates in the alveoli. Where the inflammation is confined to the whole of one or more lobes it is referred to as lobar pneumonia, or bronchopneumonia when spread more widely throughout the lungs. Similarly pneumonia can be caused by a range of pathogenic organisms including bacteria and viruses, following the aspiration of vomit or mucus and occasionally following treatment such as radiotherapy. Examples of microorganisms that cause pneumonia include:

- *Streptococcus pneumoniae*
- *Mycoplasma pneumoniae*
- *Influenza A viruses*
- *Haemophilus influenzae*
- *Chlamydia pneumoniae*
- *Legionella pneumoniae*
- *Pneumocystis carinii.*

Host factors (e.g. individual resistance) and agent factors (e.g. virulence of organism) should be taken into account when considering individual susceptibility to infection. Although fit healthy people can develop pneumonia the following may increase risk:

- smoking;
- excessive alcohol intake;
- presence of other conditions such as COPD, cancer and heart failure;
- being very young or very old;
- having a weak immune system;
- recent respiratory viral infection;
- malnutrition/poor hydration;
- treatment in intensive care;
- increased susceptibility to inhalation – impaired consciousness, swallowing difficulties.

In previously fit, healthy people who develop pneumonia involving a single lobe, treatment at home may be appropriate.

Patients with pneumonia typically present with a cough (with or without sputum) breathlessness (respiratory rate is greater than 30/minute) and chest pain and in some there is fever, agitation and confusion. Very often a chest X-ray will reveal abnormalities. Pneumonia can result in rapid deterioration within a short time frame where the ventilation perfusion relationship is seriously compromised and where shunting results in profound hypoxaemia and respiratory failure. Indeed the degree of shunt may be so severe that high-concentration oxygen fails to improve saturations and transfer to intensive care for positive pressure ventilation is necessary.

Respiratory failure

Acute cardiac and respiratory problems can result in a failure to maintain effective gaseous exchange across the alveolar capillary membrane. Acute respiratory failure is the outcome of one of the following.

Lung failure

This is where there is inadequate gaseous exchange across the alveolar capillary membrane so that arterial oxygenation cannot be maintained. The PaO_2 will fall (reduced saturations) but effective ventilation (inspiration and expiration) will continue to remove carbon dioxide. Indeed, in the early stages of acute respiratory problems (e.g. pneumonia and asthma) hyperventilation may result in low arterial carbon dioxide levels.

Ventilatory failure

The anatomical structure of the thorax is designed so that the lungs can effectively 'pump' air in and out (i.e. ventilate). This requires the chest wall, ribs, nerves and muscles to work together in order that this can be achieved. There are a number of disorders that can affect this mechanism which will result in the inability of the lungs to function as a ventilatory pump. When this occurs carbon dioxide cannot be removed from the lungs effectively and therefore levels become elevated in arterial blood (hypercapnia). As a result arterial oxygen levels will also start to fall.

Causes of ventilatory failure:
- fatigue of ventilatory muscles;
- problems with the chest wall (e.g. chest injury/deformity);
- neuromuscular problems;
- central nervous system depression.

When gas exchange is compromised in the lungs the body must compensate to maintain homeostasis. The work of breathing will increase as a result of increased airway resistance, reduced compliance or both. As a consequence the cardiovascular system will also attempt to restore balance by increasing heart rate, blood pressure

and cardiac output. This altered physiology will be reflected in the patient's changing vital signs and ongoing assessment is crucial so that these developments can be detected early and appropriate corrective measures taken. (See Respiratory assessment.)

Where there is deterioration in respiratory status with a progressive fall in saturations (SpO_2) arterial blood gas analysis is required to establish whether or not the patient is in respiratory failure. The following values would confirm the diagnosis.

Type I respiratory failure (lung failure)
Profound hypoxaemia with a PaO_2 of less than 8kPa (SpO_2 less than 90%) with normal or low $PaCO_2$ (less than 6.1kPa).

Type II respiratory failure (pump or ventilatory failure)
Profound hypoxaemia, with a PaO_2 of less than 8kPa (SpO_2 less than 90%) and an elevated $PaCO_2$ above 6.0kPa (hypercapnia).

In respiratory failure, intervention is aimed at reducing the work of breathing and restoring arterial blood gas values to within appropriate parameters agreed by the health care team. Where this is not achieved by oxygen administration positive pressure ventilation will be required.

Respiratory assessment

In acute care settings, nurses have a crucial role to play in assessment so that deterioration in respiratory status is detected as early as possible. Concerns regarding competence in this area led to the development of physiological 'track and trigger' systems in order to promote patient safety. A systematic approach should be adopted to undertake a respiratory assessment and involves the gathering of subjective and objective data.

Initial assessment will involve using the ABCDE framework and local protocol should followed regarding the use of early warning scoring systems. The following discussion has focused on assessment of breathing. Where the patient's condition dictates it may be necessary to perform cardiopulmonary resuscitation (see Chapter 7).

Subjective data

The patient's perspective is important and if possible they should be asked what they think the current problem is. A great deal of information can be obtained contributing to data analysis and identification of likely problems.

Table 5.1 History taking

• Personal biography	• Medication
• Patient perception of major problem	• Symptom/systems review
	• Psychosocial history
• Medical history – illness, surgery/recent trends	• Risk, e.g. smoking, alcohol
• Allergies	• Functional ability – self-care deficits

This is where a patient history can be taken including the exploration of each symptom that the patient may be experiencing (see Table 5.1). Information should be obtained for each symptom (e.g. pain, breathlessness, cough) the patient has and PQRSTU can assist here:

P – Provocation and palliation
Q – Quality
R – Region/radiation
S – Severity
T – Timing
U – Understanding.

Time available for history taking will depend on the condition of the patient: it may be necessary to move swiftly on to obtaining objective data where there is significant respiratory and haemodynamic instability.

Objective data

Objective data obtained should be relatively accurate, depending, of course, on the skill of the nurse and any electronic equipment used. Vital signs including pulse, blood pressure and respiratory rate will be recorded and a physical examination performed with additional diagnostic and laboratory data requested as appropriate.

> **Signs of respiratory deterioration:**
> • increased respiratory rate;
> • decreased SpO_2;
> • increased oxygen needed to keep SpO_2 in target range;
> • increased physiological trigger score;
> • CO_2 retention;
> • drowsiness;
> • headache;
> • flushed face;
> • tremor.
>
> O'Driscoll et al. (2008)

Nurses spend a great deal of time measuring and recording vital signs and this is often seen as a routine aspect of nursing care. However, observations need to be contextualised and interpreted as part of a more detailed respiratory assessment. The ability of nurses to recognise early signs of illness, and start appropriate and timely management of those who are at risk of clinical deterioration or require emergency care is crucial (NMC 2010). The frequency of monitoring will depend on the stability of the patient's condition as well as any perceived risk of complications developing during or following diagnostic/ therapeutic interventions. Where values obtained fall outside of the normal range or agreed parameters senior staff should be alerted. No matter how often measurements are recorded ongoing monitoring of the patient's condition is important as this can change within a very short time frame (i.e. in between recording observations!).

Pulse oximetry is established as soon as possible. Oxygen saturation is considered the 'fifth vital sign' and measurements (SpO_2) are obtained with a probe attached usually to the finger. Values in health are 97–100% with downward trends reflecting worsening hypoxaemia. For readings there must be capillary blood flow and this may not be the case where there is haemodynamic instability. Recordings should indicate whether measurements were taken on room air or with oxygen. Saturations alone give no information regarding oxygen delivery and where there are normal saturations the patient can still develop hypoxia. Nevertheless saturation values assist in diagnosis and monitoring during interventions to treat hypoxaemia.

> **Factors affecting pulse oximetry readings:**
> • poor peripheral perfusion;
> • carbon monoxide levels (e.g. smokers) – overestimates!
> • probe site (finger/ear lobe most accurate);
> • nail varnish and false nails.
>
> NB Saturations normal in anaemia so haemoglobin should be checked.

Although the pulse rate is usually displayed on the oximeter it is important to palpate the pulse to obtain further information. During breathlessness with increased work of breathing, heart rate can increase significantly with tachycardia, further increasing oxygen demand with compensatory increases in heart rate and cardiac output. Profound hypoxaemia may result in bradycardia and abnormal heart rhythms which may be reflected by an irregular pulse. Cardiovascular compensatory changes may cause additional problems where there are cardiac problems resulting in a weak, thready pulse. Having taken the pulse and with fingers still on the radial pulse the nurse can then count the respiratory rate, noting the depth of breathing and chest expansion (see the section 'Inspection' regarding respiratory assessment).

Blood pressure is recorded and in the early stages where there is respiratory compromise there may be a rise in blood pressure due to activation of the sympathetic nervous system. However, where there is deterioration in respiratory status this can result in haemodynamic instability with a fall in blood pressure.

Physical examination

Inspection

During the recording of vital signs the nurse is observing the patient (also using the sense of hearing) and this can provide a great deal of information about respiratory status. During inspection the nurse may hear a stridor if there is an upper airway obstruction, a cough or may hear wheezes. The level of consciousness and degree of orientation is noted and whether the patient is unable to complete a sentence in one breath. In a well-lit room, bluish discoloration of mucous membranes in the mouth (central cyanosis) and of the fingers, nose and ear lobes (peripheral cyanosis) may be visible if there is desaturation (although this alone is an unreliable sign). Where work of breathing is increased there may be signs of distress and the patient will prefer to sit upright, leaning forward where possible. If there is any sputum being expectorated then this should be observed. Blood-streaked sputum may suggest haemoptysis and green sputum bacterial infection.

> **Physical examination**
>
> Involves the following:
> - Inspection (look)
> - Palpation (feel)
> - Percussion (feel)
> - Auscultation (listen).
>
> Skills utilising look, listen and feel are important throughout any patient assessment.

Note should be made of any accessory muscles used including the neck muscles (sternomastoids) and scalenes for inspiration and abdominal muscles during expiration. As well as counting the respiratory rate the nurse should observe the depth of breathing. Remember that for adequate gaseous exchange alveolar volume is important and determined by respiratory rate and tidal volume. Poor chest expansion will result in reduced tidal volumes therefore alveolar ventilation (hypoventilation) and will increase the $PaCO_2$. Symmetry of chest movement is also important and reduced expansion on one side may indicate pneumothorax or pneumonia, for example. An increase in the anterior–posterior (A–P) diameter of the chest is usually seen in patients with chronic obstructive pulmonary disease. Nicotine-stained fingers may be seen in heavy smokers and chronic hypoxaemia may result in

clubbing of the fingers. Patients who are taking bronchodilators such as salbutamol (beta 2 agonists) may have a fine tremor of the hands and in those with carbon dioxide retention (hypercapnia) a flapping tremor of the outstretched arms is occasionally seen.

Palpation

Using touch will also provide a great deal of information during the physical examination and the nurse will already have made a few observations whilst palpating the pulse. The skin including extremities may feel warm suggesting good perfusion, while cool skin may indicate reduced cardiac output. Gently palpating the anterior and posterior chest may identify swelling and areas of localised pain. Air can sometimes escape from the lungs and accumulate in the superficial skin layers (following puncture wounds or surgery). This is called subcutaneous or surgical emphysema and gives rise to a crackling sensation during palpation.

Experienced practitioners may also palpate the position of the trachea just above the suprasternal notch in the neck. The trachea is usually central but can shift to one side if air accumulates, as in a tension pneumothorax. Finally, palpation can be used to feel for the vibrations caused by transmission of sounds from the voice. By palpating the chest on both sides and asking the patient to say 'ninety-nine' vibrations may be felt on the practitioner's hands (tactile fremitus). Solid tissue such as consolidation in pneumonia can transmit sounds well (increased tactile fremitus) where as increased air in a pneumothorax cannot (decreased tactile fremitus).

Percussion

This is where the anterior and posterior chest is percussed. The technique involves placing the middle finger firmly over the surface to be percussed (all other fingers should be off the chest) and then striking it with the middle finger of the other hand. This transmits vibrations through to the underlying chest wall and a note is produced. One side of the chest is compared to the other. Characteristics of the percussion note are as follows:

- *resonant* – over normal lung;
- *hyperresonant* – over a pneumothorax;
- *tympanic* – over a tension pneumothorax;
- *dullness* – over liver and in consolidation, e.g. pneumonia.

Auscultation

The areas previously percussed are then auscultated using the diaphragm of the stethoscope to listen for breath

Table 5.2 Physical examination: findings in specific disorders

Disorder	Inspection	Palpation	Percussion note	Auscultation
Pneumonia	Flushed Respiratory rate ↑	Fremitus ↑ Expansion ↓ on affected side	Dull over consolidation	Bronchial breath sounds over consolidation Crackles Broncophony ↑
Atelectasis	Respiratory rate ↑	Absent fremitus Expansion ↓ on affected side	Dull over affected area	Absent
Pneumothorax	Breathless Respiratory rate ↑	Fremitus ↓ or absent Trachea may shift towards the opposite side Expansion ↓ on affected side	Hyperresonant or tympanic	Breath sounds decreased or absent over pleural air Broncophony ↓
Asthma	Breathless Respiratory rate ↑ Cough/tenacious sputum	Fremitus ↓	Resonant to hyperresonant	Breath sounds obscured by wheezes, possibly crackles Broncophony ↓
Acute COPD	Cough/purulent sputum Breathless Pursed lip breathing Respiratory rate ↑ Barrel chest	Fremitus ↓	Hyperresonant	Breath sounds Crackles/wheezes Broncophony ↓

sounds. The sounds produced on one side of the chest are compared to the other side. Normal breath sounds over the anterior and posterior chest wall are vesicular, which are soft, low-pitched sounds where the inspiratory phase is longer than the expiratory phase. If bronchial sounds are heard then this may suggest an area of consolidation. Bronchial breath sounds are loud and high-pitched with the inspiratory phase shorter than the expiratory phase. As well as breath sounds there may be additional breath sounds (adventitious sounds) such as crackles and wheezes. Coarse crackles are heard in pulmonary oedema (fluid in the alveoli as a result of left ventricular heart failure) and fine crackles in pulmonary fibrosis. Wheezes can be heard in acute asthma and in chronic obstructive pulmonary disease. Differences in the transmission of voice sounds can also be heard during auscultation. Where there is consolidation the sounds produced by asking the patient to say 'ninety-nine' will be heard more loudly through the stethoscope compared to the healthy side: this is called broncophony. Conversely, where there is air then broncophony is diminished or even absent.

Nurses mostly use the skills of inspection and palpation, although increasingly specialist nurses are developing their clinical skills in percussion and auscultation to enhance their assessment of patients. However, while nurses practise independently they must be able to recognise the limits of their competence and knowledge, seeking advice from or referring to other professionals when necessary (NMC 2010). See Table 5.2 for key findings during physical examination relating to specific disorders.

Arterial blood gases

Where there is trend of worsening respiratory status with falling oxygen saturations the doctor will usually request arterial blood gas analysis where respiratory failure is suspected. A specimen of arterial blood is obtained from either the radial or femoral artery using a needle and heparinised syringe. An arteriolised blood sample may be obtained from the ear lobe and is useful for measuring pH and $PaCO_2$ (underestimates PaO_2 by 0.5–1kPa). In critical care settings, the patient may have an arterial line temporarily inserted in the radial artery and this avoids repeated

CASE STUDY 5.1 Mrs Proctor, a patient with COPD – Part 1

INITIAL ASSESSMENT

It is 11.00h and Mrs Proctor, aged 71 and a lifelong smoker, has been admitted following referral by her GP with a history of breathlessness. Despite three courses of antibiotics and steroids there has been no improvement and for the last few days she has been feeling generally unwell with increased breathlessness, initially on exertion but now at rest.

Airway

On arrival on the ward the nurse notes that although Mrs Proctor is very breathless and distressed she is fully conscious and has a patent airway with no stridor audible. The nurse offers reassurance and assists the patient in adopting the most comfortable position, which is sitting upright and leaning forward.

Breathing

Responding to questions asked during the initial assessment it is evident that the degree of breathlessness is quite severe as Mrs Proctor cannot complete sentences without stopping and gasping for air. Coughing is intermittent with the expectoration of green, tenacious sputum indicating possible dehydration and/or infection although the temperature recorded earlier was 37°C. The respiratory rate is 30 breaths per minute and although breathing is regular and chest movement symmetrical, contraction of the sternomastoids and abdominal muscles, along with poor chest expansion and pursed lip breathing confirms the increased respiratory effort required for breathing.

The nurse decides to limit the number of questions asked so as not cause further distress at this stage and explains to Mrs Proctor that she would like to assess her breathing status and perform a chest examination. Before proceeding the nurse notes that pulse oximetry shows an SpO_2 of 94% with 2 litres of oxygen delivered by nasal cannulae although the level has been falling to 87% without oxygen. On further inspection it is noted that there is pallor although no signs of cyanosis of the extremities (peripheral cyanosis) or of the tongue/buccal cavity (central cyanosis). The absence of central cyanosis is particularly reassuring as this indicates that arterial saturation is likely to be satisfactory and the nurse continues with the assessment in a systematic fashion.

On palpation, Mrs Proctor's equal chest expansion and normal tracheal position are noted. It is therefore unlikely that a tension pneumothorax is contributing to the current pulmonary compromise. Using palpation skills the nurse asks Mrs Proctor to repeat '99' and notes that tactile

fremitus is decreased bilaterally. Given that transmission of sound is poor through air, this conveys to the nurse that reduced vibration on palpation (fremitus) is possibly due to air trapping in the lungs. Percussion elicits hyperresonance over the anterior chest.

On auscultation there are reduced vesicular breath sounds over the anterior and posterior lung fields and there are some early inspiratory crackles which again could indicate infection.

Circulation

Although the nurse palpated the pulse earlier during the initial assessment, Mrs Proctor's heart rate remains at a regular 120 beats per minute and the nurse notes the bounding quality. The peripheries are warm and the capillary refill time is 2 seconds. The cardiac monitor reveals sinus tachycardia possibly caused by the sympathetic activation as a result of hypoxaemia, the stress response to critical illness or perhaps elevated carbon dioxide. However, there are no ectopic beats or other arrhythmias. The nurse reflects on these findings and how unpredictable the overall effect of carbon dioxide on the cardiovascular system can be and that although hypercapnia and acidosis can have a direct cardiovascular depressant effect, this can often be overshadowed by a sympathetic response resulting in tachycardia as in Mrs Proctor's case. Elevated $PaCO_2$ levels can also result in a systemic vasodilator effect, giving a flushed appearance and bounding pulse.

Mrs Proctor's blood pressure is elevated at 154/89mmHg with a mean arterial pressure (MAP) of 110mmHg. There is no pedal oedema, skin is dry with decreased turgor and she has not passed urine since admission. She is also complaining of feeling thirsty. Although renal blood flow and glomerular filtration rate (GFR) are likely to be reduced as a result of hypercapnia, dehydration is also likely to be a contributing factor.

Disability

The Glasgow Coma Scale (GCS) is 15/15 (E4, V5, M6). Neurological status is important as this can be affected by hypoxaemia and hypercapnia leading to drowsiness, confusion and coma. The blood glucose level is checked as the nurse is aware that this can rise as a result of sympathetic activation, but it is within normal limits at 5mmols/L.

Exposure

The nurse observes that Mrs Proctor looks underweight and calculates her BMI to be 16, which is below normal. She is

CASE STUDY 5.1 Mrs Proctor, a patient with COPD – Part 1 (continued)

aware that respiratory status can be affected by poor nutrition and dehydration and that although breathlessness may have prevented dietary intake, improved nutrition and fluid replacement would be important goals. Weight loss further increases risk and can be a poor prognostic sign. A referral to the dietician will be needed later to optimise nutritional status. Skin, however, is intact and there are no other abnormalities noted.

Diagnosis

Given Mrs Proctor's history and presentation, a provisional diagnosis of chronic obstructive pulmonary disease (COPD) is made. Given the hypercapnia a low oxygen concentration of 24% is prescribed at 2 litres per minute via nasal cannulae to achieve saturations between 88–92%. The doctor also prescribes the following drugs:

- Nebulised salbutamol 5mg 4-hrly
- Nebulised ipratropium bromide 500micrograms
- Hydrocortisone 200mg IV.

Ongoing monitoring will be necessary as bronchodilators may have already contributed to Mrs Proctor's tachycardia. As a result myocardial oxygen demand will have been increased and this may cause further compromise resulting in a reduced cardiac output with decreased tissue perfusion, further increasing risk in an already critically ill, hypoxaemic patient.

It is not unusual for older patients to have an infection without an increase in temperature and therefore a sputum sample is sent for culture and sensitivity and a broad-spectrum antibiotic commenced intravenously.

The nurse documents her findings carefully and is aware that although an initial assessment has been completed ongoing monitoring of Mrs Proctor is necessary. Once the patient is stabilised and less distressed the nurse will be able to complete a more comprehensive assessment. Although an initial systems review was undertaken additional data will be required regarding usual self-care ability and possible factors which may need to be considered in preparing the patient for discharge later.

Table 5.3 Normal blood gas values

Normal values	Arterial blood	Venous blood
pH	7.35–7.45	7.31–7.41
Hydrogen ions	35–45mmol/L	
PO_2	12–14kPa	4.6–5.8kPa
PCO_2	4.6–6.0kPa	5.5–6.8kPa
HCO_3^-	22–26mmol/L	22–26mmol/L
O_2 saturation	95% +	70–75%
Base excess/deficit	−2 to +2	

Table 5.4 Acid-base imbalance

Respiratory acid-base imbalance	Causes
↑ $PaCO_2$ = acidosis ↑ Hydrogen ions	• Chronic obstructive pulmonary disease (COPD) • Depressed respiratory centre, e.g. sedation/head injury • Neuromuscular disorders • Acute respiratory infection
↓ $PaCO_2$ = alkalosis ↓ In hydrogen ions	• Hyperventilation, e.g. psychogenic

Metabolic acid-base imbalance	Causes
↓ HCO_3 = acidosis ↑ Metabolic acids Loss of HCO_3 from the body	• Ketoacidosis • Shock • Diarrhoea • Renal disease
↑ HCO_3 = alkalosis Loss of H^+ ions (acid) from the body	• Vomiting • Gastric aspiration • Excessive bicarbonate intake

arterial stabs which are somewhat painful. (See Table 5.3 for normal values.)

If the values obtained from the gas analyser are abnormal, the problem must be identified (see Table 5.4). In respiratory problems, abnormal blood gas values often reflect a respiratory acidosis where the $PaCO_2$ is elevated above 6.0kPa (type II respiratory failure). The hydration of excess CO_2 in the body results in carbonic acid which liberates hydrogen ions and increases acidity in the blood. If the patient has ventilatory difficulty they will not be able to blow off CO_2 during expiration. In acidosis, the pH will be less than the mean of 7.4 and there will be an increase in hydrogen ion concentration (normal range 35–45nmol/L). If the pH or hydrogen concentration is

within normal limits despite an elevated $PaCO_2$ then compensation is partial or complete and the bicarbonate level (HCO_3) is likely to be elevated (is greater than 26mmol/L). Accompanying the elevated $PaCO_2$ is often hypoxaemia (PaO_2 less than 8kPa). If the PaO_2 is less than 8kPa but the $PaCO_2$ is normal (or low) then this is respiratory failure type I.

If the abnormal blood gas values reveal a $PaCO_2$ within the normal range (or low) with a decreased HCO_3 (less than 24mmol/L) then this is likely to be a metabolic acidosis. The pH or hydrogen ion concentration may reflect this acidotic state, but if within the normal range then once again the body is compensating. The body will remove some of the hydrogen ions by increasing the ventilatory drive so that more CO_2 excreted as minute ventilation is increased. In a metabolic acidosis it is other acids (not carbonic acid) that cannot be removed by the lungs which accumulate, such as lactic acid (cellular hypoxia), or hydroxybutyric acid (ketoacidosis in diabetes). Another cause of metabolic acidosis is a loss of bicarbonate from the body as in severe diarrhoea where alkaline intestinal fluid is lost.

An alkalosis occurs where either too much CO_2 is expired (e.g. hyperventilation) resulting in a respiratory alkalosis, or where either acids are being lost from the body (e.g. hydrochloric acid through vomiting) or there is a net gain in bicarbonate (intravenous sodium bicarbonate or oral bicarbonate of soda taken as an antacid) resulting in a metabolic alkalosis.

As outlined earlier, acidosis and alkalosis can affect the release of oxygen from the haemoglobin, thus affecting oxygen delivery to the cells. It is important therefore that these acid-base disorders are corrected.

Maximising respiratory status

In the acutely ill patient, care is aimed at correcting hypoxaemia by optimising gaseous exchange in the lungs and achieving normal or near normal oxygen saturations other than in those at risk of hypercapnic failure. Attempts should also be made where possible to reduce the work of breathing by increasing compliance or reducing airway resistance.

Position

Ideally the patient in acute respiratory distress is nursed in an upright position, well supported with pillows where the condition allows this (in skeletal or spinal trauma this may not be possible). This facilitates effective chest expansion and improves lung volumes. It is important to remember that ventilation and perfusion is affected not only by disease processes but also by gravitational forces. Moving the patient where possible to a high side-lying

position on alternate sides may improve saturations by encouraging perfusion in healthy lung regions. Where there is disease on one side of the chest then positioning with the affected side uppermost may improve perfusion through the dependent (healthy) lung.

Frequent re-positioning by the nurse is essential as the patient may slip down the bed and this will compromise pulmonary status further by reducing functional residual capacity (FRC) and PaO_2 (Hardie et al. 2002). FRC can reduce significantly in patients who are supine and can lead to collapse of small airways with loss of surface area for gaseous exchange.

Oxygen therapy

Oxygen is administered to correct hypoxaemia with the correct inspired oxygen concentration given to achieve a target saturation: the British Thoracic Society has published guidelines (O'Driscoll et al. 2008). In critical illness where saturations are below 85% in patients without risk of hypercapnia failure high-flow oxygen should be administered using a reservoir mask at 15 L/min. In serious illness with milder degrees of hypoxaemia oxygen can be administered through nasal cannulae at 2–6 L/min or by a simple face mask at 5–10 L/min (a simple face mask must not be used at flow rates less than 5 L/min as this may result in carbon dioxide rebreathing). The aim is to achieve normal or near-normal oxygen saturations for all acutely ill patients (apart from those at risk of hypercapnic failure) with a target oxygen saturation of 94–98%.

> Oxygen should be prescribed and saturation target identified by medical staff but administered immediately in emergencies.
>
> A prescription should show:
> - Target saturation
> - Delivery device
> - Flow rate.

In patients with risk of hypercapnic failure low-dose oxygen is administered. In those with COPD, for example, with no previous history of carbon dioxide retention with acidosis a 28% Venturi mask at 4 L/min is used with a target oxygen saturation of 88–92%. Where the patient has a history of hypercapnic failure (requiring ventilation) in hospital a 24% Venturi mask at 4 L/min should be given (28% at 4 L/min prehospital care). A Venturi mask is a fixed performance mask which provides an accurate concentration of oxygen where a low dose is important. Where the diagnosis is not known in a patient over 50 years of age but who is a long-term smoker and has a history of chronic breathlessness a diagnosis of COPD should be assumed and low-dose oxygen given until further diagnostic tests are completed (British Thoracic Society 2008).

Oxygen therapy

If saturation less than 85% then:

- non-rebreather reservoir mask at 10–15 L/min.

Otherwise:

- nasal cannulae 2–6 L/min; or
- simple face mask 5–10 L/min.

If risk of hypercapnic failure:

- venturi mask 28%;
- venturi mask 24% (if history of respiratory acidosis).

Ongoing evaluation of the effectiveness of oxygen therapy is important and ongoing monitoring of oxygen saturations and regular arterial blood gas analysis performed in order to titrate oxygen flow. Where hypoxaemia is not corrected or where there is hypercapnia it may be necessary to establish ventilatory support. Nurses need to always practise safely by being aware of the correct use, limitations and hazards of common interventions including the use of medical devices and equipment (NMC 2010).

Humidification not necessary for:

- Low-flow oxygen
- High-flow oxygen for short-term use (less than 24h).

CASE STUDY 5.2 Mrs Proctor, a patient with COPD – Part 2

RECOGNISING EARLY DETERIORATION

Following initial assessment a provisional diagnosis of COPD was made and initial treatment included oxygen administration and nebulised bronchodilators. However, Mrs Proctor's increased respiratory rate, heart rate and breathlessness with accessory muscle contraction reflect the increased work of breathing and the nurse is concerned that there is ongoing respiratory compromise. She informs the doctor and arterial blood gas (ABG) analysis is performed at 12.00 and repeated at 12.30.

Normal values	Time	
	12.00	12.30
pH (7.35–7.45)	7.31	7.29
PaO$_2$ (11–13.5kPa)	8.6kPa	8.4kPa
PaCO$_2$ (4.5–6.1kPa)	8.0kPa	8.7kPa
HCO$_3^-$ (24–26mmol/L)	32mmol/L	33mmol/L
BE (−2 to +2)	+5	+6
SaO$_2$ (96–100%)	**94%**	91%
Oxygen	2 litres NS	1 litre NS
Mode	SV	SV

The above ABG analysis reveals a worsening trend. Initially there is a partially compensated respiratory acidosis (pH 7.31/PaCO$_2$ 8.0kPa) and there is an elevation in PaCO$_2$ with more carbonic acid generated (more hydrogen ions). Hypercapnia has resulted in renal compensation, and bicarbonate is reabsorbed in an attempt to reduce hydrogen ions and acidosis. This renal compensation over

time is typical in patients with COPD who often have an increased bicarbonate (HCO$_3^-$) level and a base excess (greater than +2).

With an acute rise in PaCO$_2$ levels incomplete renal compensation probably accounts for the ongoing acidosis and symptoms of hypercapnia. An elevated PaCO$_2$ with increased levels in alveolar air can result in falling PaO$_2$ levels. Given that Mrs Proctor's PaO$_2$ and SaO$_2$ are high, the oxygen is titrated down to 1 litre per minute.

As Mrs Proctor is acutely unwell the nurse uses a physiological 'track and trigger' system (NICE 2007) as part of her ongoing clinical assessment, which includes six physiological parameters where significant change to the derived score demands medical and specialist nursing review. The current early warning score (EWS) triggers a RED Code so the medical SpR and critical care outreach team are alerted regarding the necessity for urgent review. The team notes the increasing respiratory rate and distress, widespread inspiratory wheezes and a fall in the GCS to 13 (E3, V4, M6) and with the ABG analysis at 12.30 (worsening respiratory acidosis) confirm the deteriorating respiratory status. The team decide to transfer Mrs Proctor to a level 2 bed (ICS) for non-invasive ventilation (NIV) and closer observation. This is in keeping with current guidelines urging such a move within the first 60 minutes of hospital arrival for all patients with an acute exacerbation of COPD who remain acidotic despite maximum standard medical treatment.

Further nebulisers are given and bilevel positive airway pressure (BiPAP) is initiated with an IPAP of 14 and EPAP OF 4 (14/4) and 0.5 litres of oxygen entrained. After an hour of

CASE STUDY 5.2 Mrs Proctor, a patient with COPD – Part 2 (continued)

treatment on BiPAP, in conjunction with the medical treatment, the next ABG analysis shows a fully compensated respiratory acidosis. The nurse continues to record hourly observations, noting a reduction in her respiratory rate, heart rate and EWS, and is somewhat reassured that Mrs Proctor is less distressed, stating that she feels a little better. Prompt recognition and appropriate intervention has prevented a medical emergency occurring.

	Time
	13.30
pH	7.41
PaO_2	9.6
$PaCO_2$	6.1
HCO_3	29.7
BE	+4
SaO_2	95%
Oxygen	0.5 litre
Mode	BiPAP

Additional diagnostic data become available and the nurse is able to check these with earlier findings. The chest X-ray reveals hyperinflated lungs and a flattened diaphragm, both characteristic of COPD. From the FBC and U&Es she notes a raised WBC (20 $\times 10^{(9)}$/L) and elevated CRP (14.9mg/L),

confirming the likelihood of a chest infection. Although potassium can rise in metabolic acidosis, this is normal at 4.9mmol/L. She notes a compensatory rise in haemoglobin of 17g/dl as a result of the hypoxaemia. Blood urea is slightly elevated at 10.6mmol/L and with a sodium of 146mmol/L seems to confirm the possibility of dehydration. Fortunately, creatinine is within normal limits at 84μmol/L and the nurse is therefore reassured that renal function is most likely to be normal. Magnesium and phosphate are important electrolytes for respiratory muscle function but these are within the normal range with magnesium at 0.8mmol/L and phosphate 1.4mmol/L.

A 12-lead ECG is recorded to rule out possible cardiac involvement, in particular cor pulmonale, but the ECG trace is normal.

There is no single diagnostic test for COPD. Therefore making a diagnosis relies on clinical judgement, based on a combination of history, physical examination and confirmation of airway obstruction. Once Mrs Proctor is more stable she will require further lung function tests including spirometry to confirm the diagnosis. Although the initial focus was on restoring physiological stability, nurses must be able to carry out a comprehensive systematic nursing assessment that takes into account not only physical but social, cultural, psychological, spiritual and environmental factors in partnership with the patient, relatives and other professionals (NMC 2010).

Drug therapy

Bronchodilators are often prescribed where there is increased airflow obstruction. Although these are given via a hand-held inhaler in acute care situations it is often necessary to administer these through a nebuliser.

Drugs such as salbutamol and terbutaline are beta 2 adrenergic agonists that stimulate beta 2 receptors on the cell membrane of smooth muscle cells throughout the airways. Activation of these receptors results in relaxation and dilatation of the airway lumen. Additional receptor sites can also be stimulated, however, and this results in a tachycardia with palpitations (beta 1 receptors) muscle tremor (beta 2 receptors in skeleta l muscle) as well as anxiety, headache and nervousness. Another group of bronchodilators is the anticholinergics (ipratropium bromide) which block receptors (cholinergic) on the smooth muscle cell membrane resulting in relaxation. Both groups are used for their rapid onset.

Bronchodilators will increase lumen size and therefore decrease both airway resistance and the work of breathing. They will also help with airway clearance and facilitate expectoration. By using a nebuliser, drugs can be administered in larger doses by inhalation as an aerosol over a short period of time. Usually a jet nebulising chamber is used and the aerosol is generated by using a flow rate of 6–8 litre/minute using piped air or oxygen (in hospital) or an electrical compressor (domiciliary use). Where there is a risk of hypercapnic failure nebulisers should be driven with air and if necessary low-dose oxygen given at the same time through nasal cannulae.

In adults with acute asthma when high doses of inhaled beta 2 agonists are required there is no difference in delivery between nebulisers or a holding chamber (volume spacer) with a metered dose inhaler (Cates et al. 2006).

Ongoing evaluation of prescribed medication is important and where agreed parameters including respiratory rate/depth, SpO_2, PaO_2 and $PaCO_2$ are not achieved the doctor should be informed so that the treatment plan can be reviewed.

Chest drains

A tension pneumothorax is a medical emergency and once diagnosed a needle is inserted without delay on the affected side (midclavicular line/second intercostal space) to allow the air to escape (with an audible 'hiss'). Where a chest drain is inserted into the pleural cavity to remove air, pus or blood, this is connected to an underwater seal drainage system. There are a number of devices available for this but all provide a one-way valve allowing the movement of air and fluid in one direction only. Conventionally, a drainage bottle is filled with sterile water and the tube must be below the water level (2cm) otherwise air will enter the pleural cavity during inspiration (see Figure 5.8). In a pneumothorax, air bubbles will be seen as air is displaced from the pleural cavity during expiration and coughing. The doctor may request low-level suction (e.g. 5kPa) to facilitate removal of air and/or fluid. The drainage bottle must be kept below the level of the chest and clamping of drains avoided as this can result in a tension pneumothorax. Clamps should be available, however, in case the system becomes disconnected. Pain is experienced on insertion, during drainage and on removal of a chest drain and adequate pain relief must be offered.

Following insertion it is important to observe the following:

- respiratory status;
- fluid level and amount of any drainage fluid level swing;
- underwater bubbling (air is removal) dressing and site of insertion;
- patency of drainage tubing.

For further information on intrapleural drainage, see Dougherty and Lister (2011).

Chest physiotherapy

The nurse and physiotherapist will work collaboratively to reduce breathlessness, the work of breathing, improve ventilation and the expectoration of secretions. A number of techniques may be employed but the efficacy of physiotherapy may vary depending on the clinical context. Ongoing evaluation is crucial as some interventions can lead to worsening hypoxaemia. Patients will need encouragement to expectorate and effective pain relief may be necessary before this can be achieved. Active cycle of breathing techniques are often utilised by the physiotherapist and the nurse should be able to encourage the patients with some of the exercises:

- Thoracic expansion
- Breathing control
- forced expiratory technique ('huffing').

Where there is difficulty in the expectoration of sputum nebulised isotonic saline is often effective.

Non-invasive ventilation

Where hypoxemia and/or hypercapnia are not controlled by other means non-invasive ventilation (NIV) such as continuous positive airway pressure (CPAP) or BiPAP may be beneficial. In health, expiration involves muscle relaxation and elastic recoil with zero airway pressure. By applying positive pressure during expiration (called positive end-expired pressure or PEEP) oxygenation can be improved significantly. These techniques utilise a nasal or oral/nasal mask (see Figure 5.9) rather than

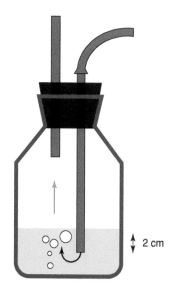

Figure 5.8 Underwater seal drainage

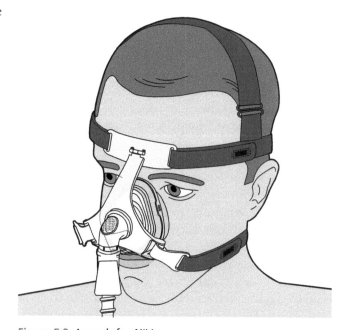

Figure 5.9 A mask for NIV

tracheal tubes and tracheostomy, thus minimising the risk of complications.

> **Situations where NIV may be beneficial:**
> - Pulmonary oedema with hypoxaemia
> - COPD (with respiratory acidosis)
> - Hypercapnic failure
> - Obstructive sleep apnoea
> - Pneumonia
> - Postoperative hypoxaemia.

CPAP

Although CPAP does not offer any ventilatory support, by applying positive pressure throughout both inspiration and expiration there is an increase in alveolar recruitment and functional residual capacity. As a result, there is an increase in surface area for gaseous exchange and a reduction in the work of breathing.

> **Advantages of NIV:**
> - increase in tidal volume;
> - recruitment of alveoli;
> - increase in FRC;
> - increased surface area for gaseous exchange;
> - improved oxygenation;
> - increase in lung compliance;
> - reduced work of breathing;
> - reduced risk of infection;
> - sedation avoided.

CPAP systems all have a flow generator which delivers a constant pressure throughout the respiratory cycle. The generator is usually adjusted to reach an end expiratory pressure of around 10cm H_2O as this facilitates the recruitment of alveoli.

BiPAP

BiPAP enables different pressures to be delivered during inspiration and expiration and provides ventilatory support. A BiPAP machine will not only sense the patient's inspiratory effort and provide an inspiratory volume but will apply PEEP. As a result, partial pressures of arterial oxygen and carbon dioxide can be improved with the work of breathing reduced (Stoltzfus 2006). Inspiratory positive airway pressure (IPAP) is adjusted up to 14cm H_2O to facilitate effective tidal volumes and expiratory positive airway pressure (EPAP) applied up to 6cm H_2O. Given the amount of dead space in the tubing an EPAP of less than 4cm H_2O may result in rebreathing with an increase in arterial carbon dioxide.

Patients selected for NIV must be conscious and able to cooperate, have a cough and be free from excessive secretions and severe haemodynamic instability. Application of positive pressure during breathing can be a little claustrophobic for some and the patient will need support and encouragement if treatment is to be effective. Increased positive pressure can also affect the haemodynamic status and while this may offer benefit in some it can cause deterioration in others. In one meta-analysis the risk of cardiac complications (e.g. myocardial infarction) was greater in patients receiving BiPAP for pulmonary oedema (Peter *et al.* 2006).

Ongoing monitoring of the patient during non-invasive ventilation is very important and the following parameters must be observed:

- Heart rate and respiratory rate
- Blood pressure
- Oxygen saturation
- Cardiac monitoring where necessary
- Degree of respiratory distress
- Accessory muscle use
- Presence of cyanosis
- Orientation
- Risk of aspiration.

If effective then NIV should result in an improvement in oxygenation and a reduction in respiratory acidosis without an increase in carbon dioxide. In patients with severe COPD saturations of 88–92% will be acceptable. Guidelines on the use of non-invasive ventilation in patients with COPD have been published by the Royal College of Physicians, British Thoracic Society and the Intensive Care Society (2008).

Nutrition and fluid balance

Insensible water loss will be greater with an increased respiratory rate, pyrexia and an increase in ambient temperature. This can result in decreased mucociliary clearance and secretion retention which can also be caused by the administration of oxygen. Where low-flow oxygen is given humidification is not required, neither is it necessary for short-term use of high-flow oxygen (less than 24 hours). However, it is important that fluid intake and hydration status is monitored carefully including skin turgor, urine output and the condition of oral mucous membranes and tongue. Unless contraindicated fluid intake should be increased with regular sips encouraged and swallowed during expiration. Poor nutritional status and electrolyte imbalance can also affect respiratory status and measures should be taken to correct any imbalance.

Psychological care

Breathlessness is extremely frightening and can generate increased anxiety and stress which, in turn, will increase the demand for oxygen. Care providers must convey a sense of calmness and efficiency around the bed area as this will increase patient confidence. Therapeutic touch as well as procedural touch is important when offering reassurance and reduces fear, as does ongoing effective communication and education. Indeed all nurses must build partnerships and therapeutic relationships through safe, effective and non-discriminatory communication, taking into account individual differences, capabilities and needs (NMC 2010). Information-giving to patients, and wherever possible including them in the decision-making process, will enable them to remain in control.

Conclusion

The respiratory system is very efficient in ensuring that oxygen delivery is facilitated effectively to meet the cells' demand for oxygen. However, in the acutely ill patient, respiratory compromise may occur very quickly resulting in profound hypoxaemia and possible life-threatening cellular hypoxia. Although primary respiratory disease can be responsible for respiratory compromise, pathology outside the respiratory system can also contribute to problems with oxygen delivery. Physiological responses activated as a result of disease or surgical intervention trigger complex neurohormonal adaptive pathways including the stress response. This will result in increased

global oxygen consumption and the respiratory system may have limited reserves to mobilise an effective response.

The skilled nurse has a sound theoretical knowledge of respiratory physiology and the many factors possibly contributing to respiratory problems. A comprehensive, holistic assessment will facilitate early detection and through ongoing vigilance in monitoring the patient, potential problems can be anticipated and appropriate measures taken to prevent further deterioration. Before changes are seen in oxygen saturation values there are often earlier signs of respiratory compromise and ongoing inspection of the patient and recording of observations is paramount.

Individual risk in relation to the development of respiratory problems can be affected by a host of different factors. Patients admitted into hospital bring with them risk as a result of for example their general physical health, smoking history, primary diagnosis, age, gender, ethnicity as well as socio-economic and mental health status. Following admission additional contextual and environmental factors can increase risk further. Immobility, poor positioning, suboptimal hydration and nutritional status, increased ambient temperatures, use of sedation, prolonged oxygen administration, invasive procedures, infection control practices and poor communication with increased stress can all increase risk significantly. The nurse has a key role to play in not only assessing individual risk and identifying those who are particularly vulnerable, but also through skilled nursing intervention and management of the care environment in the prevention of respiratory complications.

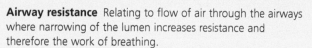

Glossary

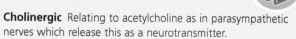

Airway resistance Relating to flow of air through the airways where narrowing of the lumen increases resistance and therefore the work of breathing.

Anatomical dead space The anatomical sections of the respiratory tract down to and including terminal bronchioles where air is not available for gaseous exchange (conducting zone).

Atelectasis Collapse of alveoli which results in loss of surface area for gaseous exchange.

Atmospheric pressure Also called barometric pressure, which is 101kPa at sea level and falls with increasing altitude.

Carbonic acid Formed by carbon dioxide in solution and also referred to as a volatile acid which can be removed from the body by increasing ventilation.

Cholinergic Relating to acetylcholine as in parasympathetic nerves which release this as a neurotransmitter.

Compliance work Relating to the work involved in distending the lungs and chest wall during inspiration.

Fibreoptic bronchoscopy A bronchoscope is passed through the nose or mouth into the air passages. The scope has many small glass fibres which transmit light and enable visual inspection.

Heliox Helium and oxygen mix (e.g. 70/30). Helium has a density less than nitrogen so at any given gas flow there is less turbulence and is beneficial where there is increased airway resistance.

Hypercapnia A rise in carbon dioxide in arterial blood as a result of reduced ventilation.

Hypoxaemia A reduced oxygen partial pressure in arterial blood.

Hypoxia A reduced partial pressure of oxygen in the cells.

Immunoglobulin There are five subclasses of immunoglobulins or antibodies – IgA, IgG, IgD, IgM and IgE – which are released by B lymphocytes.

Macrophages Mature monocytes (type of leucocyte or white blood cell) which mature and leave the circulation.

Medulla oblongata Lower portion of the brainstem which contains the vital centres.

Neurohormonal Relating to nerves and hormones released from endocrine glands. Important communication system in the body.

Ondine A water nymph who, according to German folklore, curses her unfaithful husband so that breathing stops if he should ever fall asleep again.

Oxygen consumption (VO$_2$) The oxygen utilised by the cells which will vary according to metabolic demand. This is 250 mL/minute at rest.

Oxygen delivery (DO$_2$) The oxygen delivered to the cells which is dependent on oxygen saturation, haemoglobin and cardiac output. This is 1000mL/min at rest.

Parasympathetic Division of the autonomic nervous system which results for example in narrowing of bronchioles and slowing of the heart rate.

Pathogenic Resulting in disease, e.g. pathogenic microorganisms.

Peak expiratory flow The greatest flow rate on forced expiration starting with a maximum inspiration and measured in litres per minute.

Pulmonary capillaries Tiny blood vessels where the walls are only one cell thick, therefore facilitating gaseous exchange in the lungs.

Pulse oximeter Probe attached to the finger or ear lobe which monitors the percentage of haemoglobin (Hb) saturated with oxygen.

Respiratory centre Located in the medulla oblongata of the brainstem close to the fourth ventricle of the brain which contains cerebrospinal fluid.

Surfactant Substance secreted by alveolar cells which helps to stabilise the alveoli, preventing collapse.

Sympathetic Division of the autonomic nervous system which results, for example, in dilatation of bronchioles and increase in heart rate.

Tracheal intubation Insertion of an endotracheal tube between the vocal cords into the trachea for the administration of oxygen and assisted ventilation.

Tracheostomy An opening made into the front of the trachea so that a tube (temporary or permanent) can be inserted.

Test yourself

1 Oxygen is required by the cells for which of the following:

   a. anaerobic metabolism
   b. aerobic metabolism

2 The anatomical relationship between the visceral and parietal pleural membranes creates a pleural pressure which is:

   a. negative (subatmospheric)
   b. positive (atmospheric)

3 The inspiratory muscles include:

   a. abdominals
   b. internal intercostals
   c. diaphragm
   d. external intercostals

4 The respiratory centre is found in the _____ _____ of the brain and is stimulated by rising levels of _____ _____.

5 Cholinergic nerves in the lungs stimulate cholinergic receptors resulting in:

   a. reduced airway lumen size
   b. increased airway lumen size

6 Oxygen delivery to the cells is dependent on:

   a. oxygen saturation
   b. carbon dioxide
   c. water vapour
   d. haemoglobin

7 The following respiratory disorders result in increased airway resistance:

   a. pneumonia
   b. COPD
   c. pleurisy
   d. asthma

8 Atopy results in a hypersensitivity reaction involving which of the following immunoglobulins?

   a. IgD
   b. IgM
   c. IgE
   d. IgA

9 A young patient aged 30 presents acutely ill with an oxygen saturation of 84%. Which one of the following oxygen devices would be appropriate:

   a. simple mask at 5L/min

   b. nasal cannulae at 6L/min

   c. non re-breather reservoir mask at 12L/min

   d. venturi mask at 4L/min

10 Effective positioning of the patient will help to facilitate improved gaseous exchange by increasing the following:

   a. tidal volume

   b. inspiratory reserve volume

   c. functional residual capacity

   d. residual volume

References

British Thoracic Society (2010) *BTS Pleural Disease Guideline 2010. A quick reference guideline.* Available from http://www.brit-thoracic.org.uk/Portals/0/Clinical%20Information/Pleural%20Disease/Pleural%20Guideline%202010/PleuralDiseaseQFG_web.pdf, accessed 19 March 2011.

Cates, C. J., Crilly, J. A. and Rowe, B. H. (2006) *Holding Chambers (Spacers) versus Nebulisers for Beta-agonist Treatment of Acute Asthma.* Cochrane Patabase Systematic Review CD000052. Available from http://ww2. cochrane.org/reviews/en/ab000052.html, accessed 16 October 2011.

Dougherty, L. and Lister, S. (2011) *The Royal Marsden Hospital Manual of Clinical Nursing Procedures.* Oxford: Wiley-Blackwell.

Hardie, J. A., Morkve, O. and Ellingsen, I. (2002) Effect of body position on arterial oxygen tension in the elderly. *Chest* 69, 123–8.

National Institute for Health and Clinical Excellence (NICE) (2007) *Acutely ill Patients in Hospital* (GCSO). London: NICE.

National Institute for Health and Clinical Excellence (NICE) (2010) *Chronic Obstructive Pulmonary Disease. Management of chronic obstructive pulmonary disease in adults in primary and secondary care (partial update).* Available from http://www.nice.org.uk/nicemedia/live/13029/49397/49397.pdf, accessed 17 October 2010.

National Institute for Health and Clinical Excellence (NICE) (2011) *Anaphylaxis: Assessment to Confirm an Anaphylactic Episode and the Decision to Refer After Emergency Treatment for a Suspected Anaphylactic Episode.* Available from www.nice.org.uk/cg134.

Nursing and Midwifery Council (NMC) (2010) *Standards for Pre-registration Nursing Education.* London: NMC. Available from http://standards.nmc-uk.org/PublishedDocuments/Standards%20for%ple_registration%20nursing%20education%2016082010.pdf.

O'Driscoll, B. R., Howard, L. S. and Davison, A. G. (2008) *BTS Guideline for Emergency Oxygen Use in Adult Patients.* London: British Thoracic Society. Available at from http://www.brit-thoracic.org.uk/Portals/0/Clinical%20Information/Emergency%20Oxygen/Emergency%20oxygen%20guideline/THX-63-Suppl_6.pdf, accessed 16 October 2010.

Peter, J. V., Moran, J. L., Phillips-Hughes, J., Graham, P. and Bersten, A. D. (2006) Effect of non-invasive positive pressure ventilation (NIPPV) on mortality in patients with acute cardiogenic pulmonary oedema. *Lancet* 367, 1155–63.

Resuscitation Council UK (2008) *Emergency Treatment of Anaphylactic Reactions. Guidelines for healthcare providers* Available from http://www.resus.org.uk/pages/reaction.pdf, accessed 19 March 2011.

Royal College of Physicians, British Thoracic Society, Intensive Care Society (2008) *The Use of Non-invasive Ventilation in the Management of Patients with Chronic Obstructive Pulmonary Disease Admitted to Hospital with Acute Type II Respiratory Failure (with particular reference to Bilevel positive pressure ventilation).* Available from http://www.brit-thoracic.org.uk/Portals/0/Clinical%20Information/NIV/Guidelines/NIVinCOPDFullguidelineFINAL.pdf, accessed 19 March 2011.

Scottish Intercollegiate Guidelines Network/British Thoracic Society (2011) *British Guideline on the Management of Asthma. Updated 2009.* Available from http://www.brit-thoracic.org.uk/Portals/0/Clinical%20Information/Asthma/Guidelines/sign101%20revised%20June%2009.pdf, aaccessed 21 January 2012.

Stoltzfus, S. (2006) The role of noninvasive ventilation. *Dimensions of Critical Care Nursing* 25 (2), 66–70.

Further reading

Bickley, S. (2007) *Bates' Guide to Physical Examination and History Taking.* London: Lippincott Williams & Watkins.

Davies, A. S. (2010) *The Respiratory System.* Edinburgh: Churchill Livingstone.

Spathis, A., Davies, H. E. and Booth, S. (2011) *Respiratory Disease: From advanced disease to bereavement.* Oxford: Oxford University Press.

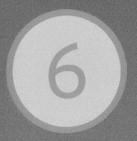

The patient with acute cardiovascular problems

Helen Dutton, Sharon Elliott and Andrew Sargent

Aims

This chapter aims to give a clear understanding of the normal anatomy and applied physiology of the cardiac and circulatory systems and to explain how altered physiology can lead to acute deterioration. An improved understanding of these principles will enhance nursing assessment and recognition of acute problems, and enable an appropriate response to medical emergencies caused by cardiac and circulatory disorders.

Objectives

At the end of this chapter you will be able to:

→ Describe the major structures and components of the cardiovascular system, the heart, coronary artery circulation and conduction system, and understand the physiological processes that generate and maintain cardiac output

→ Describe the structure and function of blood, mechanisms of clotting and the ABO and rhesus systems

→ Describe the arterial and venous system and the peripheral circulation and understand common problems of the circulatory system

→ Describe the nurse's role in assessing the cardiovascular system

→ Identify common medical emergencies related to the cardiovascular system, and understand how these are identified and managed

→ Consider the role of heamodynamic monitoring in assessing and managing therapies that optimise cardiac output and the functioning of the cardiovascular system

Introduction

The cardiovascular system is responsible for the circulation of blood to and from the organs and tissues of the body. Blood must be transported under a sufficient pressure to facilitate adequate movement of oxygen, nutrients, hormones, electrolytes, water and other blood products to their target locations. In addition to being a transportation system to the tissues of the body, the cardiovascular system facilitates the removal of waste products from cellular activity.

Applied physiology

The cardiovascular system is a continuous circuit that is comprised of three principle components:

- The heart
- The blood
- The arterial and venous system.

The heart

The heart is responsible for providing the continuous motion of blood as it travels around the arterial and venous system. The pumping action of the heart is generated by the contraction of the muscle fibres that surround the heart's four chambers. The force of this contraction will remain relatively constant during periods of rest and activity; each time the heart contracts, a volume of blood (**stroke volume**) will leave the heart and either be distributed around the arterial system, or to the lungs for oxygenation, depending on which side of the heart the blood leaves. The heart has a right and a left side. The right side of the heart collects blood that returns from the organs and tissues of the body via the venous system. This blood is deoxygenated and has a relatively high concentration of carbon dioxide. Therefore, the principal function of the right side of the heart is to move this venous blood back to the lungs where it can remove its carbon dioxide and take on more oxygen from inspired air. After this process, the blood then moves back into the left side of the heart so that it can be distributed around the body via the arterial system. Figure 6.1 provides an overview of the cardiovascular system.

Each side of the heart is comprised of two chambers, an atrium and a ventricle. The atria are the smaller chambers

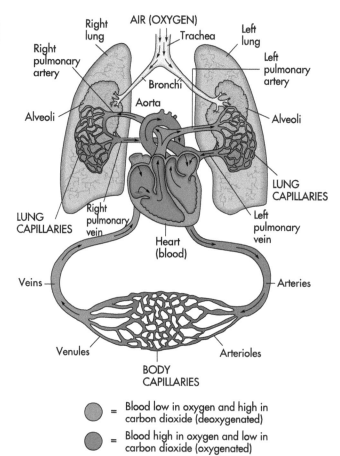

Figure 6.1 Overview of the cardiovascular system

and act as a conduit for blood to be collected and transferred into the ventricles. The ventricles are the larger chambers and move the blood out of the heart. The right ventricle is smaller than the left as it is only required to eject the blood into the pulmonary circulation, whereas the left ventricle is required to send the blood out to the peripheries of the body under sufficient pressure to facilitate the tissue perfusion. Hence, the left ventricle has a considerable muscle mass in comparison to the right.

The ventricles are each enclosed by two heart valves. These valves are responsible for ensuring that blood is not displaced backwards during ventricular contraction (**systole**) (see Figure 6.2).

These valves are:

- *Triscuspid* – which separates the right atrium and the right ventricle;
- *Mitral* – which separates the left atrium and the left ventricle;
- *Pulmonic* – controls outflow of blood from the right ventricle to the pulmonary artery;
- *Aortic* – controls the outflow of blood from the left ventricle to the aorta.

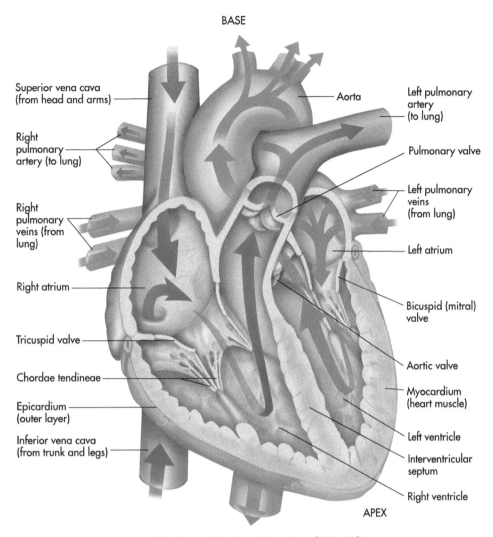

BASE

Superior vena cava
(from head and arms)

Aorta

Left pulmonary
artery
(to lung)

Right
pulmonary
artery (to lung)

Pulmonary valve

Left pulmonary
veins
(from lung)

Right
pulmonary
veins (from
lung)

Left atrium

Right atrium

Bicuspid (mitral)
valve

Tricuspid valve

Aortic valve

Chordae tendineae

Myocardium
(heart muscle)

Epicardium
(outer layer)

Left ventricle

Inferior vena cava
(from trunk and legs)

Interventricular
septum

Right ventricle

APEX

Figure 6.2 The anatomy of the heart showing direction of blood flow

Layers of the heart

The heart is primarily a muscular pump and possesses many muscle fibres. However, there are other structures that allow it to keep its shape and location in the thorax. The heart has three primary layers:

- The endocardium
- The myocardium
- The pericardium.

Endocardium

The innermost layer of the heart is a thin layer of endothelium and connective tissue that is continuous with the blood vessels that supply, and are supplied by, the heart. The endothelial layer is responsible for expressing antithrombotic factors to prevent blood from adhering to the endocardium.

Myocardium

The middle layer of the heart is the myocardium. This is the thickest layer of the heart and is responsible for providing muscular contraction so that blood can be ejected from the chambers that it surrounds. There is a layer of myocardium around the atria and the ventricles. The muscle fibres of the myocardium are laid end-to-end so that they can contract in a wave-like motion when stimulated. The myocardium requires a constant supply of oxygenated blood which is provided by the coronary arteries.

Pericardium

The outermost layer of the heart is the pericardial sac. This is a rigid structure that prevents the heart from overstretching during systole and helps the heart to maintain its shape. The pericardium is also attached to the chest wall to prevent excessive movement of the heart during activity.

Between the pericardium and the myocardium is the epicardial layer which covers the surface of the myocardium. These layers are not attached to one another and there is a small amount of pericardial fluid between them.

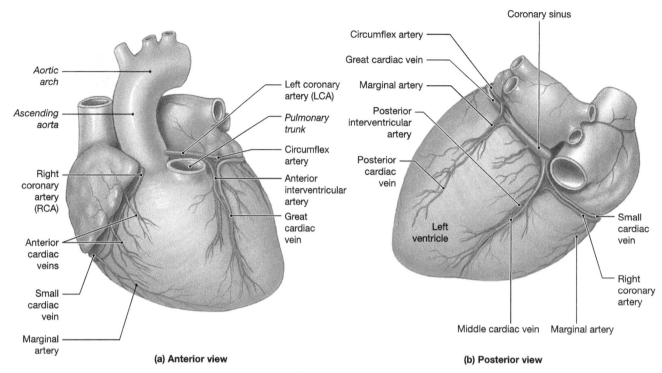

Figure 6.3 Coronary artery circulation (a) anterior and (b) posterior views
Source: Martini, F. H. and Bartholomew, E. F. (2009) *Essentials of Anatomy & Physiology*, 5th edn, San Francisco: Pearson Benjamin Cummings, Fig. 12.7, p. 414.

This fluid prevents friction damage from the rigid peri-cardium when the myocardium contracts and relaxes.

The coronary circulation

The myocardium and the conduction system require a continuous supply of blood for normal function. The heart supplies itself with blood directly from the aorta as it leaves the left ventricle. Two small openings (ostia) are located just above the aortic valve leaflets, and blood flows into the coronary circulation during diastole, the relaxed phase of the cardiac cycle. The two main coronary arteries are the right coronary artery (RCA) and the left coronary artery (LCA) (see Figure 6.3).

The right coronary artery tree

The RCA extends round inferiorly and posteriorly across the right ventricle and around to the posterior surface of the heart. Branches called the marginal arteries supply the anterior and lateral surface of the right ventricle. The posterior surface of the heart is supplied by the posterior descending artery (PDA).

Individual variance in coronary artery blood supply to the posterior surface of the heart:

● for approximately 70% of the population this is provided by the RCA;
● for 20% of the population, this is provided by the LCA;
● for the remaining 10% supply is provided by both.

The left coronary artery tree

The LCA divides into two main arteries: the left anterior descending artery (LAD) and the circumflex (CX). The LAD extends down across the surface of the heart supplying the left ventricle. The LAD has a number of branches that supply the interventricular septum (the septal arteries) and the anterior surface of the left ventricle (the diagonal arteries). The LAD terminates at the apex of the heart.

Remember:

● Inferior = underneath
● Posterior = back
● Anterior = front
● Lateral = side.

The circumflex extends around towards the lateral and posterior surfaces of the left ventricle, and in some cases may supply the posterior descending artery.

Cardiac conduction system

The cardiac conduction system is responsible for the maintenance of the correct sequence and timing of events that lead to the movement of blood through the heart. For the cardiac cycle to result in adequate cardiac output, the heart's muscular walls need to be activated in the appropriate direction to make sure that the displacement of blood from the atria and ventricles are efficient.

The cardiac conduction system is comprised of conduction cells. These cells are able to generate their own impulse, known as autorhythmicity. They are responsible for the production and transmission of electrical waves that cross the heart and stimulate the myocardium to contract. The conduction cells do not contract themselves but purely provide the stimulus for adjacent myocardial cells to do so. The conduction system is illustrated in Figure 6.4.

Each cell of the conduction system has the ability spontaneously to generate electrical potentials that move in a wave-like motion across the heart. However, the sino-atrial (SA) node is the primary source of all normal electrical activity in the heart.

Sino-atrial node

The SA node is the pacemaker of the heart and can spontaneously become activated (depolarise) at a fixed rate. This inbuilt heart rate is around 100 beats per minute and is referred to as the rate of automaticity. Each cell of the cardiac conduction system has its own rate of automaticity, but the further down in the conduction system the cell is, the slower its rate of automaticity. In order for the heart

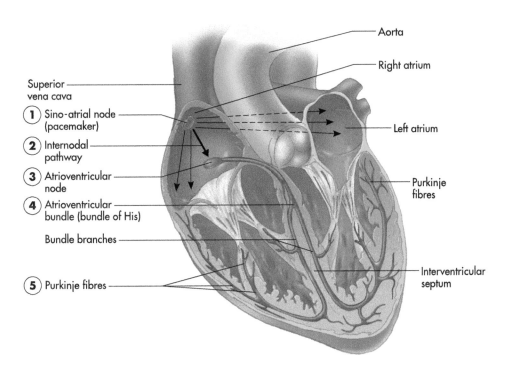

1. The sino-atrial (SA) node fires a stimulus across the walls of both left and right atria, causing them to contract.

2. The stimulus arrives at the atrioventricular (AV) node.

3. The stimulus is directed to follow the AV bundle (bundle of His).

4. The stimulus now travels through the apex of the heart through the bundle branches.

5. The Purkinje fibres distribute the stimulus across both ventricles, causing ventricular contraction.

Figure 6.4 The conduction system of the heart

rate to be increased in times of need and for it to slow down at times of rest, the SA node is controlled externally by the sympathetic and parasympathetic branches of the autonomic nervous system. The sympathetic nervous system has an excitory effect on the heart, making it beat faster during exercise, stress, pain or increased metabolic need.

The SA node's rate of automaticity is slightly too fast for normal resting activity, or when sleeping. Therefore, the SA node is constantly being slowed down according to the metabolic requirements, by the parasympathetic nervous system. So, despite the intrinsic rate of automaticity of the SA node being 100 beats per minute, the heart rate that we accept as being normal (60–100) is actually maintained mostly by the autonomic nervous system.

Once the SA node depolarises, the wave of depolarisation spreads across the atria via internodal pathways. These ensure that the atria both depolarise at the same time and that the contraction of the atria occurs in a downward direction (allowing the blood to be pushed down into the ventricles).

Atrioventricular node

The atrioventricular (AV) node is the only conduit for electrical stimulation to move from the atria through to the ventricles. In this respect the AV node has an important regulatory function when the SA node depolarises too quickly or when there is an atrial arrhythmia.

When the wave of depolarisation completes its journey across the atria it reaches the AV node. Here there is a small delay before the ventricles become depolarised. This delay lasts only around 0.1 seconds but is sufficient time for the blood to be ejected from the atria and into the ventricles. The AV node is also under the control of the parasympathetic nervous system to slow down the heart rate by increasing the period of delay.

Ventricular conduction system

The conduction of the ventricles is coordinated by the bundle branches. There are three main conduction fibres that distribute the wave of depolarisation across the ventricular myocardium: the right bundle branch; the left anterior fascicle and the left posterior fascicle. When these fibres are depolarised normally, the two ventricular masses contract simultaneously. However, if there is a block or delay in any of these pathways there will be a degree of disynchrony in the timing between the ventricles, causing an ineffective ejection. The Purkinje fibres are the most distal part of the conduction system. When the wave of depolarisation reaches these fibres they activate the myocardial cells to contract.

The ECG complex

As the cardiac conduction system becomes activated, the respective parts of the atria and ventricles contract accordingly. As the wave of depolarisation spreads through the muscle fibres of each chamber an exchange of positively charged ions move in and out of the muscle cells (myocytes). This creates a voltage change that can be recorded on a cardiac monitor as an ECG complex.

> **Cardiac monitoring**
> The cardiac monitor is used for continuous monitoring of heart rate and rhythm of patients that require close observation.
>
> **The 12-lead ECG**
> The 12-lead ECG is performed intermittently and provides a view of the heart from 12 different perspectives (see more in the Assessment section).

An ECG complex (see Figure 6.5) is comprised of three main components:

- P wave
- QRS complex
- T wave.

P wave. This is a small rounded wave that occurs during atrial depolarisation. A P wave should always be present as this indicates that the SA node is depolarising and that the subsequent wave of depolarisation is simultaneously spreading across the atrial myocardium. The PR interval is the time between the beginning of the P wave, and the first deflection of the QRS complex and is 0.2 seconds (5 small squares on ECG paper).

QRS complex. The largest part of the ECG complex is the QRS. This represents the movement of depolarisation as it spreads across the ventricular myocardium. Providing that the bundle branches are both conducting normally, the QRS should be narrow and should not have any notches in it. The QRS may be upright (positive) or downward

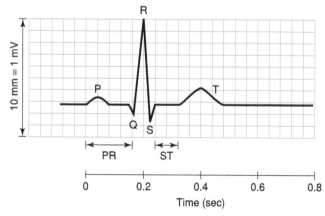

Figure 6.5 The normal PQRST complex

(negative) depending on the surface of the heart that is facing the ECG lead. The QRS complex is rapid at less than 0.12 seconds (3 small squares on ECG paper).

T wave. Once the cells of the ventricular myocardium have been depolarised they begin the process of returning to their normal resting state. This repolarisation phase lasts longer than depolarisation, hence the T wave is wider than the corresponding QRS complex that precedes it. The ST segment sits on the isoelectric line.

The cardiac cycle

The cardiac conduction system is responsible for initiating the chain of events that enables the heart to cycle between systole and diastole, maintaining a forward flow of blood through the pulmonary and systemic circulation. The ionic changes that occur during depolarisation and repolarisation increase calcium availability in the cardiac myocyte, enabling the sarcomere (the basic unit of cardiac muscle) to shorten and contract. Thus the electrical events are essential for the mechanical events of myocardial contraction to ensue.

The cardiac cycle is the period of time between one contraction and another. The cycle lasts for about 0.8 seconds, with the systolic (contraction phase) being slightly shorter at 0.3 seconds, than the diastolic (relaxation phase) at 0.5 seconds. This slightly longer diastolic phase enables flow of blood down the coronary arteries to the relaxed myocardium.

The following describes stages of the cardiac cycle and is illustrated by Figure 6.6. In *ventricular diastole* the atria and ventricles are relaxed, the atrioventricular (AV) valves are open and blood is flowing from the atria to the ventricles. Towards the end of ventricular diastole the SA node and then atria depolarise, (viewed as the P wave on the ECG) causing the atria to contract, starting *atrial systole*. The ventricles have received about 80% of their blood already, but the contracting atria push the final 20% through the AV valves: this is sometimes referred to as the 'atrial kick'. The pulmonary and aortic valves remain closed during this phase. The amount of blood in the ventricles at the end of diastole in known as the end diastolic volume (EDV).

Rhythm problems where 'atrial kick' is lost include:

● Atrial fibrillation
● Atrial flutter
● Third-degree heart block.

This may reduce the cardiac output, with ABCDE assessment revealing breathlessness, hypotension, tachycardia or bradycardia.

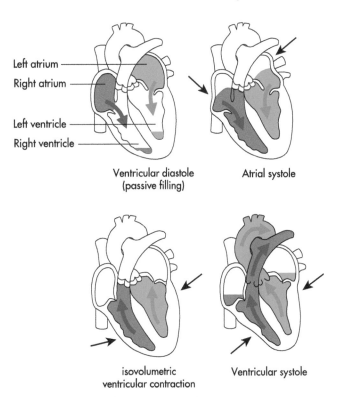

Figure 6.6 Stages of the cardiac cycle

The electrical impulse passes down the AV node, and then through the ventricular conduction system and Purkinje fibres (viewed as the QRS complex on the ECG). This signals the start of *isovolumetric ventricular contraction* as the ventricles begin to contract. The rising pressure in the ventricles forces the closure of the AV valves generating the first heart sound, 'lub'. In the isovolumetric phase, there is a change in ventricular pressure but no change in ventricular volume, because the pressure generated is not yet sufficient to open the pulmonary and aortic valves. At this point then, all four valves in the heart remain closed. This phase of the cardiac cycle consumes the most energy and therefore oxygen, and represents the greatest work of the myocardium. Eventually the pressure in the ventricles exceeds the pressure in the aorta and pulmonary vessels, the valves are forced open, and *ventricular systole* begins.

In ventricular systole, the contents of the ventricle are ejected into the pulmonary and systemic circulation. About 60–70% of the volume of blood in the ventricle at the end of diastole is ejected. End diastolic volume is typically about 120mL and the amount ejected (stroke volume) 70mL. This leaves 50mL of blood in the ventricle at the end of systole, which can be ejected if the force of contraction is increased, acting as a cardiac reserve to be used if a greater output is needed. Once the ventricles have finished their contraction, they begin to relax. Pressure in the ventricles falls rapidly, and when it falls below aortic and pulmonary pressure, the aortic and pulmonary valves close. This can be heard as the second heart sound, 'dub'. The closure of these valves, and then the opening of the AV valves, signals the beginning of ventricular diastole, and the cycle starts once again.

> **Some useful definitions**
> **Stroke volume** = amount ejected in each beat (70mL).
>
> **End diastolic volume** = the amount in the ventricle at the end of diastole (120mL).
>
> **Ejection fraction** = the percentage of blood ejected from the left ventricle
>
> (SV/EDV × 100) (60–70%).

Cardiac output

The amount of blood pumped by the ventricles in one minute is the cardiac output.

Cardiac output = heart rate (beats per minute) ×
stroke volume (mL per beat)

> An average person has a resting heart rate of 70 beats/minute and a resting stroke volume of 70mL/beat.
>
> The cardiac output for this person at rest is:
>
> Cardiac output = 70 (beats/min) × 70 (mL/beat) = 4900mL/minute.

Cardiac output decreases in sleep and rises during vigorous exercise, increasing in a trained athlete by up to seven times (up to 35L/minute). In illness, the demand may increase, as with sepsis; or the ability to maintain cardiac output may reduce, as with heart failure, and a mismatch of demand and supply may ensue. The cardiac reserve enables the output to increase by increasing the ejection fraction and therefore stroke volume and increasing heart rate. Stroke volume depends mainly on three factors:

1 Preload
2 Contractility
3 Afterload.

> An increase in heart rate will raise cardiac output but as the rate increases above about 130 there is a reduction in time available for the ventricle to fill (diastole), and cardiac output may fall.
>
> A shortened diastolic time also reduces the time for coronary artery filling, just when the myocardial oxygen demand is increasing.

These three factors are crucial for the maintenance of cardiac output and are influenced by the sympathetic nervous system.

Preload

Preload is related to the volume of the blood in the ventricle at the end of diastole, or end diastolic volume. The blood is returned to the heart by the venous circulation, and is reduced by problems such as hypovolaemia and vasodilation, and increased by hypervolaemia and vasoconstriction. Compliance refers to the ease with which the muscle can distend or stretch to accommodate the volume returned to the ventricle. A poorly compliant or stiff ventricle will not stretch easily, and therefore the ventricular end diastolic volume is reduced.

Preload is important because there is a relationship between the amount of blood in the ventricle at the end of diastole, and the amount of blood ejected during systole (stroke volume). This relationship is described by Starling's law of the heart, which states that as the amount of blood returning from the veins to the ventricle at the end of diastole increases, the stretch of the ventricular myocardium increases and therefore the strength of the next contraction is greater (Stanfield 2011). A useful analogy is an elastic band: the further it is stretched, the harder it springs back. Therefore the greater the end diastolic volume the greater the stroke volume.

The ventricular preload can be estimated in clinical practice by inserting a cannula into the internal jugular or subclavian vein and measuring the central venous pressure (CVP). A low CVP reading would be consistent with a low ventricular preload, or low blood volume returning to the heart and a fluid challenge may be needed to increase the ventricular preload. In Figure 6.7, it can be seen that as the ventricular preload (end diastolic volume) increases, so does the stroke volume. If the stroke volume increases, cardiac output and blood pressure will normally increase as well (assuming heart rate remains constant).

> **Fluid challenge**
> This involves giving an intravenous bolus of fluid, usually about 500mL, rapidly as prescribed.
>
> • Clinical response should be carefully evaluated.
> • Increasing ventricular preload (end diastolic volume) should lead to improved stroke volume, cardiac output.
> • This should lead to an improved blood pressure, and reduced heart rate.

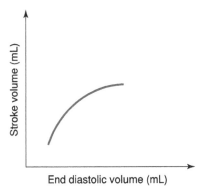

Figure 6.7 A Starling curve showing how the amount of blood ejected from the heart (stroke volume) increases as the amount of blood in the ventricle at the end of diastole (preload) increases

Contractility

Contractility refers to the ability of the myocardium to contract. Healthy myocardium will contract effectively according to how much stretch the volume in the ventricle is causing. As with the elastic band, if the myocardium becomes overstretched it may not spring back so effectively and so a damaged or failing heart, one with decreased contractility, may not have the capacity to contract so strongly. This is discussed in more detail later when considering heart failure. Factors that effect contractility are summarised in Table 6.1.

Table 6.1 Factors that affect myocardial contractility

Increased contractility	• Sympathetic stimulation
	• Positive **inotropic** drugs
Decreased contractility	• Parasympathetic stimulation
	• Ischaemia
	• **Hypoxaemia**
	• Acidosis
	• **Electrolyte** imbalance

Afterload

Afterload is the force opposing ventricular ejection; in the left ventricle this is the opposition given by the aortic diastolic pressure. Changes in systemic vascular resistance (SVR) caused by peripheral vasoconstriction or dilation will affect afterload. Systemic vascular resistance will increase with peripheral vasoconstriction and the patient who feels cool to touch will have an increased left ventricular afterload. The myocardium has to work harder to push the blood out of the ventricle, and will therefore require more oxygen as it uses more energy. In health, this is not a problem but in the failing heart pharmacological

therapy is aimed at reducing the left ventricular afterload by enabling arteriolar vasodilation, in order to reduce the oxygen requirements of the myocardium.

Blood pressure

Blood pressure measurement is a familiar activity for the nurse, but it is worth pausing to consider exactly what it is that is being measured.

Blood pressure = cardiac output × systemic vascular resistance

Blood pressure is the pressure the blood exerts on the inner walls of the arteries and is determined by cardiac output (CO) and systemic vascular resistance (SVR). It gives the nurse a good insight into the functioning of the left ventricle's ability to pump blood into the aorta. Blood pressure is a product of cardiac output and systemic vascular resistance. Blood pressure is expressed as a systolic over a diastolic pressure. Normal blood pressure varies but an ideal value is between 120/85mmHg, to a high normal of 139/89 (NICE 2011). Systolic blood pressure is generated by the strength and the volume of blood pumped by the ventricular contraction. Diastolic blood pressure is related to the tone of the blood vessels. The relationship between the factors that contribute to cardiac output are shown Figure 6.8. It can be seen that if one of these factors changes (for example preload), then stroke volume, cardiac output and blood pressure will all be affected. The sympathetic nervous system can influence each of these factors, and contributes to maintaining CO and BP.

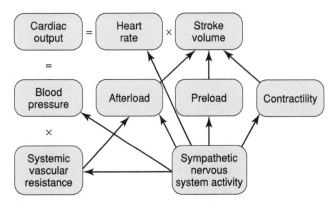

Figure 6.8 Factors contributing to cardiac output

Regulation of blood pressure

You may remember that cardiac output varies greatly to meet the physiological demand for oxygen at cellular level. Despite the wide fluctuation in cardiac output, the blood pressure remains relatively constant to ensure the required perfusion pressure is maintained throughout the system without causing organ damage.

Neural and hormonal mechanisms of blood pressure control

Neural mechanisms of blood pressure regulation lie predominately within the pons and medulla of the brain. The cardiovascular centre (CVC) controls both vessel tone, through the vasomotor centre, and heart rate, through the cardiac centre. Changes in the internal environment are detected by sensors which communicate with the cardiovascular centre via neural pathways. The cardiovascular centre responds by activation or inhibition of the sympathetic and parasympathetic branches of the autonomic nervous system, to maintain homeostasis. (The autonomic nervous system is explained in more detail in Chapter 9.) Sensor mechanisms include baroreceptors, which are sensitive to stretch and are situated in the walls of the aortic arch and bifurcation of the common carotid arteries, in an ideal position to detect pressure changes. Information from the baroreceptors is transmitted via the carotid sinus and vagus nerves to the CVC and a falling mean arterial pressure will reduce the information flow. A corresponding increase in sympathetic outflow from the CVC causes vasoconstriction via stimulation of alpha adrenergic receptors in the systemic vasculature and an increase in heart rate and contractility via beta adrenergic

---

Adrenergic receptors are receptors of the sympathetic nervous system that respond to the neurotransmitter noradrenaline:

- Beta 1 receptors are located in the heart and when activated cause an increase in contractility and heart rate.
- Beta 2 receptors are located in bronchial and vascular smooth muscle. Sympathetic nervous system (SNS) activity causes bronchodilation and dilation of vessels supplying skeletal muscles.
- Alpha receptors are located in peripheral vasculature, and cause vasoconstriction when activated by the SNS.

Pharmacology

Beta adrenergic receptor-blockers (beta-blockers) antagonise the receptors and blunt the sympathetic response:

- heart rate is decreased;
- contractility is decreased;
- renin production is decreased;
- blood pressure will be reduced.

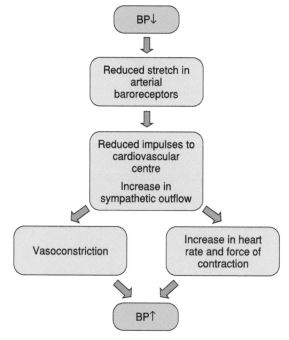

Figure 6.9 Baroreceptor reflex in response to reduced blood pressure

receptor stimulation in the heart. These responses will cause an increase in cardiac output and blood pressure (see Figure 6.9).

Conversely an increase in blood pressure would cause the opposite response; an increase in impulses down the carotid sinus and vagus nerves will inhibit the sympathetic outflow, allowing vessels to dilate, and an increase in parasympathetic activity lowers heart rate, thus reducing cardiac output and blood pressure. This regulatory system is rapid and maintains homeostasis during everyday activities, such as moving from a lying to a standing position. Figure 6.10 shows the pathways of transmission to the CVC and the effect of the sympathetic response on the heart (increase in contractility and rate) and blood vessels (vasoconstriction).

Information from chemoreceptors (see Chapter 5) also influences the activity of the cardiovascular centre and the sympathetic response is initiated in response to hypoxaemia. Emotional stress or fear perceived by higher centres in the brain will also be communicated to the CVC, activating the stress response of the SNS, raising heart rate and blood pressure, common physical manifestations of stress. When assessing cardiac status it is important to note clinical signs that indicate SNS activity, as these may be early signs of clinical changes that may lead to acute deterioration.

A number of humoral mechanisms contribute to blood pressure regulation; these are the renin angiotensin aldosterone system (RAAS) and antidiuretic hormone (ADH). Other hormones such as adrenaline are released from

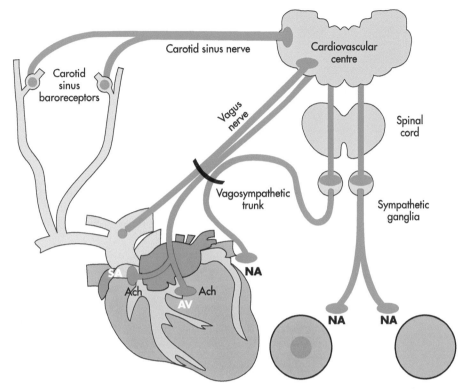

Figure 6.10 Autonomic control of blood pressure

NA = noradrenaline: neurotransmitter of the sympathetic nervous system
Ach = acetlycholine: neurotransmitter of the parasympathetic nervous system

adrenal glands and have the effect of directly stimulating an increase in heart rate, contractility and vascular tone of the gut and skin, but vasodilation of cardiac and skeletal arterioles.

The RAAS is central to blood pressure regulation and involves a chain of events that are activated if mean arterial blood pressure falls. (This is discussed in more detail in Chapter 8.) The enzyme renin is secreted from the juxta glomerular cells in the nephron in response to reduced blood flow. Renin converts angiotensinogen, a naturally occurring plasma protein, into angiotensin 1. Angiotensin-converting enzyme (ACE), present in the pulmonary endothelium, converts angiotensin 1 to angiotensin 2. Angiotensin 2 is a very powerful vasoconstrictor which increases systemic perfusion, but also activates aldosterone production from the adrenal cortex, to reabsorb sodium and therefore water in the distal convoluted tubule of the kidney, increasing blood volume.

Pharmacology

Angiotensin-converting enzyme inhibitors (ACEI) block the conversion of angiotensin 1 to angiotensin 2, this causes:

- vasodilation reducing blood pressure;
- reduction in aldosterone, increasing urine output.

ADH is released by the posterior pituitary in response to decreased blood pressure and increasing osmolality of the blood. ADH is a vaspressor (increases blood pressure by causing vasoconstriction), but also acts on the collecting ducts in the kidney to increase absorption of water back into the circulation.

Having considered the anatomy and physiology of the heart which provides the pumping force of the circulation, the blood which the heart propels and the vessels through which the blood travels will be discussed.

The blood

The importance of blood in the preservation of life has been a source of interest to scientists, philosophers, writers and artists over many centuries. Due to the relative ease in which blood can be obtained it has become one of the most studied components of the body (Pallister 1994).

Blood is an organ and is unique because it comprises the only fluid tissue of the body. It supports the functions of all other body tissues and is in turn dependent on other organs such as the lungs, heart, kidneys and liver. Blood is also one of the body's largest organs: an average 70kg man will have a total blood volume of approximately 5 litres weighing around 5.5Kg.

> Total blood volume is 5–6L depending on weight. The average adult cardiac output is around 5L therefore the severing of a major blood vessel can result in the loss of the entire circulating volume with 1–2 minutes.

Blood is a complex connective tissue and is essentially made up of formed elements (red blood cells, white blood cells and platelets) suspended in a liquid called plasma. When a sample of blood is placed in a centrifuge and spun at high speed the plasma and formed elements are separated out (see Figure 6.11).

Plasma

Plasma is 90% water and has many elements dissolved within. Approximately three litres of the total blood volume is plasma, which is pale yellow in colour, often described as straw coloured. It contains a small amount of dissolved oxygen, and organic compounds such as glucose, electrolytes and proteins. When blood samples are obtained for analysis, the values produced are those of the plasma.

Electrolytes (salts) are substances that when in solution conduct an electrical current. This is because when dissolved they separate into ions. Ions carry an electrical charge that may be either positive (cations) or negative (anions). Plasma contains extracellular electrolytes, the

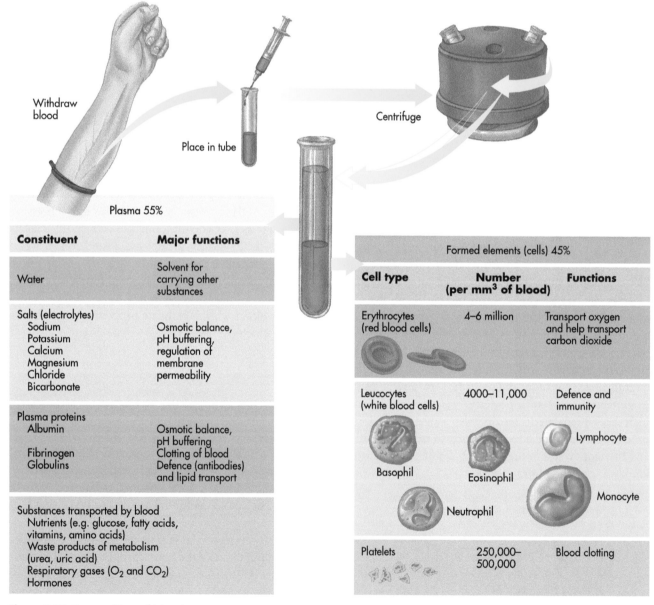

Constituent	Major functions
Water	Solvent for carrying other substances
Salts (electrolytes) Sodium Potassium Calcium Magnesium Chloride Bicarbonate	Osmotic balance, pH buffering, regulation of membrane permeability
Plasma proteins Albumin Fibrinogen Globulins	Osmotic balance, pH buffering Clotting of blood Defence (antibodies) and lipid transport
Substances transported by blood Nutrients (e.g. glucose, fatty acids, vitamins, amino acids) Waste products of metabolism (urea, uric acid) Respiratory gases (O_2 and CO_2) Hormones	

Formed elements (cells) 45%

Cell type	Number (per mm^3 of blood)	Functions
Erythrocytes (red blood cells)	4–6 million	Transport oxygen and help transport carbon dioxide
Leucocytes (white blood cells)	4000–11,000	Defence and immunity
Platelets	250,000–500,000	Blood clotting

Figure 6.11 Composition of blood

Table 6.2 Values of common cations and anions

	Chemical symbol	Normal value in plasma
Cations		
Sodium	Na+	135–145mmol/L
Potassium	K+	3.6–5.1mmol/L
Calcium	Ca++	2.1–2.6mmol/L
Magnesium	Mg++	0.75–1.0mmol/L
Hydrogen	H+	35–45nanomol/L
Anions		
Chloride	Cl-	95–107mmol/L
Phosporous	P-	2.5–4.5mmol/L
Bicarbonate	HCO3-	22–26mmol/L

Table 6.3 Protein composition of plasma

	Functions
Albumin	Colloid oncotic pressure, binds with drugs, hormones
Globulins	Forms antibodies (immunoglobulins) which attack foreign proteins and pathogens
Fibrinogen	Essential for the process of blood clotting

a summary of the protein composition of plasma see Table 6.3.

> Albumin is the most abundant of the plasma proteins. If albumin levels are low, there is a fall in colloid oncotic pressure resulting in fluid leaking out of the circulation into the tissues. This is one cause of oedema.

levels of which are carefully balanced relative to the levels in intracellular fluids. If this balance is upset it causes major disruption to virtually all body functions. The small electrical currents generated by ions are vital for muscle contraction and nerve function. For example low levels of potassium can result in cardiac arrhythmias and ectopic beats as the myocardium becomes more irritable. Plasma is always electrically neutral, in other words, the number of positive charges exactly balances the number of negative ones. Table 6.2 shows the common cations and anions in the body.

> Sodium chloride (NaCl) dissolves in water and separates into sodium (Na+), a cation, and chloride (Cl-), an anion. A solution containing charged particles is an electrolyte.
>
> Glucose is a non-electrolyte as the molecules do not dissociate in water.
>
> Glucose therefore has no effect on the electrical charge of a solution but provides an energy source.

Water, ions and electrolytes are constantly being exchanged between the plasma and the interstitial fluid (the fluid bathing the cells) and therefore the composition of the two is very similar. The main difference is the presence in the plasma of plasma proteins. They do not leave the circulation easily due to their large size and irregular shapes. Each 100ml of plasma contains 7.6g of protein. Plasma proteins are essential for maintaining colloid oncotic pressure which in turn is crucial for ensuring fluid stays within the circulation. Plasma proteins perform additional functions; some act as carrier molecules for drugs and other substances, and some have an important role in blood clotting and the immune response. For

Red blood cells (RBCs) – erythrocytes

These are the most numerous cells in the blood, the principle functions of which are carriage of respiratory gases as discussed in detail in Chapter 4. Haemoglobin molecules account for more than 95% of the composition of a RBC, and transports oxygen to the tissues and carbon dioxide back to the lungs. Haemoglobin is an iron-containing protein. If iron is deficient in the body then adequate amounts of haemaoglobin can not be made, resulting in anaemia and an inability of the blood to carry sufficient oxygen to the tissues (for causes and types of anaemia see Table 6.4). Erythrocytes do not have a nucleus and so are not able to divide to form new cells. They are formed through the process of haemopoeisis, principally in the red bone marrow – myeloid tissue. Erythrocytes are among the most abundant cells in the body accounting for about one-third of all body cells.

> Men have 4.5–6.3 million RBCs per mm³ of whole blood women 4.2–5.5 per mm³. This is the red cell count reported on a full blood count (FBC) report.
>
> Also reported in the FBC is the haemoglobin (Hb) level.

Whatever the cause of anaemia, there will be a reduced oxygen-carrying ability and the potential for reduced oxygen delivery to the tissues. For example sickle-cell disease results from an abnormality in the haemoglobin causing the red blood cell to become fragile with a tendency to change shape and become crescent or 'sickle' shaped. A sickle-cell crisis occurs when large numbers of RBCs

Table 6.4 Types of anaemia

Direct cause	As a result of	Type
Decrease in number of RBCs	• Sudden haemorrrhage	Haemorrhagic
	• Destruction (lysis) of RBCs	Haemolytic
	• Lack of vitamin B^{12}	Pernicious anaemia
	• Bone marrow depression dues to cancer, drugs or radiation	Aplastic anaemia
Reduced haemoglobin content of RBC	• Lack of iron in the diet necessary for RBC formation	Iron deficiency anaemia
	• Slow prolonged bleeding which depletes stores of iron, e.g. heavy menstrual flow	
Abnormal haemoglobin present in red cells	• Abnormal haemoglobin in the RBCs becomes sickle shaped when oxygen use increases. Sickle-cell trait is genetic and mainly occurs in people of African descent	Sickle-cell anaemia
	• Large amounts of abnormal haemoglobin present in RBCs due to a genetic abnormality resulting in a low overall level of Hb	Thalassaemia

assume this sickle shape and is a medical emergency. Sickled cells have a reduced ability to carry oxygen and due to their abnormal shape obstruct the capillaries, leading to reduced blood flow to organs and therefore ischaemia and organ damage. The most common sites for the action of sickled cells are the lungs, liver, brain, spleen and kidneys, although other parts of the body can be affected. The presenting symptoms are severe pain related to the affected organ(s) and extreme breathlessness. Immediate management includes oxygen and analgesia. A crisis may happen spontaneously with no apparent cause, however, precipitating factors can be hypoxia, hypovolaemia, hypothermia, stress and co-existing illness.

Haemoglobin (Hb) level in the blood is measured in gm per decilitre (100ml). Normal range is 13–18gm/dL in men and 11.5–16.5gm/dL in women.

People with chronic anaemia often develop quite a high tolerance for the low Hb levels: however, they have no reserves if they become ill and their oxygen demand increases. In acute situations, a patient with anaemia will commonly display symptoms of breathlessness and pallor. In the immediate term oxygen saturations should be maximised, while the underlying cause can be found and treated. It is important to remember that an oxygen saturation probe measures the amount of oxygen on the available haemoglobin. Therefore, although the level of haemoglobin may be low, it may be fully saturated with oxygen, so the saturation readings would be within the normal range. However, the overall amount of oxygen transported to the tissues would be significantly compromised. This is a good example of needing a number of

parameters when assessing clinical status, rather than just one. Assessment needs to take into account many factors in order to make an accurate interpretation. In contrast to anaemia some individuals suffer from a condition known as polycythaemia that causes an abnormally high red cell count resulting in the blood becoming so viscous that it doesn't flow properly. This reduces tissue perfusion and may increase blood pressure and the likelihood of a stroke or myocardial infarction due to thrombus formation.

The hormone erythropoietin, which is produced mainly by the kidneys, controls the rate of RBC production. People with renal failure often suffer from anaemia due to the lack of this hormone.

White blood cells (WBCs) – leucocytes

WBCs have an equally vital function to red blood cells in that they defend the body from invading pathogens and are central to the immune response. There are several different types of WBC which are grouped under two headings: *polymorphonuclear granulocytes* originating from the red bone marrow and *mononuclear granulocytes* also originating from the red bone marrow, but they mature in the lymphoid tissue.

WBCs are like a mobile defence force or army protecting the body from bacteria, viruses parasites and tumour cells. Damaged tissues give off certain chemicals that act as 'homing beacons' to the affected area. The ability of WBCs to migrate in response to these chemical signals is known as chemotaxis.

There are three types of polymorphonuclear granulocyte:

- **Neutrophils**
- **Eosinophils**
- **Basophils**.

And two types of mononuclear granulocyte:

- Monocytes
- Lymphocytes.

Neutrophils and monocytes engulf invading organisms and incorporate them into their cell bodies, destroying them by a process called phagocytosis. Neutrophils are the most numerous of the phagocytes and arrive at the site of invasion first. Monocytes arrive later and stay longer so a raised neutrophil count may indicate a chronic infection. Unlike red blood cells, which carry out their function entirely within the blood, WBCs use blood only as the means of transport to the site where their functions are needed. They are then able to move in and out of the blood vessels.

The normal WBC count in adults is $4-11 \times 10^9$/L and when an infection is present the WBC count may be significantly raised. A white cell count above 11×10^9/L is known as leucocytosis. An abnormally low WBC count below 4×10^9/L is known as leukopenia and can be caused by factors such as corticosteroids and chemotherapy drugs. Leukopenia renders the individual vulnerable to infections of all types. Problems related to infection and sepsis are discussed in Chapter 12.

> **Leukaemia**
> A cancer of the bone marrow that results in huge numbers of immature and ineffective white cells being produced. This makes the patient susceptible to infection and also causes other cells to be 'crowded out', often resulting in severe anaemia and bleeding.

Platelets – thrombocytes

Platelets are responsible for the ability of the blood to clot, and are the smallest of the formed elements of the blood. Platelets also produce a substance called serotonin that causes constriction of the smooth muscle of the blood vessels. This vasoconstriction reduces blood flow and combined with clotting helps to minimise bleeding and to achieve haemostasis; stopping the bleeding. Platelets, although a vital part of the clotting process, are just one of a number of factors in a complex series of events known as the clotting cascade. The clotting mechanism is initiated by an injury or damage to the blood vessel wall: this roughens the lining of the blood vessel (normally

> **Disseminated intravascular coagulopathy (DIC)**
> In DIC, thrombin becomes abnormally active. This may occur due to severe inflammation, infection, or cancer. Small clots form in the blood vessels. Some of these clots impede the blood supply to organs such as the liver, brain, or kidney. These organs will then be damaged.
> Over time due to the increased activity of the clotting system the clotting proteins are consumed or 'used up'. As a result, although the primary problem is abnormal clotting the most obvious clinical sign is bleeding. The risk then is serious bleeding from a minor injury or even without injury.

extremely smooth). What follows can be simplified into three essential steps:

1 Platelets become 'sticky' in response to factors released by the injured tissue. The sticky platelets join together or aggregate to form a soft plug at the site of injury. The injured tissue also releases clotting factors that speed up this process.
2 A series of chemical reactions occur culminating in the formation of thrombin. Thrombin forms from pro-thrombin which is produced by the liver and requires vitamin K.
3 The final stage in the reaction is between thrombin and fibrinogen (a plasma protein) causing fibrinogen to be converted to fibrin. Fibrin looks like a tangled mass of threads and forms a net in which red blood cells and platelets are trapped: this forms a stable clot.

> **Prothrombin time (PT)** Animal tissue factors are added to the blood sample and the time taken for the sample to clot is the PT. Normal range is 11–16 secs.
> **Partial prothrombin time (PTT)** Activators are added to the sample without tissue factor and the time taken for clotting is measured. Normal range is 25–39 secs.

When we apply pressure with gauze or similar to a bleeding wound the roughened surface of the gauze encourages platelet aggregation and the pressure fractures cells releasing the tissue factors that further speed the process. If it is possible to raise the site of injury above the level of the heart this will slow blood flow to the area and reduce bleeding.

As the damaged tissue is repaired the clot is slowly broken down. This process is called fibrinolysis and occurs as a result of an enzyme called plasmin which causes the fibrin strands to dissolve and the clot to erode. Figure 6.12 summarises the clot formation and dissolution process.

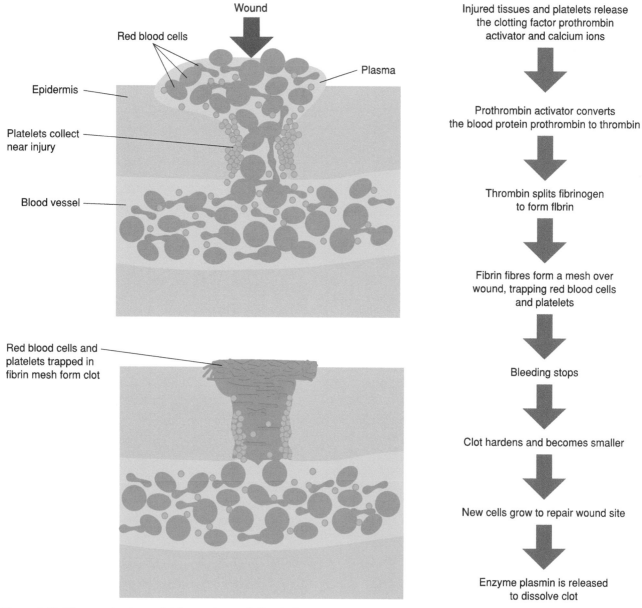

Figure 6.12 Diagram to show clot formation and dissolution

Anticoagulant therapy

Aspirin – inhibits the circulating factors which cause platelet aggregation.

Warfarin – inhibits the production of prothrombin.

Heparin – inhibits the conversion of prothrombin to thrombin. Heparin is a substance which occurs naturally in the body to ensure clots do not form inappropriately.

Clopidogrel – prevents platelets aggregating and inhibits the ability of fibrin strands to bind the clot together.

Thrombolytic therapy 'clot-busters' – e.g. streptokinase these enzymes cause plasmin to be activated and the clot to break down. They are most effective on recently formed clots and are used in the treatment of heart disease and strokes. However there are side effects and contraindications so the treatment is not suitable for all (NICE 2002).

Clots can sometimes form inappropriately in blood vessels that are not broken through injury but damaged in some way, usually due to the presence of atheroma (discussed in more detail later in this chapter). Clots may form in the coronary arteries (causing a myocardial infarction), the cerebral arteries (causing a stroke), or travel to the pulmonary vasculature (causing a pulmonary embolus), which leads to a potentially catastrophic cessation of blood supply to these organs. A clot that forms and stays in one place is known as a thrombus. A clot that forms and then moves, circulating through the bloodstream either in total or in part, is known as an embolus.

Blood groups ABO and rhesus factor

There are between 30 and 50 antigens on the plasma membranes of red blood cells, however, the main focus in relation to matching blood for patients who need transfusions is the AB and rhesus antigens. Everyone has only one of the following blood groups

- Group A (surface antigen A present on plasma membrane)
- Group B (surface antigen B present on plasma membrane)
- Group AB (no surface antigens present on plasma membrane)
- Group O (surface antigens A and B present on plasma membrane).

The majority of the population in the United Kingdom are group O (47%) and group A (40%). Group AB is the least common (3%). There are fluctuations in this among certain ethnic groups, for example persons of Asian descent are more likely to be group B and in those originating from China and Japan the incidence of group AB is higher, around 10%.

In early childhood a person with blood group A will develop antigens to blood group B, conversely those with blood group B will develop antigens to blood group A. Persons with blood group AB have no antigens where as those with blood group O have antigens to both A and B. This is illustrated in Figure 6.13.

Recipient's blood		Reactions with donor's blood			
RBC antigens	Plasma antibodies	Donor type O	Donor type A	Donor type B	Donor type AB
None (Type O)	Anti-A Anti-B				
A (Type A)	Anti-B				
B (Type B)	Anti-A				
AB (Type AB)	(None)				

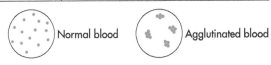

Figure 6.13 Blood groups and results of donor–recipient combinations

Rhesus factor

In addition to the AB antigens there is one further antigen that is of significance when matching blood for transfusion.

> **Rhesus problems in pregnancy**
>
> There can be serious consequences for the foetus if the father is Rh positive and the mother Rh negative.
>
> If the first pregnancy produces a child who has developed the father's Rh positive trait, the mother will develop anti-Rh antibodies during her pregnancy.
>
> During the second pregnancy if that baby is also Rh positive the mother's antibodies will cause agglutination of the foetal RBCs resulting in the death of the foetus. This is called erythroblastosis foetalis.
>
> Pregnant women are screened to identify this risk and can then be given medication to prevent the production of antibodies.

This is known as the rhesus factor (Rh): 85% of the population in the UK possess the Rh factor and are therefore termed Rh positive, those that in whom it is absent are Rh negative. In practice when blood types are talked about the term rhesus is omitted and therefore a person's blood group is described, for example, as O positive or negative. Anti-Rh antibodies will not be automatically produced by the body, as is the case for anti-A and anti-B, they are produced in response to a transfusion of Rh positive blood into a Rh negative person. The process of producing antibodies takes time and therefore the first transfusion is likely to be uneventful but any subsequent transfusion will result in a typical incompatibility reaction.

> If donated blood contains **no** A or B antigens agglutination **cannot** occur, therefore blood group O is often referred to as the **universal donor**.
>
> Those with blood group AB do not have antibodies to **either** A or B and therefore agglutination **cannot occur** with any donated blood and group AB is often referred to as the **universal recipient**.
>
> In practice, however, all blood is matched carefully to that of a recipient although in an extreme emergency such as massive blood loss due to trauma, O positive blood may be given.

Blood transfusion

The plasma membranes of RBCs carry proteins, as do those of all body cells. These proteins identify us as unique and are known as 'self-antigens'. Antigens that enter the body through wounds, transfusions etc. are 'non-self-antigens'. Because they differ from our self-antigens they are recognised as foreign by antibodies. Antibodies are produced by the immune system in response to the presence of foreign antigens, or they may be present in the plasma already. The reaction that occurs between the antigen and antibody is the basis of all immune responses. In the case of red blood cells, the antibody antigen reaction that occurs following an incompatible transfusion causes the cells to 'clump' together or agglutinate. This may result in a blockage of small vessels, causing hypoxia and tissue damage. More devastating is the rupture of red blood cells that also occurs, a process known as lysing. Lysing of red blood cells causes the release of free haemoglobin into the circulation. These freely circulating molecules travel to the kidney and block the glomerulus, resulting in renal failure and possible death.

Transfusion of blood can be a life-saving procedure, however everyone's blood is different and transfusing blood that is incompatible with the recipient's can be fatal. The hazards of transfusion not only relate to incompatibility, blood is a complex liquid tissue and transfusion also carries the risk of:

- reactions to bacterially contaminated blood;
- transfusion-related acute lung injury (TRALI);
- acute fluid overload;
- severe allergic reaction or anaphylaxis.

Thankfully serious or life-threatening acute reactions are rare, however any new symptoms or signs appearing whilst a patient is being transfused must be reported, they could be the first warnings of a serious reaction. It can be difficult to determine the type of reaction in the early stages so all those receiving a blood transfusion are monitored carefully and observations of vital signs are recorded frequently according to local protocols (usually every 30 minutes). Symptoms of transfusion reactions and appropriate actions are detailed in Figure 6.14.

Following a reaction the unit of blood must be returned to the blood bank and an incident form completed. Severe adverse reactions or events must be reported to SABRE (Serious Adverse Blood Reactions and Events) and SHOT (Serious Hazards of Transfusion), www.shotuk.org. This is done via the blood bank.

The arterial and venous systems

So far we have discussed the heart, cardiac output and the blood. We now move on to how blood is transported around the body from the heart through the systemic circulation to the tissues, and returning back to the heart.

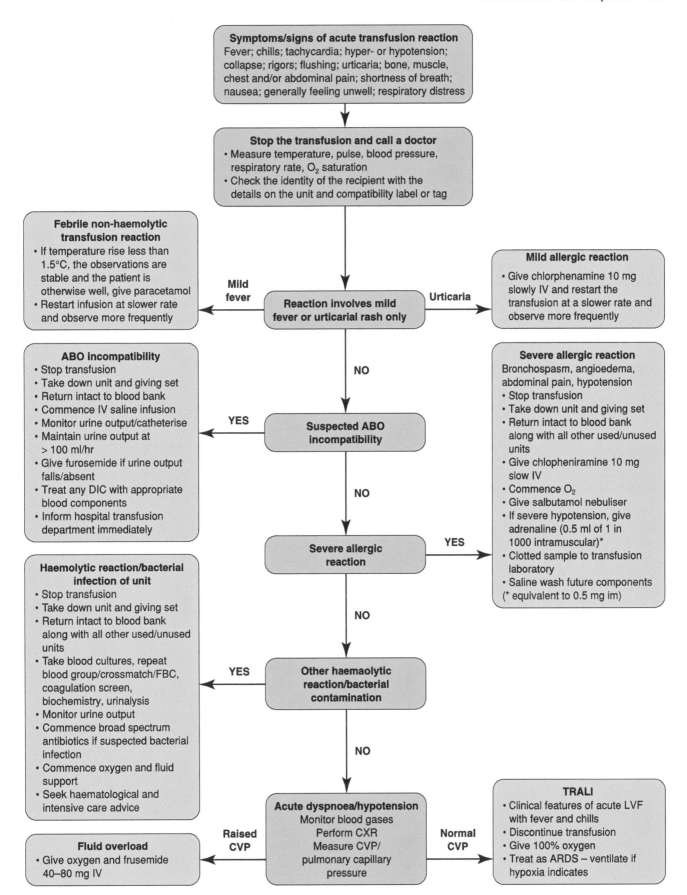

Figure 6.14 Transfusion reactions

Source: McClelland, D. B. L. (ed.) (2007) *Handbook of Transfusion Medicine*, Figure 10, p. 61. Copyright © Joint UKBTS/HPA Professional Advisory Committe (JPAC), NHS Blood and Transplant.

This is the circulatory system, a network of blood vessels that can be thought of as having two main components: the systemic circulation and the pulmonary circulation.

Blood is transported away from the heart via arteries, the largest of which is the aorta. Arteries become progressively smaller the further they are from the heart, finally becoming very small vessels known as arterioles. Arterioles feed into capillaries in the capillary bed of all body tissues. Whilst arterioles are very small, capillaries are microscopic with very thin walls. It is at the capillary bed that the exchange of nutrients and oxygen occurs from the blood to the tissues and waste products are exchanged to the blood from the tissues. Blood leaves the capillary bed via small venules that join with others to become veins, the largest of which are the superior vena cava (SVC) and the inferior vena cava (IVC). Veins transport blood to the heart.

The flow of blood down the arterioles can be controlled by regulating the diameter of the vessel. Contraction (vasoconstriction) of the vessels narrows the lumen and reduces blood flow, relaxation causes dilation of the lumen, increasing the diameter and allowing an increase in blood flow. Control of vascular tone occurs both centrally and peripherally. The autonomic nervous system (ANS) utilises hormones such as adrenaline and noradrenaline which cause vasoconstriction and antidiuretic hormone (ADH) that regulates fluid loss via the kidneys. Vasoconstriction and dilation may occur locally to preserve blood flow to vital organs such as the heart, brain and lungs, but in doing so divert blood flow from other less essential areas. In addition to collecting blood from the capillary beds and returning it to the heart, veins and venules can expand to act as reservoirs for blood, or constrict in order to divert the flow of blood elsewhere.

Structure of blood vessels

The walls of arteries and veins have three layers (see Figure 6.15). The *tunica interna* or *intima* is the innermost layer of the vessels. The surface in contact with the blood is the *vascular endothelium* and this is present throughout the heart and the vessels of the circulatory system. It is composed of completely flattened cells providing a very smooth surface to allow uninterrupted blood flow. However, it is not simply an inert lining but has a number of vital functions which are controlled by release of vasoactive substances. These functions include regulation of coagulation and platelet adhesion, immune function, fluid distribution through vasoconstriction and dilation and the mediation

---

Vascular endothelium

Actively synthesises and releases vasoactive substances:

- **angiotensin-converting enzyme** converts angiotensin 1 to angiotensin 2 in the lungs;
- **nitric oxide vasodilator**: also inhibits platelet activation and clotting;
- **prostacyline**: inhibits platelet activation and clotting;
- **endothelin**: vasoconstrictor.

Stanfield (2011)

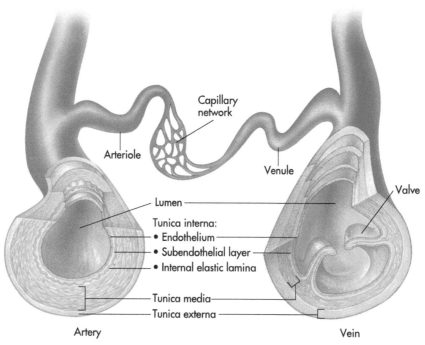

Figure 6.15 Blood vessels and connecting capillaries

of the electrolyte content of the intravascular and extra-vascular spaces. Endothelial dysfunction can result from environmental factors, for example smoking, nutritional imbalances and exposure to airborne pollutants and contribute to several disease processes such as septic shock, hypertension, hypercholesterolaemia and diabetes.

The middle layer, the *tunica media*, is composed of smooth muscle and elastic fibrous tissue that is much thicker in arteries than in veins. This is to enable the arterial wall to expand and contract in response to the pressures generated by the contraction of the left ventricle and plays a crucial role in the control of blood pressure. The venous system is a much lower pressure system and therefore the elastic muscular middle layer does not need to be as thick.

The outermost layer, the *tunica externa* or *adventitia* is made of connective fibres and provides support and protection to the vessel.

A major difference between arteries and veins in terms of structure is that the larger veins, particularly in the legs, contain valves to prevent blood flowing in the wrong direction. The low pressure in the venous system means that blood needs some assistance on the journey back to the heart. In addition to the valves preventing backflow the muscles in the legs 'squeeze' the veins and help to push the blood towards the heart. The wall of the capillaries consists solely of the tunica interna and is only one cell thick to allow exchange of substances between the blood and extracellular fluid.

> Venous return to the heart has to defy gravity so is aided by:
> - the muscular skeletal pump;
> - decreased venous capacitance (vasoconstriction);
> - respiratory pump.

Capillary bed and sphincters – tissue fluid formation and reabsorption

Capillaries, in addition to having very thin walls, have a lumen that is only slightly larger in size than the diameter of a red blood cell. These properties facilitate the efficient movement of substances in and out of the blood at a cellular level. Many capillaries join together to form a web of capillaries supplying all organs and tissues of the body: this web is known as the capillary bed.

> Even at rest the body requires 250ml oxygen and will produce 200ml carbon dioxide *per minute* so efficient movement at the capillary level is vital.

The capillary bed is composed of two types of vessel (see Figure 6.16). The vascular shunt is the main route into the network of capillaries and true capillaries where exchange of substances occurs. Within this network are structures

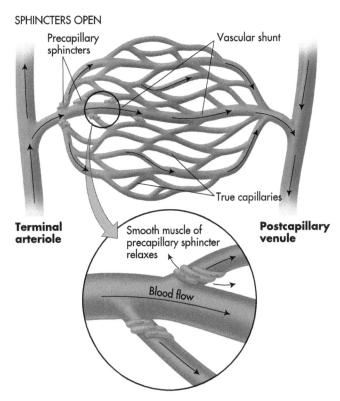

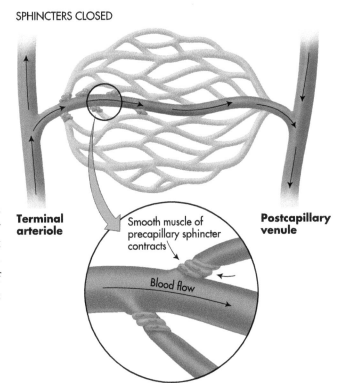

Figure 6.16 Capillary beds and sphincters

known as precapillary sphincters that control the flow of blood from the vascular shunt through into the capillaries. If the blood is stopped at the precapillary sphincters it continues through the vascular shunt, bypassing the tissues. If the sphincter is open blood will flow from the vascular shunt into the capillary bed. For example a muscle at rest may not need blood flowing through the entire capillary network because its demands for oxygen and nutrients are reduced as are the production of waste products. If the muscle becomes active due to exercise, the sphincters will open allowing flow of blood into the capillary networks.

Movement of water as well as nutrients and oxygen occurs at the capillary bed to ensure the hydration of cells. This movement is dependent upon two pressures:

1 *Hydrostatic pressure* – this is best thought of as the 'pushing force' of water and is the pressure generated by the liquid component of the blood against the vessel wall. It therefore tends to force fluid out of the capillary.

2 *Osmotic pressure* – this is generated by the presence of the plasma proteins in the blood and creates a 'pulling' or 'holding' force which attracts water to and holds it inside the capillary.

> Oedema is an abnormally large amount of fluid in the interstitial space and is evidence of fluid imbalance. It may be due to:
>
> - imbalance of electrolytes especially sodium (Na^+);
> - increase in capillary blood pressure due to venous congestion, for example right-sided heart failure;
> - decreased concentration of plasma proteins. This may be due to poor nutrition or 'leakage' into the tissues that can occur in septic shock.

At the arterial end of the capillary bed hydrostatic pressure exceeds osmotic and therefore fluid is forced out of the capillary. At the venous end osmotic pressure tends to be higher and fluid from the interstitial spaces is therefore drawn back into the circulation. Changes in either of these pressures can result in oedema as either too much fluid is forced out or not enough is drawn back in.

In health, the movement of water solutes and respiratory gases between the intravascular space (blood) the interstitial space (around the cells) and finally the intracellular space (inside the tissues cells) is controlled by this mechanism.

Fluids that may be given to patients by intravenous (IV) infusion may be:

- isotonic (having the same concentrations as body cells)
- hypertonic (having a higher concentration than body cells)

- hypotonic (having a lower concentration than body cells).

Most fluids given to patients are isotonic, for example 0.9% saline (normal saline) and 5% dextrose. Hypertonic solutions are sometimes given to patients who have oedema, as due to their high concentration they will tend to draw fluid out of the tissues and back into the circulation. Hypotonic solutions are rarely given intravenously but may be used in cases of extreme dehydration. Taking these fluids orally is more usual – most rehydrating sports drinks are hypotonic.

IV fluid therapy may be:

- *Crystalloid fluids* – solutions containing molecules which pass freely through the semipermeable membranes of the body fluid compartments, for example 0.9% saline, 5% dextrose and Hartmann's solution.
- *Colloid fluids* – these contain large protein molecules that tend to remain in the circulation longer. Vascular fluid loss can be replaced with smaller volumes than if crystalloids are used. Colloids tend to be more expensive and do have a higher incidence of adverse effects than crystalloids.
- *Blood and blood products* – these include whole blood packed red cells, fresh frozen plasma (FFP) and human albumin solution. These should be used to replace the loss of specific fluids and not for general fluid resuscitation. Caution should be exercised due to their high potential for causing adverse reactions and their expense.

Having reviewed the components and normal functioning of the cardiovascular system, an overview of some common disorders of this system – atheroclerosis, coronary artery disease, aneurysm and heart failure – will be given.

Common disorders of the cardiovascular system

Atherosclerosis

Atherosclerosis is a potentially serious condition where there is a progressive build-up of fatty deposits in the subintimal layer of medium and large arteries. It is a chronic condition and it can take several decades for these deposits to reach a level where there is significant disruption to the blood flow along the arteries. Atherosclerosis is a major risk factor for many different conditions involving a reduced blood flow. Collectively, these conditions are known as cardiovascular disease (CVD). Examples of CVD include:

- Coronary artery disease and myocardial infarction
- Peripheral artery disease
- Stroke.

Coronary artery disease

During the early stages of this disease, lipids are deposited into the subintimal space where they combine with monocytes to form large bulky cells called foam cells. As the cells proliferate they slowly start to force the endothelial layer of the arterial wall out into the lumen of the artery. As a result the diameter of the lumen becomes slowly more narrow (stenosis) (see Figure 6.17). The patient might be asymptomatic throughout the early phases of atherosclerosis build-up. By the time symptoms of chest pain

(angina) and breathlessness occur during activity, the disease will already be quite advanced.

Atherosclerosis alters the efficiency with which the endothelium prevents blood cells and platelets from adhering to the wall of the arterial lumen. In addition to this, the narrowing of the lumen slows down the flow of blood through the artery making the blood more likely to clot and form thrombi in the areas of the slowest flow. Where this occurs in coronary vessels it is the formation of the thrombus that turns coronary heart disease from a chronic disease into an acute coronary event. The sudden development of the thrombus in the coronary artery might cause either a partial or complete occlusion. Where there is a partial occlusion there might be a small residual blood flow that causes the myocardium to have reduced oxygen supply (ischaemia), in this case the myocardium is not likely to be permanently damaged but should recover once blood flow is re-established. If the thrombus in the coronary artery causes a complete occlusion then all of the myocardium that lies beyond the occlusion will first become damaged (myocardial injury) and, should the occlusion not be removed quickly, the myocardium will die (causing necrosis) and lead to myocardial dysfunction and possibly death. It is this sudden development of a partial or total occlusion by a thrombus that defines acute coronary syndrome (ACS), which is discussed in detail later in this chapter.

Aneurysm

This is an area of the arterial wall that has become weakened, possibly by atherosclerosis or sometimes due to congenital defects. This develops into a sac-like protrusion on the vessel wall that may predispose thrombus formation or may burst. If an aneurysm bursts it has potentially catastrophic consequences due to excessive loss of blood in the case of an abdominal aortic aneurysm, or if a vessel in the brain is affected (a form of stroke) a fatal rise in intracranial pressure can occur.

Acute heart failure

Heart failure is a complex clinical syndrome of symptoms and signs that suggest impairment of the heart as a pump supporting physiological circulation (NICE 2010b). Therefore the heart is unable adequately to perfuse the organs and tissues of the body. The term heart failure should not be confused with cardiac arrest (which is an emergency situation), or 'heart attack' (which normally refers to myocardial infarction). There are many reasons why the heart loses the ability to adequately supply oxygenated blood to the target organs and this is reflected by the type

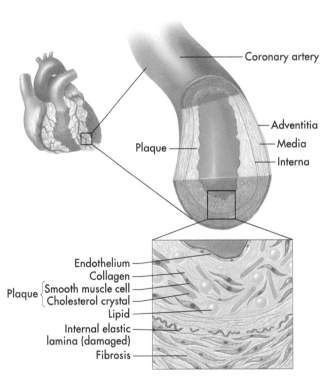

Figure 6.17 Atherosclerosis

of heart failure that exists and which side of the heart has failed.

Common causes of heart failure are ischaemic heart disease, hypertension, heart valve disease and other structural changes to the myocardium (such as cardiomyopathy). There are essentially two types of heart failure: systolic and diastolic. Other terms such as 'forward' and 'backward' heart failure are still occasionally used to describe this classification.

Systolic heart failure

Systolic heart failure is characterised by a falling ejection fraction as the ventricular myocardium is unable to contract effectively. This can be due to:

- reversible causes: including ischaemic heart disease and angina, where blood flow can be restored;
- irreversible causes: including myocardial infarction where necrosis of myocardial tissue has occurred, causing a permanent degree of residual heart failure;
- aortic stenosis and obstructive cardiomyopathy which make it difficult for the blood to be pumped from the ventricle into the aorta.

Diastolic heart failure

This happens when the heart is unable to fill adequately with blood during diastole. This can be due to:

- stenosis of the mitral or tricuspid valve, preventing blood from flowing into the ventricle;
- changes in the compliance (or distensibility) of the ventricular myocardium, so that it does not expand as the ventricle fills with blood. A poorly compliant ventricle will have a reduced volume of blood at the end of diastole, and therefore will eject a smaller amount during systole, leading to a reduced cardiac output;
- ventricular hypertrophy which happens when the ventricular wall becomes thicker and less compliant. Hypertrophy can occur in patients with a history of hypertension and/or renal failure, as the myocardium adapts to increased stress on the ventricular wall.

Left ventricular failure

In left ventricular failure (LVF), the forward flow of blood from the left ventricle into the systemic circulation is reduced. As a result of this impairment, blood pressure and tissue perfusion will decrease. The lowered ejection fraction means that pressure builds up in the ventricle (as more blood is left behind after the ventricular contraction) creating an increase in pressure in the left atrium

and pulmonary circulation. Pulmonary oedema is a common sequalae of LVF and hence breathlessness is a frequently observed symptom.

In advanced cases, the pulmonary congestion will extend back to the right ventricle, creating a dysfunction in both sides of the heart. This is commonly referred to as congestive cardiac failure (CCF) or biventricular failure.

Right ventricular failure

When the right side of the heart fails to provide adequate forward flow, the congestion extends back into the venous circulation. This might be observed as raised jugular venous pressure (JVP) and peripheral oedema. However, because the pulmonary circulation is unaffected there will be an absence of pulmonary oedema, as seen in LVF. The reduced flow of blood from the right to the left side of the heart (via the pulmonary circulation) leads to a reduction in the preload pressure in the left ventricle. Reduced cardiac output is thus a consequence of both LVF and RVF.

Symptoms
Common symptoms of heart failure are given in Table 6.5.

We have looked at some of the common conditions of the cardiovascular system that affect the lives of many people. Often these problems are monitored and managed in primary care, with occasional visits to hospital for additional investigations, or medication management. However, the disordered physiology may give rise to acute deterioration and require urgent or emergency intervention. The nurse uses assessment skills to evaluate health status and to identify possible problems.

Table 6.5 Common symptoms of heart failure

Symptom	Left ventricular failure	Right ventricular failure	Biventricular failure
Dyspnoea	Yes	No	Yes
Reduced cardiac output	Yes	Yes	Yes
Raised JVP	No	Yes	Yes
Pulmonary oedema	Yes	No	Yes
Peripheral oedema	No	Yes	Yes
Pallor	Yes	Yes	Yes
Reduced exercise tolerance	Yes	Yes	Yes

Cardiovascular assessment

In the acute care setting, the nurse has a pivotal role to play in performing a comprehensive assessment of cardiovascular status, so that deterioration can be detected as early possible. Good communication skills are necessary to build a therapeutic relationship with the patient to ensure that care is person centred and that all nursing activities are understood by the patient (NMC 2010). These skills are necessary for a sound and comprehensive clinical assessment, and Bickley (2007) advises that all nursing and medical personnel should have the skills necessary to take a medical history and perform a physical examination. A medical history involves asking questions ranging from identifying the present complaint, through to family and social history. The physical examination involves skills of inspection, palpation and auscultation, and will be performed if the patient's clinical condition is sufficiently stable. This is determined by the ABCDE assessment.

Valuable information can be gained by taking account of both subjective and objective data. The patient's experience and perspective is important and can contribute to the nurse's understanding and identification of likely problems. Taking a brief history can identify relevant past medical history, allergies, risk factors and medication taken. Symptoms should be explored systematically to help identify underlying physiological disturbances.

Objective data include the vital signs recorded by the nurse, as well as information gathered by physical examination, and diagnostics test such as electrocardiograms (ECG), serum electrolyte levels and cardiac biomarkers. The cardiovascular system is uniquely adapted to maintain homeostasis, ensuring that perfusion of vital organs such as the heart, lung and brain are maintained for as long as possible. The nurse therefore needs to be aware of subtle changes which indicate that compensation is occurring, in order to maintain oxygen delivery. Track and trigger tools have been developed in response to concerns regarding competence in this area, and have been discussed at some length in Chapter 1. Whilst these are useful tools the nurse needs to be cognisant of trends over time in order to ascertain whether clinical signs of compensation are increasing, signalling deterioration in clinical status that may give rise to a medical emergency.

Assessment utilising the ABCDE framework and incorporating basic physical assessment skills of Look (inspect) Listen (auscultate) Feel (palpate/percuss), identifies the patient at risk. The focus of the following discussion on cardiovascular assessment has integrated aspects of physical assessment. For further information on physical examination please see Bickley (2007).

Airway

Any problems identified in the airway assessment should be treated and resolved before moving on to breathing assessment.

Breathing

Cardiac problems can cause changes in respiratory status, with the sensation of breathlessness or dyspnoea being a key feature of cardiac failure. Looking at the patient can reveal signs of increased work of breathing, such as use of accessory muscles or the inability to complete sentences in one breath. The New York Heart Association classification of heart failure classifies patients' heart failure according to the severity of their symptoms. Symptoms of dyspnoea should be assessed in relation to level of activity, with dyspnoea at rest being consistent with Class 4 failure (see Table 6.6).

Orthopnoea, difficulty in breathing when lying flat, is also often a symptom of heart failure. This may be noticed at night (paroxysmal nocturnal orthopnoea). The patient may complain of being woken at night with extreme breathlessness, which may occur when the patient slips down the bed whilst sleeping. Sitting up, or out of bed in a chair may help alleviate the symptoms.

Central cyanosis, a bluish discolouration of the mucous membranes of the mouth, is a late sign of hypoxaemia and not always reliable, so pulse oximetry should be assessed as soon as possible. Pulse oximetry gives valuable information regarding capillary oxygen saturation levels, which in health would be between 97–100%, and is recorded in conjunction with the percentage of inhaled oxygen.

Table 6.6 New York Heart Association (NYHA) classification of heart failure

Class I: asymptomatic	No limitations of ordinary physical activity. Ordinary activity does not cause undue fatigue, dyspnoea, palpitation or angina
Class II: mild	Comfortable at rest. Slight or moderate limitation of physical activity. Ordinary physical activity results in symptoms
Class III: moderate	Although comfortable at rest, marked limitation of physical activity with less than ordinary activity causing symptoms
Class IV: severe	Symptoms at rest. Inability to carry on any physical activity without discomfort, symptoms of cardiac insufficiency

Peripheral cyanosis, seen as a bluish discolouration of the fingers and toes, indicates vasoconstriction and is related to poor cardiac output, rather than hypoxaemia.

Pulmonary auscultation may reveal pulmonary crackles. Crackles are non-musical sounds heard during inspiration caused by the re-opening of occluded airways, or by air moving through fluid. Crackles could be a sign of pulmonary oedema, secondary to acute left ventricular failure. The expectoration of pink frothy sputum is also a feature of pulmonary oedema and is a sign of acute deterioration, normally accompanied by tachypnoea, distress and hypoxaemia, requiring urgent medical review. Respiratory rate is counted over one full minute to ensure accuracy and enable the detection of small changes, which can be clinically significant.

Circulation

Skin colour and temperature

Observation of skin for colour and warmth can give a good indication of cardiovascular function. A reduction in perfusion will cause diversion of blood flow from the peripheral circulation, rendering the skin pale and cool to touch. Feeling along a limb for example from the toes, to foot, to calf, detects the degree of vasoconstriction. It may be that just the toes are cool, which would be mild, but if the leg felt cool up to mid-calf this would signify more compromise.

Blood pressure

Blood pressure is kept relatively constant with homeostatic mechanisms described earlier in this chapter. The nurse needs to be able to interpret blood pressure in the context of a range of parameters, such as heart rate, peripheral warmth and blood flow, level of consciousness and urine output. Changes in all of these parameters may occur prior to significant changes in blood pressure. Normal ranges of blood pressure have been discussed previously, when assessing clinical status the variation from the patient's normal pressure may be as significant as the actual value. A systolic blood pressure that has fallen suddenly by more than 20mmHg or by 30% since the last reading, or falls below 90mmHg is indicative of circulatory failure and tissue oxygen delivery will be impaired (Macintosh 2011). Though the systolic blood pressure is often the pressure that triggers on early warning systems, the diastolic pressure is important as it determines coronary artery blood flow. Diastolic blood pressure needs to be greater than 50mmHg for adequate coronary artery flow and myocardial perfusion. Pulse pressure has been discussed in relation to palpating the pulse, but can be objectively determined by subtracting diastolic pressure

from systolic blood pressure, with the normal range between 35–45mmHg (Smith 2003). A trend of decreasing pulse pressure signifies worsening cardiac output, and the cause should be ascertained early, to maximise appropriate interventions.

> **Pulse pressure**
>
> Systolic pressure – diastolic pressure
>
> Example: 120/80
>
> pulse pressure = 40mmHg
>
> Example: 110/90
>
> pulse pressure = 30mmHg
>
> This reduction in pulse pressure may indicate hypovolaemia or heart failure.

The majority of people with high blood pressure experience no symptoms, therefore monitoring of blood pressure is vital to detect and treat people early before secondary health problems are experienced.

Mean arterial pressure (MAP) is now commonly recorded in patients who are acutely unwell. Adequate perfusion pressure is essential to enable oxygen delivery at tissue level and MAP is the best way of determining perfusion pressure throughout the cardiac cycle. You may remember that the time the heart spends in diastole is longer than the time spent in systole, and therefore MAP is skewed towards the diastolic value.

A normal MAP is approximately 70–105mmHg (Morton *et al.* 2009). There is some debate as to the lowest acceptable MAP: Woodrow (2009) suggests 70mmHg is necessary for brain, kidney and major organ perfusion. Dellinger *et al.* (2008) also recommend a target MAP of 65mmHg for management of severe sepsis (discussed further in Chapter 12). MAP of over 110mmHg signifies hypertension that could have major consequences for the patient and therefore requires close monitoring and pharmacological intervention. MAP is calculated by both invasive and non-invasive blood pressure measurement devices and if requested, should be recorded on the chart with the systolic and diastolic pressure. Invasive haemodynamic monitoring is discussed briefly later in this chapter.

> MAP can be calculated by the following equation:
>
> MAP = 1/3 pulse pressure + diastole
>
> For example: for a patient with a BP of 100/61
>
> MAP = (1/3 × 39) + 61
> = 13 + 61
> = 74mmHg

Pulse

Palpation of pulses gives valuable information regarding cardiac output. It involves physical contact which can be reassuring for the patient, but also aids assessment of peripheral temperature and diaphoresis (sweating). A cold and clammy patient is indicative of sympathetic activation and is a sign of serious circulatory compromise: help should be sought immediately.

The pulse should be assessed for:

- Rate
- Volume
- Rhythm.

A normal heart rate will vary between 60–100 beats per minute but changes, even within this normal range, can indicate deteriorating circulatory status. This makes heart/pulse rate an important early warning sign. A steadily rising heart rate is indicative of circulatory problems such as hypovoleamia, cardiogenic shock or sepsis. Heart rate will normally be lower than systolic blood pressure, so if it rises beyond this point (or systolic blood pressure falls below heart rate), this is a cause for concern. A falling heart rate is the result of increased vagal tone, such as when sleeping, but could be a sign of a conduction problem. Heart rate and rhythm can be continuously assessed with ECG monitoring, so a knowledge of sinus rhythm and the PQRST complex discussed earlier in the chapter, is required if abnormalities are to be detected.

Pulses can be palpated at a number of sites
- Radial
- Brachial
- Carotid
- Femoral
- Dorsalis pedis
- Posterior tibialis
- Popliteal.

When palpating the pulse, the strength of the pulse wave has clinical significance. Pulse pressure is the difference between the pressure in systole (peak pressure) and diastole (lower pressure). A pulse with a large differential will be felt as full, or bounding. Vasodilation increases the pulse pressure and is associated with sepsis and anaphylaxis. A weak and thready pulse has a low pulse volume caused by vasoconstriction and is a sign of poor cardiac output. A pulse pressure which falls significantly during inspiration is called pulsus paradoxus and could be a sign of pericardial effusion or cardiac tamponade.

The rhythm of the pulse should be regular, though there may be slight variations within the respiratory cycle. An irregular pulse should always be further assessed with a *12-lead ECG*, to ascertain the exact rhythm. People with

irregular heart rates may also need to be placed on a cardiac monitor, so the rhythm can be continuously viewed. Problems such as atrial fibrillation, ectopic beats and conduction abnormalities will be felt as an irregular pulse, and may need urgent treatment.

The 12-lead ECG

Electrocardiograms (ECG) are used as diagnostic tools for visualising the electrical activity of the heart. The cardiac monitor is commonly used for real-time monitoring of heart rate and rhythm of patients that require close observation for changes in the heart's function. However, the cardiac monitor will usually only show the activity of the heart from one view point at a time. The 12-lead ECG provides 12 different views of the heart from standardised positions, and would be taken as part of the ABCDE assessment if the patient complains of chest pain, palpations, or an irregular pulse is felt. It is recorded intermittently, as it requires the patient to lie still while 10 electrodes are attached to the chest and limbs. Often, a series of 12-lead ECGs are needed to observe the changes to the conduction pattern that may occur during acute coronary syndromes or following the administration of antiarrhythmic drugs.

Recording a 12-lead ECG

Six electrodes are placed across the front of the chest on the left side. These electrodes give us a series of views of the left ventricle as observed from the right side of the heart around to the left side (see Figure 6.18).

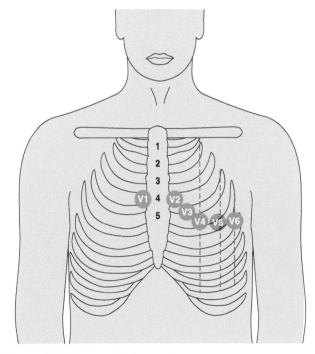

Figure 6.18 Chest lead placement

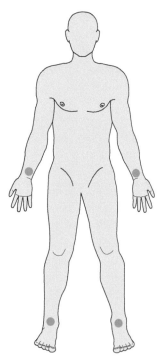

Figure 6.19 Limb lead placement

Four electrodes are placed on the limbs. These electrodes may be placed either on the extremities (ankles and wrists) or on the torso (upper chest and lower abdomen). The important point to note is that these electrodes should be placed symmetrically (see Figure 6.19).

Twelve views of the heart are obtained from these ten electrodes: six are views of the heart from the sides, top and bottom (on the vertical plane); six views of the anterior surface of the left ventricle (on the horizontal plane).

A normal ECG has been included in Figure 6.20. Recordings should be checked for the following characteristics:

- QRS complexes should be upright in leads I, II, III, aVF.
- QRS complexes should be downwards in leads aVR, V1 and V2.
- In the chest leads (V1 to V6), there should be a progressive increase in the height of the QRS complexes (V1 negative and V6 positive, with a smooth transition from one to the other). This tells us that the conduction through the ventricles is following the normal conduction pathways through the bundle branches and Purkinje fibres.
- The ST segment and the T wave should be level with the baseline in all of the ECG in all leads.

> Before recording a 12-lead ECG:
>
> - explain procedure to patient;
> - ask for consent to proceed (NMC 2008);
> - check each electrode is attached and correctly placed;
> - ask the patient to lie still and not speak for a short while whilst the recording is made.

After the ECG has printed, check, before disconnecting the cables, that you have an ECG that is free from artefact (usually appearing as a 'fuzz' through the ECG). Artefact can be caused by any electrical activity such as shivering and nearby electrical equipment. If necessary replace electrodes and repeat the tracing. Check the

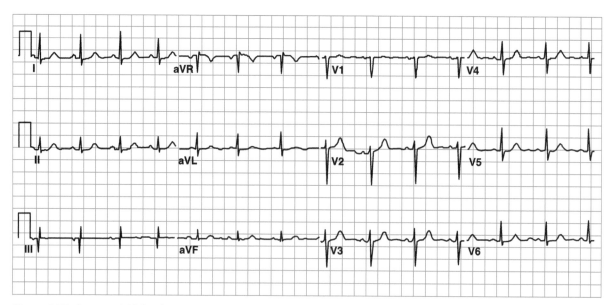

Figure 6.20 A normal 12-lead ECG

progression of the R waves in the chest leads; if this is interrupted, recheck the lead placement. Write the date, time and patient identity on the printout (if not automatically completed by the machine) and record any clinical information, such as recent chest pain, and/or any medications given (Woodrow 2009). Refer to a health care professional who is competent in 12-lead ECG interpretation as necessary.

Capillary refill time

Other clinical signs such as capillary refill time (CRT) are important indicators of cardiac output. A delayed CRT is consistent with a poor cardiac output that has led to reduction in perfusion of the peripheral circulation and may be associated with hypovoleamia and heart failure. Warm dilated peripheries with a brisk CRT may be an indication of the increased peripheral flow associated with sepsis.

Capillary refill time (CRT)

CRT can be used to give an indication of cardiac output:

- hold hand to level of heart;
- press the tip of the finger nail for five seconds, and the nail bed will blanch;
- release the pressure and observe reperfusion (will turn pink);
- normal refill time will be < 2 seconds.

Remember factors such as temperature will affect capillary refill.

Urinary output

Urinary output is one of the best indicators of circulatory function, as kidneys receive about 25% of the cardiac output. For accurate hourly measurements a urinary catheter is required and as most patients do not have catheters, urine output may not form part of the early warning score. Homeostatic mechanisms such as the sympathetic nervous system will reduce blood supply to the kidney in times of low cardiac output, so a reduced urine output is an early sign of cardiovascular compromise. Nurses caring for acutely unwell patients need to closely monitor urine output. Volumes of less than 0.5mL/per Kg per hour are a cause for concern, as renal impairment could ensue. Renal impairment is discussed more fully in Chapter 8.

Skin turgor

Assessing for skin turgor can give information regarding the degree of hydration of the patient. The skin on the back of the hand or forearm is gently pinched, then released. The skin should fall back almost immediately to its previ-

ous state. If the fold takes a little time to relax, this could indicate dehydration. Skin elasticity does decrease with age, so this is not always a reliable sign. Other indicators such as a furrowed tongue should also be assessed.

Oedema

Oedema is the accumulation of fluid in the interstitial spaces and occurs when interstitial fluid exceeds absorptive capacity. The tissue fluid is mobile and can be moved by finger pressure. Peripheral oedema is assessed for by pressing fingers gently but firmly for five seconds on the lowest part of the body where fluid may accumulate, normally the ankles. On release of finger pressure an indentation or pit is left and is evaluated on a scale of +1 (minimal) to +4 (severe). Oedema does not become evident until interstitial volume has increased by 2.5–3L (Porth 2007). Right-sided heart failure, fluid/electrolyte imbalance, low albumin levels, venous obstruction, kidney disease and sepsis should be considered if peripheral oedema is present.

Disability

A poor cardiac output will cause alterations in cerebral perfusion. This may manifest itself as a feeling of discomfort, restlessness, or even a sense of impending doom. Verbalisation of these feelings should be encouraged by the nurse so that possibly significant changes can be assessed. However, anxiety and stress are a normal response when acutely unwell and questions should be answered honestly and promptly to try and allay fears. Cardiac pain is intense and swift nursing intervention is required and is discussed with acute coronary syndromes later in this chapter. Neurological assessment tools such as AVPU and the Glasgow Coma Score detect deterioration in neurological status.

Exposure and physical assessment

Cardiac and circulatory assessment includes an inspection of the patient looking for signs that indicate cardiovascular problems. Chest wall inspection reveals scars that may indicate previous cardiac surgery or pacemaker implantation. Inspection of the nails may reveal splinter haemhorrages, a sign of endocarditis, or xanthomata, which are fatty deposits under the skin associated with raised cholesterol levels. Signs of cardiovascular disease can be observed round the eyes with xanthelasma formation (yellow cholesterol deposits linked to hyperlipidemia) and a ruddy face flush known as Malar flush suggestive of mitral stenosis. Inspection of the jugular venous pulse and pressure (JVP) gives information regarding right-sided heart function, but requires practise to visualise. It can be seen as a double pulsation in the neck, but unless raised will not be visible above the clavicle.

You may see experienced practitioners using skills of cardiac auscultation. This can identify abnormalities of blood flow through the valves in the heart. Blood flow through the heart and the closing of the heart valves generate sounds that can be heard when placing a stethoscope in key areas of the chest (see Figure 6.21, p. 138). The clearest sounds are S1, (first heart sound) generated by the closure of the mitral and tricuspid valve, signalling the onset of systole, and S2, (second heart sound) generated

by the closure of the aortic and pulmonary valves, signalling the beginning of diastole. Damaged and leaky valves cause turbulent flow and produce murmurs that can be heard in the quiet time between systole and diastole (Jones *et al.* 2010).

Nurses mostly utilise skills of observation and measurement, although you will see specialist nurses use skills in physical assessment and auscultation. By comprehensively assessing cardiovascular status and identifying problems early, nurses can instigate appropriate interventions and escalate care in a timely manner to prevent further deterioration, or transfer to a higher level of care as necessary.

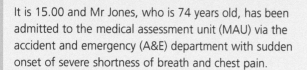

CASE STUDY 6.1 Mr David Jones

It is 15.00 and Mr Jones, who is 74 years old, has been admitted to the medical assessment unit (MAU) via the accident and emergency (A&E) department with sudden onset of severe shortness of breath and chest pain.

BACKGROUND

Mr Jones is a non-smoker who is generally fit and well. He has had extensive orthopeadic surgery in the past including three hip and one knee replacements.

ASSESSMENT

Airway

On arrival to MAU the nurse notes that Mr Jones is extremely breathless and is finding talking difficult as a result of this. There is no indication of stridor or airway obstruction. He is currently receiving oxygen via a 60% Venturi mask.

Breathing

Talking in complete sentences is impossible due to Mr Jones' breathlessness. The nurse notes that the respiratory rate is 32 breaths per minute and these are shallow but regular, Mr Jones chest movement is symmetrical but there is evidence of activation of the sternomastoid and abdominal muscles. There is no wheezing or additional respiratory sounds and no secretions on coughing. Mr Jones is clearly distressed and frightened, the nurse explains what she will be doing in order to make a full assessment and reassures him that this is being done to determine what the problem is and then deal with it. She discourages Mr Jones from talking too much as this is difficult and makes him

more breathless. The nurse attaches a pulse oximeter probe to his finger that reveals an SpO₂ of 93%. This reading is lower than it should be especially considering the amount of inspired oxygen that Mr Jones is receiving, his elevated respiratory rate reflects his respiratory distress. There is some peripheral cyanosis present at the nail beds. The nurse assists Mr Jones into an upright position well supported by pillows.

Circulation

Mr Jones' pulse is regular but fast at 124 beats per minute. While palpating the radial pulse the nurse notes that the skin feels cool and clammy. The blood pressure is 165/90mmHg with a mean of 112. His capillary refill time is three seconds No oedema is noted. Mr Jones passed 450mls of urine in A&E and is complaining of a dry mouth. The nurse offers Mr Jones a mouthwash but on removal of the mask the SpO₂ drops to 84% and he becomes very distressed, so it is replaced quickly. She commences fluid balance recording.

Disability

Although anxious and distressed Mr Jones is fully conscious and oriented with a Glasgow Coma Score of 15/15. Blood glucose was recorded at 4.7mmol/L. Although there is no known history of diabetes blood sugars may become elevated due the increased sympathetic activity caused by stress and anxiety.

Exposure

The nurse notes that Mr Jones appears to be of average weight and build and assesses his skin, she finds this to be

CASE STUDY 6.1 Mr David Jones (continued)

intact with no areas of redness. Immobility and hypoxaemia are factors that increase the risk of skin breakdown. She notes that Mr Jones has varicose veins in both legs but no areas of broken skin. She measures his calf circumference in order to fit the correct anti-embolic stockings.

RESPONSE

Having completed and documented her assessment the staff nurse calculates the EWS as a medium risk trigger, which requires a medical review. She uses SBAR to guide her discussion findings with the medical SpR who is present on the ward. In her view the relatively low SpO_2 warrants urgent arterial blood gas (ABG) analysis. She inserts an IV cannula in order to be able to administer IV fluids as Mr Jones is unable to drink at present because of his breathlessness and tendency to de-saturate when the mask is removed.

The SpR agrees and informs the nurse that the most likely diagnosis is a pulmonary embolism (PE) due to a fragment of clot which has formed in the deep veins of the leg, breaking off and circulating to the lungs, where it has become lodged in the pulmonary circulation. This has blocked part of the pulmonary circulation causing a reduction in gas exchange and hypoxaemia. Mr Jones feels breathless as he tries to increase his oxygenation by breathing faster. His heart rate is increased as his sympathetic nervous system is activated due to anxiety but also as a compensatory response to increase the delivery of oxygen to the tissues. His skin is cool, clammy and cyanosed with a delayed capillary refill time, as blood is being diverted to vital organs to ensure their supply of oxygen. Mr Jones varicose veins and extensive joint replacement surgery have predisposed him to thrombus formation, despite the lack of clinical evidence on assessment. The SpR prescribes a subcutaneous dose of low molecular weight heparin to be given immediately to prevent further clot formation and Mr Jones is prepared for a computerised tomography pulmonary angiogram (CTPA) to provide a definitive diagnosis. The nurse continues close ongoing observation and documentation of findings as further deterioration of Mr Jones's cardiac, circulatory and respiratory status is a possibility.

Following the initial diagnosis of a PE, further investigations are ordered and initial arterial blood gas analysis has been performed at 15.00. The nurse continues to observe Mr Jones carefully and uses a 'track and trigger' system (NICE 2007) as part of her assessment. At 15.30 she notes that Mr Jones seems less responsive and somewhat confused, his respiratory rate has decreased to 16 and his SpO_2 is now

87% on 60% oxygen. She changes the Venturi mask for a non-rebreathe mask using a flow rate of 15L/minute and ensuring the reservoir bag is filled before applying the mask. The early warning score is triggering a red code so she calls the SpR and the critical care outreach team asking for urgent review. A second set of ABGs are taken and analysed.

| | Time | |
Normal values	15.00	15.30
pH (7.35–7.45)	7.46	7.33
PaO_2 (11–13.5kPa)	10.6kPa	8.8kPa
$PaCO_2$ (4.5–6.1kPa)	4.0kPa	6.7kPa
HCO_3 (24–26mmol/L)	24mmol/L	26mmol/L
BE (−2 to +2)	+2	+1
SaO_2 (96–100%)	**93%**	**87%**
Oxygen	60% Venturi mask	60% Venturi mask
Mode	SV	SV

The 15.30hrs ABG analysis indicates further deterioration. Initially (at 15.00hrs) there is evidence of type I respiratory failure. Although the PaO_2 is only just outside normal limits it must be remembered that the patient is receiving 60% oxygen and considered in the light of his elevated respiratory rate. This high rate and increased minute ventilation, a compensatory mechanism for his lung failure, is resulting in a reduced $PaCO_2$ and a pH that is just to the alkalotic side of normal due to the loss of CO_2. The second set of gases is now showing type 2 respiratory failure, as the work of breathing has become overwhelming. Mr Jones's respiratory muscles are tiring, it is no longer possible to maintain his PaO_2, and he is too tired to hyperventilate. The $PaCO_2$ is starting to climb as Mr Jones's respiratory rate drops and his breathing becomes less effective. The non-rebreathe mask has brought Mr Jones's SpO_2 up to 90%. The likely causes of his deterioration are exhaustion leading to type 2 respiratory failure as the respiratory muscles are unable to maintain the work required and/or a further embolus has occurred. The decision is made to intubate and stabilise Mr Jones and transfer him to the intensive care unit for level 3 care and ventilation. Once intubated the CTPA is performed and demonstrates several pulmonary emboli. Supportive ventilatory therapy and anticoagulation are required to try and ensure adequate oxygenation and prevent further thrombus formation. The clots will dissolve over time but fibrinolytic therapy to help break down the existing clot may be considered if there are no contraindications.

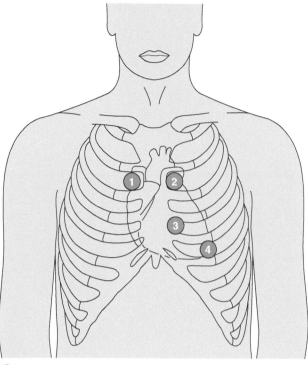

(1) Aortic area – second intercostal space, right sternal border

(2) Pulmonic area – second intercostal space, left sternal border

(3) Tricuspid area – fourth (or fifth) intercostal space, left sternal border

(4) Mitral area or apex – fifth intercostal space, left midclavicular line

Figure 6.21 Locating the assessment points

Acute cardiovascular problems: recognition and treatment

Acute coronary syndromes

Acute coronary syndrome (ACS) (see Figure 6.22) is an umbrella term encompassing a spectrum of clinical presentations all caused by the same disease process, namely the rupture of an atherosclerotic plaque, platelet clumping and thrombosis formation diminishing blood flow. These clinical presentations can be categorised as:

- unstable angina, ischaemic pain without myocardial death;
- non-ST segment elevation myocardial infarction (NSTEMI);
- ST segment elevation myocardial infarction (STEMI).

The aim of treatment for this group of patients is focused on alleviating symptoms, restoration of blood flow to relieve myocardial ischaemia and reduce the risk of cardiac arrest. The patient will usually present with severe chest pain which is 'crushing' or 'heavy' in nature and may cause the patient to experience breathlessness and a drop in blood pressure.

Assessing chest pain

Chest pain is a symptom that is associated with a number of other clinical pathologies; therefore a thorough assessment of any chest pain is essential to exclude the presence of a non-cardiac cause.

Classically, cardiac chest pain is visceral, which means that it is a deep and diffuse pain rather than a localised and superficial pain. The patient, when asked to locate the pain, will normally indicate a wide area of the chest and will be very unlikely to point to a specific point on the chest. Cardiac chest pain does vary in location from person to person but is generally experienced in the centre of the chest (or just to the left of the sternum). It may extend down to the epigastrium or up to the neck and jaw. There is a pattern of referred pain that may extend down the left arm in some cases. It should be noted that not everyone experiences chest pain in ACS. Patients with diabetes mellitus are particularly likely not to complain of chest pain as a result of the neuropathy that accompanies the disease.

NSTEMI and unstable angina

The myocardium cannot survive for long without oxygen and the demand for oxygenated blood is always high in order to maintain adequate myocardial contraction. As the amount of available oxygen in blood diminishes in the presence of even a partial occlusion, the ECG will immediately show signs of ischaemia. ECG changes associated with ischaemia are ST depression and/or T wave inversion. Evidence of heart muscle damage is assessed by measuring troponin levels. If the troponin levels are elevated, a non-ST segment elevated MI is diagnosed (NSTEMI). If adequate blood flow is not re-established then the myocardium may start to break down. The thrombus is likely to increase in size and progress onto a total occlusion. If troponin levels are normal, then unstable angina is the likely diagnosis.

> **Patient assessment for suspected ACS should include:**
>
> - full clinical history (including age, previous MI and previous medical or surgical intervention for coronary heart disease);
> - physical examination (including heart rate and blood pressure);
> - 12-lead ECG;
> - blood tests (such as troponin T or I, glucose, creatinine and Hb).
>
> (NICE 2010c)

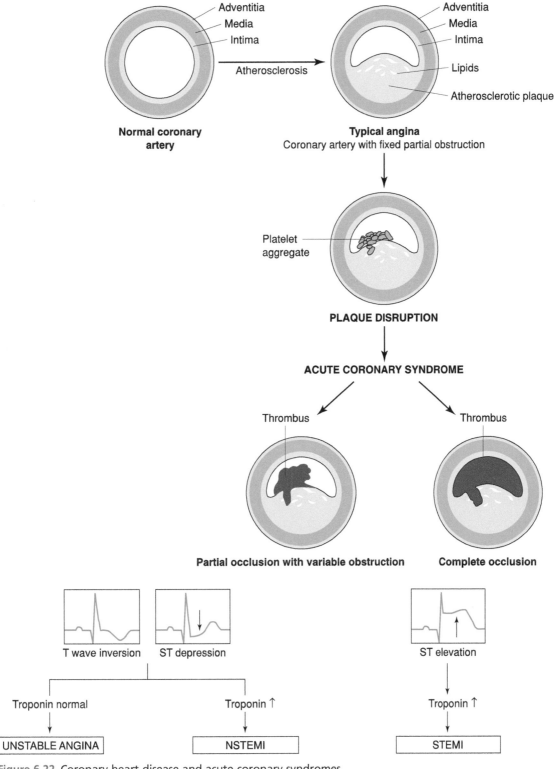

Figure 6.22 Coronary heart disease and acute coronary syndromes

Source: Adapted from Harrison, R. and Daley, L. (2011) *A Nurse's Survival Guide to Acute Medical Emergencies*, 3rd edn. Churchill Livingstone, Edinburgh. Copyright © Elsevier 2011.

The National Institute for Health and Clinical Excellence issued guidance for the assessment and management of unstable angina and NSTEMI (NICE 2010b). This guidance assists practitioners to make quick accurate assessment of the patient with suspected ACS when ST elevation is not present on the ECG, and to initiate immediate interventions. The treatments for unstable angina and NSTEMI are essentially the same and focus on pain relief and anticoagulation, which is given according to bleeding risk and planned angiography. Priorities of ACS management include:

- performing a rapid ABCDE and EWS score and seeking medical advice as appropriate;
- sitting the patient upright and giving oxygen to maintain target saturations of 94–98% (if COPD excluded);
- obtaining a 12-lead ECG;
- assessing chest pain using an objective scale;
- establishing IV access and giving diamorphine 2.5–5mg IV (the preferred analgesic), with an anti emetic as required;
- giving anticoagulation as prescribed, normally fondaparinux, or unfractionated heparin according to bleeding risk and likelihood of angiography;
- giving antiplatelet therapy as prescribed, normally aspirin, clopidogrel, or glycoprotein IIb/IIIa inhibitor (NICE 2010c).

STEMI

A total occlusion of a coronary artery starves the myocardial cells of oxygen and causes myocardial infarction (MI). The extent of the myocardial infarction depends on where the occlusion occurs, the more proximal the occlusion in the coronary artery, the larger the area of myocardial injury. For example, an occlusion of the left coronary artery at its origin (near the aorta) will affect the entire left ventricle. An occlusion at the distal end of the coronary artery will cause a small, more localised infarction. In both cases, the tissue beyond the occlusion will quickly become necrotic if reperfusion is not re-established.

Myocardial infarction

Myocardial infarction is therefore categorised in one of two ways:

1 Non-ST elevation MI (NSTEMI)
2 ST elevation MI (STEMI).

In *NSTEMI*, the infarcted area is within the ventricular wall, but does not extend through the entire wall. In this case, there is some tissue surrounding the infarcted area that is ischaemic and hence the ECG leads facing this area will show ischaemic changes. NSTEMI can easily be mistaken for unstable angina, as the ECG changes are the same, until troponin levels are received. In *STEMI*, the full thickness of the ventricle wall is affected and will show up as ST segment elevation in the ECG leads facing the infarcted ventricular wall. In both STEMI and NSTEMI, there will be biochemical (raised serum troponin levels) evidence of tissue injury in addition to the symptoms of cardiac chest pain and ECG changes.

Biochemical markers of myocardial infarction

Troponin T and troponin I markers are important in the diagnosis of MI. They appear in serum 3–6 hours after onset of symptoms.

Higher levels of troponin T and troponin I are predictive of poor outcomes.

In unstable angina troponin is not significantly raised.

The 12-lead ECG in ACS

A 12-lead ECG should be recorded at the earliest opportunity and will almost immediately show the tell-tale signs of ischaemia and infarction. This is one of the essential criteria for diagnosing ACS. The ECG changes will evolve as the coronary event progresses, so it is important to take a series of ECGs at 5–10 minute intervals, or as the patient's condition improves or deteriorates. This will give detailed information about the extent, location and evolution of the coronary event.

STEMI

The 30-day mortality for STEMI is about 50%, and of this group 50% will die in the first 2 hours. Many die before reaching hospital.

ST segment elevation occurs when the myocardium is being starved of oxygen and is starting to break down. At this point, the condition is reversible providing that early intervention to open up the affected artery is established. The location of the myocardial infarction (and hence the artery that is occluded) can be seen by looking at the leads in which the ST elevation occurs. The 12-lead ECG features of STEMI include:

- ST elevation will be present in at least two adjacent leads, depending on the extent of the infarction.
- Q waves greater than 25% of the overall height of the QRS complex. These may be seen simultaneously with the ST segment elevations and indicate that the myocardial injury is progressing on to permanent, irreversible myocardial damage.

STEMI: restoring perfusion

Reperfusion therapy either by

- primary percutaeneous coronary intervention (PCI); or by
- thrombolytic therapy (if PCI) contraindicated.

Rescue angioplasty within 2–3 hours may be required if thrombolysis fails and complete occlusion remains.

If significant occlusion remains after thrombolyisis may require angioplasty after 1–7 days.

The 12-lead ECG features of NSTEMI include:

- ST segment depression or T wave inversion located on the leads that are adjacent to the affected area. This shows reduced myocardial perfusion and is reversible: the sooner coronary flow is restored, the less the damage incurred.

Arrhythmias

The electrical conduction system is responsible for initiating and coordinating the muscular contraction that pushes the blood through the chambers of the heart, generating the cardiac output. Problems with the conduction system can occur and these are important because they can directly affect the ability of the heart to maintain adequate blood pressure, cardiac output and organ perfusion. Rhythm problems therefore need to be detected so that action can be taken to treat the arrhythmia, or reduce the affects of the arrhythmia on the cardiac output.

Before examining common arrhythmias it is important that you are confident in recognising sinus rhythm. While the study of arrhythmias can be interesting and challenging, the essential requirement of the nurse is the ability to recognise deviation from the patient's normal rhythm and evaluate the clinical affect of the arrhythmia (such as changes in blood pressure, breathlessness and/or onset of chest pain), so that early medical review can be requested in the event of rhythm change. For this reason sinus rhythm and only the most common arrhythmias of sinus tachycardia, sinus bradycardia and atrial fibrillation, will be discussed in this section.

The arrest arrhythmias of ventricular fibrillation, ventricular tachycardia (without a pulse), asystole and pulseless electrical activity, have such a devastating affect that the patient becomes unresponsive with no breathing or pulse (RCUK 2011). These are discussed in Chapter 7.

Sinus rhythm

The PQRST complex has been described earlier in the chapter. Sinus rhythm has the following characteristics (see also Table 6.7):

- rate of between 60–100 beats per minute;
- regular;
- P wave is present;
- P–R interval is normal (between 0.12–0.2 seconds or three to five small squares on ECG paper);
- QRS complex follows the P wave (duration less than 0.12 seconds or three small squares on ECG paper;
- T wave.

Sinus arrhythmia refers to the normal increase in heart rate that occurs during inspiration. This is a normal response seen more in children than adults, and is not a cause for concern. The rate of sinus rhythm will vary according to parasympathetic and sympathetic activity and will generally change over a period of time, rather than suddenly. You may notice a patient's heart rate rise when talking to relatives or after moving from bed to the chair, but this should fall back to the resting rate within a few minutes. The complexes look identical and originate from the sinus node. An example of sinus rhythm is given in Figure 6.23.

Sinus bradycardia

Sinus bradycardia is a regular heartbeat that originates from the sino-atrial node, but at a rate lower than 60 beats per minute (see Figure 6.24). While in a healthy heart this may not cause problems with cardiac output because there is a corresponding increase in stroke volume, in the diseased heart sinus bradycardia may cause circulatory compromise. If the patient becomes symptomatic, feeling dizzy, fainting, experiences chest pain, has a low blood pressure or becomes breathless, treatment will be required.

Supplemental oxygen to maintain saturations between an agreed target range of 94–98% should be commenced. IV access will be needed and atropine 0.5–3 mg IV may be prescribed as this inhibits the effect of the parasympathetic vagus nerve and allows the sinus node to increase the heart rate. If the bradycardia is extreme, a temporary pacemaker may be indicated. It is important that medications the patient is taking are reviewed: common cardiac drugs such as beta-blockers, digoxin and calcium antagonists such as diltiazam can cause a reduction in heart rate.

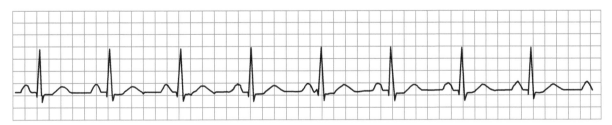

Figure 6.23 Sinus rhythm

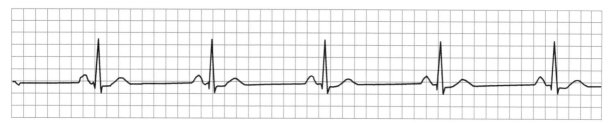

Figure 6.24 Sinus bradycardia

Causes of sinus bradycardia

- Myocardial infarction
- Hypothryoidism
- Digoxin, beta-blockers
- Increased intercranial pressure
- Athletic heart
- Sleep
- Hypothermia.

Abnormal parasympathetic stimulation such as:

- carotid sinus pressure;
- tracheal suctioning;
- valsalva manoeuvre (breath-holding and bearing down);
- reflex actions from the stimulation of PNS terminations in arteries; sometimes seen when arterial cannula sheaths are removed from the femoral artery following cardiac catheterisation.

Sinus bradycardia will contain the features listed in Table 6.7, it is similar to sinus rhythm in all but rate. If a slow rhythm does not have the features of sinus bradycardia, for example the PR interval is prolonged, or not every P wave is followed by a QRS complex, then the patient has other conduction problems such as heart block, which may require intervention even if the patient is not symptomatic; urgent medical review should be sought. Medical practitioners are guided by the Resuscitation Council (RCUK 2010a) Adult Bradycardiac Algorithm (see Figure 6.25) when selecting treatment.

Sinus tachycardia

Sinus tachycardia is a regular heartbeat that originates from the sino-atrial node, but at a rate faster than 100 beats per minute (see Figure 6.26). The resting heart rate will not normally be above 100 beats per minute so the patient should be carefully assessed to determine the cause of the tachycardia. Sinus tachycardia is non-paroxysmal, that is it doesn't start or end abruptly, which is a feature of other tachyarrhythmias. It would seem logical that an increased heart rate would always improve cardiac output and tissue perfusion, but this is not always the case. You may remember that the heart spends a larger proportion of the cardiac cycle in diastole, the filling phase. As the heart rate increases it is the diastolic phase which shortens, and as the rate moves towards 140, the time for ventricular filling may be significantly reduced, so cardiac output actually falls. Shortened diastole can also lead to a reduction in coronary artery blood flow, resulting in angina, increasing areas of myocardial ischaemia and infarction as the oxygen supply cannot meet the demand of the rapidly contracting myocardium. Oxygen therapy may be required while the cause of sinus

Table 6.7 Features of selected rhythms

	Sinus rhythm	Sinus bradycardia	Sinus tachycardia	Atrial fibrillation
Heart rate	60–100	< 60bpm	> 100bpm	Any rate but usually 100–180bpm
Heart rhythm	Regular	Regular	Regular	Irregularly irregular
P wave	Present precede each QRS complex	Present precede each QRS complex	Present precede each QRS complex	None Fibrillating wave seen
P–R interval	Normal (3–5 small squares)	Normal (3–5 small squares)	Normal (3–5 small squares)	None
QRS complex	Normal duration (less than 3 small squares) Preceded by P wave	Normal duration (less than 3 small squares) Preceded by P wave	Normal duration (less than 3 small squares) Preceded by P wave	Normal duration (less than 3 small squares)

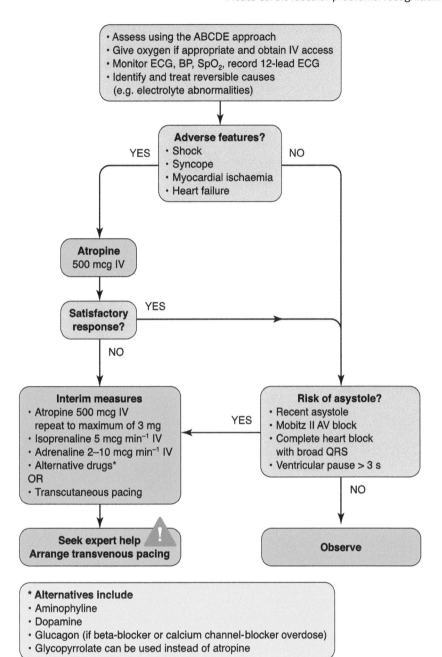

- Assess using the ABCDE approach
- Give oxygen if appropriate and obtain IV access
- Monitor ECG, BP, SpO₂, record 12-lead ECG
- Identify and treat reversible causes
  (e.g. electrolyte abnormalities)

Adverse features?
- Shock
- Syncope
- Myocardial ischaemia
- Heart failure

YES   NO

Atropine
500 mcg IV

Satisfactory response?   YES

NO

Interim measures
- Atropine 500 mcg IV
  repeat to maximum of 3 mg
- Isoprenaline 5 mcg min⁻¹ IV
- Adrenaline 2–10 mcg min⁻¹ IV
- Alternative drugs*
OR
- Transcutaneous pacing

YES

Risk of asystole?
- Recent asystole
- Mobitz II AV block
- Complete heart block
  with broad QRS
- Ventricular pause > 3 s

NO

Seek expert help
Arrange transvenous pacing

Observe

* Alternatives include
- Aminophyline
- Dopamine
- Glucagon (if beta-blocker or calcium channel-blocker overdose)
- Glycopyrrolate can be used instead of atropine

Figure 6.25 Adult bradycardia algorithm

Source: Resuscitation Council UK (2010) *2010 Resuscitation Guidelines*, p. 88. Reproduced with the kind permission of Resuscitation Council UK.

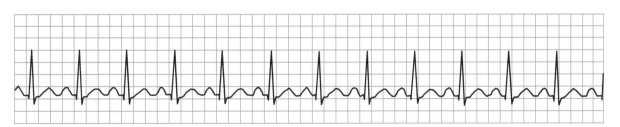

Figure 6.26 Sinus tachycardia

Table 6.8 Action to be taken on detecting cardiac arrhythmia

ABCDE assessment performed:

- If patient is unresponsive – initiate BLS/ALS
- If patient is asymptomatic – no immediate treatment indicated (refer for expert advice)
- If patient is symptomatic – treatment required to control rate and rhythm using RCUK (2010) algorithms as a guide

Sources: Adapted from Foxall (2010), Cardiac Rhythm Recognition M&K Update Cumbria.

tachycardia is detected and rectified. Ensuring that the patient not hypoxaemic and is adequately filled or not dehydrated, is a good starting point.

Causes of sinus tachycardia

- Fever
- Stress and anxiety, pain
- Vagus nerve inhibition
- Sympathetic stimulation
- Anaemia
- Hypovolaemia
- Sepsis
- Anaphylaxis
- Increased thyroxine levels
- Heart failure
- Caffeine
- Salbutamol.

Sinus tachycardia contains all the features of sinus rhythm apart from the rate, which will be above 100 beats per minute (see Table 6.8). If the patient has a fast heart rate but the features of sinus tachycardia are *not* present, for example from any of the following, no P waves are visible, P–R interval is shorter than three small squares, QRS complexes are wider than three small squares, the rhythm is irregular, or perhaps it has started abruptly, this will not be sinus tachycardia. A rapid assessment should be performed to detect cardiovaslucar compromise, oxygen therapy should be initiated to maintain saturations between 94–98%, IV access gained as appropriate and urgent medical review is indicated. Treatment for tachycardia (other than sinus tachycardia) will be guided by the RCUK (2010b) adult tachycardia with a pulse algorithm (see Figure 6.27).

Atrial fibrillation

Atrial fibrillation (AF) is the most common sustained cardiac arrhythmia (NICE 2006). AF is an atrial arrhythmia that does not originate from the sinus node. It consists of chaotic atrial impulses, firing at a rate of 400–600 per minute, from different ectopic foci. P waves

are absent, and fibrillatory waves can be seen, often with a wandering baseline (see Figure 6.28). The AV node receives these impulses, but only allows 120–180 of these to proceed to the ventricles, to produce the QRS complex and ventricular contraction. The transmission of impulses through to the ventricle is unpredictable, giving rise to a very irregular ventricular response, resulting in an irregularly irregular pulse being palpated on assessment. Diagnosis will be confirmed by a 12-lead ECG. The atria have no coordinated contraction, and therefore do not expel their contents into the ventricle in ventricular diastole. This leads to a reduced ventricular preload, especially when the ventricular response rate is high. AF then can give rise to serious haemodynamic problems in the short term, particularly when the ventricular response rate is rapid. Rate control may be the preferred management option: as the rate decreases, ventricular filling increases and cardiac output improves.

Factors contributing to atrial fibrillation

- Hypoxaemia
- Hypertension
- Heart failure
- Obesity
- COPD
- Infection
- Ischaemic heart disease
- Age
- Sympathetic stimulation
- Drugs
- Electrolyte disturbance
- Mitral valve disease
- Coronary artery disease
- Diabetes.

Immediate management involves ensuring adequate oxygenation, if necessary by giving supplemental oxygen to maintain the target saturation. Serum electrolytes should be replaced as necessary. NICE (2006) has developed guidance, with treatment options including rhythm control or rate control. Chemical cardioversion using medications such as amiodorone or digoxin is aimed at restoring sinus rhythm, as is electrical cardioversion by a synchronised electrical shock (used when AF onset is less than 48 hours). Beta-blockers or calcium channel-blockers may be the agents of choice for rate control, to reduce rate and improve cardiac output. Response to treatment should be evaluated clinically and by 12-lead ECG recordings.

Atrial fibrillation: serum electrolytes

- Check serum K⁺ (normal range 3.5–5mmol/L replace as necessary.
- Check serum Mg⁺ (normal range 0.75–1mmol/L) and replace as necessary.

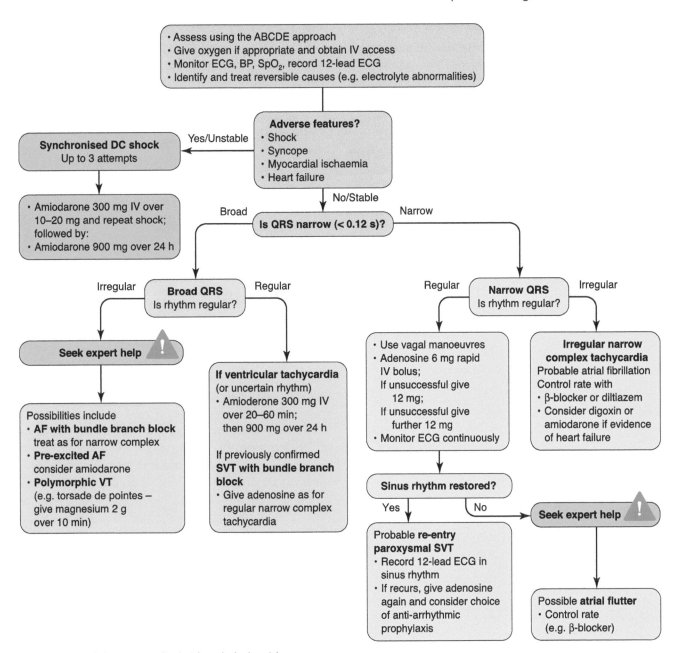

Figure 6.27 Adult tachycardia (with pulse) algorithm

Source: Resuscitation Council UK (2010) *2010 Resuscitation Guidelines*, p. 83. Reproduced with the kind permission of Resuscitation Council UK.

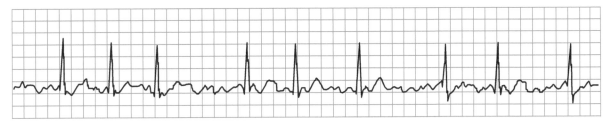

Figure 6.28 Atrial fibrillation

The formation of clots in the atria, due to the stasis of atrial blood in persistent AF (longer than 48 hours) can give rise to serious embolic problems. Though embolic episodes can effect many organs such as the kidney, the gut or even the peripheral circulation, the most serious is a thrombus travelling to the brain causing a cerebral infarction, or stroke. Anticoagulation using low molecular weight heparin in the short term, and aspirin or warfarin in the longer term, is an integral part of AF management, particularly if other relevant risk factors are present (ESC 2010).

General management of cardiac arrhythmias

If a cardiac arrhythmia is detected then a full assessment of the patient's condition is required. Often, when the arrhythmia does not affect the patient's cardiovascular status, no immediate treatment is indicated. However, if the arrhythmia results in any change to the patient's cardiac or neurological status, appropriate treatment must be initiated, the action to be taken in the event of a cardiac arrhythmia is detected is given in Table 6.8. Oxygen therapy should be used to maintain SpO_2 between 94–98% (O'Driscoll et al. 2008). A full assessment of the patient's airway, breathing and circulation (ABC) must be performed immediately, with a focus on circulation to assess compromise. The early warning score will help identify the urgency with which to call for medical evaluation and treatment. The extent to which the patient is affected by the arrhythmia will inevitably guide the subsequent management. If the patient loses consciousness, then cardiopulmonary resuscitation is required (see Chapter 7).

Severe acute LVF

Severe acute LVF can be frightening and distressing for patients and their families and is potentially a life-threatening event. The left ventricle is suddenly overwhelmed with the amount of blood returning to it from the pulmonary circulation, giving rise to increased hydrostatic pressures in the pulmonary vasculature and the formation of pulmonary oedema. Symptoms of breathlessness, tachypnoea, acute anxiety, tachycardia, confusion and the production of frothy sputum are a cause for serious concern, and usually occur in those with long-term heart failure as an acute exacerbation. Acute LVF may be caused by cardiac trigger such as ACS, or respiratory triggers such as a recent chest infection, but may also be linked with non-compliance with medications (Macintosh 2011). Management of LVF is directed at supporting airway breathing and circulation and includes the following:

- High-flow oxygen therapy to maintain SpO_2 between 94–98% (as per prescribed target oxygen saturation).
- Positioning patient upright to reduce venous return and reduce work of breathing (take care if the patient is hypotensive, they may need to be in the supine position).
- Administering IV diamorphine 2.5–5mg as prescribed to reduce the sympathetic stimulus, thereby reducing anxiety. Diamorphine also causes vasodilation and therefore reduces the work of the left ventricle.
- Administer a diuretic (often furosemide 40–80mg IV) as prescribed, to reduce pulmonary oedema and breathlessness.
- Consider using CPAP or BiPAP to reduce alveolar fluid, reduce work of breathing and improve oxygenation.
- Administer GTN, sublingually, or as an infusion as prescribed to increase venous capacitance, and reduce pulmonary capillary pressure (Dickstein et al. 2008).

Venous thromboembolic (VTE) disorders

A venous thromboembolism (VTE) is sometimes referred to as a deep vein thrombosis (DVT) and pulmonary embolism (PE). VTE is a condition in which a blood clot (thrombus) forms in a vein, most commonly it occurs in the deep veins of the leg as a DVT. If the thrombus dislodges from its site of origin to travel in the bloodstream a phenomenon called embolism develops. Thrombi may occur due to damaged blood vessel walls such as varicose veins, due to stasis of blood in the veins caused by immobility or abnormalities of the clotting mechanism. Signs of a DVT may include:

- a red, swollen calf of affected limb;
- increase in temperature of affected limb;

Risk factors for VTE

- active cancer or cancer treatment;
- age over 60 years;
- critical care admission;
- dehydration;
- known thrombophilias;
- obesity (body mass index [BMI] over 30kg/m²);
- one or more significant medical co-morbidities (for example: heart disease; metabolic, endocrine or respiratory pathologies; acute infectious diseases; inflammatory conditions);
- personal history or first-degree relative with a history of VTE;
- use of hormone replacement therapy;
- use of oestrogen-containing contraceptive therapy;
- varicose veins with phlebitis.

(NICE 2010d)

- pain in lower limb on dorsiflexion;
- distal venous dilation;
- pyrexia.

It should be noted that many people with DVT have no symptoms at all. Diagnosis can be made by ultrasound, contrast venography and D dimers. D dimers is a blood test for abnormal levels of clot breakdown products, indicating a clot is present (Humphrey 2008).

Part or all of the thrombus in the vein can move through the vena cavae and lodge in the pulmonary vasculature, the likelihood of this occurring has been estimated at around 50%. Pulmonary embolus is a life-threatening medical emergency, therefore prevention and early recognition of DVT is essential. Clinical guidance issued via NICE (NICE 2010d) requires that all patients on admission are assessed for their risk of developing a venous thromboembolism. This risk should be reassessed within 24 hours and whenever there is a change in clinical condition. All those at risk should have prophylactic therapy initiated. Preventive therapy may be mechanical devices with any one of:

- anti-embolic stockings thigh or knee length;
- intermittent pneumatic compression devices;
- foot impulse devices.

In addition to one pharmacological therapy such as:

- fondaparinux sodium;
- low molecular weight heparin injections.

Pharmacological prophylaxis should continue until the patient is no longer at risk.

Pulmonary embolism can lead to rapid onset respiratory failure and in cases of massive PE, sudden cardiorespiratory arrest. It has been suggested that half of those who develop a PE will do so while an inpatient (Heit *et al.* 2002) with mortality rates of between 6% and 15%. Symptoms of PE become apparent when greater than 30–50% of the pulmonary arterial bed becomes occluded (Torbicki *et al.* 2008). A PE should be suspected in those with sudden otherwise unexplained shortness of breath, particularly in the presence of known risk factors. The priorities of care are to maximise oxygenation through

---

Signs and symptoms of pulmonary embolus

- Breathlessness and tachypnoea
- Chest pain
- Haemoptysis
- Collapse
- Hypotension
- Hypoxaemia.

---

positioning to facilitate lung expansion, oxygen therapy, comfort to minimise anxiety and to ensure expert help is summoned.

According to both NICE (2010d) and the British Thoracic Society Guidance (BTS 2003) diagnosis of PE other than by clinical signs, which can be non-specific, should be established by Computerised Tomography Pulmonary Angiogram (CTPA). First-line treatment for a non-massive PE is heparin, either IV unfractionated heparin, subcutaneous low molecular weight heparin, or subcutaneous fondaparinux. If the suspicion that this is a PE is high, then unfractionated heparin may be given prior to confirmation by CTPA. Otherwise low molecular weight heparin is preferable as it is safer and easier to use. The clotting test, activated partial thromboplastin time (aPPT), is used to adjust unfractionated heparin doses, with a target of 1.5–2 times the control. Once PE is reliably confirmed oral anticoagulation (warfarin) can be started with a target international normalised ration (INR) of 2.0–3.0 (Torbicki *et al.* 2008). In the case of massive PE with circulatory collapse, thrombolysis is the first-line treatment.

International normalised ratio (INR)

This is a measure of coagulation. It is a value derived from the ratio between the patient's actual prothrombin time and the normal value (11–16 secs).

The normal range for INR is 0.8–1.2.

A high INR means there is a likely chance of bleeding while a low reading means there is a likely chance of clot formation.

Acute circulatory collapse

The functioning cardiovascular system requires that the heart works as an effective pump, that there is sufficient circulatory volume in the form of blood, a systemic vasculature that enables flow and can constrict/dilate to maintain perfusion pressure. If one of these components fails, then circulation is impaired and acute circulatory collapse will develop. Acute circulatory collapse is a life-threatening medical emergency in which the oxygen supply to the tissues at cellular level is insufficient to meet their demands. The hypoxic tissues metabolise anaerobically leading to acidosis, organ damage and cellular death (cellular hypoxia is discussed in Chapter 3). The nurse's assessment will help to identify which one of the components of circulation is the likely cause of the circulatory collapse, and this will help guide treatment accordingly.

The problems that can lead to circulatory failure can be categorised according to the aetiology (or mechanism):

- Hypovolaemic
- Obstructive
- Distributive
- Cardiogenic.

Classification of shock

Hypovolaemia: loss of blood, plasma or extracellular fluid.

Obstructive: inability of the heart to fill effectively, e.g. tamponade, or obstruction to outflow e.g. PE.

Distributive: lack of sympathetic tone, sepsis, anaphylactic reaction.

Cardiogenic: problem with the pumping ability of the heart.

Whatever the aetiology of shock, it will normally progress through three distinct phases which, unless the causes are identified and successfully treated, will result in an inevitable pathway to death. These stages of shock can be classified into:

- Compensated
- Progressive
- Irreversible (refractory).

A summary of these stages is given in Table 6.9.

Hypovolaemic shock

As the name suggests, hypovolaemic shock is a problem with the blood or volume component of the circulation. Hypovolaemia is the most common cause of shock and the most easily reversed (Smith 2003, Jevon *et al.* 2008). Volume can be lost from the circulation in a number of ways. External blood loss can easily be identified as long as a comprehensive assessment is performed, internal bleeding is not so easily discernible and information gained from the past medical history and pharmacological therapy contributes to diagnosis. Fluid can also be lost from the circulation into the gut as with paralytic ileus, or the peritoneal space as with liver failure (see Chapter 10). Dehydration can occur from excessive vomiting, diarrhoea, sweating, infection, burns and wound exudate/drainage. Hidden losses are not always easy to estimate and may not be obvious even when accurate fluid balance monitoring is recorded. Insensible losses in health can be around 900mL per day (Porth 2007). As they increase with pyrexia, increased respiratory rate and diarrhoea they need to be taken into account when calculating fluid requirements.

Compensatory mechanisms to regulate blood pressure are effective at preserving pressure in the initial stage of blood/fluid loss. Many people donate about 500mL of blood with few if any adverse clinical affects, and usually feel fine after a drink and a few minutes rest, however as the volume loss increases, compensatory mechanisms are

Table 6.9 Summary of physiological and clinical changes in the three stages of shock

Stage of shock	Response	Assessment findings
Compensated	- Baroreceptor and chemoreceptor activity activates sympathetic nervous system - RAAS activated - ADH secreted	- Blood pressure, heart rate, respiratory rate may have changed, but could still be within normal ranges - Patient's hands, feet and nose may feel a little cool - Patient may feel thirsty
Progressive	- Neurohormonal mechanisms increase their activity - Non-vital areas may suffer hypoxia - Impaired flow to vital organs causing organ dysfunction - Ventilation perfusion mismatch in the lungs as pulmonary circulation impaired - Anaerobic metabolism in hypoxic tissues, production of lactic acid - Cellular function impaired	- Heart rate and respiratory rate raised, urine output decreasing - Blood pressure and SaO_2 falling - Altered level of consciousness - Further changes in peripheral perfusion (cold in hypovolaemic and cardiogenic, warm in septic, neurogenic and anaphylactic shock) - Metabolic acidosis - Raised lactate - Possible pulmonary oedema
Irreversible	- Severe tissue hypoxia, ischaemia and necrosis Release of vasoactive mediators and toxic metabolites	- Severe refractory hypotension, cold clammy skin, tachycardia, respiratory failure, renal failure, alterations in blood clotting. Severe metabolic acidosis

not adequate to maintain tissue perfusion. Early warning tools differ in their ability to alert the nurse to subtle clinical change, therefore significant deterioration may occur prior to key indicators such as systolic blood pressure start to fall.

The compensatory response occurs within seconds of volume loss, sympathetic nervous system-mediated vasoconstriction mobilises blood stored in the venous circulation and spleen to increase blood return (preload) to the heart. Over a brief time, fluid from the interstitial spaces moves to the vascular space, enhancing circulating volume. At 10–15% loss (up to 750mL) ADH from the posterior pituitary stimulates the thirst reflex, constricts peripheral arteries and veins, and increases water retention in the kidneys. A decrease in renal blood flow will activate the renin angiotensin aldosterone system (RAAs) increasing sodium reabsorption and increasing vasomotor tone. Losses of 15–30% cause physiological parameters such as heart rate and respiratory rate to move outside their normal range, pulse pressure may narrow, the skin feel cool and urine output decrease. It is essential that these signs are spotted, as even at this stage the systolic blood pressure may still be within the normal range.

> **Early signs of hypovolaemic shock**
>
> - a trend in rising respiratory rate;
> - changes in peripheral perfusion, hands and nose may feel cool to touch;
> - a reduced urine output (If measured hourly);
> - a trend in rising heart rate;
> - postural hypotension;
> - patent appears restless and fidgety.

As hypovolaemic shock progresses with a volume loss of greater than 30%, the severity of the vasoconstrictive response reduces blood flow and oxygen delivery, and cells convert to anaerobic metabolism, producing lactic acid. As blood pH decreases, the respiratory rate increases to reduce the acid load by exhaling CO_2. Arterial blood gas analysis at this time will reveal a metabolic acidosis with a lowered pH, reduced HCO_3^-, and increased base deficit. Deprived of oxygen the cell cannot maintain the sodium potassium pump, sodium enters the cell causing it to swell, and potassium leaves contributing to a raised serum potassium level. Histamine release increases capillary permeability causing fluid to leak into the interstitial space and further deplete the circulating volume.

The refractory stage is reached as cellular breakdown and acidosis rise to critical levels, reperfusion may lead to reperfusion injury, during which oxygen free radicals damage remaining cells and cause microvascular damage (Strickler 2010). Organ dysfunction and failure will quickly ensue in this refractory stage of shock. The damage

sustained by the kidneys, gastrointestinal tract and blood clotting profiles will eventually lead to an irreversible decline and death.

Treatment for hypovolaemic shock is centred on oxygenation, fluid resuscitation to re-expand circulating volume and treating the underlying cause (Johnson and Henry (2009). Critically ill hypoxaemic patients should receive oxygen via a non re-breathe bag at 15L to maximise oxygen delivery (O'Driscoll et al. 2008). If bleeding is overt then stemming the flow of blood is the immediate priority: this may be achieved by direct pressure, or procedures such as angiography or surgical intervention. Insertion of two wide-bore cannulae enables rapid fluid administration. Smith (2003) advocates a rapid fluid bolus of 500–1000mL of crystalloid (such as 0.9% sodium chloride or Ringer's lactate solution), to be given over 5–10 min as an initial response to hypotension. While crystalloids are generally recommended colloids can be used to expand the intravascular space, though recent studies have failed to consistently demonstrate their benefit to offset the expense of their use (Perrel and Roberts 2007). Patients with blood loss will need blood replacement, a haemoglobin level of about 8g/dL is generally the threshold for blood transfusion, but this may vary according to age or co-morbidities such as significant coronary artery disease (Strickler 2010). Caution should be exercised if there is any history or suspicion of cardiac problems, a reduced fluid challenge of 250mL may be appropriate for this group of patients. The fluid challenge should generate a good clinical response with a decreasing heart rate, respiratory rate and increasing peripheral perfusion. Giving the fluid quickly enables rapid normalisation of clinical parameters and reduces the risk of organ damage. The fluid challenge may need to be repeated but the nurse should be aware of early signs of fluid overload such as a rise in heart rate, a decrease in oxygen saturations and hearing new crackles on lung auscultation. A urinary catheter helps evaluate the renal response to fluid therapy.

> **Crystalloids**
>
> - clear solutions containing electrolytes;
> - move freely into interstitial space;
> - only 1/3 to 1/4 remain in the vascular space, so large volumes needed;
> - cheap, easy to store, no adverse reactions.
>
> **Colloids**
>
> - opaque solutions containing large molecules, surrounded by water;
> - stay within the intravascular space longer;
> - smaller volumes needed;
> - more expensive, higher incidence of adverse reactions.

A central venous catheter is helpful to enable estimation of right atrial filling pressures and this will be inserted by an experienced medical practitioner. Central venous pressure would normally be between 2–8mmHg, but is best interpreted as a series of readings in conjunction with assessment of vascular tone. When hypotension does not respond to fluid alone it may be necessary to consider vasoactive drugs such as noradrenaline. Haemodynamic monitoring and vasoactive support are discussed later in the chapter.

Obstructive shock

Obstructive shock occurs when there is impedance to the flow of blood through the central circulation. A number of conditions can cause obstructive shock, and treatment is focused on the correction of the disorder causing the obstruction. Dissecting aortic aneurysm requires urgent surgical intervention. A large pneumothorax and as a medical emergency, a tension pneumothorax, obstructs venous return to the heart by increasing intrathoracic pressure. Treatment is with high-concentration oxygen and emergency needle decompression, a cannula usually being introduced in the second anterior intercostal space at the mid-clavicular line (MacDuff *et al.* 2010) quickly followed by chest drain insertion (see also Chapter 5).

> **Causes of obstructive shock**
> - Dissecting aortic aneurysm
> - Cardiac tamponade
> - Pneumothorax
> - Pulmonary embolism.

Cardiac tamponade (see also Chapter 7) occurs when the normal 30–50mL of fluid between the layers of the pericardium increases to such an extent that diastolic filling is impeded due to the pressure exerted on the heart. A rapid accumulation of as little of 50mL can be sufficient to cause cardiac arrest, though a gradual build up of a pericardial effusion can accommodate up to 1000mL. Immediate medical intervention of pericardiocentesis is required to relieve the pressure so the ventricle can fill, and cardiac output be maintained.

> Suspect cardiac tamponade with a patient who has:
> - restlessness, confusion;
> - decreased sats, raised RR;
> - cool peripheries, tachycardia hypotension, raised CVP or JVP, pulsus paradoxus, low urine output;
> - recent history of cardiac surgery or trauma;
> - recent history of MI.

Distributive shock

Distributive shock is caused by a lack of ability of the vessels to maintain sympathetic tone, thus systemic vascular resistance falls dramatically, and perfusion pressure is not maintained. Clinically a patient with distributive shock may feel warm, but the perfusion pressure is not adequate to deliver oxygen to the tissues, so anaerobic metabolism and acidosis swiftly follows. Categories of distributive shock are septic, anaphylactic (discussed in Chapter 12) and neurogenic (discussed in Chapter 9).

CASE STUDY 6.2 Mr Peter Fisher

Mr Fisher is a 62-year-old patient on the medical ward recovering from an acute myocardial infarction. He has been on the ward for about 12 hours. The nurse notices that since transfer to the ward, he has only asked for the bottle once and passed 100mls of urine. He is complaining of worsening shortness of breath.

BACKGROUND

Mr Fisher has been transferred from CCU to a general medical ward 48 hours following admission with central chest pain. He had been diagnosed as having an anterior myocardial infarction. At that time the 12-lead ECG had shown ST elevation in leads V1–V4. Following successful reperfusion by stent insertion to his left anterior descending artery, Mr Fisher made an uneventful recovery and was

transferred to the ward 12 hours later. He has no past medical history of note. He is normally a fit and active man who plays golf regularly.

His medications currently are: Simvostatin 40mg daily, Ramapril 2.5mg daily, Aspirin 75mg daily, Clopidogrel 75mg daily, 4L/min oxygen via nasal cannula.

ASSESSMENT

Airway

The nurse notes that Mr Fisher has developed a slight cough, which has started only recently, he is not clearing any secretions. His airway is clear, there is no stridor or wheezing. He is complaining of feeling short of breath, but is able to talk in complete sentences.

CASE STUDY 6.2 Mr Peter Fisher (continued)

Breathing

He is sitting upright, breathing 4L/minute via nasal specs maintaining and SpO$_2$ of 93%, which is below the target range set by the medical staff of 94–98%. His respiratory rate has increased from 22 to 28 breaths per minute. His breathing is regular with normal bilateral chest expansion but some use of accessory muscles indicating increased work of breathing. The nurse hears basal crackles on chest auscultation, and wonders if he may be developing a chest infection. She changes the nasal specs to a venturi mask at 40%, and is pleased to see his SpO$_2$ rise to 95%.

Circulation

His fingers have a blue tinge and the nurse notices that they feel cool. The change in his peripheral temperature is due to vasoconstriction and she notes that this could be due to a problem with cardiac output. His heart rate has increased from 90–100 beats per minute and triggers on the early warning score. He is on a cardiac monitor and a couple of broad large complexes are seen, which she thinks are ventricular ectopics. The nurse plans to check his serum potassium levels as she knows altered levels can contribute to cardiac arrhythmia. He is not complaining of any chest pain. His blood pressure has reduced from 120/70 to 105/65 since his last set of observations. His pulse pressure is calculated to be within the normal range at 40mmHg. His mean arterial pressure is 78mmHg, within normal limits. The nurse notes the trends of rising heart rate falling BP and peripheral cooling and is now a little more concerned. She doubts her first thoughts of a chest infection and starts thinking about his deterioration in cardiovascular status. Capillary refill is sluggish at three seconds. A quick check of the fluid balance chart reveals only 100mL of urine has been passed in 12 hours, and a positive balance of 1000mL. She checks his ankles for pitting oedema, none is present. His central temperature is recorded at 36.5°C. She completes a 12-lead ECG and is pleased to note there are no new changes, but after labelling it clearly puts it aside for the doctor to check.

Disability

Mr Fisher is restless, but fully conscious and orientated scoring A on AVPU scale. Blood glucose is assessed and recorded at 5.2mmol/L.

Exposure

The nurse notes that Mr Fisher has not been weighed this morning, and reflects that this would have been useful information. As he feels breathless Mr Fisher does not want to be weighed now, and as his weight would not have been at the same time of day as his previous weight recording, she does not try to persuade him further. She checks his calves for tenderness or pain, and that the anti-embolic stockings are correctly fitted. He has a venflon *in situ*.

The nurse checks the blood results and notes the serum K$^+$ is 3.4mmols/L.

RESPONSE

After completing and documenting her assessment, the EWS scores 4 (HR 1, RR, 2 and oxygen saturations 1), requiring that the doctor reviews Mr Fisher. She uses SBAR to guide her discussion with the doctor, and she agrees to come and see him within 30 minutes. The doctor agrees that he needs potassium supplements, and possibly an arterial blood gas taken when she arrives. The nurse is asked to arrange a chest X-ray to check whether Mr Fisher is developing pulmonary oedema secondary to heart failure.

Mr Fisher's doctor arrives and reviews the CXR which shows evidence of interstitial pulmonary oedema, and the 12-lead ECG which shows no new changes. She examines Mr Fisher and explains to him that she thinks his heart is not pumping as effectively as it could, probably due to some of the damage that occurred when he had his heart attack.

Arterial blood gasses are taken. The results are:

pH	7.31
PaCO$_2$	4.6kPa
PaO$_2$	8.9kPa
HCO$_3^-$	19
BE	−5.2

The acidosis is noted, and coupled with the reduced bicarbonate and BE indicates a metabolic acidosis. This would be consistent with an altered cardiac output, with not all the tissues receiving enough oxygen delivery to ensure aerobic metabolism of glucose. Action needs to be taken to improve cardiac output.

An echocardiogram is arranged to assess the degree of heart failure and the doctor discusses with the nurse that the immediate aim now is to try and reduce Mr Fisher's symptoms of breathlessness and improve his oxygen saturations by reducing some of the extra fluid in the circulating volume and reducing the amount of work the heart has to do by:

- giving 40mg IV ferusomide, to increase urine output, to reduce the accumulated fluid in Mr Fisher's lungs, to reduce the preload and afterload by reducing the volume

---

CASE STUDY 6.2 Mr Peter Fisher *(continued)*

of blood returning to the failing heart thereby relieving pulmonary oedema;

- reducing the preload of the heart by starting an infusion of nitrocine (glyceryl trinitrate);
- giving some oral potassium supplements as the ferusomide is likely to reduce his serum potassium levels further.

The nurse administered the ferusomide, and commences the nitrocine infusion at 20micrograms per minute as per prescription. The plan is to start at a low dose and up-titrate as Mr Fisher's blood pressure allows. This drug is a potent venodilator and reduces the preload pressure by dilating the pulmonary veins. This also has the additional benefit of reducing hydrostatic pressure in the pulmonary circulation, hence reducing pulmonary oedema. She is concerned that the vasodilatory effects of the nitrocine may cause Mr Fisher's blood pressure to drop, so she stays with him and checks his observations after 15 minutes. She is reassured that his blood pressure and heart rate are stable, and his respiratory rate has reduced a little from 28 to 24 breaths per minute.

Thirty minutes later Mr Fischer asks for a bottle and passes 500mls of urine, he says he is feeling better, and this is confirmed by a quick ABC assessment. His oxygen saturations have now improved to 98%, respiratory rate reduced to 21 breaths per minute. The nurse was pleased that she can no longer hear the crackles at the base of his lungs. His heart rate has reduced back down to 90 per minute with his blood pressure stable at 120/80, his hands feel warm, and his capillary refill time is now less than 2 seconds. She checked the early warning score, and finds that it is now 0. The nurse informs the doctor of Mr Fisher's progress, feeling pleased that his deteriorating status was detected and acted upon promptly, otherwise he may have experienced an episode of acute severe pulmonary oedema, which as a medical emergency is extremely distressing for the patient.

Later echocardiography revealed a reduced ejection fraction of 45%. The doctor explained to Mr Fisher that he would need to have some additional medications for a while to improve his recovery, and reduce the chance of complications. She explains to the nurse that she will come back later when he is fully stable, to consider increasing the ACEI dose, adding a beta-blocker, and maybe later spironolactone to try and reduce the risk of the heart failure as per NICE (2007) and ESC (2008) guidelines.

Cardiogenic shock

Cardiogenic shock occurs when the heart is structurally damaged to the extent that it is no longer able to adequately perfuse the organs of the body. This commonly occurs as a result of major myocardial dysfunction following a myocardial infarction, particularly when a large section of the left ventricle is involved. Cardiogenic shock is a major medical emergency and carries a poor prognosis unless the major organs can be supported until a time when heart function can be restored. Causes of cardiogenic shock have been summarised in Table 6.10.

Signs and symptoms of cardiogenic shock:

- chest pain;
- tachycardia;
- tachypnoea;
- peripheral shutdown (cold and clammy skin);
- reduced mental status;
- reduced or loss of consciousness;
- hypotension;
- oliguria or anuria;
- weak thready pulse.

Investigations required for the patient with cardiogenic shock are based upon the evaluation of the extent of the damage to the heart and the effect that this has on the major organs of the body. They include:

- *Echocardiography* – reveals the amount of ventricular damage that exists and whether heart valves are also affected. The flow of blood through the heart can also be ascertained by this method to show whether the forward flow of blood from the ventricles is impaired. In addition to this, the presence of blood in the pericardium can be seen.
- *Chest X-ray* – useful for visualising the presence of pulmonary oedema that will inevitably occur following left ventricular dysfunction. Where right ventricular dysfunction is present, the signs and symptoms will be similar, but the lung fields might not be oedematous.
- *12-lead ECG* – will show ST segment elevations in the region of an infarction, which is important for the consideration of the complications that might arise from it. For example, ST segment elevations in the leads V1 to V3 indicate an antero-septal MI; which is implicated in septal wall rupture.

Table 6.10 Common causes of cardiogenic shock

Myocardial infarction	Where a large area of the myocardium has been damaged, or has become necrotic. This leads to reduction in ventricular wall movement (hypokinesia) or complete absence of ventricular wall movement (akinesia). Echocardiography reveals the extent of the myocardial dysfunction and the structures involved
Valvular dysfunction	Where the patency of the heart valves has been severely compromised (allowing blood to be regurgitated during systole) the forward flow of blood from the ventricles is reduced. Mechanisms of valvular dysfunction vary, but sudden acute changes occur as a consequence of damage to the structures that normally prevent the valve leaflets from prolapsing into the atria during systole. These structures are the chordae tendonae that attach the valve leaflets to the endocardium, and the papilliary muscles that keep the chordae under tension when they are closed
Rupture of the heart muscle	A complication of myocardial infarction where the ventricular wall becomes so weak that the pressure from within the ventricle during systole forces the wall to disintegrate. Depending on the location, the rupture will either lead to cardiac tamponade whereby the heart becomes constricted by the accumulation of blood in the pericardium. If the rupture occurs in the ventricular septum (between the ventricles) then a shunting of blood from one ventricle to the other will exist, reducing the cardiac output
Bradyarrhythmias	A slow heart rate reduces the cardiac output if there is no corresponding increase in ventricular contractility. These bradyarrhythmias may be a consequence of AV node block, sino-atrial node disease or overdose of heart-rate-lowering drugs

- *Cardiac monitoring* – used continuously to quickly identify changes to the heart's rhythm. Arrhythmia might occur because of the damage to the ventricular wall, or as a result of changes in blood chemistry caused by renal hypoperfusion.
- *Cardiac catheterisation* – a commonly used technique for the evaluation of coronary artery blood flow to the affected region of myocardium.

Management of cardiogenic shock

The priorities are to restore adequate perfusion to the vital organs and to reduce the workload of the heart. As the primary problem is the inability of the heart to provide sufficient cardiac output to achieve organ perfusion, these priorities are interrelated. By improving cardiac output there should be a corresponding increase in perfusion pressure. However, the restoration of myocardial function might require a number of supportive therapies that can only be provided in a critical care environment, such as:

- Inotropic drugs
- Intra-aortic balloon counter pulsation
- Ventricular assist device (VAD).

Cardiogenic shock is a complex condition to manage and requires a wide range of monitoring techniques to guide its management. Inotropic drugs to increase ventricular contractility are essential to restore cardiac output in the short term, but careful titration of these drugs is needed. These measurements and treatments require invasive haemodynamic monitoring systems that would normally only be found in an intensive care (level 3) setting.

Interventions to monitor and support cardiovascular status

Haemodynamic monitoring

Assessment of cardiovascular status is looking for clinical indicators of adequate tissue perfusion, and can usually be obtained by non-invasive means such as clinical observations and the measurement of vital signs using equipment such as pulse oximetry sphygmomanometers or automated blood pressure devices. Patients who are acutely ill may benefit from a continuous display of information so that trends can be more easily observed and adverse events can be predicted and averted in a timely manner. Those who require vasoactive support, to maintain cardiac output and perfusion pressure, require continuous real-time monitoring to enable optimum titration of therapy to meet clinical need. Invasive haemodynamic monitoring involves the placement of a cannula into an artery (normally the radial) and/or a central vein (often internal jugular), connecting it to a transducer system and then a monitor which displays the pressure waveform. The advantages of continuous monitoring have to be weighed against the risks, such as dislodgement, bleeding, inappropriate drug administration, air emboli and sepsis, all of which have the potential to cause severe harm, or even death. Nurses are required to be aware of hazards of common treatments including the use of technology such as invasive monitoring devises (NMC 2010), careful observation and higher staff/patient ratios are required to ensure safe and effective care. Therefore patients who require this level of support to maintain cardiovascular status will normally be nursed in a bed designated for level 2 or level 3 care (ICS 2009). (Please see further reading for more information on haemodynamic monitoring.)

Central venous pressure

Patients who present with cool peripheries and tachycardia are likely to be hypovolaemic. If there is poor response to fluid challenge, obtaining a central venous pressure can help evaluate fluid status and right ventricular function. The fluid challenge may need to be repeated if the CVP is low or normal, to ensure circulating volume is adequate. Central venous pressure is normally between 3–8mmHg, but in clinical practice it may be maintained up to 12mmHg to ensure optimum ventricular preload. Factors that may cause a rise in CVP include:

- heart failure;
- cardiac tamponade;
- tension pneumothorax;
- vasoconstriction (caused by drugs such as adrenaline or as part of the sympathetic response to poor cardiac output).

Fluid challenge

- Measure CVP (also SaO$_2$, resp rate, heart rate, BP urine and peripheral temp).
- Administer 200ml bolus of colloid over 10 mins (or 500ml crystalloid over same period, though caution to be exercised if there is a suspicion of heart failure).
- Transient rise in CVP < 3mmHg (more fluid required?).
- Rise of 3–5mmHg with clinical improvement, normovolaemia achieved.
- > 5mmHg rise with no clinical improvement, or deterioration (Inotropic therapy required as there may be a problem with myocardial contractility).

Factors that may cause a fall in CVP include:

- dehydration;
- vasodilation caused by drugs such as nifedipine, or by distributive shock.

It is important to note that one-off readings for CVP may not be that useful because vasoconstriction can raise CVP and mask hypovolaemia. Trends and response to a fluid challenge, evaluating CVP in conjunction with other clinical parameters such as respiratory rate, oxygen saturation, heart rate, blood pressure and urine output are necessary for managing the patient with poor cardiac output.

Arterial monitoring

Arterial monitoring enables accurate measurements even in low-flow states such as hypovolaemia and sepsis. Real-time monitoring allows for rapid evaluation of circulatory compromise that may occur with ectopics and rhythm disturbances, and also enables titrating of vasoactive medication. Arterial lines have the added benefit of giving access for arterial blood gas sampling, without the need for an arterial stab. This is not only useful for assessing oxygenation and ventilatory requirements but also metabolic problems. An insight into the degree of tissue hypoxia and subsequent anaerobic metabolism can be gained by evaluation of acid-base status (pH), metabolic derangement (BE and HCO$_3^-$) and lactate levels. Trends in acid-base status are useful for evaluating response to interventions such as fluid therapy (given for hypovolaemia) or inotropes and vasoactive therapies.

Vasoactive support therapies

Patients with deteriorating cardiac output who do not respond to initial therapy may require the additional support of vasoactive and/or inotropic agents. It is possible that these drugs may need to be commenced in an acute ward area, in order to stabilise the patient prior to transfer to a higher level of care. Some acute wards have designated level 2 beds and are able to provide care for patients who require single vasoactive or inotropic support therapy.

Vasoactive: affecting vasodilation or vasoconstriction of blood vessels.

Inotropic: affecting the heart's ability to contract.

Vasoactive drugs affect the degree of constriction (vasoconstrictors) or relaxation (vasodilators) of vessels, thereby eliciting varying effects on vascular resistance. Ventricular preload is increased by constricting agents, increasing stroke volume and cardiac output, ventricular afterload is also increased, which will raise the MAP. Dilators will reduce preload and afterload, reducing heart work and MAP, but often resulting in an increase in cardiac output as peripheral resistance falls. In practice, the choice of inotropic agent varies between centres and specialities; the following discussion gives an insight only into the mechanisms and use of this complex group of agents.

Inotropic substances are those that alter myocardial contractility. A positive intotrope increases contractility, thereby increasing stroke volume and cardiac output, and a negative inotrope decreases contractility. Many inotropic

Table 6.11 Summary of effects of sympathomimetic inotropic drugs

Agent	Inotropic effect beta 1 adrenergic receptors	Vascular effect alpha and beta 2 adrenergic receptors	Major use
Adrenaline (low)	β-1	β-2 Dilatation	SBP < 90 despite fluids
High dose	β-1	α Constriction	
Dobutamine	β-1	β-2 Dilatation	Low CO, heart failure, cardiogenic shock
Dopamine			
medium dose	β-1	Low CO	
high dose	β-1	α Constriction	SBP < 90 despite fluids
Noradrenaline		α Intense constriction	Sepsis SBP < 90 despite fluids

Sources: Adapted from Cooper and Salsi (2008) and Coons and Seidl (2007).

agents also have chronotropic properties (affecting heart rate), and vasoactive properties, therefore they can be somewhat complex to manage. For a summary of inotropic agents and their action see Table 6.11. The evidence for improved outcomes with choice of **vasopressor** for problems such as hypovolaemic shock is not clear and a recent Cochrane review was unable to demonstrate mortality differences between six different vasopressors (Havel *et al.* 2011). Specific agent choice is by practitioner preference. You may find it helpful to refer back to the section on blood pressure control, to check refresh your memory on beta 1, beta 2 and alpha adrenergic receptors before looking at Table 6.11.

Intravenous vasoactive and inotropic drugs are normally only administered in areas that are designated for nursing patients of level 2 or 3 dependency (DH 2000, ICS 2009). This is due to several factors, not least of which is that patients who require this type of support are potentially or actually very sick and require frequent/continuous observations of haemodynamic parameters. Nurses are required by the NMC to act within the limits of their own competence (NMC 2010), close supervision and additional preparation may be necessary to equip the nurse with the skills required to safely care for patients requiring vasoactive support, and those of level 2 and level 3 dependency. These intravenous drugs are very potent and have very short half-lives, so plasma concentrations can fall very rapidly. The short life is advantageous in that it allows the experienced clinician to titrate the dose on the basis of required effects (e.g. increase in BP) against the non-required effects (e.g. tachycardia). The nurse needs to understand these physiological effects so that they can be monitored closely, in order for the

Half-life

The half-life of a drug is the time it takes for the plasma concentration to reach half of its original concentration.

Catecholamine (sympathomimetic) inotropic drugs have a short half-life of 1–2 minutes, and reach maximum plasma concentration in about 10 minutes.

Catecholamine inotropes include:

- Adrenaline
- Noradrenaline
- Dobutamine
- Dopamine.

health care team to make appropriate decisions regarding treatment. Doses are calculated and prescribed in micrograms per kilogramme per minute, to ensure they are tailored precisely to patient needs. The calculations can be challenging so even experienced nurses may need to update their numeracy skills to ensure that correct doses are given. To ensure the delivery of a consistent even infusion, inotropes will always be administered via a volumetric pump or syringe driver and through a clearly labelled dedicated lumen on a central line to prevent accidental bolus doses. Peripheral lines are not appropriate due to the high risk of necrosis if extravasation occurs. Continuous monitoring of blood pressure via an arterial line will alert the nurse to any changes in flow rate and drug delivery, which may result in significant deterioration. It is important that patients with hypovolaemic or distributive shock have an adequate circulating volume prior to commencement of inotropic support, to ensure organ perfusion is optimised, as many inotropes cause vasoconstriction at higher doses which could actually reduce organ perfusion.

Inotropes and vasopressors can be extremely effective at restoring adequate oxygen to the tissues in the shocked state. However, there are a number of issues of which the nurse should be aware when caring for a patient receiving such therapy. Vasoconstrictive agents can cause reduced peripheral blood flow, causing ischaemia which can be a problem for patients with existing peripheral vascular disease. Sympathomimetic agents may increase myocardial ischaemia and myocardial irritability, rendering the patient vulnerable to cardiac arrhythmias, so continuous ECG monitoring and maintenance of electrolytes within normal limits is a priority. These agents also decrease serum potassium levels and increase the risk of arrhythmia further. Sympathomimetic agents raise serum glucose levels, so these need to be closely monitored and treated as necessary.

Vasodilators such as glyceryl trinitrate (GTN) reduce preload and afterload, and increase myocardial perfusion through dilating coronary arteries and improving collateral flow. GTN is used in decompensated heart failure and ACS.

Inodilators such as milrinone belong to a group of drugs called phosphodiesterase inhibitors (PDI). This group of inotropes have a much longer half-life, and also have profound vasodilator properties. PDIs are ideal for management of severe congestive heart failure, and are often used in conjunction with other vasoactive/inotropic medication.

Conclusion

A functioning cardiovascular system is crucial to ensure that oxygen and nutrients are delivered to the body tissues adequate to their needs and to remove potentially harmful waste products. Acute exacerbation of chronic cardiovascular disease and circulatory failure are common and potentially serious problems. This chapter has reviewed physiological concepts of the cardiovascular system and considered some common cardiovascular problems and those that may lead to a medical emergency. The nurse's role in assessment and management has been explored, and concepts relating to the more highly dependent patient with deteriorating cardiovascular function have been introduced. Nurses are required by the *Code* of Conduct (NMC 2008) to provide a high standard of care at all times. The code opens with the line 'The people in your care must be able to trust you with their health and wellbeing' (NMC 2008). In order to ensure this, care delivered to patients needs to be underpinned by a sound knowledge base to ensure competent practice. As can be seen from the case studies presented, problems which are primarily of a circulatory nature can have a profound effect on the respiratory system as the two systems work closely together to ensure adequate oxygen supply to the tissues. Without this understanding, it is not possible to interpret what you observe and therefore to make the full assessment necessary to ensure the safety and well-being of the patient.

Glossary

Action potential An event in which the electrical membrane potential of a cell rapidly changes due to ionic movement in and out of the cell. In the cardiac cell, this starts the wave of depolarisation giving rise to the PQRS complex.

Acute coronary syndrome (ACS) An umbrella term encompassing unstable angina, NSTEMI and STEMI.

Adrenergic receptors Receptors of the sympathetic nervous system, subdivided into alpha beta 1 and beta 2.

Afterload The load the (normally left) ventricle has to work against to open the aortic valve and eject its stroke volume. It can also be seen as ventricular wall stress in systole.

Aldosterone A hormone produced by the adrenal cortex. Aldosterone increases sodium and water reabsorption from the distal convoluted tubule in the kidney and increases potassium excretion.

Alpha receptor Receptor of the sympathetic nervous system mainly located in the peripheral vasculature.

Anaemia A lower than normal number of red blood cells which depletes the ability to transport oxygen.

Angiotensin-converting enzyme inhibitors (ACEI) A hormone necessary for the conversion of angiotensin 1 to angiotensin 2.

Anion Negatively charged ion.

Antidiuretic hormone (ADH) Also known as vasopressin, ADH is a hormone secreted from the posterior pituitary which promotes reabsorption of water back into the circulation via the collecting ducts of the kidney. It also causes widespread constriction of arterioles, which leads to increased arterial pressure.

Atherosclerosis Disease of large and medium-sized muscular arteries where the lumen of the vessel is narrowed by build-up of lipid, cholesterol and calcium. This build-up results in plaque formation, abnormalities of blood flow and eventually diminished oxygen delivery.

Atrial fibrillation Common cardiac arrhythmia in which multiple ectopic foci in the atria cause them to fibrillate, rather than contracting in a coordinated manner. AF is characterised by an irregular pulse and lack of p waves on the ECG.

Atrial flutter Cardiac arrhythmia in which a single ectopic focus in the atria fires rapidly causing abnormal atrial conduction. Atrial flutter is normally regular (or regularly irregular) and is characterised by 'saw tooth' waves replacing the P wave on the ECG.

Atrioventricular node The conduit of the electrical impulse from the atria to the ventricles.

Automaticity The capacity of a cell to initiate an impulse without an external stimulus, i.e. to spontaneously generate an impulse.

Autonomic nervous system The nervous system is divided into the somatic (voluntary) and autonomic (involuntary). The autonomic regulates individual organ function and homeostasis.

Baroreceptors Sensory nerve endings in the carotid bodies and aortic arch that detect stretch and therefore blood pressure changes.

Basophil A type of white blood cell that contains histamine and heparin.

Beta adrenergic receptor A receptor of the sympathetic nervous system subtypes; beta 1 (in myocardium) and beta 2 (in smooth muscle).

Cardiac output The amount of blood ejected by the ventricle in one minute:

$$CO = SV \times HR$$

Cardiovascular centre An area in the medulla of the brain that regulates the cardiovascular system. It responds to sensory information from the autonomic nervous system, and acts to maintain cardiac output via the sympathetic and parasympathetic nerves.

Cation Positively charged ion.

Centrifuge A device that separates the components of a liquid, by spinning the liquid at a high speed.

Colloid oncotic pressure The pressure exerted by plasma proteins that pulls water back into capillaries.

Compliance When referring to the heart: the ease with which the ventricle expands or stretches to accommodate ventricular filling.

Conduction system Specialised conducting tissue of the heart which transmits an electrical wave across the heart, causing myocardial contraction.

Contractility The ability of the myocardium to contract.

Coronary circulation Arterial supply for the heart, arising from behind the aortic cusps of the aortic valve.

Depolarisation A rapid movement of ions across the cell membrane causing a change in voltage, that leads to the action potential. In cardiac muscle this initiates myocardial contraction.

Diastole The resting phase of the cardiac cycle in which ventricular filling occurs.

Diastolic pressure The pressure exerted (usually in the vessels) during the relaxation phase of the cardiac cycle.

Ejection fraction The amount of blood ejected from the ventricle in systole, divided by the amount of blood that was in the ventricle at the end of diastole.

Electrolyte A solution containing solutes that can conduct an electrical charge.

Embolism Circulating foreign object such as air, fat or a blood clot which can lodge in and block a vessel.

End diastolic volume The amount of blood in the ventricle at the end of diastole.

Endocarditis An infection, usually caused by bacteria, of the inner lining of the heart which can damage the cardiac valves.

Endocardium The innermost layer of the heart.

Endothelium A thin layer of cells that lines the blood vessels.

Eosinphils Type of white blood cell so called because they can be stained with a dye called eosin.

Erythrocyte A red blood cell.

Fibrinogen A substance in the plasma activated by thrombin to produce fibrin, necessary for clot formation.

Fibrinolysis The breakdown of a clot also know as thrombolysis.

First heart sound Heard as 'lub', this is the sound of the atrioventricular valves closing in the onset of systole.

Foam cells Foam cells are found in atheromatous plaques and are made up from both macrophages and smooth muscle.

Haemoglobin A red pigment present in red blood cells made of haem, a molecule containing iron and globin, a protein with oxygen-carrying properties.

Haemolytic Destruction of red blood cells.

Haemopoesis Production of red blood cells and platelets from the bone marrow.

Haemostasis The stoppage of bleeding following the formation of a clot.

Hypoxaemia A low level of oxygen in the blood, measured by arterial blood gas analysis or by SpO_2 in pulse oximetry.

Inodilators A drug which has both inotropic and vasodilator properties.

Inotropic (also inotrope) Has an effect on myocardial contractility. A positive inotrope increases contractility, a negative inotrope decreases contractility.

Interstitial fluid Fluid around and between tissue cells.

Intracellular fluid Fluid inside the cell walls.

Isovolumetric ventricular contraction Phase of the cardiac cycle after ventricular depolarisation. All four valves are closed as the pressure in the ventricle is increasing, but not yet sufficient to open the aortic and pulmonic valves.

Jugular venous pressure (JVP) The pressure in the jugular veins which can be seen as a pulsating column in the neck. It can be used to estimate whether cardiac filling pressures are high.

Juxta glomerular cells A group of cells situated in the afferent arteries of the nephrons in the kidney that store renin.

Leucocyte A white blood cell containing a nucleus but no haemoglobin.

Leukaemia A malignant disease of the blood in which large numbers of leucocytes are present.

Lysis Destruction of a cell or the process of breaking up or destruction.

Malar flush A high colour over the cheekbones, often with a bluish tinge. May be indicative of mitral stenosis.

Mean arterial pressure (MAP) The average pressure in the circulation throughout the cardiac cycle.

Mitral valve Valve which separates the left atria from the left ventricle.

Myocardium The thick muscle layer of the heart which contracts in a wave-like motion.

Neutrophil A type of white blood cell that can attack and destroy bacteria.

Parasympathetic nervous system A branch of the autonomic nervous system.

Pericardiocentesis A procedure in which fluid from the pericardial sac is removed by a needles.

Pericardium Rigid sac-like structure surrounding and protecting the heart.

Peripheral cyanosis A blue tinge in fingers or extremities, due to inadequate circulation.

Plasma Yellow watery liquid that makes up the fluid component of blood.

Plasma protein A protein found in plasma, e.g. albumin, gamma globulin, fibrinogen.

Platelet A small blood cell which multiplies rapidly following injury and encourages clotting of blood.

Pneumothorax A collection of air in the pleural space (between the lung and the chest wall) resulting in collapse of the lung on the affected side.

Preload Left ventricular end diastolic pressure/volume. It can be thought of as the amount of blood returning to the heart from the circulation into the ventricle.

Pulse pressure The difference in pressure between systole and diastole.

Repolarisation Movement of ions back across the cell membrane causing the resting potential to be re-established.

Sarcomere The basic functional unit of striated muscle made up of muscle fibres.

Second heart sound Heard as 'dub', this is the sound of the aortic and pulmonic valves closing at the beginning of diastole.

Sino-atrial node The heart's primary pacemaker which spontaneously depolarises 100 times per minute.

Splinter haemorrhages Tiny line haemorrhages that can be seen under the nails, indicative of bacterial endocarditis.

Stroke volume The amount of blood ejected by the ventricle during systole, normally about 70mL.

Sympathetic nervous system A branch of the autonomic nervous system.

Sympathomimetic A substance that mimics the sympathetic nervous system (used to categorise inotropic pharmacology).

Systemic vascular resistance The resistance offered to the circulation by the peripheral circulation.

Systole Phase of the cardiac cycle when contraction occurs.

Systolic pressure Pressure, usually systemic, exerted on the walls of the arteries during systole.

Tamponade Compression of the heart by the accumulation of fluid in the pericardial space.

Tension pnuemothorax Presence of air in the pleural space that occurs when air escapes into the pleural cavity from a bronchus but cannot regain entry into the bronchus. As a result, continuously increasing air pressure in the pleural cavity causes progressive collapse of the lung tissue.

Thalassaemmia A hereditary disorder that causes an abnormality in the protein component of haemoglobin.

Thrombin A substance which converts fibrinogen to fibrin to enable blood clotting.

Thrombocyte Another name for **platelet**.

Thrombus A blood clot.

Tricuspid valve Valve which separates the right atrium from the left ventricle.

Vagal tone The level of activity in the parasympathetic nervous system, for example the vagus nerve has an inhibitory affect on the heart rate.

Vasopressor A substance (often a drug) which increases the degree of vasoconstriction of the blood vessels.

Ventricular assist device (VAD) A mechanical device which can be used to assist the pumping action of the heart.

Ventricular hypertophy A thickening of the muscle layer of the heart, the ventricular myocardium, usually in response to disease, high blood pressure, or problems that increase ventricular afterload.

Venturi mask Type of disposable oxygen face mask which delivers a precise consistent mixture of air and oxygen regardless of the patient's inspiratory flow rate.

Xanthelesma Yellow/white fatty bumps under the skin around the eye lids, often the upper lid.

Xanthomata A bump in the skin caused by fats building up under the surface. They appear as small white, or larger yellow bumps, and may be associated with a high level of lipids in the blood.

Test yourself

1 Name the two systems that are circulations within the cardiovascular system:

a. splenic and hepatic
b. pulmonary and mesenteric
c. renal and systemic
d. systemic and pulmonary

2 Blood flows round the heart in the following order:

a. right atrium, right ventricle, pulmonary artery, pulmonary vein, left atria, left ventricle, aorta
b. right ventricle, right atrium, pulmonary artery, pulmonary vein, left ventricle, left atria, aorta
c. left atria, left ventricle, pulmonary vein, pulmonary artery, right atria, right ventricle, aorta
d. right atrium, right ventricle, pulmonary vein, pulmonary artery, left atria, left ventricle, aorta

3 The pressure of 120/80, known as blood pressure is consists of a systolic and diastolic pressure. Which of the following statements is true?

a. the systolic pressure is generated in the left ventricle as it fills
b. the diastolic pressure is the best guide to organ perfusion
c. the systolic pressure is pressure generated by the blood on the vessels after ventricular contraction
d. the diastolic pressure needs to be below 50mmHg for coronary artery perfusion to occur

4 There are three layers to the heart: endocardium, myocardium and pericardium. Which of the following statements is true?

a. the pericardial sac is important for the conduction pathway of the heart
b. the myocardium is the muscle of the heart, and is thickest in the left ventricles
c. the endocardium has a rough surface to help the blood to clot if there are any bleeding problems
d. the valves of the heart are made out of myocardial tissue

5 What name is given to acute severe central chest pain, due to a decreased blood supply to the heart?

a. stroke
b. myocarditis
c. angina
d. hypertension

6 What percentage of your blood volume is plasma?

a. 1
b. 55
c. 70
d. 90

7 In the ECG, the P wave represents:

a. depolarisation of the ventricle
b. depolarisation of the atria
c. repolarisation of the ventricle
d. repolarisation of the atria

8 If a patients heart rate is 80 and their stroke volume in 60mL what would their cardiac output be?

a. 4200ml
b. 5600mL
c. 3200mL
d. 4800mL

9 Increased venous return to the heart causes increases in which of the following:

a. preload
b. cardiac output
c. strength of contraction
d. all of the above

10 Increased sympathetic stimulation of the heart causes:

a. increased force of contraction
b. increased heart rate
c. increased cardiac output
d. all of the above

11 When arterial blood pressure increases, it is detected by the baroreceptors. These communicate with the cardiovascular centre and the response initiated causes:

a. increase in sympathetic outflow to the heart
b. increase in parasympathetic outflow to the heart
c. increase in sympathetic outflow to the peripheral vasculature
d. decrease in sympathetic outflow to the peripheral vasculature
e. a and c only
f. b and d only

12 Clinical findings of raised respiratory rate, raised heart rate, cool peripheries and low blood pressure are consistent with:

a. hypovolaemic shock and cardiogenic shock
b. septic shock
c. early neurogenic shock
d. late hypovolaemic shock and early anaphylactic shock

13 Which of the following is not a reason for a cardiac arrhythmia to develop?

a. hypoxia
b. hypokalaemia
c. central venous pressure below 5mmHg
d. infection

14 On noticing a cardiac arrhythmia, the nurse should:

a. put out an arrest call immediately

b. check ABCDE assessment and refer for medical help quickly if the patient is compromised

c. not be overly worried; cardiac arrhythmias are very common

d. give oxygen, do a 12-lead ECG and wait for the doctor to review on the next ward round

15 Acute coronary syndrome refers to:

a. a situation where there is disrupted blood flow down the coronary artery due to obstruction of a thrombus

b. a situation where there has been death of the heart muscle due to lack of blood flow

c. a rapid irregular heart beat which requires emergency action

d. a situation where the patient has chest pain, but no changes on the 12-lead ECG recording

16 Which of the following is a function of plasma proteins?

a. They are important electrolytes

b. They provide energy

c. They help maintain colloid oncotic pressure

d. They contribute to the transport of oxygen

17 The following are true of erythrocytes:

a. they contain haemoglobin

b. they have a large nucleus and can divide rapidly

c. there are only a few cells functional at one time

d. they are phagocytes and help engulf pathogens

18 Which blood group is described as the universal donor and which the universal recipient?

a. O positive is the universal recipient and B negative the universal recipient

b. O negative is the universal recipient and O positive is the universal donor

c. O negative is the universal donor and AB positive the universal recipient

d. A positive is the universal recipient and AB negative the universal recipient

19 Which type of shock may be characterised by vasoconstriction and tachycardia?

a. septic and hypovolaemic

b. cardiogenic and anaphylactic

c. obstructive and cardiogenic

d. neurogenic and hypovolaemic

20 The ABCDE approach to assessment is important because:

a. it is a recognised pain assessment tool

b. it helps to identify problems with breathing and circulation

c. it provides a systematic approach to assessment

d. it provides a systematic approach to assessing neurological status

References

Bickley, S. (2007) *Bates' Guide to Physical Examination and History Taking*. London: Lippincott, Williams & Wilkins.

British Thoracic Society Standards of Care Committee Pulmonary Embolism Guideline Development Group (2003) British Thoracic Society guidelines for the management of suspected acute pulmonary embolism. *Thorax* 58, 470–84.

Coons, J. and Seidl, E. (2007) Cardiovascular pharmacotherapy update for the intensive care unit. *Critical Care Nursing Quarterly* 30 (1), 44–57.

Cooper, A. and Salsi, G. (2008) Review and update on inotropes and vasopressors. *AACN Advanced Critical Care* 19 (1), 5–15.

Dellinger, R., Levy, M. and Carlet, J. (2008) Surviving sepsis campaign: International guidelines for the management of severe sepsis and septic shock. *Critical Care Medicine* 36 (1), 296–327.

Department of Health (2000) *Comprehensive Critical Care: A review of adult critical care services*. London: The Stationery Office.

Dickstein, K., Cohen-Solal, A., Filippatos, G., McMurray, J. J. V., Porikowski, P., Poole-Wilson, P. A., Strömberg, A., van Veldhuisen, D. J., Atar, D., Hoes, A. W., Keren, A., Mebezaa, A., Nieminen, M.,

Priori, S. G. and Swedbergm, K. (2008) ESC guidelines for diagnosis and treatment of acute and chronic heart failure. *European Heart Journal* 29, 1682–8.

ESC (2010) *Guidelines for the Management of Atrial Fibrillation*. The Task Force for the Management of Atrial Fibrillation of the European Society of Cardiology (ESC). Developed with the special contribution of the European Heart Rhythm Association (EHRA). Endorsed by the European Association for Cardio-Thoracic Surgery (EACTS). *European Heart Journal* 31, 2369–429. Available from http://www.escardio.org/guidelines-surveys/esc-guidelines/GuidelinesDocuments/guidelines-afib-FT.pdf.

ESC (2008) *ESC Guidelines for the Diagnosis and Treatment of Acute and Chronic Heart Failure 2008*. The Task Force for the Diagnosis and Treatment of Acute and Chronic Heart Failure 2008 of the European Society of Cardiology. Developed in collaboration with the Heart Failure Association of the ESC (HFA) and endorsed by the European Society of Intensive Care Medicine (ESICM). *European Heart Journal* 29, 2388–42. Available from http://www.escardio.org/guidelines-surveys/esc-guidelines/GuidelinesDocuments/guidelines-HF-FT.pdf.

Foxall, F. (2010) *Cardiac Rhythm Recognition*. Keswick: M&K Update.

Harrison, R. and Daley, L. (2011) *A Nurse's Survival Guide to Acute Medical Emergencies*, 3rd edn. London: Churchill Livingstone.

Havel, C., Arrich, J., Losert, H., Gampes, G., Müllner, M. and Herkner, H. (2011) *Cochrane Database Systematic Reviews* 11 (5), CD003709.

Heit, J. A., O'Fallon, W. M., Petterson, T. M., Lohse, C. M., Silverstein, M. D., Mohr, D. A. and Melton, J. (2002) Relative impact of risk factors for deep vein thrombosis and pulmonary embolism: A population-based study. *Archives of Internal Medicine* 162, 1245–8.

Intensive Care Society (2009) *Levels of Critical Care for Adult Patients*. London: Intensive Care Society.

Jevon, P., Humphreys, M. and Ewens, B. (2008) *Nursing Medical Emergency Patients*. London: Wiley-Blackwell.

Johnson, L. and Henry, K. (2009) Shock, systemic inflammatory response syndrome and multiple organ dysfunction syndrome. In Morton, P. and Fontaine, D. (eds) *Critical Care Nursing: A holistic approach*, 9th edn. London: Lippincott, Williams & Wilkins.

Jones, B., Higginson, R. and Santos, A. (2010) Critical care: Assessing blood pressure, circulation and intravascular volume. *British Journal of Cardiac Nursing* 19 (3), 153–9.

MacDuff, A., Arnold, A. and Harvey, J. (2010) Management of spontaneous pneumothorax: British Thoracic Society pleural disease guideline 2010 on behalf of the BTS Pleural Disease Guideline Group. *Thorax* 65 (Suppl 2), ii18–31. Available from http://www.brit-thoracic.org.uk/Portals/0/Clinical%20Information/Pleural%20Disease/Pleural%20Guideline%202010/Pleural%20disease%20 2010%20pneumothorax.pdf.

Macintosh, M. (2011) Cardiovascular assessment and management. In Macintosh, M. and Moore, T. (eds) *Caring for the Seriously Ill Patient*, 2nd edn. London: Hodder Arnold.

Morton, P., Reck, K. and Tucker, T. (2009) Patient assessment: Cardiovascular system. In Morton, P., Fontaine, D. (eds) *Critical Care Nursing: A Holistic Approach*, 9th edn, London: Lippincott, Williams & Wilkins.

NICE (National Institute for Health and Clinical Excellence) (2011) *Hypertension. Clinical management of primary hypertension in adults*, CG 127. London: NICE.

NICE (National Institute for Health and Clinical Excellence) (2010a) *Chest Pain of Recent Onset. Assessment and diagnosis of recent onset chest pain or discomfort of suspected cardiac origin*. NICE guideline 95. Available from http://guidance.nice.org.uk/CG95.

NICE (National Institute for Health and Clinical Excellence) (2010b) *Chronic Heart Failure National Clinical Guideline for Diagnosis and Management in Primary and Secondary Care*. NICE Clinical Guideline No 108. Available from http://www.nice.org.uk/nicemedia/live/13099/50514/50514.pdf.

NICE (National Institute for Health and Clinical Excellence) (2010c) *Unstable Angina and NSTEMI: The early management of unstable angina and non-ST-segment-elevation myocardial infarction*, CG 94. London: NICE. Available from http://www.nice.org.uk/nicemedia/live/12949/47921/47921.pdf

NICE (National Institute for Health and Clinical Excellence) (2010d) *Venous Thromboembolism: Reducing the risk of venous thromboembolism (deep vein thrombosis and pulmonary embolism) in patients admitted to hospital*. London: National Clinical Guideline Centre – Acute and Chronic Conditions (formerly the National Collaborating Centre for Acute Care) at The Royal College of Physicians.

NICE (National Institute for Health and Clinical Excellence) (2007) *Clinical Guideline 50: Recognition of and response to acute illness in adults in hospital*. London: NICE. Available from http://guidance.nice.org.uk/CG50.

NICE (National Institute for Health and Clinical Excellence) (2006) *Atrial fibrillation National Clinical Guideline for management in primary and secondary care*. NICE Clinical Guidelines No 36 Royal College of Physicians of London. Available from http://www.nice.org.uk/CG36.

NICE (National Institute for Health and Clinical Excellence) (2002) *Technology Appraisal No. 52: Guidance on the use of drugs for early thrombolysis in the treatment of acute myocardial infarction*. London: NICE. Available from http://guidance.nice.org.uk/TA52.

NMC (Nursing and Midwifery Council) (2010) *Standards for Pre-registration Nursing Education*. Available from http://standards.nmc-uk.org/PublishedDocuments/Standards%20for%20pre-registration%20nursing%20education%2016082010.pdf.

Nursing and Midwifery Council (2008) *The Code: Standards of conduct, performance and ethics for nurses and midwives*. London: NMC.

O'Driscoll, B. R., Howard, L. S. and Davison, A. G. (2008) *BTS Guideline for Emergency Oxygen Use in Adult Patients*. London: British Thoracic Society. Available from http://www.brit-thoracic.org.uk/Portals/0/Clinical%20Information/Emergency%20Oxygen/Emergency%20oxygen%20guideline/THX-63-Suppl_6.pdf

Pallister, C. (1994) *Blood Physiology and Pathophysiology*. Oxford: Butterworth-Heinemann.

Perrel, P. and Roberts, I. (2007) Colloids versus crystalloids for fluid resuscitation in critically ill patients. *Cochrane Database Systematic Reviews* 4 CD000567.

Porth, C. (2007) *Essentials of Pathophysiology, Concepts of Altered Health States*, 2nd edn. London: Lippincott, Williams & Wilkins.

RCUK (Resuscitation Council UK) (2011) *Advanced Life Support*, 6th edn. London: Resuscitation Council (UK).

RCUK (Resuscitation Council UK) (2010a) *Adult Bradycardia Algorithm*. Available from http://www.resus.org.uk/pages/bradalgo.pdf.

RCUK (Resuscitation Council UK) (2010b) *Adult Tachycardia (with Pulse) Algorithm*. Available from http://www.resus.org.uk/pages/tachalgo.pdf.

Smith, G. (2003) *ALERT Acute life-threatening Events, Recognition and Treatment: A multi-professional course in care of the acutely ill patient*. Portsmouth: University of Portsmouth.

Stanfield, C. (2011) *Principles of Human Physiology*, 4th edn. London: Benjamin Cummings.

Strickler, J. (2010) Traumatic hypovolaemic shock. *Nursing* October, 34–9. Available from http://journals.lww.com/nursing/Fulltext/2010/10000/Traumatic_hypovolemic_shock__Halt_the_downward.13.aspx.

Torbicki, A., Perrier, A., Konstantinides, S., Agneli, G., Balie, N., Pruszczyk, P., Bengel, F., Brady, A., Ferreira, D., Janssens, U., Klepetko, W., Mayer, E., Remy-Jardin, M. and Bassand, J. (2008) Guidelines on the diagnosis and management of acute pulmonary emobolism of the European Society of cardiology (ESC). *European Heart Journal* 29, 2276–3215.

Woodrow, P. (2009) An introduction to electrocardiogram interpretation: Part 2. *Nursing Standard* 24 (13), 48–56.

Further reading

Bickley, S. (2007) *Bates' Guide to Physical Examination and History Taking*. London: Lippincott, Williams & Wilkins.

Casey, A. and Elliot, T. (2010) Prevention of central venous catheter-related infection: Update. *British Journal of Cardiac Nursing* 19 (2), 78–86.

Fern, T., Harris, J., McMahon, T. and Wright, K. (2010) Mean arterial pressure and the assessment of acutely ill patients. *Nursing Standard* 25 (12), 40–4.

Jevon, P. (2010) Procedure for recording a standard 12-lead electrocardiogram. *British Journal of Nursing* 19 (10), 549–651.

Levick, J. R. (2011) *Cardiovascular Physiology: Questions for self-assessment*. London: Hodder Arnold.

Nobel, A. (2011) *The Cardiovascular System*. Edinburgh: Churchill Livingstone.

Rosaire, G. and Pack, L. (2011) *Cardiovascular Disease in the Elderly: A practical manual*. Oxford: Oxford University Press.

Sargent, A. and Rowlands, A. (2011) *The ECG Workbook*, 2nd edn. Cumbria: M&K Publishing.

Scales, K. (2010) Arterial catheters: Indications, insertion and use in critical care. *British Journal of Nursing Intravenous Supplement* 19 (19), S16–S21.

Woodrow, P. (2009) An introduction to electrocardiogram interpretation: Part 1. *Nursing Standard* 24 (12), 50–57.

Woodrow, P. (2009) An introduction to electrocardiogram interpretation: Part 2. *Nursing Standard* 24 (13), 48–56.

Woodrow, P. (2002) Central venous catheters and central venous pressure. *Nursing Standard* 16 (26), 45–51.

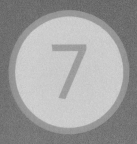

Recognition and management of cardiopulmonary arrest

Sharon Elliott

Aims

The aim of this chapter is to improve your recognition and management of the patient who has problems with maintaining airway patency and/or cardiopulmonary arrest and to explore the issues surrounding the end of life that accompany many of these emergencies in acute care.

Objectives

At the end of this chapter you will be able to:

→ Recognise partial and complete airway obstruction, and identify appropriate airway support manoeuvres

→ Understand in detail the chain of survival, its application to in-hospital resuscitation and the advanced life support algorithm

→ Differentiate between shockable and non-shockable rhythms and explain the safe use of defibrillation

→ Identify the drugs most commonly used during a cardiac arrest

→ Identify the important aspects of post-resuscitation care and staff debriefing

→ Describe the role of the nurse in caring for the family during and after a resuscitation attempt and explore and evaluate the ethical issues involved in resuscitation attempts and do not attempt resuscitation (DNAR) orders

Introduction

Most people who experience a cardiopulmonary arrest will die (RCUK 2011). This is particularly true in the hospital setting where approximately 80% of patients who arrest have shown a slow deterioration in their recorded clinical signs, usually associated with progressive hypoxia and hypotension (Schein *et al.* 1990, Smith and Wood 1998, NCEPOD 2005).

The preceding chapters in this book have aimed to equip you with the knowledge needed to recognise and identify changes in a patient's condition that could precede a cardiac arrest. Early recognition and effective management will prevent cardiac arrest from occurring in many instances (Hodgetts *et al.* 2002), however, even with optimal assessment and monitoring, some patients will suffer cardiopulmonary arrest. This chapter outlines airway management and the actions required along with the underpinning rationale in the event of a cardiopulmonary arrest, based on the latest guidance from the Resuscitation Council (Resuscitation Council UK 2010).

Airway assessment and management

Airway assessment and management requires assessing whether the airway is open or closed or at risk and includes the measures taken to reduce the risk of obstruction or to relieve it.

A partially obstructed or completely obstructed airway may be the primary event leading to a cardiopulmonary arrest. A reduced level of consciousness is often the cause, but loss of gag reflex and inability to clear secretions are also important factors. In order to ensure the best chance of a successful outcome prompt assessment, protection of the airway and adequate oxygenation are essential.

Recognising airway obstruction

The best approach is to **look**, **listen** and **feel**:

- **look** for chest and abdominal movement;
- **listen** for breath sounds;
- **feel** for air movement at the nose and mouth.

Partial airway obstruction is **noisy** and may be indicated by:

- *inspiratory stridor* – caused by obstruction at, or above, the larynx;
- *expiratory wheeze* – suggests constriction or spasm of the lower airways;

- *gurgling* – suggests liquid in the upper airway;
- *snoring* – the pharynx is semi-occluded by the tongue;
- *crowing or stridor* – caused by laryngeal spasm or obstruction;
- partial airway obstruction will involve the use of accessory muscles such as those of the neck, shoulders and abdomen as well as the intercostal and subcostal muscles.

Complete airway obstruction is **silent** and may result in paradoxical or 'see-saw' breathing. As attempts are made to draw in air, the chest is drawn in and the abdomen distends. The opposite occurs on exhalation.

> **Causes of airway obstruction**
>
> Obstruction can occur at any level from the nose/mouth to the bronchi. Potential causes are:
>
> - lack of muscle tone of the epiglottis, soft palate and tongue may be the cause in a person with reduced conscious levels;
> - vomit, blood, foodstuff or other foreign bodies;
> - oedema due to burns, anaphylaxis or inflammation;
> - inhalation of irritant or stimulation of the upper airway, such as during intubation, may result in laryngeal spasm;
> - obstruction below the level of the larynx is less common but can occur due to excessive secretions, bronchospasm, pulmonary oedema.

Obstruction of the airway with a foreign body

This can occur due to inhalation of foodstuffs. Sudden airway obstruction results in choking. Foreign body airway obstruction (FBAO) is very frightening and occurs very acutely so the patient is often unable to explain what is happening to them. If the obstruction is severe, it can result in rapid loss of consciousness and death. Therefore effective life-saving measures are required quickly. Immediate recognition and response are of the utmost importance.

The Resuscitation Council UK (2010) have compiled the adult choking treatment algorithm (see Figure 7.1) which is a helpful guide in the recognition and treatment of airway obstruction.

The key stages are:

- Recognition
- Assessment of the severity of the obstruction
- Management.

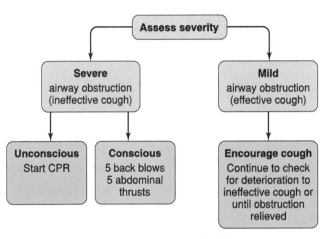

Figure 7.1 Adult choking treatment algorithm

Source: Resuscitation Council UK (2010) *2010 Resuscitation Guidelines.* Reproduced with the kind permission of Resuscitation Council (UK).

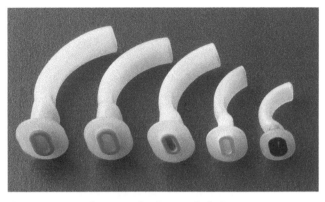

Figure 7.2 Oropharyngeal colour-coded airways

Opening the airway

The basic techniques of head tilt and chin lift and the jaw thrust manoeuvre are discussed later. Simple airway adjuncts such as the oropharyngeal airway (OPA) and nasopharyngeal airway (NPA) can be helpful in maintaining an open airway but should only be inserted if you have been trained to do so.

Oropharyngeal airways come in a variety of sizes from infant to adult and ensuring the correct size is important. If it is too big it can obstruct the airway or cause trauma. Figure 7.2 shows the OPA which is colour-coded according to size.

To ensure the correct size the bite block should be placed at the level of the incisors, and should reach to the angle of the jaw (see Figure 7.3).

The airway is inserted upside down and then turned 180° once contact has been made with the back of the throat (see Figure 7.4).

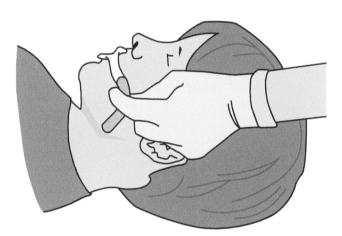

Figure 7.3 The correct sizing of OPA

OPAs should only be used in an unconscious casualty. In a conscious person, their insertion can stimulate the gag reflex and induce vomiting.

Nasopharyngeal airways are inserted into the nasal passageway to secure an open airway (see Figures 7.5

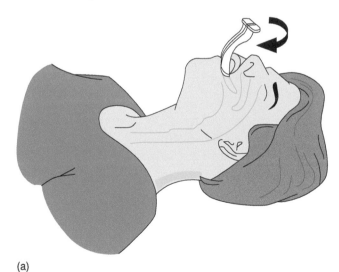

(a)

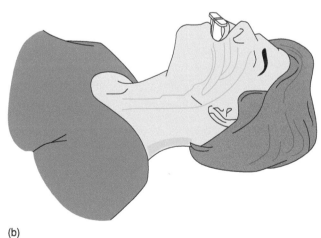

(b)

Figure 7.4 (a) Inserting the OPA; (b) The OPA *in situ*

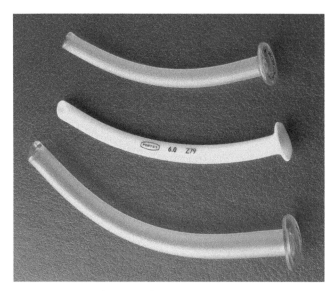

Figure 7.5 Nasopharyngeal airways

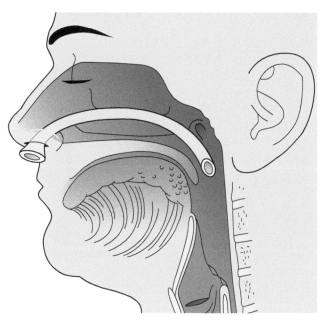

Figure 7.6 NPA *in situ*

and 7.6). An NPA can facilitate removal of secretions as a suction catheter can be passed down it. They can be used in a conscious casualty but should not be used in case of head trauma until a fractured base of skull has been ruled out.

> **Remember**
> Once the airway is open the priority is to maintain it and ensure adequate ventilation and oxygenation. Obstruction of the airway and/or lack of oxygen for more than a few minutes can cause injury to the brain and other vital organs.

Once inserted oropharyngeal or nasopharyngeal airways can be used to help maintain the airway and can be used in conjunction with the pocket mask or bag valve mask devices as an aid to ventilation. Even with an OPA or NPA *in situ* the airway can obstruct if the head is not correctly positioned.

Suction

A wide-bore rigid suction device (Yankauer) can be used to remove blood, vomit and secretions from the mouth. Caution should be used if the patient is semi-conscious as it can stimulate the gag reflex and therefore vomiting. Fine-bore flexible suction catheters can be passed via an oropharyngeal or nasopharyngeal airway to remove secretions.

Chain of survival

In a hospital setting, it could be patients or relatives who are the victims of a cardiac arrest. Ideally, patients at high risk should be cared for in an area that enables monitoring and facilities for immediate resuscitation, however, cardiac arrests may occur in non-clinical areas such as bathrooms, corridors and car parks. In the event of a cardiac arrest time is of the essence. If the person who has collapsed is not found quickly and/or cardiac arrest is not recognised the chances of survival diminish significantly as each minute passes. There will be varying skill levels amongst staff and you should only attempt what you have been trained to do. However, there is a public and professional expectation that all clinical staff can carry out CPR and ensure that expert help and equipment is summoned immediately. This basic requirement is the minimum expected of student nurses and newly qualified staff nurses.

When a patient suffers a cardiac arrest there are four priorities needed to provide the best chance of a successful outcome. These are:

1 early recognition of cardiac arrest and call for help;
2 early basic life support (BLS) also termed cardiopulmonary resuscitation (CPR);
3 early defibrillation, if appropriate;
4 post-resuscitation care aimed at restoring quality of life.

> In all UK hospitals, there is now a standard number to use in the event of a cardiac arrest: **2222**.

These are often conceptualised as the chain of survival (see Figure 7.7).

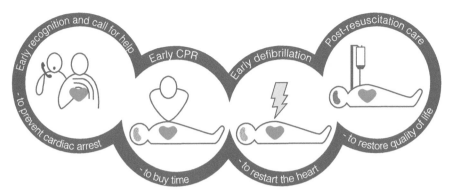

Figure 7.7 The chain of survival

Source: Nolan, J., Soar, J. and Elkeland, H. (2006) Chain of Survival. *Resuscitation*, 71, 270–1.

Each of the four links in the chain is essential – if any one of them is weak the whole chain is weakened. Basic life support (BLS) is integral to advanced life support (ALS).

> Cardiac arrests are relatively rare events. It is therefore essential that clinical staff have the opportunity to rehearse and practice the algorithms on a regular basis to ensure the response is effective.

To help ensure that the collapsed patient receives the best chances of survival, it is necessary that clinical staff are familiar with the procedures to follow and techniques to use. The Resuscitation Council UK (RCUK) sets the standards in relation to these procedures and techniques. The Council was established in 1981 with the objective of ensuring both lay and health care professionals are educated in the most effective methods of resuscitation appropriate to their needs. The guidance is reviewed every two to three years to ensure it is in line with the latest evidence. The RCUK has produced a series of algorithms. These are diagrammatic representations of the steps to follow in the event of a cardiac arrest (see Figure 7.8). Emergency situations require a coordinated team response to enable the best outcome. This is better achieved if everyone is following the same agreed process.

The chain of survival underpins the in-hospital resuscitation algorithm.

The sequence of events to follow for a collapsed person can be easily remembered by acronym DRS ABC.

D = Danger

Check that the area around the patient is safe. Although there are relatively few documented cases of first responders to a cardiac arrest suffering adverse effects your safety and that of the other members of the team is always the first priority.

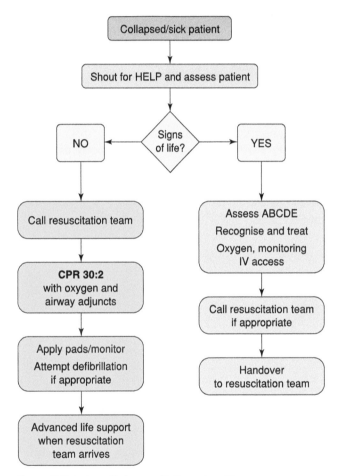

Figure 7.8 In-hospital resuscitation algorithm

Source: Resuscitation Council UK (2010) *2010 Resuscitation Guidelines*. Reproduced with the kind permission of Resuscitation Council (UK).

Use appropriate personal protective clothing as soon as possible. In most cases, this will be non-sterile gloves and aprons, although masks and eye protection may be required in some circumstances, for example major trauma.

R = Response

Gently shake the shoulders and shout the name of the person who has collapsed to assess if there is a response.

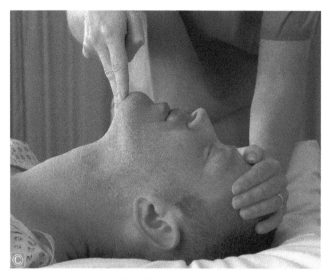

Figure 7.9 Head tilt chin lift manoeuvre

Source: Resuscitation Council UK (2011) *Advanced Life Support*. Photographs reproduced with kind permission of Michael Scott and the Resuscitation Council (UK).

S = Shout

Or summon help. In reality, checking for response and getting help will usually occur simultaneously, as in most cases, if a patient appears to have collapsed, additional help of some kind will be required. As soon as it is apparent that a cardiac arrest has occurred the resuscitation or medical emergency team *must* be called.

A = Airway

The airway should be opened by tilting the head back and lifting the chin up. This will cause the tongue to move away from the back of the pharynx, creating a patent airway (see Figure 7.9).

If necessary, the patient may need to be moved to enable opening of the airway, but if other injuries are suspected this should be minimised until further help arrives. Despite the presence of other injuries, opening the airway is the priority in a collapsed unconscious casualty, because if the airway remains closed there is no chance of survival regardless of the cause of collapse. It may be easier for you to open the airway without moving the casualty too much by employing the jaw thrust manoeuvre (see Figure 7.10).

B = Breathing

With the airway open the unconscious casualty may breathe spontaneously. To check if this is the case it is necessary to:

- *Look* – at the chest for movement, coughing or other signs of life
- *Listen* – for breath sounds with your face close to the casualty's
- *Feel* – for movement of air against your face

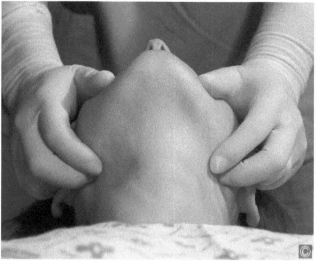

(a)

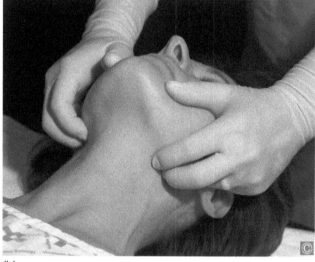

(b)

Figure 7.10 Jaw thrust manoeuvre

Source: Resuscitation Council UK (2010) *Advanced Life Support*. Photographs reproduced with kind permission of Michael Scott and the Resuscitation Council (UK).

This should be done for no more than 10 seconds.

> Occasional gasps, slow laboured or noisy breathing known as agonal breathing is common in the immediate stage following cardiac arrest. This must not be confused with normal breathing.

If the casualty remains unconscious and there is no normal breathing, assume that a cardiac arrest has occurred and commence chest compressions.

If there are signs of life assess the patient using the ABCDE approach whilst waiting for assistance.

C = Compressions

Ensure help has been summoned and commence CPR (see Figure 7.11). This is achieved by:

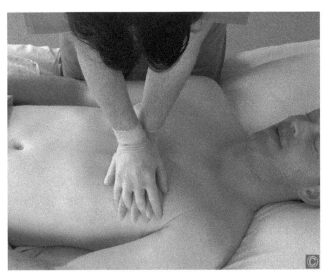

Figure 7.11 Chest compressions

Source: Resuscitation Council UK (2011) *Advanced Life Support*. Photograph reproduced with kind permission by Michael Scott and the Resuscitation Council (UK).

- locating the sternum;
- interlocking the fingers;
- applying downward pressure to the lower half of the sternum with straight arms (see Figure 7.11);
- 30 compressions should be performed;
- the pressure applied to the sternum should compress the chest one-third of its depth (approximately 5–6cm);
- the rate of compression should be 100–120 per minute.

> Two people should alternate cycles of chest compressions to ensure they remain effective. However, this should occur without long pauses in compressions as even minor delays have been shown to adversely effect the outcome of resuscitation.
>
> (Resuscitation Council UK 2010)

> There should be minimal delay between cycles of compressions. Compressions generate a pressure in the arterial system which enables the flow of oxygenated blood. Delays result in the pressure falling, reducing the oxygen supply to vital organs and tissues.

Two rescue breaths then immediately follow the 30 chest compressions.

Remember your safety. In a clinical setting, rescue breaths should never be attempted without using a pocket mask (Figure 7.12) at the very least to protect the first responder from contamination from exhaled air and body fluids. These should be readily available in all areas and the time taken to complete the 30 compressions gives someone else time to get one for you. You should deliver the breath over one second and ensure you see the chest

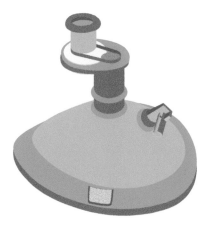

Figure 7.12 Pocket mask

rise. If it does not, you may need to adjust the head position to ensure the airway is fully open.

Adjuncts to aid ventilation

A pocket mask (Figure 7.12) is used to safely deliver rescue breaths during a cardiac arrest. It can easily be used by one person as both hands are free to hold the mask firmly to the face maintaining an airtight seal. It should be used in conjunction with an appropriately sized Guedel airway. Pocket masks are often situated in key areas and, as such, are often available before the crash trolley arrives. They have the benefit of ease of use.

> Using only your expired air for rescue breaths is much better than nothing but this should be enriched with oxygen as soon as it is available. Set the oxygen flow to 15 litres per minute and either attach to the port on the pocket mask or place the oxygen tubing under the mask.

A bag valve mask (see Figure 7.13) is a hand-held device designed to provide rescue breaths for a casualty who is not breathing or breathing inadequately. The device consists of an air chamber, which can attached to a reservoir bag and oxygen supply and a face mask. It can be used with air but oxygen supply should be attached as soon as it is possible to do so at a flow rate of 15L/min. The device then has the benefit of giving high percentages of oxygen, without the rescuer using her own breaths. However, normally two people are required to use this effectively, one to hold the mask to maintain an airtight seal, and the other to squeeze the bag in between the cardiac compressions. The ratio of 30 compressions to rescue breaths is continued until a request is made to stop is made by the resuscitation team.

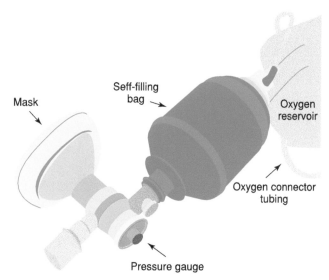

Figure 7.13 Bag valve mask

> **Remember!**
>
> The priority here is to ensure that effective rescue breaths are given.
>
> If you find this easier to do with a pocket mask then stick with that rather than trying to use the bag valve mask device.
>
> Don't forget to use an OPA if possible and add supplemental oxygen.

Having followed these steps, you have ensured the first two links of the chain of survival have occurred: early recognition, calling for help and commencement of CPR. *You have already given the patient a significantly improved chance of survival.*

Defibrillation

The next link in the chain is early defibrillation, the purpose of which is to re-establish a rhythm capable of producing an adequate cardiac output.

When a cardiac arrest occurs the heart rhythm will be in one of two categories:

- Those that are amenable to reversal by defibrillation: shockable – ventricular fibrillation and pulseless ventricular tachycardia.
- Those that aren't amenable to reversal by defibrillation: non-shockable – asystole and pulseless electrical activity (PEA).

> Defibrillation consists of delivering a controlled amount of electrical energy to the heart using a **defibrillator**. The aim is to depolarise the myocardium and terminate the arrhythmia. This allows normal sinus rhythm to be re-established by the sino-atrial node.

As soon as the defibrillator arrives the pads should be attached in order that the rhythm can be assessed. Chest compressions should continue whilst the pads are applied. As soon as the pads are applied the rhythm must be assessed and chest compressions will need to stop whilst this occurs. It is at this point that we move from the in-hospital resuscitation algorithm to the ALS algorithm (Figure 7.14).

> For rhythms that are amenable to defibrillation the best chance of survival will be achieved if the first shock is delivered within three minutes of collapse.

It is important to understand the probable sequence of events in advanced life support (ALS) as nurses form an essential component of the resuscitation team. This may involve drawing up, checking and recording drugs given, or communicating with the patient's relatives as the process continues. Knowledge of the patient's history, immediate problems and laboratory results are crucial to decision-making during this stage. The patient's notes need to be available to the resuscitation team.

Rhythm assessment is vital to determine whether the patient has a shockable or non-shockable rhythm. If shockable, this needs to be performed without delay. Shockable rhythms include:

- VT (without a pulse) (see Figure 7.15)
- VF (see Figure 7.16).

Shocking asystole or PEA is of no value and could reduce the chances of survival by increasing the pause in chest compressions.

> **Remember!**
>
> Stopping compressions to assess the rhythm should be for the shortest time possible.

Shockable rhythms

- Once the rhythm has been identified as shockable the first shock should be delivered as soon as possible.
- As soon as the first shock has been given chest compressions must recommence and CPR resumed for another two minutes.
- After two minutes the rhythm is reassessed and, providing the rhythm remains shockable, a further shock

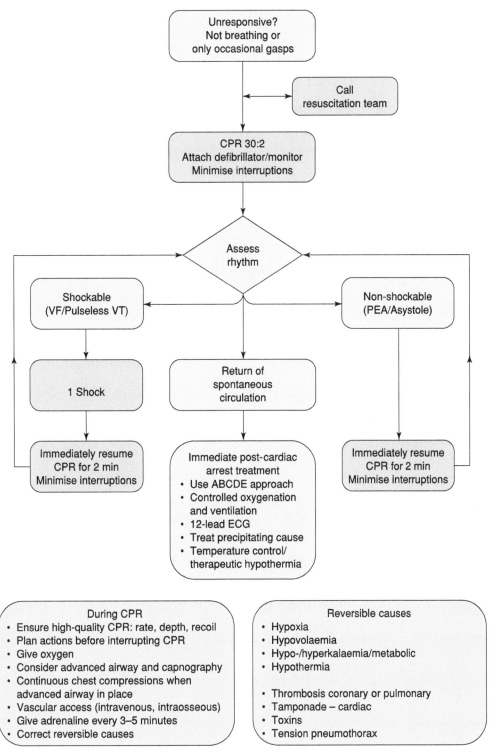

Figure 7.14 Adult advanced life support algorithm

Source: Resuscitation Council UK (2010) *2010 Resuscitation Guidelines*. Reproduced with the kind permission of Resuscitation Council (UK).

is given followed by another two minutes of CPR. This cycle continues unless the rhythm changes.

- Before the third shock is delivered 1mg of adrenaline is given intravenously (IV).
- After this further doses of adrenaline at the same dose is given before each alternate shock.

CPR commences immediately after defibrillation without checking for a pulse. This is because even if a perfusing rhythm has been restored it is unlikely that a pulse will be felt immediately and the delay would be harmful if the defibrillation has not been successful.

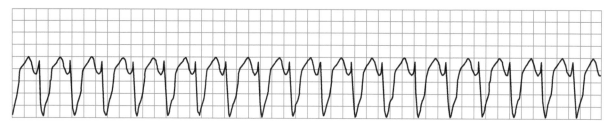

Figure 7.15 Ventricular tachycardia (VT) (without a pulse)

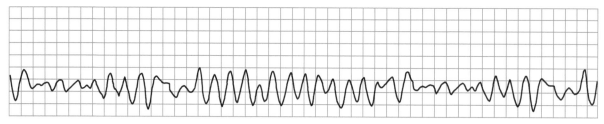

Figure 7.16 Ventricular fibrillation (VF)

CASE STUDY 7.1 Staff nurse Jane – Part 1

Jane, a staff nurse returning from her break, passes a visitor waiting area and sees a lady collapsed on the floor.

ASSESSMENT

She checks the area is safe and approaches the lady, calling for assistance from John, a porter at the other end of the corridor, as she does so. The lady appears to be unconscious. Jane kneels beside her and gently shakes her shoulders and asks her in a loud voice 'are you alright?' There is no response. There are no signs of any injury so Jane turns the lady onto her back and opens the airway using a head tilt chin lift manoeuvre.

Jane checks for breathing by looking, listening and feeling, while also checking for any signs of life such as movement or coughing. She tries to feel for a carotid pulse but is unable to find one. After 10 seconds there is no breathing noted or any signs of life.

John, the porter, asks Jane if he can help. Jane asks him to phone 2222 and call the resuscitation team.

RESPONSE

Daniel, a second-year student nurse on Jane's ward, has heard her call and she asks him to go to the nearest ward at the end of the corridor and to bring the emergency trolley and defibrillator. Jane commences 30 chest compressions and continues until Daniel returns with the emergency trolley.

Jane confirms that Daniel knows how to do basic life support. A pocket mask is stuck to the wall of the lift lobby, so Jane uses this to administer two breaths. She then asks Daniel to put on gloves and continue with 30 more chest compressions. Jane takes a size 3 Guedel airway from the trolley, places it in the patient's airway and adds 10L of oxygen to the pocket mask, ready for the next breath.

Jane is trained in defibrillation, so attaches the defibrillator pads onto the patient's chest and switches on the machine. The voice prompt requests that compressions are stopped whilst the rhythm is analysed.

The next voice prompt tells them the rhythm is shockable and to step away whilst the machine charges. Once charged a further prompt reminds them to stand clear as the shock is delivered. They are then prompted to commence two minutes CPR.

Jane, now wearing gloves, takes over the compressions and asks Daniel to continue the ventilation using the pocket mask and oxygen at 15L/min. At this point the resuscitation team arrives.

Types of defibrillator

There are different types of defibrillator available in clinical practice:

- Manual defibrillators: these require a high level of rhythm recognition skills on the part of the operator but have the advantage, when used in expert hands, of reducing the delay in compressions to less than 5 seconds.
- Automated external defibrillators (AEDs): these are sophisticated computerised devices that can reliably analyse the heart rhythm and through voice and visual prompts guide you through safe defibrillation. In areas where staff may not have skills in rhythm recognition and/or do not use defibrillators regularly training in the use of AEDs is achieved much more easily and quickly than manual defibrillators and offers a way of achieving the goal of delivering the first shock within three minutes of collapse.

> **Remember!**
> The use of any defibrillator should never be attempted unless you have been trained in its use.

Energy levels

The amount of electrical energy delivered is measured in joules. The number of joules delivered will depend on the type of defibrillator: most defibrillators in clinical practice are biphasic and the recommended energy level for the first shock is 150 joules. Subsequent shocks using biphasic defibrillators may stay at 150J or be escalated up to a maximum of 360J. This will depend on the device used and local protocols.

> - In older monophasic defibrillators the energy travels in one direction between the two pads on the patient's chest.
> - In biphasic defibrillators it travels from one pad through the chest to the other pad and back again, therefore two 'jolts' of energy are delivered. This means the energy level set on the machine can be lower.

Some older manual defibrillators are monophasic and the recommended energy level for these is 360 joules. Subsequent shocks using monophasic defibrillators are delivered at the same energy level.

AEDs automatically select the energy level and guide you through the delivery of the shock.

Safety considerations

Defibrillation uses live electricity that is an obvious hazard and can pose risks. The use of AEDs does reduce some of these risks but there are still important safety considerations to take into account when using any defibrillator.

- Ensure the area around the patient and the patient's chest are dry – this could be an issue if, for example, the patient has collapsed in the bathroom.
- No one should touch the patient whilst the shock is being delivered – this includes indirect contact such as touching the bed or IV stand.
- Always use self-adhesive pad electrodes.
- The combination of an oxygen-rich environment and a spark from a poorly applied pad could cause a fire. To minimise this risk oxygen should be removed to at least one metre away from the patient during delivery of a shock. Once an endotracheal tube is *in situ* the oxygen may be left connected as this is a closed system.

> It is recommended that all members of the team wear gloves. This not only protects from body fluid contamination but may provide limited protection from electrical current in the event of inadvertent contact during defibrillation.

- When using an AED the voice prompts will tell you when to stand clear.
- When a manual defibrillator is being used compresions only stop during rhythm analysis and actual shock delivery. Whilst the machine is charging compressions continue although everyone else is asked to step away.
- If you are the person doing the compressions you may feel quite vulnerable as everyone else has been asked to step away and you continue to have contact with the patient whilst the defibrillator is charging. It is important that you have confidence in the person operating the defibrillator and that you can see what that person is doing at all times.

Non-shockable rhythms

Non-shockable rhythms are asystole (see Figure 7.17) and pulseless electrical activity (PEA).

> Early data from the National Cardiac Arrest Audit (NCAA) indicate that of those people who suffer a cardiac arrest in hospital 13.5% survive to discharge.
>
> 18% of these will present with a shockable rhythm and 44% survive whilst of those who present with a non-shockable rhythm only 7% survive to discharge.

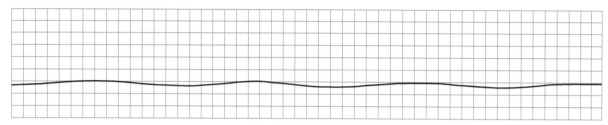

Figure 7.17 Asystole

Asystole is when there is no electrical activity detected on the monitor. Always ensure the pads/electrodes are securely attached and the correct monitoring mode and gain are selected.

Pulseless electrical activity is when some organised electrical activity within the myocardium is detected on the monitor (this could even look like a normal ECG trace) but does not result in a cardiac output sufficient to produce a pulse. Unless a treatable cause can be found quickly, survival from asystole or PEA is unlikely. Because these rhythms are not amenable to defibrillation the focus is on good-quality CPR and early identification of a possible cause.

The sequence of events is therefore:

- commencement of CPR at a ratio of 30:2;
- administration of adrenaline 1mg IV as soon as access is established;
- recheck the rhythm every two minutes, if it becomes shockable (VF or VT) then move to the shockable side of the algorithm;
- if the rhythm remains non-shockable continue with CPR and repeat the adrenaline dose on alternate cycles of CPR (every 3–5 minutes).

> The purpose of giving adrenaline repeatedly during a cardiac arrest is that it increases coronary and cerebral blood flow and may therefore improve the effectiveness of CPR.

During CPR

In both shockable and non-shockable sides of the algorithm there is much to be done to improve chances of survival.

- The most important task is maintenance of good-quality CPR.

- The gold standard for protecting the airway is tracheal intubation but this can only be performed by someone expert in the technique. Until this point ensure ventilation is achieved by whichever means you are competent to perform.
- Once tracheal intubation is achieved ventilations can be administered at a rate of 10 per minute without stopping compressions.
- Intravenous access should be obtained as soon as possible.
- If it is not possible to achieve intravenous access, intraosseous access may be considered using either the tibia or the humerus. Both drugs and fluids can be administered via this route.

> **Remember!**
> Ventilation must be supplemented with 100% oxygen as soon as possible. Avoid over-inflation as this may result in gastric regurgitation.

While you may not be able to perform some of the tasks during an arrest you still have an important part to play once the resuscitation team arrives:

- helping to keep effective CPR going which is vital;
- assisting with tracheal intubation;
- preparing drugs such as adrenaline;
- the team leader may allocate someone to document events and the drugs that were given;
- there may be relatives or other patients who need support.

Reversible causes

In all cases of cardiac arrest it is important to consider the factors that could be the primary cause or are aggravating factors and which may be reversible.

To make these easier to remember it is helpful to think of them as the four Hs and four Ts.

Four Hs

1 **Hypoxia**: this is minimised by:

- ventilating during the arrest with 100% oxygen. Oxygen saturation should be monitored aiming for a reading of 90% or above;
- ensuring adequate chest movement with each breath;
- ensuring patency and correct placement of any artificial airway.

2 **Hypovolaemia**: this may be a primary cause of PEA, often due to severe bleeding:

- bleeding may be obvious, as in severe trauma, or hidden as in the case of a gastrointestinal bleed;
- hypovoleamia may also be caused by severe dehydration, for example as a result of prolonged or excessive diarrhoea and vomiting;
- circulating volume should be restored rapidly with blood and fluids and if necessary, surgery to stop the haemorrhage.

3 **Hyperkalaemia** may be present as a result of renal insufficiency and can be treated immediately with an infusion of dextrose and insulin, but it may require renal replacement therapy in the longer term.

Other metabolic abnormalities that should also be considered are:

- **hypokalaemia**: this may happen following aggressive diuretic therapy and is treated by administering a potassium chloride infusion;
- hypoglycaemia treated with a bolus of 50% dextrose;
- hypocalcaemia treated with calcium chloride.

These disturbances may be detected on biochemical tests and from the patient's history, for example renal impairment.

> Both hyper- and hypoglycaemia post-arrest are not uncommon and both are associated with poor outcome. The aim is to keep the blood sugar between 4–6mmol/L.

4 **Hypothermia**: this should be suspected in any cases of near drowning or exposure. Attempts should be made to rewarm the patient using warmed IV fluids and warming blankets.

Four Ts

1 **Tension pneumothorax**: this could be the primary cause of PEA and is initially relieved by needle decompression and then by insertion of a chest drain.

2 **Cardiac tamponade**: this is a build-up of fluid in the pericardial sack restricting myocardial contraction resulting in PEA. It can be difficult to diagnose as the clinical signs of low blood pressure and distended neck veins are difficult to observe during an arrest but penetrating chest injury or arrest immediately post-cardiac surgery should raise suspicions.

3 **Toxic**: this may be difficult to detect unless there is history of intentional or accidental overdose or ingestion of toxic substances.

4 **Thromboembolic**: massive pulmonary embolism (PE) is the commonest cause of mechanical circulatory obstruction. If a PE is thought to be the cause thrombolytic drug therapy should be considered.

Post-resuscitation care

Following a successful resuscitation as determined by a return of spontaneous circulation (ROSC) the patient will need to be transferred to an intensive care unit or high-dependency facility for close monitoring and further management. This process usually takes some time and while awaiting transfer the patient should be monitored and managed using the ABCDE approach. The aim of this is to optimise oxygenation and tissue perfusion whilst observing for, identifying and treating any complications such as hypoglycaemia or convulsions. During this time a member of the medical team will usually remain with the patient.

> **ICU management post-cardiac arrest**
> - early coronary reperfusion and optimisation of circulatory status
> - ventilatory control
> - blood glucose control
> - temperature control
> - control of seizures
> *Standards for the Management of Patients after Cardiac Arrest (ICS 2008)*

Decisions to stop resuscitation

Sadly, the majority of people who suffer an in-hospital cardiac arrest do not survive, and therefore there will come a point during the resuscitation process where a decision to stop needs to be made. This is a difficult situation for all concerned. The most senior doctor present has the legal responsibility to take the decision to stop, but in reality when this occurs, there is a need to take into account the views of the whole team and in some cases the family. As time elapses the chances of a successful outcome decrease, however recovery can occur even after prolonged resuscitation attempts, particularly in cases of near drowning, electrocution, hypothermia or some drug overdoses. Assuming adequate oxygenation and effective CPR and the absence of an untreated reversible cause failure of repeated defibrillation and drug treatment usually signal the point has been reached to take the decision to stop.

Following a period of intense activity focused on saving the patient's life this outcome is often emotional and sometimes confusing. You may worry that as the first responder it was something you did or didn't do that resulted in this outcome. If you adhere to the principles of the chain of survival this is very unlikely to be the case. Remember it is unfortunately more likely that the person will die as a result of a cardiac arrest.

It is now considered good practice to have a team debrief after the event. This does not need to be very long but will focus on constructive feedback and learning rather than the apportioning of any blame.

Presence of relatives at resuscitation attempts

It is becoming increasingly common for relatives to be present during the resuscitation. Work by Hansen and Strawser (1992) identified that relatives would choose to remain during resuscitation if given the option. Relatives perceive advantages to being present (Awoonor-Renner 1991, Hansen and Strawser 1992, Whitlock and Adams 1994) and these include:

- it helps with coming to terms with the death and enables a healthier bereavement process;
- they have the chance to speak to their loved one for the last time;
- it is possible to see that everything that could be done was done;
- they can touch their loved one while the body is still warm;
- they believe that their presence is important both to themselves and their loved one;
- to be removed from the situation when they wished to be present would be highly distressing.

Other authors (Martin 1991, Osuwagu 1991, Crisci 1994, Schilling 1994) have cited disadvantages:

- watching the resuscitation attempt could be distressing, particularly in the absence of support;
- relatives may hinder the resuscitation attempt or may be offended by remarks made by the team;
- they may be disturbed by the memory of the events although evidence suggests that people are disturbed less by facts than by what they imagine.

In any other end-of-life scenario most health care practitioners would accept that the presence of family and loved ones is both desirable and entirely normal. Given that the majority of resuscitation attempts will result in the person's death we must ask ourselves why this should be different. In 1996 the Resuscitation Council UK published the findings of a working party which favoured relatives' attendance providing that was their wish and that they received support and information (Resuscitation Council UK 1996). By 2003 work by Grice *et al.* indicated that 56% of medical staff and 66% of nurses working in an adult intensive care unit felt that relatives should be given the option to stay. If relatives requested to stay 70% of medical staff and 82% of nurses said they would allow this.

Each situation must be judged individually, but the consensus seems to be that if a relative wishes to stay she should be allowed to do so but that someone who is appropriately qualified should stay and support her. You may be designated this task, particularly if you know the family already. There is no script to follow but there are a few principles that could help you to manage this emotional situation:

- Acknowledge how difficult this is for them.
- Make it clear that the choice to stay or go is entirely theirs and that either choice is fine.
- Let them know that they will be looked after whatever their choice. If the family decide to leave, then go with them if possible.
- Give clear explanations about what has happened, for example, 'John's heart has stopped beating and we are doing everything we can to re-start it' and also what to expect, 'we are giving John oxygen through a special mask and pressing down on his chest to pump the oxygen around the body while his heart is not beating.'
- Offer them the chance to touch the patient when this is appropriate and be clear about when and why it is not appropriate, for example during defibrillation.
- Answer any questions honestly. Some questions may be asked which you can't answer such as 'is he going to live?' 'Will he be brain damaged?' It is OK to say you can't answer those questions at present as the situation is too uncertain but offer reassurance that they will be kept informed at all stages.

- Don't be afraid of silences in these situations people often need time to take in what is happening and may not wish to, or need to, talk.

Do not attempt resuscitation (DNAR) orders

Successful resuscitation has led to many people experiencing extended and useful lives precious to them and their loved ones. Unfortunately, these success stories are in the minority, and it must be recognised that resuscitation carries the risk of causing morbidity and suffering by prolonging the process of dying.

> It is essential to differentiate between the natural process of death and a reversible cardiac arrest.

It is not always appropriate to attempt resuscitation, for example:

- where the chances of success are very slight;
- if a successful outcome would result in a reduced quality of life. This is often the most common reason given and the most difficult area to make decisions about;
- if there is a known wish expressed by the patient not to be resuscitated. This may be written or verbal but must be valid – made by a patient competent to make the decision and in full possession of the facts. It is important to bear in mind that situations change, which could affect the validity of the advanced decision.

In-depth explanation and guidance can be found in a joint statement from the Royal College of Nursing, British Medical Association and the Resuscitation Council UK (2007). This is a complex area and for detailed information this document is recommended reading. There are, however, some key points:

- Decisions related to CPR and DNAR should be made carefully and on an individual basis in consultation with the patient wherever possible, and include the family unless the patient does not wish this to be the case. In the case of a patient who lacks capacity the discussion should involve family to explore the patient's likely feelings, wishes and beliefs.
- While the final decision rests with the senior doctor in charge of the case there should be consultation with the multi-professional team involved.
- Advance care planning including making decisions about CPR is part of good-quality clinical care for persons who may be at risk of cardiac arrest, for example people with chronic heart or lung disease.
- It is not necessary to have these discussions with patients for whom there is no reason to believe they are at risk of a cardiac arrest.
- Once made, decisions should be accurately documented, communicated and reviewed.
- Any patient with the capacity to do so who refuses CPR or those who lack capacity but have a valid advance decision refusing CPR should have their wishes respected.
- A DNAR order should not override clinical judgement. For example, in the unlikely event of a patient with a DNAR order developing a sudden reversible cause of cardiac arrest unrelated to the underlying condition such as choking or anaphylaxis, the decision may be taken to attempt CPR.
- Where there is no explicit advance decision or in circumstances where this is unclear or unknown then CPR should always be attempted.
- DNAR orders only refer to CPR and not other forms of treatment.

This final point is important. The presence of a DNAR does not preclude other treatments that may include oxygen therapy, ventilation, pain relief and nutritional support among others. High-quality, safe and effective nursing care remains paramount.

CASE STUDY 7.2 Staff nurse Jane – Part 2

Jane, with the assistance of John and Daniel, has ensured the first three links of the chain of survival have been implemented before the MET arrived:

- She assessed the situation, recognised a cardiac arrest had occurred and ensured the MET was called.
- CPR was started quickly and the emergency equipment brought to the scene as soon as possible. This enabled rescue breaths to be delivered via a pocket mask, with a

Guedel airway *in situ*, supplemented with high-flow oxygen.

- Pads were applied and the rhythm analysed. By the time the MET arrived one shock had been delivered and 2 minutes of CPR was underway.
- Both Jane and Daniel applied gloves as soon as it was practical to do so, in order to protect them from any body fluid contamination.

→

As the MET arrives a second lady comes into the room carrying two cups of coffee and becomes very distressed as the lady on the floor is apparently her mother.

A member of the MET advises Jane and Daniel to continue with CPR and helps the daughter, whose name is Laura, to a chair. Two minutes of CPR are complete and the voice prompt on the defibrillator advises stopping compressions in order to analyse the rhythm.

The next voice prompt tells them the rhythm is shockable and to step away whilst the machine charges. Once charged a further prompt reminds them to stand clear as the shock is delivered. They are then prompted to commence two minutes' CPR.

Daniel continues with chest compressions and anaesthetist takes over the management of the airway and prepares to intubate the patient.

The team leader asks Jane to relate the events so far and requests that she remain with Laura and explain what has happened and what is going on now. Jane finds out that Laura and her mother Mary were visiting her father who is an inpatient following a knee replacement. Mary has had 'heart problems' for years.

Two minutes of CPR are complete and the anaesthetist has secured the airway with an endotracheal tube. A peripheral IV cannula has been inserted and a dose of adrenaline 1mg IV is given and flushed with 20mL saline. The team leader has switched the defibrillator to manual mode and requests Daniel to stop compressions to enable analysis of the rhythm. A second member of the team is designated to operate the defibrillator. The rhythm is confirmed as VT and the operator requests Daniel to recommence compressions as the machine charges. Everyone else is asked to step away. The anaesthetist leaves the oxygen connected to the re-inflatable bag and ET tube as a closed circuit. As soon as the defibrillator is charged Daniel is asked to step away and the operator discharges the shock. Once the shock is delivered a third member of the team takes over compressions for another 2 minutes' CPR.

Jane explains to Laura that she had found her mother collapsed on the floor and that her heart has stopped.

She said she realised that this was a huge shock and a lot to take in but that all efforts were now being made to restart Mary's heart. She offered Laura the option to stay or to wait in another area, reassuring her that she would stay with her throughout.

After another two minutes of CPR compressions were stopped and the rhythm analysed again. Atrial fibrillation now showed on the monitor. This is a rhythm that could be consistent with an output. The anaesthetist confirmed the presence of a weak carotid pulse.

A full ABCDE assessment was commenced and the ICU was contacted to arrange a bed for post-resuscitation care. Laura was able to come and sit next to her mother and hold her hand.

At the point of transfer to ICU:

Airway and breathing

Mary remained intubated but was making some respiratory effort. Oxygen saturations 98%.

Circulation

Her heart rate was 112 in AF with a blood pressure of 110/85, she was cool peripherally with a capillary refill time of > 3secs.

Disability

Her blood glucose level was 5.3mmol/L and she was responding to painful stimuli.

Exposure

No obvious wounds or abnormalities noted although she had been incontinent of urine.

Jane accompanied Laura to ICU and assisted in the handover to ICU staff.

Following transfer to ICU Jane and Daniel were commended for their efforts during the team brief for acting so promptly. It was likely that Mary had suffered a myocardial infarction. She had a shockable rhythm that reverted after three shocks to atrial fibrillation which could possibly be Mary's normal heart rhythm.

Caring for the bereaved

In the case study, Mary is transferred to intensive care following a successful resuscitation. Sadly, however, as mentioned in the beginning of this chapter, most people who experience a cardiopulmonary arrest will die (Resuscitation Council UK 2010). While the focus of care is very different following the death of the individual concerned, it is imperative that a high level of sensitive and practical support continues to be provided to the suddenly bereaved (Kent and McDowell 2004), some of whom may have witnessed the resuscitation attempt. This is of significance both in terms of your role in helping to facilitate a positive grieving process and also when doing so after having only just met the bereaved and in very traumatic circumstances.

Breaking bad news

When the resuscitation has been unsuccessful, news of the patient's death needs to be delivered (preferably face to face although this may not always be possible) and is generally done by a senior member of staff, preferably in a quiet and private area. You may, however, be on hand to support this process. This news can be devastating for the bereaved, although a sudden and unexpected death may carry different meanings to different families; and the responses to such news can be very diverse. This makes it very stressful for the clinicians involved who may never have met the relative before (Walker 2010).

How the bad news is broken can have a major impact on the bereaved (Edwards and Shaw 1998, Kent and McDowell 2004, Walker 2010), and if not handled well can become a traumatic memory seared into their consciousness. The language used needs to be simple, clear and unambiguous avoiding all euphemisms, and delivered at a gentle pace, outlining exactly what was done during the resuscitation. It needs to be made clear that all attempts to prevent the person's death were made and that the deceased was not left to die alone (DH 2005). Explaining how the patient may now look and small details, such as why the deceased's clothes were removed or cut, can go a long way to avoiding unnecessary distress on the part of the bereaved. Such difficult discussions require significant empathy and competence in communication skills (Wilson and White 2011).

Giving the bereaved the opportunity to view and be with the deceased in a quiet and private space is an important part of the aftercare, especially if the relatives or next of kin were not present when the patient died. The evidence shows that this can minimise any later difficulties in the grieving process experienced by the bereaved (Raphael 1984, Wright 1996).

Spiritual and cultural care

The aftercare you provide needs to be sensitive and supportive regarding any particular cultural or religious rituals that are important to the bereaved in caring for

the deceased, being careful not to make any assumptions. While some may wish to be involved in the last offices of the deceased, this needs to be dealt with on an individual basis. The bereaved may request to have a spiritual leader contacted, or be comforted to receive one of the hospital chaplaincy members as key support at this time.

Information provision

There are a number of important practical responsibilities that need to be undertaken following the death of a patient, and this also needs to be dealt with sensitively and in a timely manner. For example, all necessary paperwork, e.g. the registration of death and the death certificate, should ideally be dealt with quickly and efficiently and given to the bereaved with appropriate explanations. They should also be informed of the process that will be followed regarding a post-mortem if appropriate and when and how they might obtain the results and from whom (DH 2005). If the deceased is not known to the hospital the death may be referred to the coroner, then documentation such as the death certificate may be delayed, and this can be very stressful for the bereaved. The bereaved may also require information regarding funerals or cremation and also helpful external contacts who may be able to give information regarding support, both in the immediate term and in the longer term (Murray Parkes 1998, Pattison 2008). This may be specific local services that are available in the trust (DH 2005, Walker 2010) or through other national organisations, some of which are listed in the text box. Providing informative leaflets to the bereaved (ideally translated into other languages) about support services may be helpful (Walker 2010).

National bereavement support

CRUSE Bereavement Care
A nationwide service that provides bereavement counselling advice, information and social contact.

Website: www.crusebereavementcare.org.uk

Helpline to find details of local branches:
0870 167 1677

The Compassionate Friends
An organisation that offers grief support to partents and bereaved families after the death of a son or daughter.

Website: www.tcf.org.uk

Helpline: 08451 232304

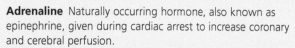

Conclusion

For many patients who experience a cardiac arrest, the efforts made do not result in survival and of those who do survive some will suffer long-term effects. However, at the outset it is often impossible to judge who will survive and make a full recovery. Following the guidance set out in this chapter will enable you to provide the best possible chances of a happy outcome. Adherence to the Resuscitation Council UK (2010) algorithms ensures that all those attending the cardiac arrest will be following the same procedures, enabling a coordinated and uniform response.

In addition to the care of the patient, the support of relatives regardless of the outcome has been discussed. A cardiac arrest may present you not only with many challenges but also the opportunity to provide high-quality care to patients and families at a very difficult time. Because of the challenges and difficulties involved in this situation it is important that following the event, whatever the outcome, you are involved in some sort of debrief. This does not need to be very time consuming but it is important to help you to put things into perspective. If you have followed the guidance given here it is very unlikely that anything you did or didn't do will have negatively affected the outcome. However, if you are left with feelings of worry and uncertainty you must seek guidance from a mentor, preceptor or more senior colleague.

Glossary

Adrenaline Naturally occurring hormone, also known as epinephrine, given during cardiac arrest to increase coronary and cerebral perfusion.

Agonal breathing Deep sighing, irregular gasping breathing, also known as Cheyne–Stokes breathing, which occurs at the end of life.

Algorithm Step-by-step procedure for problem-solving, often expressed as diagram or flow chart.

Asystole Complete absence of electrical and mechanical activity in the heart.

Bag valve mask A device used to provide artificial ventilation which consists of a manual compressible chamber with an oxygen reservoir at one end and a one-way valve and mask at the other.

Basic life support See cardiopulmonary resuscitation.

Cardiopulmonary arrest The sudden cessation of breathing and effective cardiac output.

Cardiopulmonary resuscitation (CPR) Emergency procedures to be undertaken in the event of cardiopulmonary arrest aimed at preventing irreversible brain damage caused by lack of oxygen. CPR consists of rescue breathing and cardiac compressions. CPR is also known as basic life support (BLS).

Defibrillation The reversal of fibrillation (inefficient and non-rhythmic contraction) by the delivery of a controlled electric shock.

Embolism Circulating foreign object such as air, fat or a blood clot which can lodge in and block a vessel.

Hyperkaleamia High level of potassium in the blood.

Hypokalaemia Low level of potassium in the blood.

Hypothermia Abnormally low temperature.

Hypovolaemia Low circulating blood volume.

Hypoxia Low levels of cellular oxygen.

Intraosseous The inside of a bone.

Intravenous The inside of a vein.

Pulmonary embolism The blockage of a pulmonary artery by a blood clot, fat or air.

Pulseless electrical activity (PEA) Organised electrical cardiac activity in the absence of a pulse.

Tamponade Compression of the heart by the accumulation of fluid in the pericardial space.

Tension pneumothorax Presence of air in the pleural space that occurs when air escapes into the pleural cavity from a bronchus but cannot regain entry into the bronchus. As a result, continuously increasing air pressure in the pleural cavity causes progressive collapse of the lung tissue.

Ventricular fibrillation Disorganised electrical activity in the ventricular myocardium resulting in an absence of effective cardiac output.

Ventricular tachycardia Cardiac arrhythmia originating from within the ventricles characterised by rapid ventricular complexes at a rate greater than 100/min. It may or may not be associated with a pulse.

Test yourself

1 On discovery of a collapsed unresponsive casualty who is not breathing the sequence of events you should follow is:

   a. assess for danger, assess for response, call for help, open the airway, assess breathing, commence compressions

   b. shout for help, open the airway, check for response, assess breathing assess for danger, commence compressions

   c. check for response, commence compressions, shout for help, assess for danger, open the airway, assess breathing

   d. check for danger, open the airway, assess response, assess breathing, commence compressions, shout for help

2 In *partial* airway obstruction:

   a. there will be no sound

   b. there will be paradoxical chest movement

   c. the casualty will be talking normally

   d. there will be tracheal tug with intercostal and subcostal recession

3 The interventions that contribute to a successful outcome following a cardiac arrest are known as:

   a. the weakest link

   b. the chain reaction

   c. the chain of survival

   d. the chain of resuscitation

4 Which of the following rhythms would you shock in a cardiac arrest situation?

   a. pulseless electrical activity (PEA)

   b. pulseless ventricular tachycardia

   c. atrial fibrillation

   d. asystole

5 During a cardiac arrest, adrenaline is given to:

   a. restart the heart

   b. slow the heart rate

   c. prevent further arrythmmias

   d. increase cerebral and coronary perfusion

6 When using a defibrillator you should:

   a. be trained in its use

   b. ensure oxygen is removed at least one metre away from the patient

   c. ensure everyone is clear of the immediate area before delivering a shock

   d. all of the above

7 During a cardiac arrest, chest compressions:

   a. should continue without any interruptions at all times

   b. should only stop during defibrillation

   c. should be continuous once the trachea is intubated

   d. should be delivered at a rate of 150 per minute

8 A *reversible* cause of a cardiac arrest is:

   a. hypovolaemia

   b. deep vein thrombosis

   c. myocardial infarction

   d. pyrexia

9 A reason to abandon a resuscitation attempt could be:

   a. the cardiac arrest team is called to another arrest

   b. discovery of cardiac tamponade

   c. asystole for more than 20 minutes without a reversible cause

   d. the casualty is over 80 years of age

10 A do not attempt resuscitation (DNAR) order may be put in place when:

   a. the patient has a terminal illness

   b. there is a documented request from a competent patient not to resuscitate

   c. the quality of life following a successful outcome is predicted to be very poor

   d. all of the above

References

Adams, S., Whitlock, M., Bloomfield, P. and Baskett, P. J. F. (1994) Should relatives watch resuscitation? *BMJ*, 308, 1687–9.

Awoonor-Renner, S. (1991) I desperately need to see my son. *BMJ* 302, 351.

Crisci, C. (1994) Local factors may influence decision. (Letters) *BMJ* 309, 406.

DH (Department of Health) (2005) *When a Patient Dies. Advice on developing bereavement services in the NHS*. London: DH.

Edwards, L. and Shaw, D. (1998) Care of the suddenly bereaved in cardiac care units: A review of the literature. *Intensive and Critical Care Nursing* 14, 144–52.

Grice, A. S., Picton, P. and Deakin, C. D. S. (2003) Study examining attitudes of staff, patients and relatives to witnessed resuscitation in adult Intensive Care Units. *British Journal of Anaesthesia* 91 (6), 820–4.

Hansen, C. and Strawser, D. (1992) Family presence during CPR: Foote Hospital 9-year perspective. *Journal of Emergency Nursing* 18, 104–6.

Hodgetts, T. J., Kenward, G., Vlackonikolis, I., Payne, S., Castle, N., Crouch, R., Ineson, N. and Shaikh, L. (2002) Incidence, location and reasons for avoidable in-hospital cardiac arrest in a district general hospital. *Resuscitation* 54,115–23.

ICS (Intensive Care Society) (2008) *Standards for the Management of Patients After Cardiac Arrest*. London: ICS.

Kent, H. and McDowell, J. (2004) Sudden bereavement in acute care settings. *Nursing Standard* 19 (6), 38–42.

Martin, J. (1991) Rethinking traditional thoughts. *Journal of Emergency Nursing* 17, 67–8.

Murray Parkes, C. (1998) *Bereavement. Studies of grief in adult life*. Harmondsworth: Penguin.

Osuwagu, C. C. (1991) ED codes: Keep the families out. *Journal of Emergency Nursing* 17 (6), 363–4.

Pattison, N. (2008) Caring for patients after death. *Nursing Standard* 22 (51), 48–56.

Raphael, B. (1984) *The Anatomy of Bereavement. A handbook for the caring professionals*. London: Hutchinson.

Resuscitation Council UK (2011) *Advanced Life Support*, 6th edn. London: Resuscitation Council UK.

Resuscitation Council UK (2010) *Resuscitation Guidelines*. London: Resuscitation Council UK. Available from http://www.resus.org.uk/pages/GL2010.pdf.

Resuscitation Council UK (1996) *Should Relatives Witness Resuscitation? A report from a project team of the Resuscitation Council (UK)* London: Resuscitation Council UK.

Royal College of Nursing, British Medical Association and the Resuscitation Council UK (2007) *Decisions Relating to Cardiopulmonary Resuscitation: A joint statement from the British Medical Association, the Resuscitation Council UK and the Royal College of Nursing*. London: BMA, RCUK, RCN.

Schein, R. M., Hazday, N., Pena, M., Ruben, B. H. and Sprung, C. L. (1990) Clinical antecedents to in-hospital cardiopulmonary arrest. *Chest* 98, 1388–92.

Schilling, R. J. (1994) No room for spectators. (Letters) *BMJ* 309, 406–12.

Smith, A. F. and Wood, J. (1998) Can some in-hospital cardio-respiratory arrests be prevented? A prospective survey. *Resuscitation* 37, 133–37.

Walker, W. M. (2010) Sudden cardiac death in adults: Causes, incidence and interventions. *Nursing Standard* 24 (38), 50–56.

Whitlock, M. and Adams, S. (1994) Should relatives watch resuscitation? *Proceedings of the Fourth International Conference of Accident and Emergency Medicine*.

Wilson, J. and White, C. (2011) *Guidance for Staff Responsible for Care After Death (Last Offices)*. London: The Stationery Office.

Wright, B. (1996) *Sudden Death. A Research Base for Practice*, 2nd edn. New York: Churchill Livingstone.

Further reading

Department of Health (2008) *Help is at Hand: A resource for people bereaved by suicide and other sudden traumatic death*. London: Department of Health.

Jevon, P. (2010) *Advanced Cardiac Life Support: A guide for nurses*, 2nd edn. Oxford: Wiley.

Moule, P. (2009) *Practical Resuscitation for Healthcare Professionals*, 2nd edn. Oxford: Wiley.

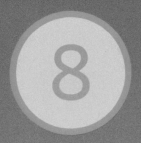

8

The patient with acute renal problems

Jacqui Finch

Aims

The aim of this chapter is to familiarise you with the functions of the kidney and the presentation and management of acute renal problems.

Objectives

After reading this chapter you will be able to:

→ Identify the major anatomical structures of the renal system

→ Identify the anatomical components of the nephron and describe the physiological properties of each section

→ Differentiate, from a physiological perspective, the three phases of urine production: tubular filtration, tubular reabsorption and tubular secretion

→ Distinguish between objective and subjective assessment data and the nurse's role in collecting this information

→ Critically discuss the nursing care and medical interventions that might be implemented in order to maximise renal status

Introduction

The renal system has a crucial role to play in maintaining homeostasis. The primary function of the kidneys is to produce urine as a waste product that can then be excreted from the body by the accessory renal organs: the ureters, the urinary bladder and the urethra. This is a complex physiological process, because as the blood plasma is filtered through the kidneys many adjustments are made to the water and solute levels in order to maintain a dynamic equilibrium within the body. Renal impairment, from a primary or secondary cause or a systemic illness such as sepsis, can quickly lead to life-threatening complications. The nurse therefore has a key role in, first, the prevention of acute renal injury in all patients (but particularly those most at risk) and, second, the early recognition and assessment of renal problems. The nurse must also effectively plan, implement and evaluate all interventions for those individuals with established renal dysfunction, effectively liaising with other members of the multidisciplinary team in the provision of quality care.

In this chapter, we will discuss four key areas: the applied anatomy and physiology of the renal system, common acute renal problems affecting patients, renal assessment and finally the ways in which renal status can be optimised through nursing care and medical management.

Gross anatomy of the kidney

The kidneys are situated on the posterior abdominal wall, outside the peritoneal cavity. Located on either side of the vertebral column, they are approximately 11cm in length, 5 to 6cm in width and 3–4cm thick. They are partially protected by the eleventh and twelfth pairs of ribs and they are capped by the adrenal glands. Each kidney is surrounded by three layers: a tough fibrous covering, the 'renal capsule', a layer of protective fat and a layer of connective tissue, the 'renal fascia', which attaches the kidney to the posterior abdominal wall (see Figure 8.1).

Each kidney has a hilum where the nerves, blood vessels, lymphatics and the ureter enter and exit. The renal artery, from the abdominal aorta, branches into interlobar, arcuate and interlobular arteries and finally the afferent arterioles which eventually form tufts of capillaries called glomeruli. Venous return is via a single efferent arteriole which branches to form a second capillary bed, the 'peritubular capillaries' and then interlobular, arcuate and interlobar veins leading to the renal vein and ultimately the inferior vena cava (see Figure 8.2). Lymphatic vessels follow the larger renal blood vessels and drain to the lateral aortic lymph nodes. The nerve supply to the kidney is via the sympathetic branch of the autonomic nervous system with afferent fibres entering the spinal cord at T10, T11 and T12. Blood flow is regulated by vasodilatation

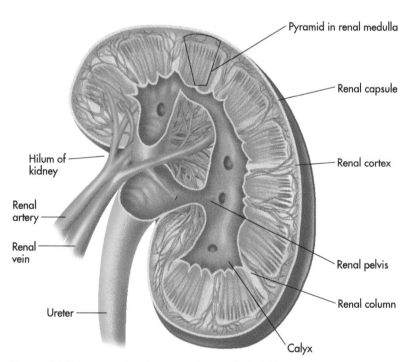

Figure 8.1 Internal and external anatomy of the kidney

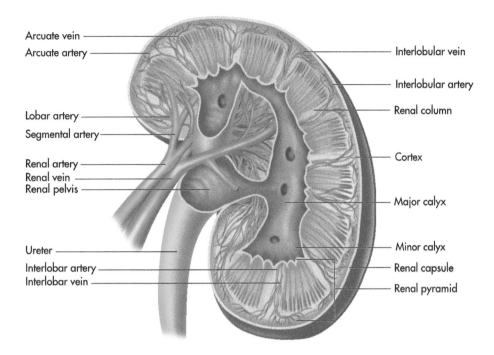

Renal artery → Segmental arteries → Lobar arteries → Interlobar arteries → Arcuate arteries → Interlobular arteries → Afferent arterioles → Glomerulus → Efferent arterioles → Peritubular capillaries → Interlobular veins → Arcuate veins → Interlobar veins → Lobar veins → Renal vein

Figure 8.2 Renal blood vessels and the pathway of blood through the renal system

and vasoconstriction, therefore controlling blood pressure in the glomerulus.

The *nephron* is the functional unit of the renal system. There are approximately one million of them per kidney and put together they would have a combined length of about 80 kilometres. Each nephron consists of two sections. First, a tubular area consisting of the glomerulus, the proximal convoluted tubule, the loop of Henle, the distal convoluted tubule and the collecting duct and secondly, a vascular area called the vasa recta (see Figure 8.3).

There are three specific areas in the kidney. There is an outer section called the *renal cortex* and this contains all of the glomeruli and portions of the tubule. The inner section is known as the *renal medulla* and this contains the straight segments of the proximal and distal tubules and the collecting ducts. Renal pyramids are found here and these cone-shaped areas have their apices ending in the papillae which open into the minor calyx. Urine passes from the collecting ducts in the pyramid to two small cavities, the minor calyces and the major calyces, and from here it enters the renal pelvis. Finally, the *renal pelvis* is formed from the expanded upper section of the ureter and it acts as a collecting space.

Accessory structures of excretion

There are several accessory structures of excretion in the renal tract (see Figure 8.4).

The ureters

These two tubes, approximately 28–34cm in length, convey urine from the renal pelvis to the bladder. In cross-section each ureter has a star shape and is composed of three layers:

- the tunica mucosa, an inner mucous lining;
- the tunica muscularis, a muscular middle layer (which propels urine by peristalsis along the ureters);
- the tunica adventitia, an outer fibrous layer.

The ureters run obliquely for a short distance within the bladder wall and this enables them to act as valves, preventing back flow of urine from the bladder into the ureters. In the female the ureters are close to the cervix and the ovaries, in the male they are adjacent to the seminal vesicles and prostate gland.

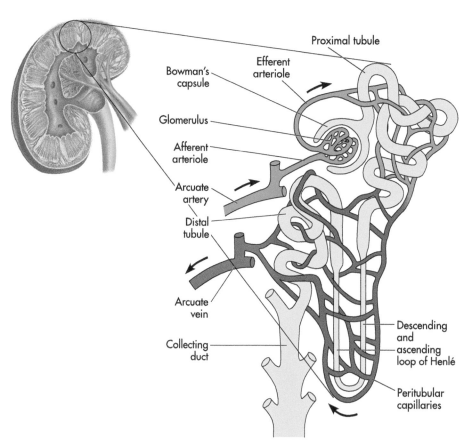

Proximal tubule

Efferent arteriole

Bowman's capsule

Glomerulus

Afferent arteriole

Arcuate artery

Distal tubule

Arcuate vein

Collecting duct

Descending and ascending loop of Henlé

Peritubular capillaries

Figure 8.3 The nephron

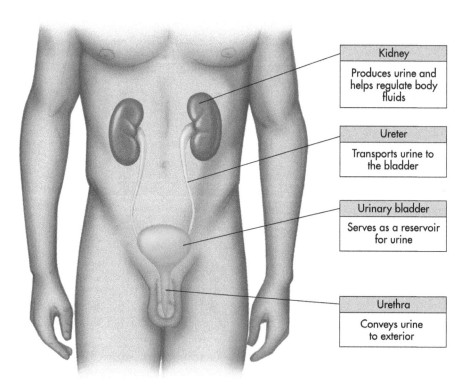

Kidney

Produces urine and helps regulate body fluids

Ureter

Transports urine to the bladder

Urinary bladder

Serves as a reservoir for urine

Urethra

Conveys urine to exterior

Figure 8.4 Anatomy of the urinary system

The bladder

This is a hollow, muscular bag located behind the symphysis pubis and in front of the rectum. In females, it rests on the anterior vagina and in front of the uterus and in males, it is situated above the prostate gland. The wall of the bladder is made up of three different layers:

- The tunica mucosa: this has folds called rugae in it and they allow the bladder to distend while acting as a reservoir for urine before it is excreted from the body.
- The tunica muscularis: this consists of three layers of meshed smooth muscle. In this area, a network of muscle fibres cross over one another in different directions and these are known collectively as the detrusor muscle.
- The tunica serosa or adventitia: this outer layer moistens tissue and lubricates surfaces so that when the bladder is full it does not compress other organs.

The average bladder can hold up to 300mL of urine before the desire to void is noted. Passing urine begins with voluntary relaxation of the external sphincter muscle of the bladder and then different regions of the detrusor muscle contract, forcing urine out of the bladder and through the urethra. Parasympathetic fibres from the autonomic nervous system transmit impulses that cause bladder contraction, therefore injury to the central nervous system can result in problems with passing urine.

Urethra

This is a small tube lined with mucous membrane leading from the floor of the bladder (trigone) to outside of the body. In the female it lies behind the symphysis pubis and in front of the vagina, extending down for approximately 3cm. In the male, the urethra is about 20cm long and it passes through the centre of the prostate gland, where it is joined by two ejaculatory ducts, thus also serving as a pathway for semen. From there it extends down and forward into the penis and ends as the urinary meatus at the tip of this organ. Urine is prevented from mixing with semen during ejaculation by a reflex closure of sphincter muscles at the bladder's opening.

Applied physiology

Functions of the kidney

The kidneys have a major role in maintaining homeostasis and when their function is impaired through disease or injury physiological effects can be seen throughout the

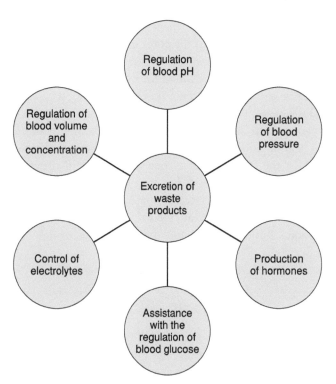

Figure 8.5 The functions of the kidney

body, affecting all organs. Through the regulation of body fluid volume, composition and pH, the subsequent production of urine to excrete waste products and the production of various hormones, the kidneys maintain equilibrium within the body (see Figure 8.5).

The regulation of body fluids and the production of urine

The tubular components of the nephron have a specific role to play in the formation of urine, which occurs in three stages: filtration, tubular reabsorption and tubular secretion.

Glomerular (Bowman's) capsule

This is where the first stage of urine production, filtration, takes place. Filtration is defined as the passage of a fluid and the substances in that fluid through a membrane under pressure. So, in this case, the blood and all of the constituents in the blood are pushed by the arterial blood pressure (at around 60–70mmHg) through the glomerular capillaries and then into the Bowman's capsule, via the glomerular-capsular membrane. This membrane has three special filtration layers in it with different size pores and the purpose of these is to retain some substances in the blood and to select others to be excreted via the renal tubules. First, the endothelial layer prevents the passage of blood cells, second, the basement membrane prevents the passage of large proteins and, third, the visceral layer prevents the passage of medium-sized proteins. Apart from the varying size of the pores in these different layers, there is another reason that blood and proteins cannot pass through from the blood into the filtrate and this is because these glycoproteins are carrying a negative electrical charge. The filtration membrane also carries a negative electrical charge and therefore repels them. Therefore, in health, blood cells and proteins should not be filtered out of the blood because they are needed in order to maintain normal blood function and to maintain the integrity of the intravascular space. Remember also, the kidney has an important role in regulating blood components through the production of erythropoietin.

> The hormone erythropoietin stimulates red blood cell production (erythrogenesis) in the bone marrow.

In contrast, whilst larger molecules cannot pass through, substances of smaller molecular weight like water, electrolytes, urea and amino acids can. Ultimately therefore, this means the kidneys are able to excrete certain amounts of these substances from the body. On average, 180 litres of plasma is filtered per day by the kidneys. Significant factors in this filtration process are, first, the arterial blood pressure and the degree of renal perfusion (especially if this is lowered). Second, the presence of proteins in the blood such as albumin, globulins and fibrinogen which may be impaired by conditions such as hypoalbuminaemia. Third, the pressure exerted by the Bowman's capsule itself which might be altered in disease processes such as glomerulonephritis. While in health, the kidneys have the ability to regulate filtration by adjusting blood flow into and out of the glomerulus through vasoconstriction or vasodilatation of the afferent arteriole, if any of the aforementioned parameters are deranged, for example, by hypovolaemia, this can affect the filtration pressure and in turn can lead to an abnormal glomerular filtration rate (GFR). The average GFR for an adult male is about 125mL per minute and for an adult female, 105mL per minute, but these parameters would be much reduced in conditions where poor renal perfusion occurs, such as in the case of dehydration (see Figure 8.6).

> Significant factors in filtration are: the arterial blood pressure, the presence of plasma proteins in the blood and the pressure exerted by the Bowman's capsule itself.

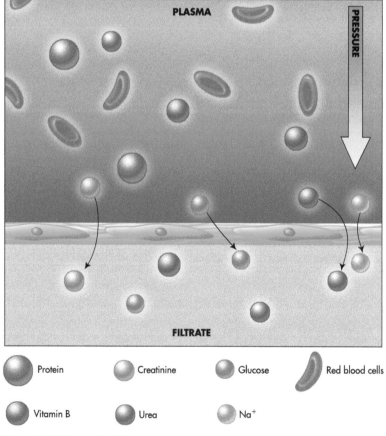

Figure 8.6 Filter selectivity

The kidney secretes an enzyme called renin from cells in the juxta glomerulus apparatus and this plays a significant role in regulating fluid balance and subsequently blood pressure. Renin is a vasoconstrictor and it leads to the release of other substances with similar properties: the chain of events that it initiates is collectively known as the renin–angiotensin–aldosterone system. Renin leads to the release of angiotensinogen produced by hepatocytes and converted in the plasma into angiotensin 1. This is then converted in the lungs into angiotensin 2, a very powerful vasopressor. The latter has two main functions:

- vasoconstriction of the afferent arterioles leading to a reduced glomerular filtration rate;
- the activation of aldosterone from the adrenal cortex which leads to the reabsorption of sodium into the extracellular space, with chloride and water following it.

The overall effect of these measures is to increase the circulating blood volume by fluid replenishment and ultimately an increase of the arterial blood pressure. Should the perfusion to the kidney continue to decrease, however, more drastic physiological responses are called for. In this case, the sympathetic autonomic nervous system will be activated and the release of norepinephrine will lead to increased vasoconstriction of the renal vasculature and a further reduction in the glomerular filtration rate.

Proximal convoluted tubule

The second stage of urine production, tubular reabsorption, begins in this section of the nephron. The filtrate coming from the glomerulus passes over the epithelial microvilli found here and is then reabsorbed back into the peritubular capillaries. In fact 99% of the plasma being filtered per day will be reabsorbed back into the blood via active transport mechanisms (using energy, adenosine triphosphate) and passive electrochemical gradients such as osmosis and diffusion. Two-thirds of this will have been reabsorbed by the time the filtrate reaches the end of the proximal convoluted tubule. A key substance to be reabsorbed is sodium, and glucose and amino acids are co-transported with it. Other substances such as potassium, calcium, phosphate, bicarbonate, magnesium, uric acid, amino acids, small polypeptides, lactic acid and water-soluble vitamins will also be reabsorbed under the influence of sodium in this part of the nephron. Reabsorption of all of these solutes increases the osmolality (concentration) of first the tubule cells, second, the

Remember

The kidneys can perform gluconeogenesis or the production of new glucose. This provides more glucose for energy production.

interstitial fluid and, finally, the blood. This in turn attracts water by osmosis and thereby ensures that the blood is osmotically balanced: in fact 65% of the filtered water is reabsorbed in the proximal convoluted tubule, at a rate of about 80mL per minute.

Calcium is needed for muscle contraction and together with phosphate it builds the extracellular bone matrix.

In this section of the nephron some tubular secretion, the third stage of urine production, also takes place. Hydrogen ions are actively exchanged for sodium ions to maintain electrochemical balance and ammonia, a toxic waste product derived from various amino acids, is filtered out into tubular fluid in the form of urea, most of which is secreted. Other agents like creatinine and some drugs such as penicillin are also secreted here.

Loop of Henlé

The loop of Henlé reabsorbs about 20–30% of the filtered sodium, potassium and calcium and there is also some bicarbonate, chloride and water reabsorption taking place here. This part of the nephron is composed of ascending and descending limbs; filtrate flows in one direction down the descending limb and then in the other direction up the ascending limb, therefore in opposing directions in parallel tubes. For this reason, this is often referred to as 'the counter-current mechanism'. Ultimately, the purpose of these limbs is to concentrate the filtrate and form an osmotically concentrated urine for excretion. This is achieved by the descending and ascending limbs having varying degrees of permeability to water and other solutes and also by having differences in their capacity to transport substances such as sodium and urea. Key factors influencing how concentrated urine becomes are active transport mechanisms and hormonal influences such as the action of the antidiuretic hormone (ADH), called vasopressin. This is made in the hypothalamus and secreted from the posterior lobe of the pituitary gland. Its role is to control the level of water reabsorption or excretion by the kidney.

Distal convoluted tubule

This structure begins with a convoluted section and this is virtually impermeable to water and so, because the water is retained in the lumen, it is able to contribute to the dilution of tubular fluid. The second, straighter segment is more permeable to water and is regulated by the antidiuretic hormone. Sodium can also be reabsorbed here and potassium actively secreted, both under the influence of the hormone aldosterone, secreted by the adrenal cortex.

The kidneys and the lungs together control acid-base balance. In the kidney, the distal convoluted tubule contributes to this process by secreting hydrogen ions. Hydrogen is very important because it maintains the integrity of cellular membranes and it facilitates enzyme action. The body produces about 50 to 100mEq of body acids per day through the metabolism of proteins, fats and carbohydrates, but the concentration of this acid in the body (in the form of hydrogen ions) must be kept within a fairly narrow range with a pH of 7.35–7.45. Even slight changes in the level of this substance can lead to cellular instability and altered biological processes in tissues. This is why in acute and critical illness, a disturbance of the acid-base balance often occurs and this can lead to organ damage.

> pH changes in the blood can lead to problems with perfusion and oxygenation.

In summary, when the blood pH decreases (becomes more acidic, for example pH 7.23) the kidneys secrete more hydrogen ions and simultaneously reabsorb more bicarbonate ions as a base substance and the net effect of this is to increase the pH back to normal. In contrast, if the blood pH increases (becomes more alkalotic, for example pH7.51) the kidneys will secrete less hydrogen ions and decrease bicarbonate reabsorption. This lowers the pH back to normal.

The collecting duct

This is a large straight tubule that extends down from the cortex of the kidney into the medullary section. On its route through the kidney it is joined by the distal tubules of several nephrons. The collecting duct then joins larger ducts and eventually forms a renal pyramid, these structures finally converge to form a tube that enters into the small calyces. From here the filtrate, now called urine, drains into the renal pelvis and then the bladder.

In summary, each of the components of the renal tubule has a key role in the production and finally excretion of the filtrate as urine (see Figure 8.7).

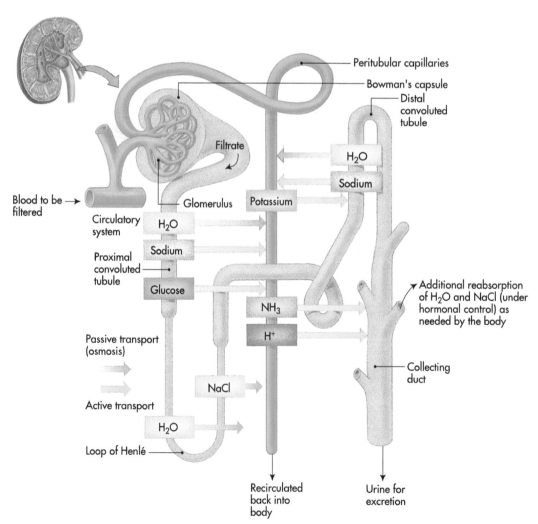

Figure 8.7 Sites of tubular reabsorption and secretion

Normal urine composition

In health urine is composed of water (approximately 95%) and various solutes, with a normal pH of 5.0–6.5 (although this may vary and become more alkaline after eating). It has a distinctive, aromatic odour (which should not be offensive) and a characteristic yellow colour and this is because it contains yellow pigments called urochromes which are produced by the breakdown of red blood cells in the liver. Bilirubin and its by product urobilinogen, also found in urine, are generated by the breakdown of old red blood cells.

> Urinalysis should always be performed at least daily on all patients in order to detect any abnormalities.

Specific gravity is the estimated level of solute in the urine and the normal range is between 1.016 to 1.022: the greater the solute level in relation to water, the greater the concentration. To illustrate this, in dehydration the reading might be high, for example 1.030, owing to reduced levels of water in the blood in comparison to solid matter. Urea constitutes the bulk of the solute in urine and this, together with other substances produced by protein catabolism, such as uric acid, ammonia and creatinine, form the nitrogenous waste products. There are also a number of electrolytes present, for example; sodium, potassium, ammonia, chloride, bicarbonate, phosphate and sulfate. In health, the amounts of these substances will vary slightly with diet. Hormones can also sometimes be found in urine if levels of these substances are high in the blood and toxins such as bacteria may also be present in the event of ill health (Thibodeau and Patton 2003).

When things go wrong – common acute renal problems

Glomerular disorders

Many disorders of the glomerulus are related to immunologic factors, but toxins such as drugs and some systemic diseases like diabetes mellitus can all contribute to the development of glomerular dysfunction. They may present initially as acute problems and while most people recover quite well, they can lead to a chronic disorder is some individuals, requiring haemodialysis and even renal transplantation.

One common complaint is glomerulonephritis, which is the collective name for all disorders that lead to inflammation of the glomerulus. Some patients presenting with this disease have what is known as a nephrotic syndrome. McCance et al. (2010) outline the characteristics symptoms of this disorder:

- a reduced glomerular filtration rate;
- haematuria and proteinuria. These abnormalities occur because the filtration membrane has been damaged. This leads to increased permeability and loss of the normal negative electrical charge, thus allowing these substances to pass into the urine when they would not usually be able to do so;
- oedema secondary to loss of plasma proteins in the urine such as albumin;
- hypertension secondary to excess fluid retention;
- hyperlipidaemia secondary to increased triglyceride and cholesterol production by the liver.

Depending on the cause, people with this problem often require pharmacological intervention in the form of diuretic or antihypertensive therapy to relieve oedema and hypertension, antibiotic administration to counteract infection, steroid administration to reduce inflammation and lipid-lowering drugs to reduce elevated blood fat levels (McCance et al. 2010). Specialist dietary advice should also be sought in order to reduce fat and replace lost proteins.

Infection

In health, urine is naturally acidic, the bladder empties completely, flushing the urethra and there is no back flow of urine into the renal tract: this means that above the urethra the urine is sterile. If, however, any part of the urinary tract is infected, a large number of microbes will be found in the urine, usually gram negative in origin (Thibodeau and Patton 2003). These infections may affect the lower urinary tract such as urethritis (inflammation of the urethra) or cystitis (inflammation of the bladder) or they may colonise the upper urinary tract involving the ureters and kidneys. One very common reason for bacterial colonisation of the urinary tract is urinary catheterisation (O'Callaghan 2006). The catheter can introduce bacteria into the bladder on insertion, it can cause damage to the urethra creating a portal for bacterial entry and it bypasses the normal voiding process. When caring for a patient with an indwelling urinary catheter the nurse must ensure that drainage bags are changed frequently, that daily meatal cleansing takes place and that good hand-washing practices are observed (Jones 2007). Samples of urine should also be sent to the microbiology department for culture and sensitivity, as ascending infection is easily introduced into the urinary tract and any infection that has occurred needs to be identified early so that appropriate treatment can be instigated.

> The insertion of a urinary catheter is a common cause of urinary tract infection.

One of the most common kidney infections is pyelonephritis. In many cases this is caused by the spread of bacteria such as *Escherichia coli* from the gut and, as with most urinary tract infection, it is more commonly seen in females due to the short urethra and the close proximity of the rectal and urethral openings. With pyelonephritis, the infection ascends into the bladder and then progresses to the ureters and eventually the kidneys, affecting the renal tubules and blood vessels. The symptoms are similar to those of all urinary tract infections in that they may include urgency and frequency of urination, pyrexia, back pain, increased leucocytes in the blood, dysuria and cloudy urine with bacteria present. If the infection becomes a chronic problem, scar tissue can form on the kidneys and lead to impaired function (McCance *et al.* 2010). Once infection is established other treatment is required in order to prevent long-term renal damage. This includes increased fluid intake to 'flush' the system (instigated for most patients unless there are specific reasons not to do so, such as fluid overload), antibiotic therapy and the prescription of antispasmodic drugs.

> Signs and symptoms of a urinary tract infection include:
> - Frequent, painful urination
> - Pyrexia
> - Back pain
> - Increased white cell count
> - Cloudy urine.

Renal calculi

These kidney stones are made up of calcium and other minerals found in urine and they can accumulate in the renal pelvis and calyces, leading to renal obstruction. Factors that predispose individuals to this problem include dehydration, excessive intake of vitamin D or calcium, high levels of uric acid and renal infection (Tortora *et al.* 2009). Small stones can pass through the ureters and urethra and be excreted in the urine, but larger stones can lead to obstruction of the ureters, especially as they may sometimes have jagged edges. When this happens it leads to intense, stabbing pain called 'renal colic', where the muscles of the affected ureter rhythmically contract in an attempt to dislodge the stone. The pain often starts in the flank of the affected side and radiates into the groin and it

may be accompanied by other urinary tract symptoms such as frequent urination or urge incontinence. If the stone cannot be moved, hydronephrosis may occur, this is when the kidney swells due to the obstructed flow of urine (Thibodeau and Patton 2003).

> Renal calculi causes severe pain as the muscles of the ureters try to pass the stones.

Renal calculi are usually diagnosed by a combination of history taking, clinical assessment and investigative procedures such as abdominal X-ray (90% of renal stones are radio-opaque), intravenous pyelogram (IVP) or a computerised tomography (CT) scan. Once diagnosed, treatment includes analgesia for the pain, an increase in water intake to help flush the stones out, an increase in dietary fibre because this binds calcium in the bowel and reduces its absorption and excretion in the urine and finally antibiotic therapy to treat any infection. Historically, surgical intervention was always required for the removal of stones that could not be passed. More recently, while this method of treatment may still be an option for very large stones, shock wave lithotripsy can be used to remove most calculi. In this radiological procedure, high-energy shock waves are used to reduce the stone to smaller fragments which can then be excreted in the urine (Tortora *et al.* 2009).

Acute urinary obstruction

Patients may present with difficulties in voiding urine owing to lower urinary tract obstruction. They can present with acute urinary retention requiring immediate catheterisation (possibly suprapubic) and then diagnosis of the cause. The common reasons for this problem include:

- In men, prostatic hypertrophy of benign or malignant origin. The passage of urine is impaired as the urethra passes through an inflamed or enlarged prostate gland.
- In women, organ prolapse. The uterus can herniate through the vaginal canal, so severely in some cases that it is visible on inspection of the external genitalia. A cystocele (when a portion of the bladder wall descends into the vaginal canal) or a rectocele (where the rectum bulges into the vaginal canal) can also develop and these disorders nearly always occur secondary to childbirth, although it is not usually until the menopause that they become evident.
- In men or women, urethral stricture may occur secondary to infection or trauma.
- In men and women, tumours of the renal tract may occur and these tend to affect individuals in the fifth

and sixth decades of life. Common symptoms include haematuria, pain in the affected area and sometimes a swelling of tissue. Kidney tumours are usually malignant in origin, metastasise early and often lead to urinary obstruction with hydronephrosis. Bladder cancers are also common, but with early intervention the prognosis is better than for kidney tumour. The development of bladder carcinoma is strongly linked to smoking and exposure to industrial chemicals. Aromatic amines, found in paints, dyes and other substances of a similar nature, have all been linked with the occurrence of the disease (Tortora *et al.* 2009).

Treatment for these disorders depends on the severity and the progression of the problem, but often surgical intervention is required to rectify the anatomical injury or disease.

Acute kidney injury

Acute kidney injury is when there is a sudden impairment of renal function leading to the accumulation of waste products in the blood. It is often a reversible condition, but if left untreated can lead to chronic renal failure. There are several predisposing factors, including age greater than 65 years, male gender, Afro-Caribbean descent and hypertension (Suleman and Rechner 2009).

> Risk factors in acute kidney injury:
> - 65 yrs
> - Male gender
> - Afro-Caribbean descent
> - Hypertension.

Acute kidney injury is classified according to the degree of blood chemistry impairment and the extent to which the urinary output is abnormal. In 2006, the Acute Dialysis Quality Initiative Group (ADQI) devised the RIFLE criteria (Suleman and Rechner 2009). This is outlined in Table 8.1.

The Acute Kidney Injury Network (AKIN) later proposed a modified version of the RIFLE criteria, called the AKIN criteria (see Table 8.2). With this classification system, there are two defining features: the serum creatinine in the blood and the degree of oliguria. If these are increasingly abnormal the acute kidney injury is said to be worsening (Davenport 2007).

The causes of acute kidney injury fall into three main categories.

Pre-renal

This volume-responsive injury occurs when there is a significant reduction in perfusion to the kidneys. It may

Table 8.1 The RIFLE criteria

Risk	Serum creatinine × 1.5 baseline or GFR > 25% Urinary output: < 0.5mL/kg/hr for 6 hours
Injury	Serum creatinine × 2 baseline or GFR > 50% Urinary output: < 0.5mL/kg/hr for 12 hours
Failure	Serum creatinine × 3 baseline or GFR > 75% or serum creatinine 352umol/L with acute rise > 44umol/L Urinary output: < 0.3mL/kg/hr for 24 hours or anuria for 12 hours
Loss	Complete loss of kidney function for more than 4 weeks
End stage kidney disease	End stage kidney disease for more than 3 months

Table 8.2 The AKIN criteria

Stage 1	Increased serum creatinine 150–200% from baseline. Urine output < 0.5mL/kg/hr
Stage 2	Increased serum creatinine >200–300% from baseline. Urine output < 0.5mL/kg/hr for > 12 hours
Stage 3	Increased serum creatinine >300% from baseline. Urine output < 0.3mL/kg/hr × 24hrs or anuria × 12 hours

happen as a result of a variety of conditions, but commonly:

- loss of circulating volume caused by dehydration, haemorrhage, burns;
- cardiac impairment leading to poor circulation;
- dilatation of peripheral blood vessels reducing the peripheral vascular resistance and therefore affecting the blood pressure (this occurs in sepsis);
- obstruction of renal blood vessels, for example, renal artery stenosis.

> **Remember**
> A lack of circulating volume leads to poor renal perfusion and a poor urine output: less than 0.5mL/kg/hr.

In all cases, the sympathetic autonomic nervous system and the renin–angiotensin–aldosterone system once activated, as part of a normal homeostatic response to changes in blood volume, contribute to the vasoconstriction and a further reduction in blood supply to the kidneys.

Acute intrinsic

This is when actual structural damage to the nephrons has occurred and it may lead to acute tubular necrosis, where tubular cells die and are shed into the tubule lumen resulting in tubular blockages. The most common causes for this are as follows:

- prolonged hypoperfusion;
- nephrotoxic drug therapy, especially the aminoglycoside antibiotics and the non-steroidal anti-inflammatory agents;
- exposure to radiocontrast agents;
- infections, for example unresolved glomerulonephritis;
- other diseases that can affect tubular function such as sickle-cell disease and certain malignancies.

> All nephrotoxic drugs should be stopped if the patient has renal impairment in order to avoid further renal injury.

Post-renal

This is where an obstruction anywhere in the renal tract is unresolved and eventually leads to kidney damage.

There are said to be three distinct phases to acute kidney injury what ever the original cause (Donald 2011). These are illustrated in Figure 8.8.

The patient's initial clinical presentation depends on the progression and severity of the disease, but commonly includes the following signs and symptoms:

- urine output less than 0.5mL/kg/hr;
- metabolic acidosis which may or may not be compensated;
- raised serum creatinine level above 111umol/L;
- raised serum potassium level above 5.1mmol/L;
- raised serum urea level above 7.0mmol/L;
- the serum sodium level may be high or low, depending on the kidney's ability to reabsorb the sodium into the blood.

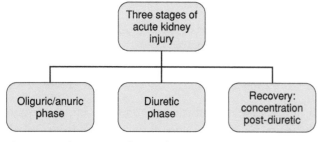

Figure 8.8 The stages of renal failure

Renal assessment

Historically, there have been problems with the late recognition and treatment of renal impairment amongst ward patients. Significantly, poor fluid balance management and unsatisfactory record keeping by the multidisciplinary team have been contributing factors. In such cases, the signs and symptoms of renal dysfunction have not been identified early enough and this has sometimes been followed by poor investigation and poor treatment of the patients' problems (Beaumont 2008, Scales and Pilsworth 2008). As late as 2009, a report from the National Confidential Enquiry into Patient Outcome and Death (NCEPOD) noted that the substandard management of individuals with a diagnosis of acute kidney injury had led to increased mortality for this patient group (Suleman and Rechner 2009).

> Clinical presentation includes:
> - Urine less than 0.5mL/kg/hr
> - Metabolic acidosis on blood gas
> - High serum creatinine, urea and potassium
> - High or low serum sodium.

In order to address these issues from a nursing perspective, a systematic approach to patient assessment must be adopted. The use of the ABCDE format and effective implementation of physiological track and trigger systems will monitor clinical parameters, identifying any significant changes. All early warning scoring systems enable recognition of patient deterioration from the onset and facilitate optimal intervention.

In previous chapters, the importance of recording subjective and objective data during the assessment process has been highlighted. A considerable amount of valuable information can be gathered about the patient's general medical history, any medication they are taking, the history of the current problem, the patient's perception of what is troubling them, their physical appearance and finally a physical examination. We also have a range of tests and investigations that can be used to determine renal status.

Subjective data

If any part of the renal tract is not working normally, the patient will probably be aware of it and report a range of unpleasant symptoms. In addition, such is the importance of the kidney to health that when problems do occur, all of the body's systems can be affected. A variety of complaints may arise if there are any abnormalities with the production and/or excretion of urine. These include among others lethargy and drowsiness, feelings of breathlessness, dizziness, palpitations, difficulties with urination, weight gain, pruritis, feeling hot or cold, nausea and vomiting and sometimes severe pain.

Objective data

Monitoring of vital signs is crucial in renal impairment. Patients with acute renal problems may exhibit changes with respiratory rate, heart rate and pattern, blood pressure, temperature and oxygen saturation, all owing to a number of physiological factors including: pain, pyrexia, dehydration or fluid overload, electrolyte disorders and acid-base imbalance. Frequent monitoring of these parameters, according to the early warning scoring system in use and the perceived severity of the patient's condition will alert nursing staff to any deterioration.

Obtaining the patient's weight gives useful information regarding fluid status.

One important issue is fluid balance. As discussed earlier, urine output should be at least 0.5ml/kg/hr, but if this volume is abnormal the patient may become dehydrated or overloaded with fluid. For this reason the patient's weight should be recorded, as this will reveal important information about fluid status. The patient may be volume depleted or alternatively the accumulation of oedema may have significantly increased their normal 'dry' weight, meaning the one they had before the onset of illness. If the severity of the patient's condition prevents them from being weighed, an estimate should be made from their physical appearance (height and body mass). Following this, strict charting of fluid gains and losses must be undertaken every 24 hours, with a calculated fluid deficit or fluid accumulation being reported to medical staff immediately. Nurses should also be aware of insensible losses, for example fluid lost through profuse sweating. All of this information needs to be taken into account when reporting fluid balance. Nurses must also always ensure that a urinary catheter is patent before assuming that the patient is oliguric or anuric – a bladder washout may be required for this purpose (Jevon 2007). In addition, bladder ultrasonography may be requested in order to establish if there is any urinary retention (Selius and Subedi 2008).

Always maintain an accurate fluid balance chart and take into account insensible losses.

Any urine that is passed must be tested for specific gravity, pH and the presence of abnormal constituents such as blood and protein, both of which can indicate malfunctioning kidneys. Remember though, it is important when testing urine to ensure that other causes of abnormal findings have been excluded, for example: haematuria secondary to menstruation or urethral trauma following catheterisation. Similarly, there may be proteinuria following contamination of a collecting receptacle. The appearance and smell of urine is also significant, for example, cloudy urine with an offensive odour is likely to indicate that a urinary tract infection is present.

A number of investigations into renal function may also be ordered by the medical staff. Nursing staff require knowledge of all invasive and non-invasive procedures so that they can work collaboratively with medical colleagues in treating the patient and act as a resource should the patient seek further information. Common renal investigations are outlined in Table 8.3.

Table 8.3 Renal investigations

Blood biochemistry	Looking at serum values of sodium, potassium, creatinine, urea and albumin amongst others
Full blood count	To diagnose whether or not the patient is anaemic, has an abnormal white cell count or low platelets – all common findings as renal function deteriorates
Arterial blood gas analysis	To measure the pH of the blood and identify metabolic acidosis consistent with renal failure
Microbiology	Cultures of blood and urine may be required in order to identify specific infections
Histology	A percutaneous renal biopsy may be needed to diagnose tumours and other causes of renal disease
Ultrasound	This test is always performed so that the size of the kidneys can be ascertained and so that any obstruction can be located
Angiography	A variety of techniques can be employed to inject contrast media into the renal tract so that its different structures can be visualised more closely. It should be noted that the radio-contrast agent that is used for this investigation can be nephrotoxic and sometimes protective pharmacology in the form of N-acetylcysteine is administered prior to the procedure being carried out (Suleman and Rechner 2009)

Physical examination

In order to identify patients at risk nurses have a professional responsibility to conduct a thorough holistic assessment using appropriate diagnostic and decision-making skills (Nursing and Midwifery Council 2010). It is important to remember however that while technology may be very useful in assisting this process, it can fail. The nurse must therefore not become complacent and rely exclusively on information gathered in this way, but instead use an array of assessment strategies to recognise and monitor the patient's condition (Browne and Cook 2011). As we have seen in earlier chapters, the ABCDE approach is a comprehensive assessment strategy to employ: this tool together with the key skills of looking, feeling and listening can reveal vital information about a patient's condition.

> **Remember:**
> - Look
> - Feel
> - Listen.

Inspect (look)

Observing a patient with renal problems can give the nurse vital information. First, when assessing the patient's ability to maintain their own airway via visual inspection and use of the Glasgow Coma Scale, the nurse should take into account the recorded levels of urea and electrolytes in the blood. As we have seen earlier, these can be grossly deranged in acute renal dysfunction and particular problems like a rising urea or a sodium imbalance can affect the level of consciousness and subsequently airway maintenance.

Even if the patient is able to maintain an airway, their breathing may be affected by the renal impairment for several reasons. Owing to a metabolic acidosis the patient may increase their respiratory rate in an attempt to excrete more carbon dioxide via the lungs and ultimately increase the pH of the blood. The arterial blood gas in this case will show a compensated metabolic acidosis, for example ph: 7.35, $PaCO_2$: 3.0kPa, PaO_2: 11.0kPa, HCO_3: 16 mmol/L and base deficit: −8 mmol/L.

It is essential to maintain a strict fluid balance chart because some patients may also have fluid overload and this can lead to the development of pulmonary oedema, where fluid fills the alveoli and prevents normal gas exchange. Hypoxaemia and eventually retention of carbon dioxide will occur and these will be evident on the arterial blood gas reading. In such cases, the work of breathing is increased and may manifest itself by an abnormal respiratory rate, changes to the pattern of breathing and use of the accessory muscles of respiration. The nurse will also be able to see the frothy, pink-tinged secretions expectorated by the patient and these are very characteristic of pulmonary oedema. If the patient is fluid overloaded they might appear oedematous, with fluid retention in the face and limbs (the latter particularly in dependent areas owing to gravity). There may also be a noticeable weight gain and as the problem progresses, changes to the vital signs may be evident in the form of hypertension and tachycardia as the workload of the heart is increased. A more detailed discussion on this is included in the cardiac chapter.

> Observe signs of anaemia, such as dyspnoea, pallor and lethargy.

Lastly, although it is more common in chronic renal impairment, the patient may be pale in appearance and very tired due to anaemia: as discussed earlier in the chapter, the kidney produces the hormone erythropoietin and this may be impaired. A blood sample should be sent for full blood count analysis to confirm a suspected anaemia and appropriate treatment started if necessary. This is a significant clinical issue, because anaemia will further increase the work of breathing for the patient owing to the lack of haemoglobin required for oxygen carriage.

While some patients with renal impairment may be fluid overloaded, some in contrast will present with fluid depletion owing to a loss of circulating volume, for example, severe haemorrhage. When assessing the circulatory function, it might be noted on inspection that the patient's skin is dry with a loss of elasticity. They may have a furred tongue, cracked lips and sometimes sunken eyes. In this case, if there is any urine output it will be diminished in volume (less than 0.5mL/kg/hr) and appear very dark and concentrated, with a high specific gravity noted on urinalysis. This patient may also present with hypotension and tachycardia due to hypovolaemia.

> Observe for signs of dehydration, such as dry skin, furred tongue, cracked lips and sunken eyes.

A problem common to all patients with renal insufficiency is electrolyte imbalance and this may lead to the

> Observe for frothy sputum – a sign of pulmonary oedema.

development of cardiac arrhythmias (the existing metabolic acidosis will further contribute to cardiac instability because of cellular disruption). If a cardiac monitor is *in situ* or a 12-lead electrocardiograph (ECG) recording is taken, specific changes may be noted, such as arrhythmias or damage to one particular area of the heart. All ECG changes need to be recognised and acted upon quickly in order to prevent life-threatening arrhythmias such as ventricular tachycardia, ventricular fibrillation and asystole from occurring. A more detailed discussion on electrophysiology can be found in the cardiac chapter.

> Monitor the patient for cardiac arrhythmias and record a 12-lead ECG.

Holistic assessment of the patient is important when renal impairment is suspected as the inability of the body to excrete waste products can affect all organs. We have already noted how the patient's conscious level may be impaired by the accumulation of urea; the higher this substance is in the blood the more likely the patient will become comatose. Individuals with deteriorating renal function can develop uraemic encephalopathy and this occurs when high levels of urea in the blood have impaired neurotransmission. Similarly, visual inspection of the skin is important not just for an estimate of the patient's fluid status, but to determine whether or not the uraemia is worsening. The skin can take on a yellow tinge as can the mucous membranes as the urea accumulates. The patient may subsequently complain of intense pruritis and this may lead to an increased risk of infection through skin trauma. As the gut is also affected by rising urea levels in the blood, the patient may have signs of gastrointestinal illness such as persistent hiccupping, vomiting and diarrhoea (O'Callaghan 2006).

Palpation and percussion (feel)

In renal dysfunction, the nurse can gather important assessment data from touching the patient. Feeling the patient's pulse can identify if it is weak as in volume depletion, bounding as in volume overload or irregular as in the presence of arrhythmias. Touching the skin can detect pyrexia, hypothermia or poor perfusion; the latter can be further assessed by testing capillary refill. Oedema and swelling can also be noted from palpation and percussion.

> Always take a patient's pulse manually so that the strength can be felt.

It is also important to remember that from a psychological perspective touch can be therapeutic for the patient, creating a means of non-verbal reassurance and comfort (Hayes and Cox 2009). Touching the patient's hand during the assessment process may relieve anxiety and instill a sense of peace, however, the nurse should always be sensitive to the appropriateness of physical contact and explain all actions. From a cultural perspective, touch may be deemed unsuitable by some patients, especially if there is a difference in gender (Giger and Davidhizar 2004).

Auscultation (listen)

Listening is an important skill for the nurse to acquire and perfect. In the first instance we need to listen carefully to our patients and note what they are actually saying. Unless a patient is unconscious, they can often report significant symptoms that will facilitate nursing care and assist medical diagnosis and treatment. Patients with renal colic for example can inform us of the location, duration and intensity of their pain: similarly patients with urinary tract infections can recall the unpleasant sensations of frequency and urgency of micturition. They can also directly evaluate therapeutic interventions and, although some patients are better historians than others, chart the progress of a disorder from onset to resolution.

> Listen for sounds of an obstructed airway or abnormal breathing such as wheezing and stridor.

The way in which a patient speaks is also significant, as there may be evidence of confusion or the patient may be very breathless and unable to complete sentences. Even if patients are unable to verbalise, nurses can still gather valuable information through listening to physiological sounds. A patient with a compromised airway due to uraemic encephalopathy may start to make a snoring noise as the muscular tone in the oropharynx is reduced. Other noises indicative of impaired airway patency include stridor caused by occlusion or the high-pitched crowing noise characteristic of laryngeal spasm (Jevon and Ewens 2007). These problems require the nurse to initiate emergency airway management, an issue discussed in more detail in the respiratory chapter.

Auscultating a patient's chest can also reveal useful information. The frothy secretions that occur in pulmonary oedema create adventitious breath sounds: fine crackles can be heard when a stethoscope is placed appropriately on the chest wall. Wheezing may also be heard if there is a degree of bronchoconstriction present.

CASE STUDY 8.1 Mr Jones with an acute kidney injury secondary to volume depletion

PATIENT HISTORY AND INITIAL ASSESSMENT

Mr Jones, a 70-year-old retired building contractor, has been admitted to the ward from the accident and emergency department accompanied by his wife. For the past 10 days he has been at home suffering from severe diarrhoea and vomiting: infective gastroenteritis is thought to be the cause as other members of his family have recently been unwell too, including Mrs Jones.

His vital signs on admission are:

Heart rate: 120 beats per minute, sinus rhythm
Blood pressure: 88/55mmHg
Respiratory rate: 28 breaths per minute
SpO$_2$: 90% on air
Temperature: 37°C.

On physical examination, the medical registrar notes that his abdomen is soft and non-tender to palpation, with no evidence of distension. A chest X-ray is taken and no abnormality is noted, the chest is clear. Blood is taken for biochemical and arterial blood gas analysis and the following results are obtained:

Biochemistry

Haemoglobin: 13.7 (range: 13.0–17.5g/dL)
White cell count: 12.5 (range: 4.5–11.0 ×10^9/L)
Platelets: 493 (range: 140–450 ×10^9/L)
Sodium: 142 (range: 135–145mmol/L)
Potassium: 6.8 (range 3.5–5.1mmol/L)
Urea: 39.2 (range: 3.2–7.0mmol/L)
Creatinine: 317 (range: 63–111umol/L)
Glucose: 7 (range: 4–8mmol/L)
Inflammatory marker C reactive protein: 200 (range 0–8mg/L).

Arterial blood gas

pH: 7.32 (range: 7.35–7.45)
PaCO$_2$: 4.5 (range: 4.5–6.1kPa)
PaO$_2$: 9.5 (range: 11–13kPa)
HCO$_3^-$: 18 (range: 22–26mmol/L)
BE: −6 (range: −2 to +2mmol/L).

These blood readings together with the history and the initial physical examination confirm that the problem is probably of infective origin. They also confirm that there is renal impairment, with the development of a metabolic acidosis and elevated serum potassium, urea and creatinine readings. Given the history and the blood analysis, dehydration is the most likely cause. Not only has Mr Jones lost body fluids through the diarrhoea and vomiting, he has also not been able to eat and drink normally. He tells the nurse caring for him that he has only had sips of water

for the past 5 days and has not drunk anything for the past 24 hours. He has not passed any urine for about 12 hours.

A lifelong smoker of up to 40 cigarettes a day, he has recently given up. He has a past medical history of hypertension and prior to this current illness he had been taking a daily dose of oral furosemide (40mg) prescribed by his GP to manage this.

Oxygen therapy is commenced at 2 litres via a face mask, intravenous access is obtained and a urinary catheter inserted and confirmed as patent. 100ml of dark, concentrated urine is drained and on urinalysis it has a specific gravity of 1.030, but no actual abnormality is detected in it. Mr Jones is then given a fluid challenge of 500ml of normal saline 0.9% over 15 minutes. In response to this, his blood pressure improves slightly to 90/60mmHg but he remains tachycardic at 110 beats per minute. He is then given a further 1.5 litres of the same crystalloid solution over the next two hours. Another priority at this time is the reduction of the serum potassium level and, in order to achieve this, an infusion of 50ml of dextrose 50% with 10 units of actrapid insulin added to it is commenced and given over 20 minutes. Close monitoring of Mr Jones' vital signs and urine output continues throughout this period.

Following the fluid administration his vital signs spontaneously revert to normal parameters:

Heart rate: 82 beats per minute, sinus rhythm
Blood pressure: 115/60mmHg
Respiratory rate: 18 breaths per minute
SpO$_2$: 98% on 2 litres of oxygen.

The serum potassium level is also rechecked and found to be 5.8mmol/L, there is however no improvement in his urinary output. A decision is made that no other immediate treatment be instigated at this time and the plan is to transfer him to the ward for further assessment and management.

WARD ASSESSMENT AND ONGOING MANAGEMENT

Airway

Mr Jones is fully conscious with a patent airway.

Breathing

His respiratory rate remains stable and regular at 16–18 breaths per minute and there is no evidence of increased work of breathing. He is not using his accessory muscles of respiration and his oxygen saturation reading remains at

98–99% on 2 litres of oxygen via a face mask. He has a cough which is dry and non-productive, but chest auscultation reveals no adventitious breath sounds.

Circulation

Mr Jones is very pale in appearance and his skin cold to the touch, particularly at the peripheries. His capillary refill time is prolonged at four seconds suggesting that perfusion is inadequate, a common finding in cases of hypovolaemia. He is emaciated in appearance, with dry skin, a furred tongue and sunken eyes, all clinical signs of dehydration. An intravenous infusion of 500ml of normal saline 0.9% is currently in progress and further fluids are prescribed. Cardiac monitoring is commenced and hourly observations taken: his heart remains in sinus rhythm with a rate of 80–90 beats per minute. The nurse is particularly aware that Mr Jones still has an elevated potassium on the last reading and that this electrolyte disorder can precipitate cardiac arrhythmias and even cardiac arrest: close observation is therefore required to detect the characteristic warning signs, such as flattened P waves, peaked T waves and ectopic beats.

At present all other vital signs are stable, but as the medical registrar has advised that there is no clinical indication for further arterial blood gas analysis the nurse is especially vigilant to monitor the heart rate, blood pressure and respiratory rate in case the patient's condition deteriorates. The presence of a metabolic acidosis will have a depressant effect on the myocardium and may precipitate further arrhythmias and hypotension, there may also be compensatory respiratory changes in the form of hyperventilation in order to excrete acid and increase the pH of the blood.

Mr Jones is weighed and found to be 78 kilograms, so the nurse takes this into account when recording the amount of urine he is passing each hour which is about 10–15ml. This is inadequate at this body weight, indicating that the patient is oliguric. The nurse is also aware that given the patient's medical history, his pre-existing hypertension will predispose him to renal impairment. Renal blood vessels can be damaged by angiotensin 2 stimulation and subsequent vasoconstriction leading to poor glomerular filtration. Mr Jones has also been taking a daily dose of furosemide which is known to have some nephrotoxic properties. She commences a fluid balance chart in order to monitor input and output closely.

Disability

In spite of Mr Jones' serum urea being elevated he is able to ask and respond to questions without any confusion or disorientation being apparent. He is weak, but able to fully mobilise and he was able to assist staff in transferring him from the accident and emergency trolley on to the ward bed. His Glasgow Coma Score is 15: E4/V5/M6.

Exposure

His temperature remains stable at 37.°C and there are no wounds or abrasions to his body other than the intravenous access that is *in situ*. In deteriorating renal function there is an increased risk of infection, so potential sources are closely monitored, such as an inflamed intravenous access site or a skin abrasion. Mr Jones already has a high white cell count and a raised C reactive protein level as a result of the gastric infection he acquired. In addition, he is dehydrated and he has not eaten for nearly two weeks, his nutritional state is therefore severely impaired which again will predispose him to infection. He is currently nil by mouth until the vomiting has completely subsided. The nurse feels that the patient requires anti-emetic medication and contacts the doctor, because apart from the gastric infection the high urea levels in his blood are making him feel nauseated. The nurse also discusses with the doctor the need to commence an infusion of dextrose 20%, in order to prevent hypoglycaemia. He is also aware that in the days to come dietary advice will need to be sought from the dietician, as Mr Jones will eventually require a carefully calculated balance of protein, fats and carbohydrates.

At the end of the assessment the nurse calculates the early warning score according to the trust's protocol. She records a score of 1 for an increased respiratory rate and 2 for a decreased urine output, making a total of 3. The trigger point according to the trust documentation is 4, so for the time being close monitoring of his condition is required without further escalation of treatment. She documents all findings and prepares to inform colleagues at the nursing handover that Mr Jones has been diagnosed with a likely volume-responsive kidney injury secondary to hypovolaemia. The initial plan is to continue with the administration of intravenous fluids to fully rehydrate him and to closely monitor his renal function over the next 24–48 hours. If this does not improve and reach the target goal of at least 0.5ml/kg/hr, further medical management of his renal dysfunction will be required.

Mr Jones does not show any significant increase in his urine output over the next 24 hours, in spite of the fluid replacement. A decision is made to insert a central venous pressure line via the left internal jugular vein so that his fluid status can be correctly ascertained and this shows

---

CASE STUDY 8.1 Mr Jones with an acute kidney injury secondary to volume depletion (*continued*)

that he has a reading of 12mmHg. As he is now fully rehydrated, the continued administration of significant volumes of intravenous fluid may be potentially harmful and predispose him to becoming overloaded with fluid, however, his urea and creatinine levels remain elevated and his potassium level is beginning to rise again. The nurse therefore contacts the doctor and a decision is made to commence a furosomide infusion at a dose of 2mg per hour (50mg/50ml) in order to stimulate renal function. The doctor also requests that Mr Jones urine output is

monitored closely for the next six hours. Unfortunately, during this time, his renal output remains very poor for his body weight and his electrolytes remain abnormal, so a specialist opinion is sought from a nephrologist who recommends that renal replacement therapy in the form of haemofiltration be commenced. Mr Jones is subsequently transferred to the intensive care unit for this intervention and while his body fluids and electrolytes are being optimised, a plan of care is formulated for future medical management.

Maximising renal status

The aims of treating a patient with acute renal impairment are the early recognition of the problem and the restoration of normal fluid and electrolyte status. All therapeutic interventions are focused on rectifying the kidneys' inability to excrete the waste products of metabolism and on preventing further kidney injury from developing. For some patients this will not be possible and they will go on to develop chronic renal dysfunction, but for a large number of individuals who have sustained a perfusion injury in acute illness, early effective medical intervention and good nursing care can prevent further deterioration and ultimately preserve renal function.

Fluid replacement

There has been some debate in recent years as to which type of intravenous fluid a hypovolaemic patient should be given to increase their circulating volume: colloid or crystalloid solutions (Younker 2007). Blood products and other colloid infusions like gelofusine contain larger molecules and are therefore able to increase blood pressure without the administration of large volumes of fluid. They do this by expanding the plasma compartment and increasing the plasma osmolality, their large molecules generate an oncotic pressure and pull water from the interstitial compartment and subsequently increase the circulating volume (Sumnall 2007). Colloids are widely used for this purpose, but they do carry the risk of allergic reaction for some patients and they can impair blood clotting and reduce haemoglobin levels through haemodilution. The latter may be a problem for patients with anaemia due to reduced erythropoietin production and blood transfusion may be required in some cases.

Crystalloid solutions like normal saline 0.9% and dextrose saline are isotonic in nature. They are also able to increase the circulating volume, but because their molecules are smaller it has been suggested that larger volumes of these solutions are required to have the same effect as colloids. They contain similar sodium concentrations to the extracellular fluid and are distributed to all body compartments, their plasma expansion being quite short-lived. Caution must be taken when administering them because of the risk of fluid overload and in some cases the potential to disrupt serum chloride levels which in turn can lead to a metabolic acidosis (Sumnall 2007, Kishen 2008).

> A 24-hour urine collection may be requested to determine fluid balance and creatinine clearance.

Which then is better – colloid or crystalloid? In fact, there is no clinical evidence to suggest that either is; both have their place in intravenous fluid replacement regimes and both have advantages and disadvantages that nursing staff need to be aware of when administering them. One useful guide to fluid restoration is to replace what has been lost from the body, for example if haemorrhage has occurred then blood will be required, in contrast if a patient has severe dehydration through persistent diarrhoea and vomiting (like Mr Jones in the case study) then crystalloid fluid replacement is usually given (Ewart and Huntington 2007, Sumnall 2007, Younker 2007).

> **Remember!**
> Pyrexia increases fluid loss through sweating and increased respiration.

Whatever is prescribed, the nurse must ensure that strict monitoring and charting of all fluids lost (including any wound and nasogastric drainage or diarrhoea) and all fluids administered is carried out in order to avoid further physiological complications. Twenty-four-hour urine collections are often requested in order to gain additional information about fluid and electrolyte balance, especially creatinine clearance. The nurse should also be aware of insensible fluid losses, particularly in the presence of pyrexia, when assessing a patient's fluid status. Ideally, a patient receiving fluid resuscitation will have a central venous catheter sited so that accurate assessment of right-sided heart function and fluid status can be determined. Fluid challenges (for example 500mL of normal saline 0.9% or a colloid solution like gelofusine given over 15–30 minutes intravenously) are often administered in the first instance so that cardiac and renal response to volume loading can be safely assessed prior to the administration of larger amounts of fluid (Leach 2009). If a patient is known to have compromised cardiac status smaller volumes of fluid, for example 250mL, would be given as a fluid challenge (Jevon 2007).

> A fluid challenge may be requested to determine response to volume loading.

Correction of abnormal electrolyte levels

In the fluid and electrolyte chapter, we learned of the significance of maintaining optimal electrolyte levels in the body. Abnormal levels, whether they are too high or too low, can be life threatening for the patient. Sodium, potassium, calcium and magnesium in particular are required for cellular stability and levels that are out of the normal range can lead to severe problems with cardiac, renal and neuromuscular function. The nurse will need to be vigilant for any signs of electrolyte imbalance, such as lethargy, muscle weakness, paraesthesia, gastrointestinal symptoms and, most significantly, hypotension and arrhythmias. Together with careful observation of fluid balance, cardiac monitoring should be in process and regular 12-lead ECG readings taken.

In acute renal impairment, the following may be seen:

- Sodium levels may be high or low depending on whether or not the kidney is able to reabsorb sodium back into the blood, a process that should naturally occur in health. In advancing states of renal dysfunction the kidney is often unable to reabsorb the sodium and the patient develops a polyuria, the ability of the

> Some patients with renal dysfunction can present with polyuria as their condition worsens.

body to conserve water being lost. In all cases, careful fluid management is required.

- Potassium reabsorption and secretion should be regulated by the kidney, but when function is impaired it will start to rise in the blood and this can lead to fatal arrhythmias amongst other problems. A significantly high potassium level (greater than 6.5mmols/L) needs to be treated urgently, usually by the administration of one of the following pharmacological interventions. First, intravenous dextrose and insulin in combination or, second, administration of the beta 2 agonist salbutamol (nebulised or intravenous). Both therapies can be used in prescribed doses to lower the serum potassium level. These agents will work by promoting potassium transport from the serum into the intracellular space. Calcium (10mls of calcium gluconate 10% by slow intravenous injection) may also be given because this has cardioprotective properties: it will prolong the plateau phase of the action potential and therefore prevent any tachyarrhythmias from occurring. Calcium resonium, an exchange resin, can also be used to extract potassium from the gut, either by oral or rectal administration. All of these drugs will have a temporary effect, but will allow time for the underlying cause to be identified and specific treatment commenced (Roseveare 2009).

> Abnormal electrolyte levels can be life threatening and require immediate correction.

- Serum calcium levels are usually normal in acute kidney injury, but patients who are developing a chronic renal impairment often present with low levels of this cation in their blood and this is due to inadequate vitamin D production by the kidneys. Calcium replacements will then be required. This problem is often accompanied by rising levels of phosphate in the blood.

- Magnesium levels may be low in patients with renal disease, especially those who consume excessive amounts of alcohol.

Other pharmacological interventions

Drugs are metabolised in different ways according to their molecular properties, some are protein bound, some lipid soluble and some water soluble. Many of them are excreted by the kidney and if there is renal impairment toxic levels of the agent can accumulate in the blood. Impaired glomerular filtration and ineffectual tubular secretion can lead to certain drugs reaching harmful levels, added to which patients with renal problems can often develop increased sensitivity to drugs, with poor tolerance of their side effects.

Two key issues to address then are, first, what is being prescribed and whether or not adjustments need to be made to the drug dosage in the interests of patient safety. Second, are any known nephrotoxic agents currently being taken by or given to the patient. Drugs such as ampicillin, gentamicin and digoxin can all reach toxic levels and need to be monitored closely. Others, like non-steroidal anti-inflammatory drugs, can lead to direct kidney injury and would need to be stopped immediately (Jevon 2007).

> The nurse should check that nephrotoxic drugs have been stopped or are being monitored very closely.

Some pharmacological agents are used in the treatment of renal impairment, the choice of which depends on the type of kidney injury and the severity of the problem:

- *Oxygen therapy* previously discussed in the respiratory chapter may be prescribed for some patients in order to optimise gas exchange. Careful monitoring of the patient's colour, perfusion and SPO$_2$ readings must be carried out and arterial blood gas analysis where required.
- *Diuretic therapy* in the form of furosemide is often prescribed if patients are deemed to be overloaded because of fluid retention, especially if there is a degree of pulmonary oedema secondary to heart failure. This drug is classified as a loop diuretic and it works by inhibiting reabsorption from the ascending limb of the loop of Henlé in the renal tubule. It has several side effects, most significantly hypokalaemia (because it is not a potassium-sparing diuretic), hyponatraemia, hypocalcaemia, hypomagnesaemia and hypotension all owing to excessive diuresis. Another side effect of furosemide, if given in large enough doses, is ototoxicity. Generally, caution must be taken with the drug because it has also been known to contain some nephrotoxic properties (Sumnall 2007).

> When diuretic therapy is prescribed, the nurse should be aware of the possibility of hypotension and excessive electrolyte loss in the urine.

- *Correction of metabolic acidosis* may be necessary. This problem is common to all types of renal impairment and cannot be left untreated because it will impair tissue perfusion and have a depressant effect on the myocardium. In the first instance, it can often be remedied by fluid therapy, as this will restore tissue and renal perfusion. However, if the patient is fluid overloaded, then diuretic therapy may be required to promote the

excretion of metabolic acid. Of more concern though is the severe acidosis (pH less than 7.10) that is resistant to these preliminary interventions, in such cases intravenous sodium bicarbonate may be administered. This solution will buffer the excess hydrogen ions that have accumulated and therefore increase the pH of the blood. Caution must be taken however, as side effects include metabolic alkalosis with respiratory compensation and an increased serum sodium level which may ultimately affect fluid balance in the body (Leach 2009).

- **Inotropic therapy** is occasionally used to manage renal impairment, although it is not widely recommended. There is sometimes a need to increase the mean arterial pressure to improve renal perfusion, in such cases norepinephrine or epinephrine may be prescribed (Leach 2009).

> **Remember!**
> For accurate, safe administration of inotropic drugs, the dose must be calculated in mcg/kg/min.

Renal replacement therapy

Finally, this therapy will be required if the acute kidney injury fails to respond to fluid therapy and pharmacological interventions. With this treatment fluid and solutes are removed from the patient's blood as it passes through a membrane or filter and then returned into the systemic circulation. It may take the form of peritoneal dialysis, haemofiltration or haemodialysis, although haemofiltration is the mode of choice for acutely ill patients as this removes substances in a slower, more continuous way which is better tolerated if there is any haemodynamic instability (O'Callaghan 2006, Leach 2009, Roseveare 2009).

Holistic nursing care for patients with renal dysfunction

Patients with a diagnosis of renal dysfunction require skilled nursing care. Continual assessment of the patient's condition and careful planning, implementation and evaluation of nursing interventions is essential if actual and potential problems are to be addressed and the patient's safety ensured. Accurate documentation and record keeping are also part of this process, as is effective communication with all members of the multidisciplinary team (Nursing and Midwifery Council 2010).

Physically, renal patients present with many signs and symptoms which may not only lead to systemic instability and a risk of further deterioration, but will leave them feeling very weak, tired and generally unwell. Full nursing care is required, with particular attention being paid to the skin which may easily break down or become infected, and oral care is needed especially if the patient has impaired consciousness, is dehydrated or receiving oxygen therapy. In most cases the patients will also have a degree of anorexia and malnutrition requiring the nurse to encourage oral intake (if oral diet is permitted) or to provide enteral or parenteral nutrition. Specialist advice should be sought from the dietician when addressing the dietary needs of renal patients, especially with regard to the protein, potassium and sodium content of food and drinks, as these need to be carefully calculated on an individual basis according to the patient's renal function. Once the diet has been reviewed the nurse then has an important role in health education and health promotion, as the patient may find it difficult to adhere to the regime (Nursing and Midwifery Council 2010).

> To effectively address the dietary needs of renal patients, specialist advice must be sought from the dietician.

Psychosocially, the patient may have other needs. They may be very concerned about the diagnosis of renal dysfunction because, unless a good response to initial treatment is seen, long-term dialysis may be required with the introduction of strict dietary and fluid restrictions. These treatments will have a considerable impact on the patient's lifestyle, in some cases raising difficulties with personal relationships or with their employment status – possibly leading to financial hardship. In addition, the patient may ultimately undergo renal transplantation if a suitable donor can be found and will then have further treatment modalities to adhere to postoperatively. If the patient (and family) wishes to discuss any concerns the nurse needs to spend time listening and, where appropriate, offer advice and guidance, with appropriate referral to colleagues such as the social worker where necessary. It is important that as a health care provider the nurse works across professional boundaries and acts as a change agent within the multidisciplinary team, providing leadership and direction to care delivery (Nursing and Midwifery Council 2010).

> A diagnosis of renal failure can have a profound psychological effect on the patient, especially if long-term dialysis is required.

Conclusion

In this chapter, we have reviewed the anatomy and physiology of the renal system and explored the ways in which acute dysfunction may manifest itself. Investigations into renal function and how the patient's clinical condition might be maximised by nursing and medical intervention has also been addressed.

In summary, the kidneys have a key role in maintaining fluid, electrolyte and acid-base balance as well as in producing and regulating several hormones within the body. When problems occur with any of these functions patients often become acutely unwell and they have an increased risk of further deterioration. Nurses must therefore have the requisite skills and knowledge to conduct a thorough assessment of each patient, collecting and recording subjective and objective data that will contribute towards accurate diagnosis, optimal management and effective evaluation of care. Through constant liaison and communication with other members of the multidisciplinary team a holistic, cohesive approach can be adopted that will ultimately enhance the delivery of quality care.

Glossary

Active transport Using energy in the form of adenosine triphosphate (ATP) to move fluid and solutes between cellular compartments.

Acute kidney injury An abrupt reduction in kidney function characterised by a rising serum creatinine level and a reduction in the urine output.

Anuria Less than 100ml of urine in 24 hours.

Colloid A solution with large insoluble molecules that can generate an osmotic pressure and expand the plasma compartment.

Computerised tomography (CT) scan A specialised X-ray where pictures are taken from a multidimensional perspective.

Creatinine A waste product of muscle metabolism secreted by the kidney.

Crystalloid An aqueous solution that contains mineral salts and other water soluble molecules.

Diffusion The movement of solutes from a state of higher concentration to that of lower concentration.

Diuretic A drug that increases urine output.

Early warning system (EWS) A scoring system that detects early deterioration in the patient's condition.

Erythropoietin A hormone produced in the kidney that promotes erythrogenesis in the bone marrow.

Filtration (renal) The forcing of blood and the substances in it through the glomerular-capsular membrane under arterial pressure.

Glomerular filtration rate (GFR) The rate at which substances pass through the filtration membrane and enter the proximal convuluted tubule.

Glomerulonephritis Inflammation of the glomerulus.

Haematuria The presence of blood in the urine.

Inotropic therapy Drugs that work on the contractility of the myocardium and ultimately improve cardiac performance.

Intravenous pyelogram (IVP) Investigation of the kidney and ureters for obstructive lesions (using contrast media).

Nephrotic syndrome An inflammatory disease of the glomerulus characterised by proteinuria, hypoalbuminaemia, oedema and hyperlipidaemia.

Oliguria 100–400ml of urine in 24 hours.

Osmolality The concentration of solutes in a kilogram of water.

Osmosis The distribution of water from a lesser area of solute concentration to an area of higher concentration.

Proteinuria The presence of protein in the urine.

Renal calculi Stones made up of calcium and minerals that can obstruct the ureters.

Renal replacement therapy An extra-corporeal circuit used to filter excess fluid and waste products from the blood.

Renin A protein produced by the juxta glomerular apparatus that leads to the formation of angiotensin 2.

Specific gravity A measurement of urine osmolality.

Tubular reabsorption Reabsorption of the filtrate back into the peritubular capillaries.

Tubular secretion Substances are filtered out of the blood into the tubular fluid for secretion.

Ultrasound The production of an image from ultrasound waves that are created by structures within the body.

Urea A waste product of protein metabolism.

Vasa recta A network of blood vessels found in the cortex and medullary regions of the kidney.

Vasopressin Also known as the antidiuretic hormone, this polypeptide controls water reabsorption and secretion.

Test yourself

1 The nephron is the functional unit of the kidney. Which of the following structures is not part of the tubular area?

   a. glomerulus
   b. proximal convuluted tubule
   c. loop of Henlé
   d. vasa recta
   e. distal convuluted tubule
   f. collecting duct

2 The ureters and bladder have three layers, name them:

   the tunica _____
   the tunica _____
   the tunica _____

3 Name the three stages of urine production:

   tubular _____
   tubular _____
   tubular _____

4 During urine production, which of the following substances are filtered out into the tubular fluid?

   a. blood
   b. albumin
   c. creatinine

5 What is the average glomerular filtration rate for an adult male?

   a. 125ml per minute
   b. 160ml per minute
   c. 180ml per minute

6 Which substance regulates water reabsorption or excretion in the body?

   a. renin
   a. erythropoietin
   c. vasopressin

7 Which of the following is not a usual symptom of a urinary tract infection?

   a. pyrexia
   b. oliguria
   c. back pain
   d. increased leucocytes in the blood

8 When diagnosing acute kidney injury which blood test result is the most significant?

   a. urea
   b. creatinine
   c. sodium
   d. albumin

9 When conducting a nursing assessment of a patient with renal dysfunction, which of the following is not a sign of a volume responsive injury?

    a. urine output less than 0.5ml/kg/hr
    b. raised serum potassium
    c. weak dilute urine
    d. metabolic acidosis

10 Which of the following drugs could be used *directly to* lower high serum potassium levels?

    a. intravenous dextrose and insulin in combination
    b. intravenous of nebulised salbutamol
    c. intravenous calcium gluconate

References

Beaumont, K. (2008) Deterioration in hospital patients: early signs and appropriate actions. *Nursing Standard* 23 (1): 43–8.

Browne, M. and Cook, P. (2011) Inappropriate trust in technology: Implications for critical care nurses. *Nursing in Critical Care* 16 (2), 92–8.

Davenport, A. (2007) What's new in acute kidney injury? *Care of the Critically Ill* 23 (4), 95–6.

Donald, R. (2011) Caring for the renal system. In Macintosh, M. and Moore, T. (2011) *Caring for the Seriously Ill Patient*, 2nd edn. London: Hodder Arnold, p. 80.

Ewart, C. and Huntingdon, S. (2007) The peri-operative phase. In McArthur Rouse, F. and Prosser, S. (eds) *Assessing and Managing the Acutely Ill Surgical Patient*. Oxford: Blackwell, pp. 32–3.

Giger, J. and Davidhizar, R. (2004) *Transcultural Nursing Assessment and Intervention*, 4th edn. St Louis, MO: Mosby.

Hayes, J. and Cox, C. (2009) The experience of therapeutic touch from a nursing perspective. *British Journal of Nursing* 8 (18), 1249–54.

Jevon, P. (2007) *Treating the Critically Ill Patient*. Oxford: Blackwell Publishing.

Jevon, P. and Ewens, B. (2007) *Monitoring the Critically Ill Patient*, 2nd edn. Oxford: Blackwell Publishing.

Jones, S. (2007) Care of urinary catheters and drainage systems. Available from http//www.nursingtimes.net/nursing-practice-clinical-research-evidence-care-of-urinary-catheters-and-drainage-systems/439075.article.

Kishen, P. (2008) Prevention of peri-operative renal dysfunction and renal failure. *Care of the Critically Ill* 24 (2), 39–43.

Leach, R. (2009) *Acute and Critical Care Medicine at a Glance*, 2nd edn. Oxford: Wiley.

McCance, K. L., Huether, S. E., Brashers, V. L. and Rote, N. S. (2010) *Pathophysiology: The biologic basis for disease in adults and children*, 6th edn. St Louis, MO: Mosby.

Nursing and Midwifery Council (2010) *Standards for Pre-registration Nursing Education*. London: MWC. Available from http://standards.nmc-uk.org/PublishedDocuments/Standards%20for%20pre-registration%20nursing%20education%2016082010.pdf.

O'Callaghan, C. (2006) *The Renal System at a Glance*, 2nd edn. Oxford: Blackwell.

Roseveare, C. (2009) *Acute Medicine*. Oxford: Wiley-Blackwell.

Scales, K. and Pilsworth, S. (2008) The importance of fluid balance in clinical practice. *Nursing Standard* 22 (47), 50–58.

Selius, B. and Subedi, R. (2008) Urinary retention in adults: Diagnosis and initial management. *American Family Physician* 77 (5), 643–50.

Suleman, R. and Rechner, I. (2009) Acute kidney injury in the critical care setting. *Care of the Critically Ill* 25 (2), 40–43.

Sumnall, R. (2007) Fluid management and diuretic therapy in acute renal failure. *Nursing in Critical Care* 12 (1), 27–33.

Thibodeau, G. and Patton, K. (2003) *Anatomy and Physiology*, 5th edn. St Louis, MO: Mosby.

Tortora, G., Gerard, J. and Derrickson, B. (2009) *Principles of Anatomy and Physiology*, 12th edn. Chichester: Wiley.

Younker, J. (2007) Commentary: Saline versus albumin fluid evaluation (SAFE) investigators (2006). Effect of baseline serum albumin concentration on outcome of resuscitation with albumin or saline in patients in intensive care units: Analysis of data from the saline versus albumin fluid evaluation (SAFE)) study. *Nursing in Critical Care* 12 (3), 168–9.

Further reading

El Nahas, A. M. and Levin, A. (2010) *Chronic Kidney Disease: A practical guide to understanding and management*. Oxford: Oxford University Press.

Reneke, H. G. and Denker, B. M. (2010) *Renal Pathology. The essentials*. Philadelphia: Lippincott.

Townsend, R. R. and Cohen-Stein, E. N. (2010) *100 Questions & Answers About Kidney Disease and Hypertension*. Bullington & Jones: Bartlett.

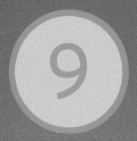

The patient with acute neurological problems

Katie Scales

Aims

This chapter aims to provide you with improved knowledge of the structure and function of the nervous system, allowing you to relate normal physiology to the pathophysiology of neurological disease or injury and understand the nurse's role in the assessment and management of patients with deteriorating neurological status.

Objectives

After reading this chapter you will be able to:

→ Describe the anatomy of the nervous system

→ Describe the structure of a neurone and the physiology of nerve impulses, and relate this to the pathophysiology of neuromuscular disease

→ Explain the normal function of the autonomic nervous system and relate this to the stress response seen in acute illness

→ Describe the techniques used in neurological assessment

→ Explain the pathophysiology and clinical management of neurological emergencies

→ Identify clinical interventions to optimise neurological function

Introduction

The nervous system communicates with and controls all other body systems. It is essential for consciousness, cognitive thought and memory, movement and manual dexterity, perception and behaviour. Together with the endocrine system it is responsible for homeostasis, the maintenance of a stable internal environment irrespective of external conditions. It is a rapid response system that responds to a crisis without hesitation yet is also essential for relaxation and sleep. This chapter focuses on the cells that make up the nervous system and the way in which the nervous system is organised. The structure and function of the central and peripheral nervous system are discussed and an overview of the autonomic nervous system is presented. Common neurological diseases and injuries are reviewed and neurological assessment described. Competence in neurological assessment is an important nursing skill and is essential for the early detection and management of neurological and medical emergencies.

Applied anatomy and physiology of the nervous system

The nervous system has two main subdivisions; the central nervous system (CNS) and the peripheral nervous system (PNS). The brain and spinal cord form the CNS and the cranial nerves, spinal nerves and their branches form the PNS. The PNS is subdivided into the autonomic and somatic nervous systems.

The function of the nervous system can be considered under three main headings: sensory, integrative and motor.

- *Sensory* – sensory receptors detect information internally and externally. For example, sensory receptors in the brain detect body temperature while sensory receptors in the skin detect environmental temperature. Sensory information is transmitted to the brain by cranial and spinal nerves.
- *Integrative* – sensory information received by the brain is analysed, some information is stored and decisions are made about the type of response that is required. This process is called integration. Perception is essential for cognitive thought and is an important integrative function.
- *Motor* – having received and integrated the sensory information the brain decides whether a motor response

is necessary and appropriate muscles or glands are stimulated via cranial and spinal nerves.

These three key activities provide a continuous mechanism of feedback and regulation to maintain homeostasis and manage emergencies.

Cells of the nervous system

There are two main cell types within the nervous system: neurones and glial cells.

Neurones

It is estimated that the central nervous system (CNS) contains 100 billion neurones. Neurones vary in shape and size depending on their location and function. All neurones have the same structure; a cell body, which is the main part of the neurone, dendrites that bring information to the cell body and an axon that carries nerve impulses away from the cell body (see Figure 9.1).

The neurone *cell body* is similar to other cells and contains a nucleus with a prominent nucleolus, mitochondria, Golgi apparatus, free ribosomes and rough and smooth endoplasmic reticulum and lysosomes, all surrounded by cytoplasm and contained by a cell membrane. Neurones synthesise vast amounts of protein to maintain cell membrane proteins, intracellular organelles and neurotransmitters and to support the neural processes that extend from the cell body. Protein is synthesised by large numbers of free ribosomes and rough endoplasmic reticulum called Nissl bodies or granules.

Dendrites increase the surface area of the cell membrane and connect with other neurones. This function is maximised by the presence of dendritic spines, small hair-like projections on the dendrites. Dendrites bring information to the cell body.

> **Dendrite** – from the Greek word for *tree*, dendrites often look like little trees extending from the cell body.

Axons transmit information away from the cell body. Axons vary in length from less than 1mm to over a metre. The proximal portion of the axon is called the initial segment and is the origin of the action potential required for nerve transmission. Action potentials are electrical signals that travel along the surface of a neurone. The signal is maintained (or propagated) by the movement of ions (electrolytes) across the membrane of the neurone.

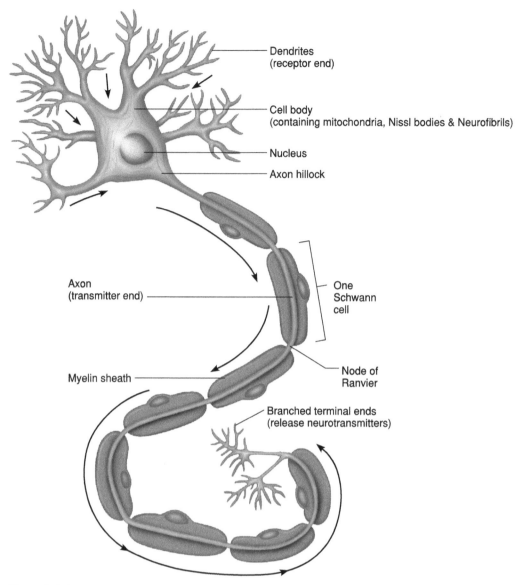

Figure 9.1 A neurone

Source: Zelman, M., Tompary, E., Raymond, J., Holdaway, P., Mulvihill, M., Steggall, M. and Dingle, M. (2011) Introductory *Pathophysiology for Nursing and Healthcare Professionals*, Harlow: Pearson Prentice Hall, Fig. 13.1, p. 302.

Axons divide to form branches with button-like endings called terminal boutons where neurotransmitters are stored in synaptic vesicles.

The connection between a terminal bouton and another tissue structure is called the synapse. Terminal boutons form the presynaptic component of the synapse and the structure it connects to forms the post-synaptic component. Neurotransmitters released from synaptic vesicles inhibit (suppress) or excite (stimulate) the post-synaptic component. When a neurone connects with a muscle fibre the synapse is termed a neuromuscular junction and the post-synaptic component is termed the motor end plate (see Figure 9.2).

When touching something hot, sensory nerves rapidly transmit information to the brain, which responds immediately by sending a motor signal to withdraw from the source of heat. This takes a fraction of a second.

Most axons are wrapped in a lipid-based substance called myelin, which insulates the axon and increases the speed of conduction along the axon. Neurones wrapped in myelin are classified as myelinated neurones, those not wrapped in myelin are classified as unmyelinated.

Neurones are classified as sensory or motor neurones according to their function. Sensory neurones detect or

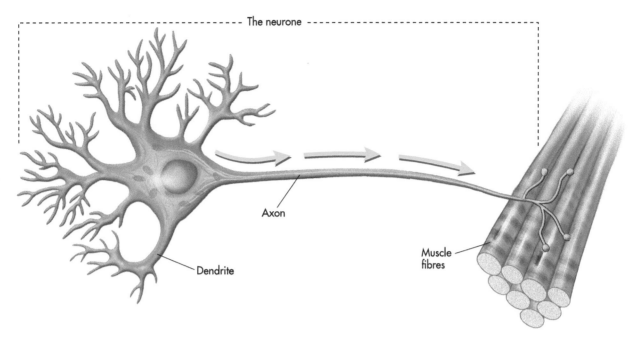

Figure 9.2 A neurone connecting to skeletal muscle fibres

sense internal or external stimuli and transmit sensory information to the brain. The brain receives and integrates sensory information and produces an appropriate motor response. Sensory neurones are also known as afferent neurones (afferent means carried towards) whilst motor neurones are termed efferent neurones (efferent means away from).

A nerve is a bundle of many hundreds of axons together with their blood vessels and connective tissue, they only occur within the PNS. Bundles of axons within the CNS are called tracts.

A ganglion is the term used to describe a cluster of neurone cell bodies within the PNS. Clusters of neurone cell bodies within the CNS are called nuclei.

Neuroglia

Neuroglia, or glial cells, are the dominant cell structure making up 90% of all cells within the CNS. Glial cells are structural cells providing support, nutrition and protection for neurones. They do not generate or conduct nerve impulses and do not form synapses but they can divide by mitosis to create new cells. Because of their ability to reproduce glial cells are the main cause of primary tumours within the nervous system.

Glial cells are classified as macroglia or microglia – big and small glial cells. There are several types of macroglia

> **Glia** – from the Greek meaning *glue*; also translates as 'holding together'.

within the CNS; astrocytes, oligodendrocytes and ependymal cells. Microglia are the macrophages of the CNS, removing cell debris and microorganisms by phagocytosis.

Astrocytes are so named because of their star-like appearance. Multiple processes extend from the cell body, some of which end in foot processes that interface with cerebral blood vessels. Astrocytes are important for the movement of molecules from the blood to the brain and form part of the blood–brain barrier.

Ependymal cells form a single layer of cells lining the ventricles of the brain and the central canal of the spinal cord. They contain microvilli and cilia and are involved with the circulation of cerebrospinal fluid.

Oligodendrocytes generate myelin within the CNS (see Figure 9.3). Schwann cells, also a type of glial cell, generate myelin in the PNS. Schwann cells wrap around axons, forming a myelin sheath. The outer layer includes the Schwann cell's cytoplasm and nucleus and is called the neurolemma. The neurolemma is thought to promote axon regeneration in the PNS. When a myelinated axon is examined microscopically there appear to be gaps in the myelin called nodes of Ranvier. One Schwann cell myelinates the segment of axon between two nodes of Ranvier, myelinated nerves will therefore have several Schwann cells (see Figure 9.1).

Myelination is different within the CNS. A single oligodendrocyte can myelinate up to 50 adjacent axons. Oligodendrocytes project multiple processes that wrap around the axons but because the cell body and nucleus are not wrapped around the axon there is no neurolemma (see Figure 9.4). This may contribute to the lack of axonal

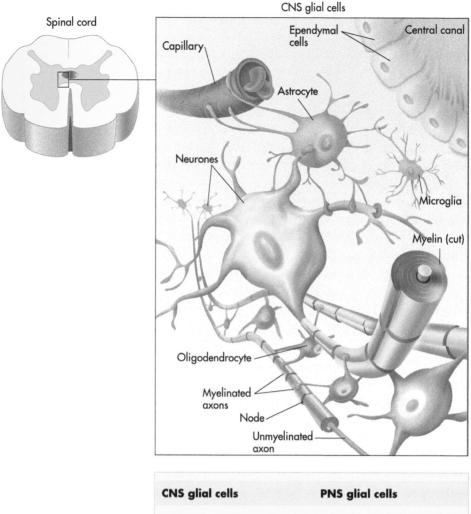

Figure 9.3 Glial cells and their functions

regeneration within the CNS. Myelinated neurones within the CNS have fewer nodes of Ranvier than neurones in the PNS.

Demyelination describes the loss or destruction of myelin. Rapid shifts in serum sodium can cause CNS demyelination and neurological injury with symptoms similar to hypoxic brain injury. Abnormal serum sodium levels must be corrected slowly at a rate not exceeding 5mmol/L per day. CNS demyelination is a side effect of some chemotherapy regimens. Inflammatory demyelinating diseases

also occur and form part of a group of diseases called polyneuropathies, for example Guillain–Barré syndrome (GBS) and multiple sclerosis (MS).

MS, a chronic demyelinating disease of the CNS, is an autoimmune disease characterised by degeneration of the myelin sheath. The name comes from the pathophysiology of the disease. In *multiple* areas, the myelin sheaths degenerate until they form hardened plaques called *scleroses*. Plaques are found in the brain and spinal cord of MS sufferers. Demyelination prevents saltatory conduction

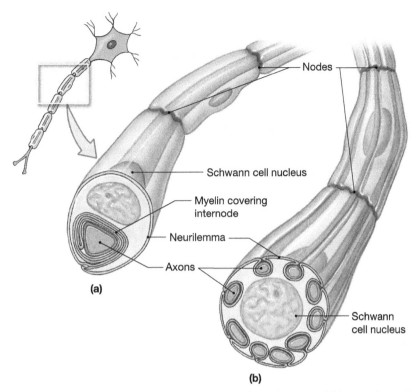

Figure 9.4 Schwann cells and peripheral axons: (a) mylinated axon and (b) unmyelinated axon
Source: Martini, F.H. and Bartholomew, E. F. (2009) *Essentials of Anatomy & Physiology*, 5th edn, San Francisco: Pearson Benjamin Cummings, Fig. 8.5, p. 252.

and reduces nerve transmission. Symptoms include muscle weakness, altered sensation and blurred vision. Acute episodes are followed by periods of remission but frequency and severity of the attacks increases with time.

> **Autoimmune** describes a disease in which the body is attacked by the patient's own immune system.

GBS, an acute demyelinating disease of the PNS, often presents after a bacterial illness. Macrophages attack myelinated axons, stripping away the myelin sheath. Treatment is directed towards the immune system using plasmapheresis (plasma exchange) and intravenous immunoglobulin therapy. Steroids have not been shown to be beneficial in GBS. In the acute phase, progressive muscle weakness starts in the periphery and progresses centrally. If respiratory muscles are affected patients may require intubation and ventilation.

Nerve impulses

A nerve impulse, or action potential, is a series of electrical events that take place sequentially along the length of an axon. An action potential has two phases: depolarisation and repolarisation. When a neurone is stimulated sodium ions (Na^+) flow rapidly across the initial segment and into the cytoplasm of the axon: this is depolarisation. Depolarisation changes the electrical charge of that section of the axon causing potassium ions (K^+) to flow rapidly out of the axon and into the interstitial space: this is repolarisation. The sequential depolarisation and repolarisation of the axon cell membrane is like a row of dominoes, once the first action potential has occurred it causes neighbouring sections of the membrane to depolarise. The Na^+/K^+ pump on the axon cell membrane ensures the Na^+ and K^+ ions are restored to their normal positions ready for the next action potential to occur (see Figure 9.5).

Nerve transmission requires a series of action potentials to be generated in sequence along the length of the axon from the initial segment all the way to the terminal boutons. Nerve impulses are transmitted more rapidly by myelinated axons. The impulse jumps between the nodes of Ranvier in a process known as saltatory conduction.

> **Saltatory** from the Latin for *leap* or *jump*.

The diameter of the axon affects nerve transmission: the bigger the neurone the faster it will transmit. Local anaesthetic agents such as lidocaine work by blocking the influx of Na^+ and preventing the action potential from being generated. If the action potential cannot be generated the impulse cannot pass along the axon, preventing transmission of pain signals to the brain.

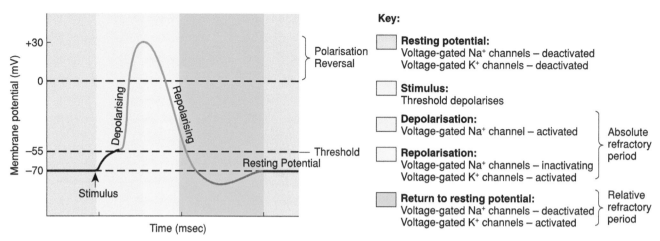

Figure 9.5 Action potential

Ice can also be used to reduce the sensation of pain by locally cooling the nerve supplying the injured tissue. Cooling slows the transmission of nerve impulses, reducing the number of pain signals transmitted to the brain.

Action potentials can be affected by electrolyte imbalances. Disturbance of action potentials within the CNS may result in altered cerebral function with symptoms ranging from irritability to seizures and coma. Disturbance of action potentials in the PNS can result in muscle weakness or excessive muscle contraction, known as tetany.

Hyponatraemia, hypernatraemia, hypocalcaemia, hypomagnesaemia and uraemia can all affect cerebral function. Hypo- and hypernatraemia are common causes of seizures. Hypocalcaemia and hypomagnesaemia can cause tingling of the hands and feet and in extreme cases tetany.

The synapse

The synapse is a collective term describing the interface between a terminal bouton and another tissue structure, which may be another nerve but could be a blood vessel, a muscle, an organ or a gland.

Synapses can be electrical or chemical. Electrical synapses are found in cardiac muscle and the smooth muscle of the gastrointestinal (GI) tract, they also occur in the CNS. Electrical synapses are special channels directly connecting the cytoplasm of neighbouring cells. This allows the flow of ions between cells and accounts for the 'wave-like' muscular activity seen in cardiac contraction and gut motility, the rapid spread of electrical information ensures the entire muscle is synchronised and produces a coordinated contraction. Electrical synapses are faster than chemical synapses.

Most synapses are chemical, neurotransmitters are used to bridge the gap between the terminal bouton and the post-synaptic structure (see Figure 9.6). Neurotransmitters released from the presynaptic terminal diffuse across the synaptic cleft and bind to the post-synaptic terminal where they inhibit or excite the post-synaptic structure. Inhibition blocks the post-synaptic structure, excitation stimulates the post-synaptic structure.

Calcium is important in chemical synapses. As the electrical impulse arrives at the terminal bouton the action potential causes calcium to flow into the terminal bouton from the interstitial space, triggering the synaptic vesicles to release the neurotransmitter into the synaptic cleft. The neurotransmitter diffuses across the synaptic cleft and binds with the receptors on the post-synaptic structure, generating an action potential in the post-synaptic cell.

Chemical synapse requires the following steps:

1 Neurotransmitter synthesised by neurone cell body and transported to axon terminal.
2 Neurotransmitter stored in synaptic vesicles within the terminal boutons ready for release.
3 Nerve impulse reaches the axon terminal and triggers the influx of Ca^{++} from the interstitial space.
4 Increase in Ca^{++} triggers the release of the neurotransmitter into the synaptic cleft.
5 Neurotransmitter diffuses across the synaptic cleft and binds to a specific receptor causing ion channels to open.
6 Influx of ions from the synaptic cleft generates an action potential at the post-synaptic component stimulating or inhibiting the post-synaptic cell.
7 Neurotransmitter is removed from synaptic cleft by enzyme inactivation, reuptake or by diffusing away from the synapse.

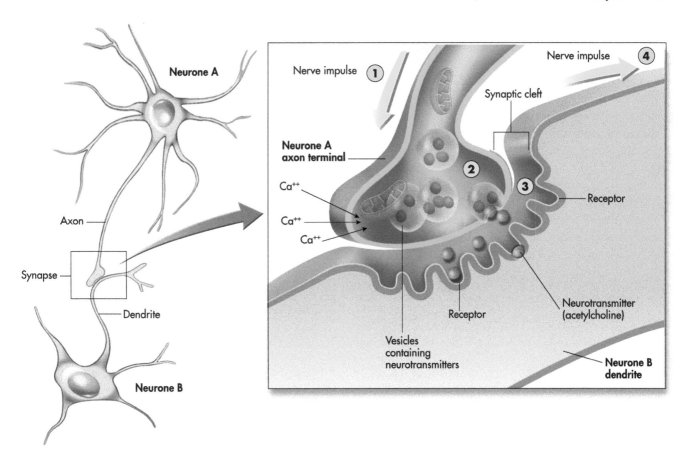

Figure 9.6 The chemical synapse. Step 1, the impulse travels down the axon. Step 2, vesicles are stimulated to release neurotransmitter (exocytosis). Step 3, the neurotransmitter travels across the synapse and binds with the receptor site of the post synaptic cell. Step 4, the impulse continues down the dendrite

In summary, the impulse begins as an electrical signal transmitted along the axon of a neurone. When the signal reaches the terminal bouton it is converted into a chemical signal that diffuses across the synaptic cleft and binds to the post-synaptic cell. The post-synaptic cell converts the chemical signal back into an electrical signal.

Once the synapse has occurred the neurotransmitter must be cleared from the synaptic cleft, otherwise the post-synaptic cell will be stimulated repeatedly. Neurotransmitters can be cleared in three ways:

- Enzyme inactivation – enzymes break down the molecular structure of the neurotransmitter, e.g. acetylcholine is inactivated by acetylcholinesterase.
- Cellular uptake – neurotransmitters are transported back to the neurone that released them and reused, e.g. norepinephrine (noradrenaline), or taken up by glial cells.
- Diffusion – neurotransmitters diffuse away from the synaptic cleft preventing contact with their receptor sites.

Neurones receive thousands of synapses. Weak synapses do not generate action potentials: if the signal is strong enough an action potential will occur and an impulse will be transmitted. This is described as an 'all or nothing' event.

Neurotransmitters

Neurotransmitters are chemicals that excite, inhibit or modify the response of another cell (Hickey 2009). They are classified by their molecular size into small-molecule neurotransmitters and neuropeptides (Tortora and Derrickson 2009).

Small molecule neurotransmitters include acetylcholine, norepinephrine, epinephrine and dopamine.

Acetylcholine (ACh), an important neurotransmitter in both the PNS and the CNS, is inactivated by the enzyme acetylcholinesterase (AChE).

Myasthenia gravis is caused by the autoimmune destruction of ACh receptors. ACh produced at the synapse is broken down by AChE before the patient's muscles have contracted. By blocking AChE the breakdown of ACh is prevented and the muscle is stimulated until it contracts. Drugs that block AChE are called acetylcholinesterase inhibitors, for example pyridostigmine, and are the main-stay of myasthenia gravis management.

Norepinephrine and epinephrine are classified as catecholamines because of their chemical structure and are both neurotransmitters and hormones. As well as being released at synapses norepinephrine and epinephrine are released directly into the bloodstream by the adrenal medulla. Norepinephrine and epinephrine are inactivated by reuptake from presynaptic neurones and are recycled or destroyed by enzymes.

Dopamine, also a catecholamine, is active in both the CNS and the PNS. In the CNS, dopamine is involved in emotion and pleasure and may be associated with addictive behaviours. In the PNS dopamine helps to regulate muscle tone: it is deactivated by reuptake in presynaptic neurones.

Parkinson's disease is caused by inadequate levels of dopamine creating an imbalance in the ratio of dopamine to ACh, resulting in involuntary muscle contractions producing the characteristic clinical feature of tremor. Involuntary movements interfere with voluntary movements, for example buttoning a shirt is difficult because the hands shake. Dopamine cannot be administered orally or by injection as it cannot cross the blood–brain barrier. L-dopa does cross the blood–brain barrier and once inside the CNS is converted to dopamine, restoring dopamine levels and controlling symptoms.

An excess of dopamine has been implicated in some forms of schizophrenia.

Neuropeptide neurotransmitters – chains of amino acids linked by peptide bonds, examples include endorphins and substance P. Neuropeptides are synthesised in neur-one cell bodies, formed into vesicles and transported to the terminal boutons, they are active in the CNS and the PNS.

Endorphins, described as opioid peptides, function as natural analgesics by binding to opiate receptors in the CNS. Endorphins can be triggered by acupuncture and acupressure, providing pain-relieving effects.

Substance P is released in the PNS by neurones responsible for the transmission of pain information to the CNS. Substance P is also found in spinal cord pathways and in parts of the brain associated with pain. Substance P increases the perception of pain. Endorphins inhibit the release of substance P and reduce the perception of pain.

The brain

The brain is surrounded and protected by the skull and the meninges. The section of skull enclosing the brain is called the cranium and is made up of eight bones. Swelling of the brain causes intracranial pressure to rise because the adult skull is unable to expand to accommodate the swelling. Swelling of the brain is termed cerebral oedema and if left untreated can be fatal.

The meninges is a collective term describing the three membranes that cover and protect the brain and spinal cord. The acronym *PAD* may help you to remember the names of the meninges. Starting from the surface of the brain and working outwards the membranes are the pia mater, the arachnoid mater and the dura mater. Inflammation of the meninges is called meningitis (see Figure 9.7).

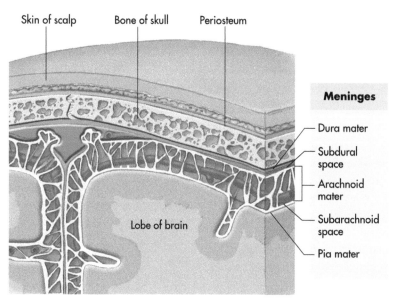

Figure 9.7 The meninges

Cerebrospinal fluid (CSF) protects the brain and spinal cord from injury. Adults have 80–150mL of CSF circulating continuously around the brain and spinal cord (Tortora and Derrickson 2009). CSF transports oxygen, glucose and electrolytes from the blood to the neurones and neuroglia of the CNS and removes waste from neural tissues. CSF makes the brain buoyant, effectively floating within the skull, ensuring the brain is not damaged from resting against the skull.

CSF is a colourless, clear liquid produced by a network of capillaries called the choroid plexus in the walls of all four ventricles within the brain. The choroid plexus is surrounded by ependymal cells (glial cells) that continuously generate CSF from the plasma of the blood by a process of filtration and secretion. As well as a blood–brain barrier the brain also has a blood–CSF barrier protecting it from harmful substances that may be carried in the plasma of the blood. Ependymal cells form the blood–CSF barrier, controlling the substances that are allowed to enter the CSF.

CSF flows from the two lateral ventricles into the third ventricle where another choroid plexus generates more CSF. CSF then flows through the cerebral aqueduct, or aqueduct of Sylvius, into the fourth ventricle where further CSF is generated. The CSF then enters the subarachnoid space, the space between the arachnoid mater and the pia mater, through openings in the ceiling of the fourth ventricle. CSF circulates in the subarachnoid space around the brain and spinal cord and also in the central canal of the spinal cord. CSF is absorbed back into the blood by arachnoid villi, finger-like projections of the arachnoid mater. If the volume of the CSF is to remain constant then the CSF must be produced and reabsorbed at the same rate. Once generated the CSF should flow unobstructed from the ventricles through the arachnoid space and into the spinal canal. The flow of CSF can be affected by tumours, inflammatory conditions like ventriculitis and by intraventricular or subarachnoid haemorrhage which can cause CSF flow to become obstructed by thrombus. If this happens CSF continues to be produced but cannot drain adequately and the pressure of the CSF increases: this clinical condition is termed hydrocephaly. Hydrocephaly can be controlled temporarily by the insertion of an extra-ventricular drain (EVD) or permanently by the insertion of a ventricular–peritoneal (VP) shunt. Because adult skull bones are fused any increase in CSF pressure will result in an increase in intracranial pressure (ICP) and is a clinical emergency.

Blood supply to the brain

The internal carotid and vertebral arteries provide most of the blood supply to the brain. The internal carotids branch

to form the anterior cerebral artery and the middle cerebral artery. Anastomoses of the right and left internal carotid arteries and the basilar artery form a special cerebral circulation at the base of the brain called the circle of Willis. Most of the brain is supplied by arteries arising from the circle of Willis. The circle of Willis equalises blood pressure across the brain and provides an alternative blood supply if an artery within the brain becomes blocked or diseased.

> The internal carotid artery supplies the eyeball, ear, most of the cerebrum, pituitary and nose.

Neurones reply on a constant supply of glucose and oxygen for normal brain function. Brief interruptions in blood flow can cause unconsciousness, for example standing up too fast and fainting, or transient ischaemic attacks (TIAs) caused by temporary obstruction of an artery by thrombus or atherosclerosis. Loss of blood flow (and therefore oxygen) for four minutes or more, for example during cardiac arrest, causes irreversible brain injury.

The brain stores very little glucose and relies on a continuous supply of glucose via the bloodstream. Hypoglycaemia can result in confusion, seizures and altered consciousness.

Because hypoglycaemia affects consciousness patients who are unexpectedly drowsy, confused or unconscious should have their blood glucose checked. Hypoglycaemia can be corrected by the use of oral or intravenous glucose preparations and by the administration of glucagon.

Alert patients with hypoglycaemia can be given a sugary drink and carbohydrates to eat. Sugar quickly raises blood glucose and carbohydrate provides a slow release supply of glucose to prevent recurrence of hypoglycaemia. Patients who are less alert can be given an oral preparation of glucose that can be rubbed on the gums. Unconscious patients are treated with intravenous glucose or intramuscular glucagon (NICE 2004). Hypoglycaemia should be investigated and blood glucose levels checked regularly, especially before the patient goes to sleep.

The blood–brain barrier

The blood–brain barrier is an important structure that prevents harmful substances in the bloodstream from entering brain tissue. The blood–brain barrier has two main components; a thick capillary basement membrane and tight junctions between the endothelial cells of the capillaries. Capillaries in other parts of the body have gaps between the endothelial cells that allow substances to diffuse across the capillary wall and enter the interstitial space. Tight junctions in brain capillaries and the thick basement membrane prevents diffusion, the brain relies

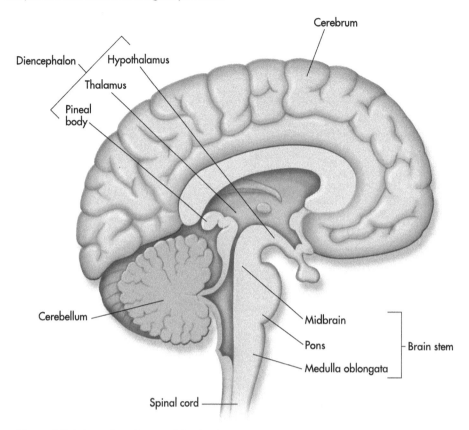

Figure 9.8 Internal anatomy of the brain

on astrocytes to control the movement of substances from blood to brain. The foot processes of astrocytes press tightly against the endothelial wall of brain capillaries, secreting chemicals that control the permeability of the capillary. Some water-soluble substances can pass across the blood–brain barrier easily, for example glucose, but most water-soluble substances cannot, for example proteins and antibiotics. Fat-soluble substances cross the blood–brain barrier relatively easily, e.g. oxygen, carbon dioxide, alcohol and most anaesthetic agents (Tortora and Derrickson 2009). The blood–brain barrier is affected by trauma and inflammation and can malfunction.

The brain is primarily divided into four parts: the cerebrum, the diencephalon, the cerebellum and the brainstem (see Figure 9.8).

The *cerebrum* is the largest part of the brain and is subdivided by the *great longitudinal fissure*: each half is called a cerebral hemisphere. In cross-section the hemispheres consist of an outer layer of grey matter and an internal area of white matter. White matter is made up mainly of myelinated axons, grey matter is mainly made of neurone cell bodies, dendrites, unmyelinated axons and neuroglia. The outer layer of grey matter is approximately 3mm thick, contains billions of neurones and is called the cerebral cortex.

The surface of the hemispheres has multiple folds called gyri which increase the surface area of the brain (see Figure 9.9). The deep grooves between the gyri are called fissures, the shallower grooves are called sulci. The two hemispheres are connected by the corpus callosum, which is a band of white matter filled with axons running between the hemispheres.

> *Sulci* is the plural of sulcus.
> *Gyri* is the plural of gyrus.

The hemispheres are subdivided into paired lobes named after the skull bones that cover them: frontal lobe, parietal lobe, occipital lobe, temporal lobe. Each lobe is separated

Gyrus

Sulcus

Cerebral cortex

Cerebral white matter

Fissure

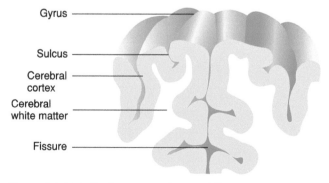

Figure 9.9 Detail of a gyrus, sulcus and fissure

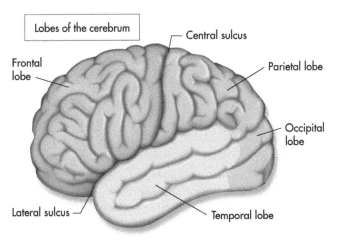

Figure 9.10 External brain anatomy

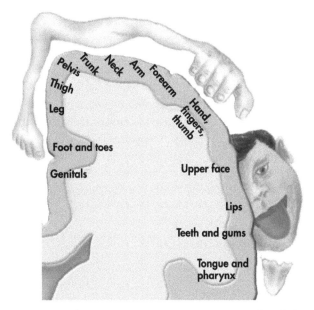

Figure 9.12 Primary somatosensory area, cross sectional view of section A in Figure 9.11, showing how different parts of the body map to different areas of the sensory cortex

by a sulcus (see Figure 9.10). One hemisphere is usually more highly developed than the other; this is known as cerebral dominance: 90% of the population have a dominant left hemisphere which results in right-handedness, an important consideration when dealing with unilateral brain injuries such as acute stroke. Motor control of speech is usually located within the dominant hemisphere.

Function of the cerebral cortex

The cerebral cortex processes sensory, motor and integrated signals. The central sulcus is an important area of the cerebral cortex because it separates the primary somatosensory area from the primary motor area in each hemisphere (see Figure 9.11).

The primary somatosensory area is a highly specialised area of the cerebral cortex containing a 'map' of the body: each point on the body surface can be mapped to a specific part of the primary somatosensory area (see Figure 9.12). The amount of cortex receiving signals from

a particular part of the body depends on the number of receptors in that body part, not the size of the body part. For example the tongue is relatively small but a relatively large part of the primary somatosensory area receives signals from the tongue, because the tongue contains large numbers of sensory nerve endings.

The primary somatosensory area is important for perception of sensation including touch, tickle, itch, pain, temperature and joint posture. Other senses are interpreted in different parts of the cortex:

- *sight and visual perception* – posterior portion of occipital lobe;
- *taste* – parietal cortex;
- *smell* – temporal cortex;
- *hearing* – temporal cortex.

The *primary motor area* of the cerebral cortex is located immediately anterior to the primary somatosensory area, in the posterior section of the frontal lobe. Stimulation of the primary motor area results in contraction of a specific skeletal muscle. Again, body parts do not map in proportion to their size but in proportion to the number of motor neurones present in that particular part of the body. Large parts of the cortex relate to muscles that are required for complex, skilled or delicate movements. For example highly dextrous parts of the body, such as the fingers, contain more motor neurones than the toes.

Speech is an important motor function and is controlled in a specialised zone of the motor cortex called Broca's speech area, in the left frontal lobe. Motor neurones connect Broca's speech area with the larynx, pharynx,

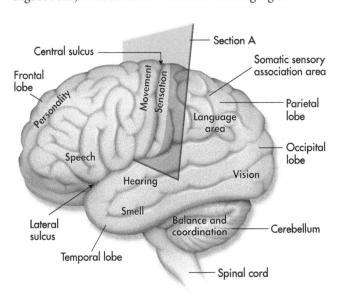

Figure 9.11 Primary somatosensory area

mouth and the respiratory muscles. Speech is the result of high-level coordination between talking, breathing and swallowing.

Wernicke's area, located broadly within the left temporal and parietal lobes, interprets speech by recognising spoken words and translating them into thoughts.

The areas in the right hemisphere corresponding to Broca's area and Wernicke's area are responsible for the emotional elements of speech.

Conversation requires integrated sensory functions; speech must be heard (auditory function), interpreted (cognitive function) and translated into speech (verbal function).

Brain injuries such as acute stroke can cause a range of communication problems. Damage to Broca's area results in expressive aphasia, where the patient is capable of thought but incapable of speech. Damage to Wernicke's area results in receptive aphasia, the inability to put words together coherently. The patient may be capable of a diverse range of words but cannot create a meaningful sentence. This is usually due to left-sided brain injuries, irrespective of hemisphere dominance.

> Aphasia from the Greek *aphatos* meaning *speechless*.

The *diencephalon* is located below the cerebrum and includes the thalamus, hypothalamus and epithalamus.

The *thalamus* is a pair of oval-shaped structures made of grey matter, in most individuals the right and left halves are joined by a bridge of grey matter. The thalamus acts as a relay station between the cerebral cortex and the spinal cord, between different areas of the cerebrum and between the cerebrum and the cerebellum. It is involved with consciousness.

The hypothalamus is beneath the thalamus and controls temperature, water metabolism, autonomic function, physical emotion and pituitary secretions such as growth hormone. The hypothalamus contains a feeding centre which contributes to the sense of hunger and a satiety centre that causes a sense of fullness and triggers individuals to stop eating. The thirst centre is also located within the hypothalamus. Osmoreceptors in the hypothalamus are stimulated by an increase in the osmotic pressure of the blood and trigger the sensation of thirst. The hypothalamus influences the circadian rhythm of the body – the sleep/wake cycle.

The epithalamus consists of the pineal gland and the habenular nuclei. The pineal gland secretes melatonin and is considered an endocrine gland. The habenular nuclei have an integrative role linking smell and emotion, for example a particular smell may evoke a specific memory.

Beneath the diencephalon are the cerebellum and the brainstem. The cerebellum lies posterior to the brainstem. The surface of the cerebellum is similar to the surface of the cerebrum, has multiple sulci and gyri and contains a rim of grey matter. The cerebellum regulates posture and balance and is important for the coordinated contraction of skeletal muscle, damage to the cerebellum affects muscle coordination and causes ataxia. Ataxia is most noticeable when walking as individuals appear to stagger or have an abnormal gait. Similar signs of ataxia can be seen after excessive alcohol consumption: alcohol inhibits cerebellar function.

The brainstem contains the midbrain, the pons and the medulla oblongata. The spinal cord is an extension of the brainstem descending into the vertebral column (see Figure 9.11).

The midbrain contains sensory and motor pathways controlling movement of the eyes, head and trunk in response to visual and auditory stimuli. The midbrain is the origin of cranial nerves III–V.

The pons also contains sensory and motor pathways and is a relay station between the cerebral cortex and the cerebellum. Together with the medulla the apneustic and pneumotaxic areas of the pons control breathing. The pons is the origin of cranial nerves V–VIII.

The medulla oblongata contains the vasomotor centre, also called the cardiovascular centre, which regulates the heartbeat and controls the diameter of blood vessels, thereby controlling blood pressure. The medulla is responsible for the rhythmical pattern of breathing. The medulla contains ascending sensory pathways and descending motor pathways connecting the spinal cord with other parts of the brain. The area where the medulla joins the spinal cord is where most of the ascending and descending pathways (tracts of axons within the CNS) cross over: as a result each cerebral hemisphere is responsible for sensation and voluntary movement on the opposite side of the body.

Nuclei (clusters of cell bodies within the CNS) within the medulla control important protective reflexes including swallowing, coughing, vomiting, sneezing and hiccoughing. The medulla also contains sensory nuclei involved in sensations of touch, pressure, vibration, taste, balance and hearing. The medulla is the origin of cranial nerves V, VII, VIII–XII.

Cranial nerves

There are 12 pairs of cranial nerves and they form part of the PNS. Each nerve is named according to its function and is identified numerically by Roman numerals.

Brainstem injuries have the potential to affect several cranial nerves because most of them originate within the brainstem. Cranial nerves l and ll are the only cranial nerves whose origins are not in the brainstem; they originate from the cerebral hemispheres.

Cranial nerves can be tested by asking the patient to perform an action that the cranial nerve usually controls.

Cranial nerves
I   Olfactory (sensory – smell)
II Optic (sensory – sight)
III Oculomotor (motor – eye movement, upper eyelid control and pupil constriction)
IV Trochlear (motor – eye movement)
V   Trigeminal (sensory and motor – face, scalp, nose and mouth)
VI Abducens (motor – eye movement)
VII Facial (sensory and motor – closing eyes, crying, smiling, grimacing, taste, salivation)
VIII Vestibulocochlear (sensory – hearing and balance)
IX Glossopharyngeal (sensory and motor – sensation and taste tongue and pharynx)
X   Vagus (motor and sensory – pharynx, larynx, heart, lungs, gut, viscera)
XI Spinal accessory (motor – shoulder and head movement)
XII Hypoglossal (motor – speech, swallowing).

The spinal cord and spinal nerves

The spinal cord lies within the spinal canal inside the vertebral column and is protected by the meninges and cushioned by CSF. The spinal cord is an extension of the brainstem running from the medulla oblongata to the top of the second lumbar vertebra, approximately 45cm long and 1cm wide.

In cross-section, the spinal cord has areas of white and grey matter (see Figure 9.13). Grey matter is arranged in an H shape and divided into regions called horns. Horns are classified as anterior (ventral) or posterior (dorsal) depending upon location. The posterior horns contain sensory axons, the anterior horns contain motor axons. The white matter is divided into regions called columns; anterior, posterior and lateral white columns. The amount of grey and white matter varies in different sections of the cord.

Spinal nerves are part of the PNS and together with the cranial nerves they connect the CNS with the rest of the body. Thirty-one pairs of spinal nerves exit the spinal column between each vertebra and are named according to the section of the vertebral column they emerge from (see Figure 9.14).

Spinal nerves are arranged as follows:

- 8 pairs of cervical nerves (C1–C8)
- 12 pairs of thoracic nerves (T1–T12)
- 5 pairs of lumbar nerves (L1–L5)
- 5 pairs of sacral nerves (S1–S5)
- 1 pair of coccygeal nerves (Co1).

Spinal nerves have two connections to the spinal cord; an anterior and a posterior root containing sensory and motor axons. Classified as mixed nerves, spinal nerves branch many times and directly innervate many peripheral structures.

Motor neurone disease (MND) is a degenerative disease affecting the ventral horns of the spinal cord and the ventral nerve roots that connect with skeletal muscle. Loss of nerve stimulation leads to muscle wasting and weakness. Because the ventral horns contain motor neurones MND affects voluntary muscle and patients become progressively unable to walk, talk, swallow and breathe.

The spinal cord does not extend below the second lumbar vertebra. Beneath L2 the spinal canal is filled with the lumbar, sacral and coccygeal nerve roots that continue down the spinal canal exiting at their appropriate level. This collection of nerve roots is called the cauda equina.

Cauda equina is Latin for 'horse's tail' – the nerve roots in the spinal canal look like a horse's tail.

Figure 9.14 shows the parts of the body supplied by spinal nerves. These areas have been mapped out and the resulting map is called a dermatome.

Spinal cord injury (SCI) describes damage to the spinal cord resulting in loss of mobility or sensation. SCI is a lifelong condition affecting over 40,000 people in the UK (Royal College of Physicians 2008). The spinal cord does not have to be severed for loss of function to occur, bruising and tearing can cause long-term injury. Fractured vertebrae do not necessarily cause spinal cord injury.

Traumatic causes of SCI include:

- Falls
- Sports injuries
- Stabbings
- Shootings
- Road traffic accidents (RTA).

Diseases that can cause SCI include:

- Spina bifida
- Polio

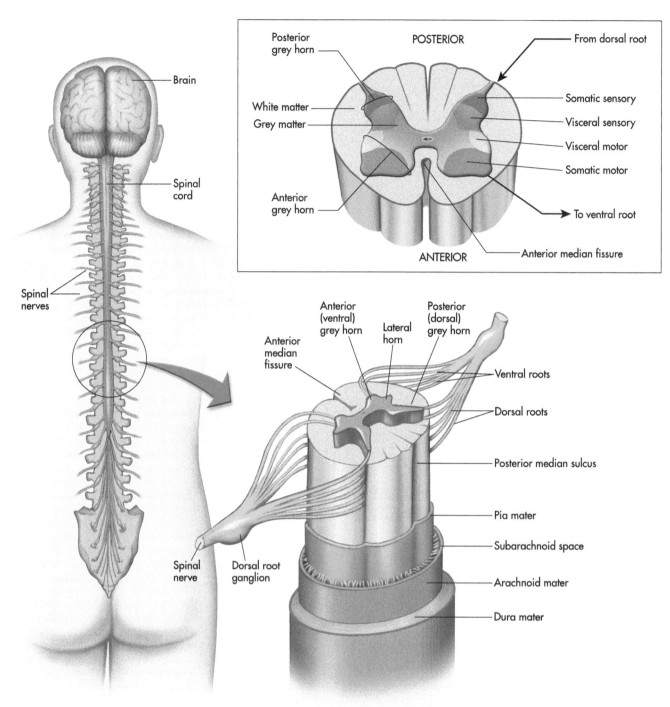

Figure 9.13 Internal anatomy of the spinal cord

- Primary or metastatic tumours
- Severe disc prolapse
- Inflammatory diseases such as rheumatoid and osteoarthritis
- Infective diseases such as TB of the spine, osteomyelitis and epidural abscess
- Haematoma
- Ageing.

Spinal cord injuries can have several phases:

- Primary injury, i.e. trauma
- Secondary injury, i.e. cord ischaemia
- Subsequent injury, i.e. additional injury from manual handling.

Primary injury is usually traumatic and damage begins at the moment of injury. The primary trauma causes

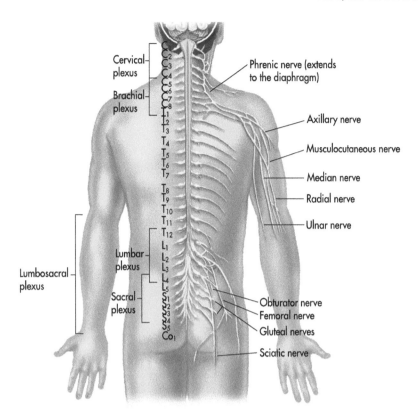

Figure 9.14 Spinal cord plexuses

SPINAL NERVE PLEXUSES

PLEXUS	LOCATION	SPINAL NERVES INVOLVED	REGION SUPPLIED	MAJOR NERVES LEAVING PLEXUS
Cervical	Deep in the neck, under the sternocleidomastoid muscle	C_1–C_4	Skin and muscles of neck and shoulder; diaphragm	Phrenic (diaphragm)
Brachial	Deep to the clavicle, between the neck and the axilla	C_5–C_8, T_1	Skin and muscles of upper extremity	Musculocutaneous Ulnar Median Radial Axillary
Lumbosacral	Lumbar region of the back	T_{12}, L_1–L_5, S_1–S_4	Skin and muscles of lower abdominal wall, lower extremity, buttocks, external genitalia	Obturator Femoral Sciatic Pudendal

vascular and chemical changes leading to secondary injury such as cord ischaemia, hypoxia and oedema. Secondary injuries may also be caused by arterial insufficiency, thrombosis or hypotension.

SCI is classified by the clinical effects of the injury:

- Quadriplegia (also called tetraplegia)
- Paraplegia.

Both types of injury may be complete or incomplete.

In incomplete SCI, the ability of the brain and spinal cord to convey messages is not entirely lost, some degree of motor or sensory function is present below the level of the injury. Patients with complete SCI have no function below the level of the injury, no sensation and no voluntary movement, both sides of the body are equally affected. Understanding the anatomy of the spinal nerves helps predict how the patient will be affected.

Cervical injuries usually cause quadriplegia and affect diaphragm control and breathing. Patients with complete high cervical injuries (C1–3) lose diaphragm function and cannot cough or breathe effectively, usually requiring a tracheostomy and often ventilator dependent. All function below the level of the injury is lost.

Injuries at thoracic level usually cause paraplegia, breathing is not as badly affected and patients usually retain the use of their arms and hands. Lesions above T6 predispose patients to autonomic dysreflexia – an excessive

Signs of autonomic dysreflexia

- Severe, uncontrolled hypertension 300/200mmHg
- Severe headaches
- Sweating or shivering
- Anxiety
- Blurred vision
- Flushing of the skin above the injury
- Coolness of the skin below the injury.

autonomic response to a stimulus below the level of the SCI, e.g. a blocked catheter, constipation.

Lumbar injuries affect leg muscles and walking. Sacral injuries affect bowel, bladder and sexual function.

Initial SCI management focuses on stabilising the spine, reducing oedema, maintaining cord blood flow and preventing further injury.

Staff caring for patients with SCI must be trained in the safe handling of SCI patients.

The autonomic nervous system

The autonomic nervous system (ANS) is regulated by centres within the brainstem and the hypothalamus, it is subdivided into the sympathetic and parasympathetic nervous systems.

The sympathetic nervous system is involuntary and maintains the body in a state of readiness to deal with any problems that arise. It is active during times of stress and generates the body's 'fright, fight and flight' response. Sympathetic fibres arise from the thoracic section of the spinal cord, T1–T12. The neurotransmitter released by the sympathetic nervous system is norepinephrine, also known as noradrenaline, consequently the sympathetic nervous system is described as *adrenergic*. Noradrenaline binds to adrenergic receptors and creates a physiological effect. Adrenergic receptors are divided into different subtypes: α_1, α_2, β_1, β_2, β_3.

The parasympathetic nervous system is also involuntary and in general counteracts the action of the sympathetic nervous system, restoring the body to its resting state: it is needed for relaxation and sleep. Parasympathetic fibres arise from cranial nerves III, VII, IX and X and also from the sacral section of the spinal cord, S2–S4. The neurotransmitter released by the parasympathetic nervous system is acetylcholine, the parasympathetic nervous system is described as *cholinergic*. Acetylcholine binds to cholinergic receptors to produce a physiological effect.

Cholinergic receptors are divided into two subtypes: nicotinic receptors and muscarinic receptors. Most organs are innervated by sympathetic and parasympathetic fibres, the major exception is the vascular system which is generally under sympathetic control. The systemic effects of the sympathetic and parasympathetic nervous system can be seen in Table 9.1.

Table 9.1 Systemic effects of the sympathetic and parasympathetic nervous system

Location	Sympathetic	Parasympathetic
Heart muscle	Increases heart rate and contractility (β_1)	Decreases heart rate and contractility (mAChR)
Coronary arterioles	Vasodilation (β_2)	Vasoconstriction (mAChR)
Bronchial smooth muscle	Bronchodilation (β_2)	Bronchoconstriction (mAChR)
Skeletal muscle arterioles	Vasodilation (β_2)	No known effect
Pupils	Dilation (α_1)	No known effect
Liver	Glycogenolysis and gluconeogenesis	Glycogen synthesis
Kidney	Secretion of renin (β_1)	No known effect
Bladder	Relaxation of bladder (β_2) Constriction of sphincter (α_1)	Contraction of bladder and relaxation of sphincter (mAChR)
GI tract	Reduced motility (α_1, α_2, β_2) Contraction of sphincters (α_1)	Increased motility Relaxation of sphincters (mAChR)
Skin arterioles	Vasoconstriction (α_1)	No known effect
Arrector pili muscle (hair follicles)	Contraction, hairs stand up (α_1)	No known effect
Sweating	Increased sweating on the palms of the hand (α_1)	No known effect
Adipose tissue	Lipolysis (β_3)	No known effect

Imagine walking home one evening and hearing footsteps in the dark. An instant decision is made either to turn to confront the person or to run away. This is the 'fight or flight' response of the sympathetic nervous system. Whichever action is taken requires the release of adrenaline and an important series of physiological events automatically occur:

- *pupils dilate* – improving environmental awareness;
- *heart rate and contractility increases* – sending more blood to the muscles, facilitating the physical response;
- *coronary arteries dilate* – delivering more oxygen to the myocardium whilst it works harder;
- *bronchi dilate* – increasing airflow and improving oxygenation;
- *arterioles supplying blood to skeletal muscle dilate* – delivering more oxygen to the muscles;
- *arterioles supplying the skin vasoconstrict* – diverting blood to essential organs, causing the peripheries to cool;
- *kidneys releases renin* – a vasoconstrictor that increases blood pressure;
- *liver breaks down stored glycogen to form glucose which is released into the bloodstream* – maintaining the supply of glucose to the brain and the muscles;
- *adipose tissue is broken down* – to provide more energy;
- *gut motility is reduced, sphincters constrict* – the gut is not essential in a crisis;
- *the trigone of the bladder relaxes allowing the bladder to fill* – reducing the urge to urinate;
- *arrector pili muscles contract* – the hairs on the skin stand on end;
- palms of the hands may begin to sweat.

The sympathetic nervous system has instantly prepared the body to deal with the crisis. When the crisis is over the parasympathetic system takes over and reverses the sympathetic effects. Parasympathetic effects can be quite noticeable. The acronym SLUDD helps to remember the five key parasympathetic responses (Tortora and Derrickson (2009):

S – salivation
L – lacrimation (tears)
U – urination
D – digestion
D – defaecation.

The parasympathetic system decreases the heart rate and constricts the bronchi and the pupils.

Stress is physiological as well as environmental. Acute and critical illness creates physiological stress and a sympathetic response occurs. Patients become tachycardic, hypertensive, tachyapnoeic, peripherally cool, clammy, hyperglycaemic and if conscious may become anxious. Acutely ill patients may experience these symptoms for days or weeks and may exhibit all the effects listed in Table 9.2, including constipation and urinary retention.

Neurological emergencies

The unconscious patient

Consciousness refers to a state of awareness of oneself and one's surroundings (Bradley *et al.* 2004). An acute episode of unconsciousness is a medical emergency irrespective of the cause. Unconsciousness has many potential causes, not all of which are neurological, but the treatment of the patient will be the same until the diagnosis has been made. Common causes of acute unconsciousness can be found in Table 9.2.

If the patient is unresponsive call for expert help immediately, in hospital it is appropriate to make peri-arrest, cardiac arrest or medical emergency calls, in the community dial 999 for an ambulance.

The first-line management of all medical emergencies is the same – ABCDE – airway, breathing, circulation, disability, exposure. For the management of cardiac arrest see Chapter 7.

Having established that the patient is not in cardiac arrest, place the patient in the recovery position to optimise the airway. Reduced consciousness is potentially life-threatening and may result in postural airway obstruction

Table 9.2 Common causes of acute unconsciousness

• Hypotension	• Seizures
• Hypoglycaemia	• Head injury
• Diabetic ketoacidosis	• Raised intracranial pressure
• Hyponatraemia	• Hypoxia
• Uraemia	• CO_2 narcosis
• Sensitivity to narcotics	• Alcohol excess
• Overdose and poisoning	• Anaphylaxis
• Hepatic encephalopathy	• Hypothermia
• Acute stroke	• Dysrhythmias
• Cerebral haemorrhage	• Cardiac arrest
• Meningitis	
• Encephalitis	

and loss of airway reflexes such as cough, gag and swallow reflexes. Without these reflexes the patient is at risk of aspirating secretions or vomit. A nasopharyngeal airway may be required if positioning alone does not maintain the airway.

Administer oxygen initially at 15L/min via non-rebreathing face mask, when stable the inspired oxygen can be titrated to maintain oxygen saturations within the normal range. A full set of vital signs should be recorded.

The cause of reduced consciousness requires formal medical diagnosis, the blood glucose should be checked to detect hyper- or hypoglycaemia. Hypoglycaemia should be treated immediately with oral or intravenous glucose.

Unconscious patients are unable to give consent to treatment but it is a professional expectation that nurses will act in the best interests of the patient and provide all necessary care until the patient regains consciousness and competence (Nursing and Midwifery Council 2008).

Care of the unconscious patient includes:

- *Psychological support* – explaining all nursing actions prior to carrying them out, not talking over patients, actively orientating patients to time and place.
- *Hydration* – intravenous or enteral fluids to meet hydration requirements including insensible losses. Maintain accurate intake and output records, calculating fluid balance at least 12-hourly (NMC, 2010).
- *Nutrition* – nasogastric (NG) feeding to meet calorie requirements as advised by dietetics, checking and recording NG position prior to use and supplementing electrolytes as indicated by blood results.
- *Oral hygiene* – oral suction if needed and toothbrush and paste to maintain oral hygiene.
- *Eye care* – if unable to blink eyes should be kept closed if possible and the corneas lubricated with eye drops or eye ointment.
- *Positioning* – to promote airway maintenance, normal limb posture and to prevent pressure injury. Pressure-relieving mattresses as indicated by regular assessment using a pressure risk-assessment tool.
- *Bowel management* – laxatives as required to prevent constipation, record bowel actions on a bowel chart and follow local policy for diarrhoea management.
- *Urinary management* – catheterisation or convene to monitor urine output and to prevent skin breakdown.
- *Skin care* – control of secretions, use of barrier creams to prevent skin excoriation, prompt incontinence management, avoidance of incontinence pads, regular washes if diaphoretic. Men should be shaved if this

is their normal practice. Fingernails should be kept clean and trimmed, toenails should be kept clean and trimmed (refer to podiatry or chiropody if patient is diabetic).

- *Observations* – frequency appropriate to the patient's condition and agreed with the nurse in charge, report abnormal observations immediately, particularly adverse changes in neurology (NMC 2010). Perform GCS assessment at shift handover to promote consistency of scoring.
- *Thromboprophylaxis* – administer anticoagulants and apply anti-emboli stockings or compression devices in accordance with local policy, regular reassessment of risk.
- *Vascular access* – regular assessment of all vascular access insertion sites utilising a phlebitis scoring tool, document findings (NMC 2010). Timely removal of devices when no longer required, timely replacement of devices that have reached maximum dwell time.
- *Medications* – administer as prescribed, monitor drug levels, electrolytes and vital signs as indicated for each particular medication (NMC 2010).
- *Support family and friends* – provide support and information appropriately whilst maintaining an appropriate level of patient confidentiality (NMC 2008, 2010).

Neurological assessment

Neurological assessment is performed for the following reasons:

- to establish baseline neurology;
- to identify change in relation to an earlier neurological assessment;
- to identify neurological abnormalities or deficits;
- to identify the impact of a neurological deficit on the activities of living (AL).

Specific elements of neurological assessment vary depending upon the patient's level of consciousness, their ability to follow simple commands and their clinical situation. The frequency of neurological assessment is dictated by the patient's clinical condition. Acutely unstable neurological patients may require observation every 5–15 minutes, the stable neurological patient may require observation every 4–8 hours. Clinical judgement is required when performing neurological assessment, if the patient's condition is deteriorating frequency of assessment should increase. Neurological assessment is recorded on a neurological observation chart, which may or may not incorporate an early warning scoring system (see Figure 9.15).

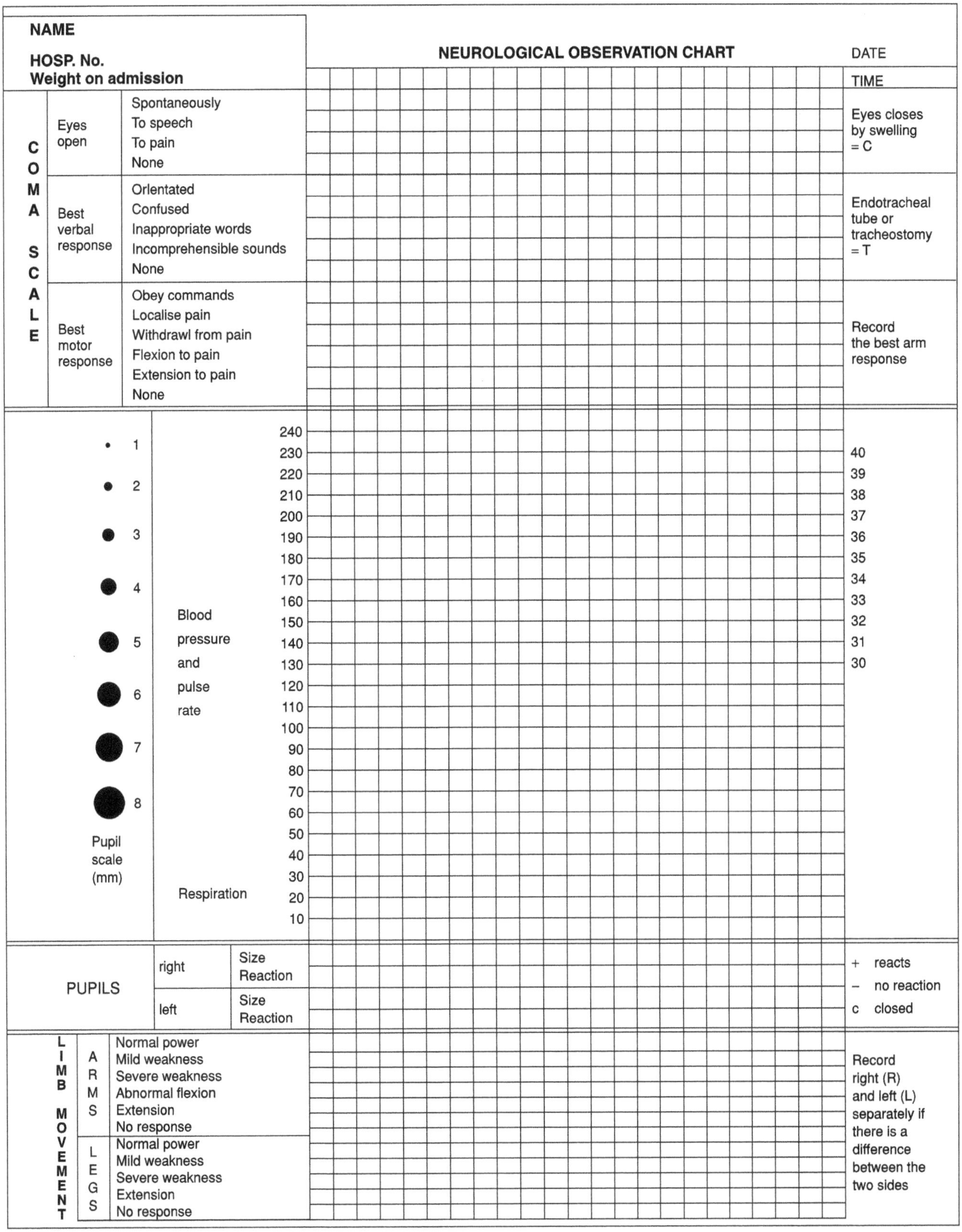
NAME
HOSP. No.
Weight on admission
NEUROLOGICAL OBSERVATION CHART
DATE
TIME
COMA SCALE
Eyes open
Spontaneously
To speech
To pain
None
Eyes closes by swelling = C
Best verbal response
Orientated
Confused
Inappropriate words
Incomprehensible sounds
None
Endotracheal tube or tracheostomy = T
Best motor response
Obey commands
Localise pain
Withdrawl from pain
Flexion to pain
Extension to pain
None
Record the best arm response
1
2
3
4
5
6
7
8
Pupil scale (mm)
Blood pressure and pulse rate
Respiration
240
230
220
210
200
190
180
170
160
150
140
130
120
110
100
90
80
70
60
50
40
30
20
10
40
39
38
37
36
35
34
33
32
31
30
PUPILS
right
Size
Reaction
left
Size
Reaction
+ reacts
– no reaction
c closed
LIMB MOVEMENT
ARMS
Normal power
Mild weakness
Severe weakness
Abnormal flexion
Extension
No response
LEGS
Normal power
Mild weakness
Severe weakness
Extension
No response
Record right (R) and left (L) separately if there is a difference between the two sides

Figure 9.15 Neurological observation chart

Neurological assessment includes:

- assessment of consciousness;
- pupil size, shape, equality and reaction to light;
- respiratory rate and pattern;
- blood pressure, pulse and temperature.

Assessing consciousness

The Glasgow Coma Scale (GCS) is probably the most widely used neurological assessment tool in the world. GCS assessment has three elements:

- Best eye-opening response
- Best verbal response
- Best motor response.

Each element contains subcategories with a score (see Table 9.3).

The maximum possible score is 15/15 the worst possible score is 3/15. Patients may be unable to speak because of intubation or a cuffed tracheostomy tube, these patients have no air flow through their vocal cords. In this situation the nurse awards the patient a verbal score of 1 and annotates the score as follows 1(T) indicating intubation as the cause of the verbal deficit. A score of eight or less indicates unconsciousness in most patients.

GCS is intended to be an objective assessment of the patient's level of consciousness, however the person performing the GCS must judge the patient's response to stimuli and therefore a certain amount of subjectivity is inevitable. For this reason it is considered good practice for nurses to jointly assess GCS at handover to ensure both agree the GCS. If the GCS deteriorates a second competent nurse should immediately check the GCS,

confirming the deterioration prior to alerting the medical team (NICE 2007).

GCS assessment commences the moment the nurse approaches the patient's bed space. In a busy ward environment, in daylight or when the lights are on, most patients will be awake. The fact that a patient is sleeping in a noisy environment may be the first indication that the GCS is not 15/15, even if there is no primary neurological problem.

If the patient wakes and opens their eyes as the nurse approaches, the eye-opening score will be 4 for spontaneous eye opening (see Table 9.3). It is now appropriate to assess the patient's verbal response. Having greeted the patient there are compulsory questions that must be asked to establish whether the patient is orientated to time and place. The nurse must ask the patient where they are, if the patient knows they are in hospital the nurse should be more specific and ask the patient to name the hospital. Next, ask the patient to state the year, if the patient answers correctly ask the patient to name the month. Correct answers indicate orientation to time and place and scores 5 for the verbal response (see Table 9.3).

If the answers are relevant to the question but incorrect the patient should be scored as confused. For example the patient may be in hospital but might think they are at home, the answer is relevant to the question but incorrect, they will score 4 for confusion.

If the patient answers with words or phrases that are irrelevant to the question the answer is classified as 'inappropriate words' and scores 3 points.

Unintelligible speech, making sounds not words, classifies the response as 'incomprehensible sounds' scoring 2 points. If there is no verbal response at all the patient scores 1 point.

After assessing verbal response the motor response is assessed. As seen in Table 9.3, motor response has six possible results. The nurse asks the patient to perform a specific action to determine whether the patient is capable of obeying commands. It is important to choose an action that the patient is unlikely to perform by coincidence. A hand squeeze can be used to assess motor function. If this is the chosen command the nurse places their fingers on the ventral side of the patient's fingers, not across the palm of the patient's hand. This avoids triggering the grasp reflex which may occur without cognitive intention. Alternatively ask the patient to raise their arms or to stick out their tongue.

Dorsal = upper, back or posterior surface.
Ventral = lower, under or anterior surface.

If the patient obeys commands the next part of motor assessment is to test the symmetry of the motor response,

Table 9.3 Glasgow Coma Scale

Best eye-opening response	Eyes open spontaneously	4
	Eyes open to speech	3
	Eyes open to pain	2
	No eye opening	1
Best verbal response	Orientated to time and place	5
	Confused	4
	Inappropriate words	3
	Incomprehensible sounds	2
	No verbal response	1
Best motor response	Obeys commands	6
	Localises to pain	5
	Withdrawal from pain	4
	Flexion to pain	3
	Extension to pain	2
	No motor response	1

identifying any limb deficits such as hemiparesis. Symmetry is assessed by simultaneously checking the bilateral strength of the hand grip or by assessing equality of arm raising. The lower limbs should also be assessed.

If the patient's eyes do not open spontaneously as the nurse approaches the bed space it will be necessary to use a stimulus to assess the patient. There are two types of stimulus – verbal and tactile stimuli.

Verbal stimuli refers to use of voice to stimulate a response. Begin by greeting the patient in a normal tone to see if their eyes open 'Hello Mr Smith'. If unsuccessful repeat the greeting more loudly. If the patient opens their eyes continue the GCS assessment. If the patient does not open their eyes speak loudly, into both ears, in case the patient is deaf. Ask the patient to open their eyes. While talking, observe for spontaneous limb movement. If verbal stimulus is unsuccessful tactile stimulus is needed.

Tactile stimuli – gently shake the patient's shoulders to see if they awaken. Neurological patients often sleep very deeply, it may be necessary to ensure the patient is fully awake before proceeding with GCS assessment.

If gentle shaking is unsuccessful a pain stimulus is required to assess GCS. A central pain stimulus should be used, peripheral pain stimuli can invoke spinal reflexes and may result in an incorrect GCS assessment. A spinal reflex is a signal that travels via a sensory nerve to the spinal cord producing a motor response from the spinal cord back to the periphery. The impulse does not travel via the brain and is not an indicator of motor function.

There are several ways to apply a central pain stimulus, not all are clinically appropriate. The application of supraorbital pressure is a type of central pain stimulus but is contraindicated in patients with facial fractures and should not be attempted unless trained to do so. A sternal rub can easily bruise the soft tissue over the sternum and is not recommended. The easiest and most common method of applying a central pain stimulus is to squeeze the trapezius muscle between the neck and the shoulder joint. If the trapezius squeeze is contraindicated, for example if the collar bones are fractured, mandibular pressure may be applied by using the index and middle finger to press upwards and inwards at the hinge of the mandible.

Nurses may be hesitant to apply a pain stimulus, concerned about hurting the patient. This misplaced concern may result in an incorrect GCS assessment which may be detrimental to the patient. Nurses caring for patients with altered consciousness have a professional obligation to assess the patient accurately in order to ensure the patient receives the most appropriate treatment. Nurses must overcome their anxiety and learn to apply a central pain stimulus correctly.

Prior to applying a pain stimulus the nurse should ensure that the patient is positioned appropriately and that the arms and the feet have been uncovered in order to observe limb responses. Arms should be placed away from the body, allowing enough space for the limbs to move freely. If the arms are too close to the patient's body it may be difficult to interpret the motor response of the upper limbs.

A trapezius squeeze is performed using the thumb and index finger to grasp about 5cm of trapezius muscle at the base of the neck, squeeze and twist the muscle while observing carefully for eye opening and for motor response of all four limbs. Pain stimulus should be maintained until the nurse is certain of the patient's response.

Having applied a pain stimulus the motor response must be interpreted and a score awarded (see Table 9.3). To achieve a motor score of five the patient must localise to pain. If the brain is intact the normal response to pain is to move away from the pain or to remove the source of the pain. Having applied a trapezius squeeze if the patient moves their arm purposely towards the source of the pain, attempting to remove the assessor's hand, they are said to be localising to pain. The patient's hand must be raised to the height of the chin to award a motor score of 5. This is a positive sign suggesting a relatively intact brain.

If the patient is unable to raise their arm to chin height but has at least reached the midline they may be awarded a score of 4 for 'withdrawal from pain'. Withdrawal suggests that the patient is unable to make a purposeful attempt to remove the source of the pain.

If the patient is unable to achieve withdrawal, but can flex the arm, bringing the hand towards the body by bending the elbow, they are scored 3 for flexion.

Patients with severe brain injuries may exhibit an extensor response to pain. There are two types of extensor response:

● Decerebrate
● Decorticate.

A decerebrate response can be easily misinterpreted if the pain stimulus is not applied for long enough to accurately assess the patient's response. When the pain stimulus is applied the shoulders appear to move upwards, the elbows appear to flex and as the pain stimulus continues arms internally rotate, fingers flex to form a fist and the arms push down and extend away from the source of pain, legs extend and toes point.

A decorticate response is often brisker than a decerebrate response. When a pain stimulus is applied spastic arm flexion occurs, legs extend and toes point.

Extensor responses score two points (see Table 9.3). If there is no response to central pain one point is awarded for motor function.

By now a score will have been generated for all three sections of the GCS. The scores are recorded and communicated to identify each section of the score as well as giving a total score. For example E2 V3 M4 gives a GCS of 9/15.

The motor section of the GCS carries the most weight. A GCS of 7/15 that is achieved by E1 V1 M5 is viewed more positively than a GCS of 7/15 that is achieved by E4 V1 M2. By presenting the information for each section it becomes clear where the patient has lost points.

When patients are unable to obey commands it is difficult to assess limb power. Muscle tone can be assessed by moving each limb through the normal range of passive movement. This reveals whether the limb is normal, flaccid or has increased tone.

When patients are able to obey commands limb power is graded from 0–5 (see Table 9.4).

Table 9.4 Grading limb power

Grade	Indicator of limb power
5	Active movement against gravity, full resistance, normal strength
4	Active movement against gravity, some resistance that can be overcome by the examiner
3	Active movement against gravity, unable to resist the examiner
2	Active movement when gravity is eliminated
1	No active movement, weak muscle contraction can be palpated
0	No muscle contraction detected

Assessing pupils

This element of neurological assessment is performed on conscious and unconscious patients unless the eyes are closed by oedema, in which case a 'C' is marked on the neurological observation chart.

Pupil size, pupil shape, reactivity to light and equality of pupil size should be assessed and recorded on the neurological observation chart.

A pupil gauge, printed on the neurological observation chart, is used to measure pupil size. Normal pupil size ranges from 2–6mm but abnormal pupils may be as large as 9mm. Extremely small pupils are described as pinpoint and may result from opiate administration. Pupils that are large, dilated and unreactive to light are described as 'fixed and dilated'. This is a severe sign of raised intracranial pressure and may indicate that death is imminent.

Pupils are normally round but pupil abnormalities do occur. An oval-shaped pupil indicates raised intracranial pressure and must be reported immediately. A keyhole pupil is the result of eye surgery and is not a neurological sign.

To assess the pupils both eyelids should be elevated simultaneously and pupil size compared. Using a pen torch, shine light into the eye, observe the pupil, it should constrict immediately as light is applied and should dilate when the light is withdrawn – this is the direct light reflex. The application of light to one pupil should cause a simultaneous response in both pupils – this is the consensual light reaction.

A plus sign (+) indicates pupil reactivity on the neurological observation chart, a minus sign (−) indicates no reaction.

Respiratory assessment

Respiration may be affected by conscious level and brain pathology. Respiration is controlled by the pons and the medulla in the brainstem, abnormal respiratory patterns suggest brainstem pathology. Brainstem injury is associated with tachypnoea, bradypnoea and apnoea.

Cheyne–Stokes breathing: a cyclical pattern of rapid breathing becoming progressively slower and shallower until apnoea occurs. The patient usually starts breathing again spontaneously but may be stimulated to breathe by tactile stimulation if apnoea is prolonged. This respiratory pattern is associated with widespread cortical lesions and thalamic dysfunction. Apnoea is an important observation and should be reported. Non-invasive respiratory monitoring is indicated if apnoea is frequent or prolonged.

Vital signs assessment

Thermoregulation may be affected by neurological disease or injury. Hyperthermia is more common than hypothermia, it may be central in origin and is associated with subarachnoid haemorrhage, blood in the CSF and in patients with posterior fossa surgery. It is important to remember that fever may not be neurological in origin, it is also seen in acute MI, PE, sepsis and local infection.

Hyperthermia increases cell metabolism which increases oxygen demand, CO_2 production and lactic acid. CO_2 is a potent vasodilator within the systemic circulation and has the potential to increase intracranial pressure (ICP). Hyperthermia in neurological patients has been shown to independently contribute to increased mortality and length of stay in neuro-critical care units (Diringer *et al.* 2004). Attempts should be made to control temperature but it is important to prevent shivering in acute or unstable patients as shivering increases ICP. Antipyretics, tepid sponging, removing blankets and increasing skin exposure all help to reduce fever.

Therapeutic hypothermia is increasingly being used to improve outcomes following cardiac arrest, traumatic brain injury and acute stroke.

CASE STUDY 9.1 Susan with drowsiness, headache, neck stiffness, vomiting and photophobia – Part 1

Susan, aged 20, is a university student. She lives in university accommodation and missed classes yesterday. That morning she did not appear as agreed for a private study session, her friends called security and entered her room. Susan was found in bed with the bedclothes over her head and the lights off, there was vomit on the floor. Susan's friends don't know her past medical history but she has been well up until now. Susan was brought to the emergency unit (EU) at 14.00 by her friends.

INITIAL ASSESSMENT

On examination Susan was lying on her side with her hands over her face, her eyes were closed, she was not moving.

Airway

Susan did not speak when spoken to but did speak when the nurse gently shook her shoulder and spoke more loudly, indicating the airway was patent and Susan was conscious. There was no evidence of stridor or paradoxical breathing.

Breathing

Susan's respiratory rate was 32bpm, her respiratory pattern was regular, oxygen saturation was 91% on air and she was not using any accessory muscles. She had no inspiratory pain and did not feel short of breath when questioned. Breath sounds were clear and air entry slightly reduced on the right, the side that Susan was lying on.

Susan spoke in short sentences or single words and only spoke when directly questioned, she said this was because talking made her head hurt. The nurse administered oxygen via a non-rebreathing face mask at 15L/min and Susan's oxygen saturation rapidly increased to 100%. Susan was reluctant to turn onto her back and the nurse was unable to palpate Susan's chest. In view of the normal breath sounds and good oxygen saturations this element of the respiratory assessment was not pursued. In the absence of any difficulty in breathing and with normal breath sounds the nurse concluded that Susan's tachypnoea was not respiratory in origin.

Circulation

Susan's pulse rate was 132bpm on palpation, the pulse was regular and the pulse volume was reduced. Susan felt centrally and peripherally hot, skin was slightly sweaty and flushed, no peripheral oedema. Temperature recorded at 39.4°C axilla, blood pressure 78/54mmHg with a MAP of 62mmHg, the CRT was two seconds. Vasodilation from fever makes CRT clinically difficult to interpret. Susan is

attached to a cardiac monitor, revealing a sinus tachycardia with occasional atrial ectopics.

The tachycardia may be due to Susan's high fever which increases cell metabolism, oxygen demand and oxygen consumption, explaining Susan's low-grade hypoxia. Increased metabolism results in increased CO_2 production, explaining Susan's tachypnoea. CO_2 dissolves in the plasma forming carbonic acid. Carbonic acid dissociates to form H^+ and HCO_3^-. The H^+ ions diffuse into the CSF crossing the blood–brain barrier where they stimulate the central chemoreceptors in the brainstem. Susan's respiratory rate is centrally driven as she tries to control her pH and CO_2 by increasing her respiratory rate. Fever, acidosis and increased metabolism create physiological stress resulting in adrenaline release by the sympathetic nervous system, also contributing to Susan's tachycardia. Susan's blood pressure is lower than expected for her age. Hypotension can result in a reflex tachycardia in attempt to maintain cardiac output. Susan's fever causes vasodilation as the body attempts to lose heat through the skin, contributing to the hypotension. Fever is usually caused by infection unless a patient has a primary neurological problem. Pathogenic microorganisms release toxins that are vasoactive and can cause vasodilation during a septic episode.

Susan doesn't know if she is thirsty or not. Fever increases insensible loss from sweating and from increased respiratory rate, causing dehydration. As Susan has been in bed for more than 24 hours oral intake is likely to have been reduced. Increased insensible loss and reduced intake can cause significant dehydration contributing to hypotension. Hypotension and dehydration result in reduced renal blood flow and will put Susan at risk of pre-renal acute kidney injury (AKI).

Disability

Susan did not wake when approached and did not speak until a light tactile stimulus was applied. She did not open her eyes when she spoke and tended to mumble. The nurse asked Susan to open her eyes, Susan said she couldn't. When questioned she said the light hurt her eyes and she had a bad headache. The nurse turned the overhead light off and asked Susan to turn her head but Susan said her neck was stiff and it hurt to move her head. Susan still couldn't open her eyes, she was photophobic. On questioning Susan whispered that she was at home, she didn't know what year it was, indicating she was confused. She was able to obey commands when asked to squeeze

---

CASE STUDY 9.1 Susan with drowsiness, headache, neck stiffness, vomiting and photophobia – Part 1 *(continued)*

the nurse's hand and her limb power was reduced but symmetrical. Her GCS was E1 V4 M6 = 11/15. Pupils were not assessed as Susan couldn't open her eyes and would not allow the nurse to open them. The nurse recorded the pupil responses as 'C' on the neurological observation chart.

Exposure

Susan denied abdominal pain or calf pain. Her abdomen was soft and non-tender on palpation, she had scanty bowel sounds, calves were soft and non-tender.

Susan had no signs of IV drug usage and denied having taken any drugs, she had a mild erythematous rash on her legs. Skin appeared intact and she was continent.

Blood glucose was 10.1mmol/L and BMI appeared normal. The nurse was unable to gain any additional information from Susan but was concerned that Susan may not have eaten or drunk for at least 24 hours. Susan was too drowsy to take nutrition and fluids orally.

The nurse realises that the elevated blood glucose level may be due to physiological stress, activating the sympathetic nervous system causing glycogenolysis and gluconeogenesis. The sympathetic nervous system may also be responsible for the quiet and infrequent bowel sounds heard. Susan requires regular blood glucose monitoring and intravenous hydration fluids.

DIAGNOSIS AND INITIAL MANAGEMENT

In view of the presentation and clinical findings, which include; headache, stiff neck, photophobia, rash, fever,

tachycardia, hypotension, tachypnoea and oliguria a provisional diagnosis of bacterial meningitis and hypovolaemia are made. This is a clinical emergency.

The doctor prescribes humidified O_2 to be titrated to maintain the oxygen saturation greater than 98%. Consent is obtained and a radial arterial puncture is performed, the arterial blood gas (ABG) sample is processed and results given to the doctor. Regular ABG analysis is needed to ensure the $PaCO_2$ does not become too low, the PaO_2 is maintained and pH is within normal range.

A large-bore peripheral cannula is inserted and 1 litre of 0.9% NaCl is given immediately. Blood is taken for blood cultures, full blood count, electrolytes, C-reactive protein, liver function tests and a clotting screen at the time of cannulation. Susan's skin is cleaned with 2% chlorhexidine in 70% isopropyl alcohol prior to cannulation and the blood culture bottles are also cleaned with a 2% chlorhexidine in 70% isopropyl alcohol wipe. The cannula is labelled with the date and time of insertion and a cannula observation chart is commenced.

Broad-spectrum intravenous antibiotics are prescribed to treat the meningitis and intravenous acyclovir is also prescribed in case the symptoms are caused by viral encephalitis. Both drug regimens will be given until the culture results become available. Susan has no known drug allergies and the drugs are administered without delay. Susan's nurse records the GCS and the vital signs, it is agreed that Susan remain on continuous monitoring with half-hourly recording of observations. An urgent CT scan of the head is requested and Susan remains nil by mouth.

Maximising neurological status

Raised ICP is damaging to brain tissue and must be prevented or managed urgently. The skull contains brain tissue, CSF and blood vessels, and strategies to reduce ICP focus on one or more of these elements.

Removal of brain tissue is not desirable unless clinically indicated and strategies to control brain tissue generally focus on the control of cerebral oedema or the relief of pressure. Cerebral oedema is managed by administration of osmotic diuretics and steroids and the restriction of fluids. Raised ICP is relieved by the creation of burr holes (holes drilled in the skull) or by craniectomy (a surgical procedure to remove a flap of bone).

Position

Patients with reduced or fluctuating levels of consciousness are at risk of aspiration if protective airway reflexes are lost. Elevating the head of the bed to 30° reduces this risk. Head elevation also increases venous drainage from the head, helping to control cerebral blood volume and reduce ICP. For patients with acute elevations in ICP extreme flexion of the hips and knees is contraindicated as this may increase intra-abdominal pressure with a resulting increase in thoracic pressure and intracranial pressure.

Optimising cerebral blood flow

The cerebral blood vessels and the blood contained within them take up approximately 10 per cent of the space within the skull. Blood vessel diameter affects the amount of space that the blood vessels occupy within the brain. Blood vessels may dilate due to increased blood volume or because of metabolic factors influencing blood vessel tone, for example, pH, PaO_2, and $PaCO_2$. Hypoxia, hypercapnoea and acidosis cause vasodilation of systemic blood vessels, increasing ICP. The reverse is also true: hypocapnoea and alkalosis cause systemic vasoconstriction, reducing cerebral blood flow. Because of the effects of blood gases on cerebral blood vessels it is normal practice to control blood gases within strict limits in order to control ICP.

Oxygen is administered to maintain the PaO_2 greater than 11 kPa. This high target PaO_2 is important in order to help optimise vasoconstriction and ICP control. Intubation and ventilation may be needed to control $PaCO_2$ and to optimise oxygenation. By preventing hypoxia and hypercapnoea the blood vessels remain in a state of partial tone and will occupy less space within the brain.

In the case study, Susan is fluid resuscitated to increase her blood pressure. Cerebral blood flow and oxygen delivery are essential for normal cerebral function. Although the brain only weighs about 1.5kg, or 2% of body weight, it receives approximately 20% of the cardiac output and 20% of available oxygen. The brain is able to autoregulate to control cerebral blood flow. Autoregulation describes the brain's ability to maintain a constant blood flow irrespective of changes to blood pressure. This phenomenon only functions correctly when mean BP is between 60 and 150mmHg. Below 60mmHg cerebral blood flow diminishes and above 150mmHg it increases. Hypotension causes cerebral ischaemia and brain injury, neurological management focuses on the maintenance of mean BP by the administration of fluids and vasopressors.

> Calculating cerebral perfusion pressure:
> $$MAP - ICP = CPP$$

In health, little notice is taken of cerebral perfusion pressure (CPP) because the brain autoregulates; for acute neurological patients CPP is considered to be important. CPP is calculated from the mean arterial blood pressure minus the ICP and should be maintained at 50–70mmHg to prevent cerebral ischaemia. From the formula it can be concluded that if MAP were to fall and ICP were to rise CPP would be significantly affected. Trauma to the vasomotor centre may cause autoregulation to fail, hypotension from failure of the vasomotor centre is termed neurogenic shock.

CASE STUDY 9.2 Susan with meningitis – Part 2

Susan's nurse prepares the equipment for catheterisation. Suddenly and without warning Susan has a projectile vomit after which she coughs for about 20 seconds. Projectile vomiting is associated with neurological disorders and can be an indication of severe neurological irritation or raised intracranial pressure: it is common in meningitis. Coughing suggests that some vomit may have penetrated the top of Susan's airway, the airway reflexes are working and Susan coughs to clear her pharynx. The nurse carries on talking to Susan but Susan is unresponsive. The nurse repeats the GCS assessment. Susan has no verbal response, even when her shoulders are gently shaken, she is no longer obeying commands. A trapezius squeeze is performed, Susan groans and raises her right arm towards her shoulder. The nurse assesses Susan's GCS to be E1 V2 M4 = 7/15. This is a significant drop and the nurse realises that a GCS of 7/15 means that Susan is no longer conscious. The nurse pulls the emergency bell for help; as she does so Susan has a seizure.

The nurse goes back to the beginning of the ABCD assessment.

Airway
Susan's mouth is shut, her teeth are clenched, there is froth around her mouth, there is no condensation on the oxygen face mask, no exhalation is detected and the airway is obstructed. The nurse selects a size 7 nasopharyngeal airway from the emergency bedside equipment. Having quickly checked to confirm the size by measuring from the nares of the nose to the tragus of the ear the nasopharyngeal airway is inserted. Airway is reassessed, there is condensation on the face mask as Susan breathes, the airway is secure. A Guedel airway is not appropriate as Susan's teeth are clamped shut. A jaw thrust is difficult during a seizure as the muscles are in spasm. A nasopharyngeal airway is the management technique of choice in seizure. Susan is positioned on her side in case of further vomiting.

Breathing
Breathing is slightly noisy and the respiratory rate is 30 bpm. Oxygen saturations are 100%. Chest movements are symmetrical. Secretions can be heard on chest auscultation.

Suction via the nasopharyngeal airway is performed and vomit obtained. Susan may have aspirated.

Circulation

The cardiac monitor displays a sinus tachycardia of 120/min and blood pressure is 100/70mmHg, pulse volume has improved a little since the fluids were administered. CRT is now three seconds and Susan's hands are a little cooler. This is probably due to the sympathetic effects of adrenaline causing vasoconstriction.

Disability

Susan is unresponsive to speech and continues to seize. The medical team arrives, prescribes IV diazemuls 5mg given immediately, the seizure terminates, Susan relaxes, she appears to be deeply asleep. This is the post-ictal phase that occurs after a seizure. Susan's pupils are round, size 3mm, equal in size and react to light. GCS is E1 V1 M3 = 5/15.

Implications

Susan is awaiting a CT scan, an important part of her diagnosis. CT scans are performed with the patient supine (on their back); however, Susan's GCS is too low and she will be at risk of postural airway obstruction or vomiting and aspirating if she is sent to CT scan with an unprotected airway. The team refers to the critical care outreach team and anaesthetics for further management. Susan is intubated and stabilised, medically escorted to the scanner with full invasive monitoring; following the scan she is transferred to ITU for further management. The scan aids diagnosis and confirms whether lumbar puncture is safe to perform. Susan's clotting will also be assessed prior to lumbar puncture reducing the risk of epidural haematoma. Timely antibiotic administration, surveillance of culture samples and supportive care of the unconscious patient are the main elements of meningitis management.

Meningitis

Meningitis is the term used to describe inflammation of the meninges surrounding the brain and spinal cord. Inflammation can be caused by bacteria, viruses, fungi, protozoa, cancer cells or by irritant drugs. Most commonly meningitis is caused by bacterial infection. Bacterial meningitis affects the subarachnoid space and the meninges either side of the space, the pia and arachnoid mater. The CSF is also affected.

Bacterial meningitis is most common in children, and adolescents and the over-55 age group. Meningococcal meningitis is particularly dangerous and is associated with outbreaks, or small epidemics. People most at risk are those living in close quarters such as student halls of residence, hostels, nursing homes or military barracks.

Bacterial meningitis can also occur following neurosurgery, lumbar puncture, skull fracture or penetrating head injury. This type of meningitis is not contagious and is caused by bacteria entering the meninges when the CNS is opened.

Severe headache and fever are early symptoms of meningitis, hyperpyrexia is common. Neck stiffness is also an early sign and may be associated with lethargy and confusion. Lethargy can quickly progress to unconsciousness. Photophobia, nausea and vomiting are also common.

The immune system responds to the bacterial invasion of the meninges and inflammation develops. Inflammation may affect blood vessels, causing thrombus or haemorrhage. Inflammation also damages brain tissue and may cause seizures, stroke and cerebral oedema. Cerebral oedema can obstruct CSF drainage leading to hydrocephaly and raised ICP. Meningococcal meningitis can lead to life-threatening septicaemia and multi-organ failure. Early diagnosis and treatment is essential to reduce mortality.

Diagnosis is primarily based on signs and symptoms and treatment should not be delayed while waiting for results of tests or investigations. Diagnosis is confirmed by CT scan and lumbar puncture but may also include physical signs such as Brudzinski's sign (when the neck is flexed the hips and knees flex simultaneously) and Kernig's sign (with the patient supine the knee is flexed and then straightened, straightening causes acute pain).

Due to the potential mortality from meningitis treatment should start immediately. Intravenous antibiotics and antivirals are given until culture results are known. Corticosteroids are also used to suppress the inflammatory response and reduce cerebral oedema.

Intravenous fluids are given to maintain hydration, intravascular volume and MAP. Insensible losses from sweating and measurable losses from vomiting must be replaced.

Anticonvulsants are usually prescribed, such as intravenous phenytoin.

If ICP is dangerously high intravenous mannitol, an osmotic diuretic, may be given. Mannitol is a large-molecule sugar solution that rapidly increases the osmotic pressure of the blood. The increased osmotic pressure draws water from the interstitial space into the blood compartment, reducing interstitial cerebral oedema. The increase in blood volume is detected by the aortic and carotid baroreceptors and the atrial diastolic stretch receptors. Increased signals are sent to the vasomotor centre indicating that the circulating volume is too high. Antidiuretic hormone is inhibited and reabsorption of water by the kidneys ceases causing an immediate diuresis. Mannitol is a potent osmotic diuretic and patients may pass several litres of urine per hour. It is essential to maintain the patient's electrolytes, particularly potassium, to prevent cardiac dysrhythmias as a complication of diuresis.

Acute stroke

Acute stroke is a common condition – someone suffers an acute stroke every five minutes in England (Markus *et al.* 2010). In the developed world approximately 15 per cent of strokes are haemorrhagic and 85 per cent are ischaemic (Markus *et al.* 2010). A number of risk factors for stroke exist: some are modifiable, some are not. Non-modifiable risk factors for stroke include age – the risk of stroke increases exponentially with age; gender – men are at increased risk when compared to women; ethnicity – individuals of black and Asian origin have a greater risk of stroke when compared to white people; genetics – a family of history of stroke in individuals under 65 years of age is a risk factor for stroke (Markus *et al.* 2010).

Modifiable risk factors (factors which the individual can influence) include smoking, obesity, socio-economic class, sedentary lifestyle, alcohol excess, hypertension, diabetes, hypercholesterolaemia, metabolic syndrome, the oral contraceptive pill and diet (Markus *et al.* 2010).

The first sign of stroke may be collapse but patients may also be aware of the following symptoms and may know that a stroke is occurring:

- facial weakness or numbness;
- difficulty walking;
- difficulty speaking;
- paralysis or numbness of one side of the body;
- visual disturbance;
- headache.

Immediate medical review is indicated: the more quickly a stroke is treated the better the outcome. Patients with an acute stroke should receive brain imaging within one hour and be admitted to a specialist acute stroke unit where they can be assessed for thrombolysis and receive the therapy appropriately (NICE 2010). The NHS FAST campaign is designed to identify the symptoms of stroke as quickly as possible, ensuring emergency medical management is provided (NHS 2011).

FAST

Face – has the face fallen on one side, can they smile?
Arms – can they raise both arms and keep them there?
Speech – is their speech slurred?
Time – time to call 999 if you see any one of the signs.

Patients with haemorrhagic stroke will be referred to a neurosurgical unit, a craniotomy may be indicated to evacuate the haematoma and control intracranial pressure.

Whatever the setting, patients experiencing an acute stroke require neurological assessment, vital sign assessment and support for nutrition and hydration until they recover their independence. It is recommended that patients with acute stroke have their swallowing assessed by a specially trained health care professional within four hours of admission to hospital and before being given food, fluid or medication (NICE 2010).

Seizures and status epilepticus

The term seizure refers to a single episode of abnormal cerebral activity resulting in a temporary state of altered consciousness. Epilepsy refers to chronic, recurrent episodes of abnormal cerebral activity accompanied by altered consciousness. Epilepsy is in effect recurrent seizures and is one of the most common neurological disorders. Anyone may potentially suffer a seizure if the right circumstances exist within the CNS. Seizures may be triggered by particular risk factors such as trauma, alcohol, brain tumour, electrolyte imbalance, Alzheimer's disease and neurodegenerative diseases. For some individuals triggers can be specific such as flashing lights, a specific smell or a particular type of music. General triggers include tiredness, lack of sleep, fever, menstruation, constipation and emotional stress.

Seizures may follow a predictable pattern (Hickey 2009):

- *Aura* – a warning sign that a seizure is imminent. Auras may be visual, auditory or gustatory (taste) and are usually consistent in their presentation.

- *Automatisms* – coordinated involuntary activities that precede the seizure, such as pacing about or lip smacking.
- *Autonomic symptoms* – physical symptoms resulting from stimulation of the ANS such as sweating, flushing and pupil dilation.
- *Tonus* – major contraction of voluntary muscles resulting in generalised stiffness and extension of the arms and legs, the jaw is clamped shut (the tongue may be bitten), apnoea and incontinence may occur.
- *Clonus* – muscular spasms with a violent rhythmic pattern of muscular rigidity and relaxation, the *clonic phase* of seizure may be accompanied by hyperventilation, eye rolling, frothing at the mouth and tachycardia.
- *Post-ictal* – the after phase when patients may be deeply asleep and difficult to rouse but the muscle spasms have ceased. This may last several hours and on waking patients may be disorientated or amnesic.

Status epilepticus usually refers to a seizure lasting at least five minutes or recurrent seizures where the patient does not regain consciousness between seizures (Lowenstein and Alldredge 1998). Because of the unpredictable nature of seizures patients may sustain secondary injuries such as falls, burns or head injuries.

Occasionally seizure activity may be seen in an isolated muscle group such as the arm or face, this is described as a focal seizure. Recurrent seizures are usually recorded on a seizure or fit chart allowing objective assessment of the frequency and duration of seizures and evaluation of management strategies.

Treatment focuses on underlying causes such as correction of electrolyte imbalance or removal of brain tumours. For chronic sufferers avoidance of triggers is important.

Drug management includes the use of traditional anti-epileptic medications such as phenytoin or more modern agents such as levetiracetam (keppra), the mode of action of which is unknown but it is thought to influence synapse transmission.

The management of an acute seizure focuses on:

- airway maintenance;
- oxygenation;
- prevention of environmental harm;
- termination of the seizure with medications;
- post-seizure care, including ABGs, electrolytes, medication review, general observations and investigations to identify the cause.

Conclusion

The nervous system is a highly integrated system that ensures an appropriate response to changes in the internal or external environment. Diseases of the nervous system may be acute or chronic. Nurses must understand the anatomy and physiology of the nervous system in order to understand neurological disease processes and to anticipate the clinical implications of neurological dysfunction. Competence in neurological assessment is a key clinical skill for nurses faced with a medical emergency in any clinical setting and is an essential skill within a neuroscience setting. Neurological emergencies have the potential to be life threatening if normal control of airway, breathing or circulation is lost. Ability to assess patients using an ABCDE approach is essential for the management of neurological emergencies.

Glossary

Abducens VIth cranial nerve, motor control of eye movements.

Acetylcholine A neurotransmitter of the parasympathetic nervous system released by many neurones within the peripheral nervous system and by a few neurones in the central nervous system.

Acetylcholinesterase The enzyme that destroys the neurotransmitter acetylcholine.

Acetylcholinesterase inhibitors Drugs that block the production of the enzyme acetylcholinesterase, e.g. pyridostigmine.

Action potential An electrical signal that travels along the surface of a neurone, the signal is propagated by the movement of ions across the cell membrane of the neurone.

Adrenaline Now called epinephrine, neurotransmitter of the sympathetic nervous system.

Afferent neurone An alternative name for a sensory neurone, carries information towards the brain.

α_1 **receptor** Receptor within the sympathetic nervous system located on the post-synaptic surface, responds to epinephrine creating a physiological effect, e.g. vasocostriction.

α_2 **receptor** Receptor within the sympathetic nervous system located on the pre-synaptic surface, detects unused or surplus epinephrine and inhibits further epinephrine secretion.

Anterior horns Section of the spinal cord, comprised of grey matter and containing motor axons.

Anticonvulsants Drugs used to control seizures.

Aphasia Absence of speech.

Apneustic centre Located within the pons, controls breathing in conjunction with the pneumotaxic centre and the medulla.

Apnoea Temporary cessation of breathing, usually self-terminating, more prevalent following brainstem injury.

Arachnoid mater Middle layer of the meninges.

Astrocyte A type of glial cell within the central nervous system, star-like in appearance, with multiple processes extending from the cell body, some of which end in foot processes that interface with cerebral blood vessels forming part of the blood–brain barrier.

Autonomic dysreflexia Extreme autonomic response that can occur in patients with spinal cord injury above the level of T6.

Autonomic nervous system Branch of the peripheral nervous system containing two major subdivisions; the sympathetic and parasympathetic nervous systems.

Axon The section of the neurone that extends away from the cell body.

β₁ receptors Part of the sympathetic nervous system, adrenergic receptors located within the heart muscle, stimulation causes increase in heart rate and contractility.

β₂ receptors Part of the sympathetic nervous system, adrenergic receptors with widespread activity including vasodilation and bronchodilation.

β₃ receptors Part of the sympathetic nervous system, adrenergic receptors located in brown adipose tissue, stimulation causes thermogenesis.

Blood–brain barrier An important structure that prevents harmful substances from entering the brain tissue. The blood–brain barrier has two main components; a thick capillary basement membrane and tight junctions between the endothelial cells of the capillaries.

Brainstem An essential structure within the brain containing the *midbrain*, the *pons* and the *medulla oblongata*.

Broca's speech area Motor control of speech within the cerebral cortex, motor neurones connect Broca's speech area with the larynx, pharynx, mouth and respiratory muscles to enable coordination of talking, breathing and swallowing.

Cauda equina A collection of lumbar, sacral and coccygeal nerve roots within the spinal canal below the height of L2.

Cell body The main part of the neurone containing cytoplasm and organelles.

Central nervous system A subdivision of the nervous system comprising the brain and spinal cord often referred to as the CNS.

Cerebellum Part of the brain that lies beneath the cerebral hemispheres and posterior to the brainstem, regulates posture and balance, important for the coordinated contraction of skeletal muscle.

Cerebral cortex Outer rim of grey matter that forms part of the cerebral hemispheres.

Cerebral dominance The development of one cerebral hemisphere more than the other.

Cerebral hemispheres The two halves of the cerebrum.

Cerebral oedema Swelling of the brain.

Cerebral perfusion pressure Or CPP, calculated from the mean arterial blood pressure minus the ICP, the pressure of the blood perfusing the brain.

Cerebrospinal fluid Also called CSF, a colourless, clear liquid that circulates around the brain and spinal cord, produced by a network of capillaries in the cerebral ventricles called the choroid plexus.

Cerebrum The largest part of the brain, divided into two parts by the *great longitudinal fissure*, each half is called a *cerebral hemisphere*.

Cervical nerves A group of eight spinal nerves that arise from the cervical section of the spinal column and are annotated C1–C8.

Cholinergic receptors Receptors within the sympathetic nervous system, divided into two subtypes; nicotinic receptors and muscarinic receptors.

Choroid plexus A network of capillaries in the walls of all four ventricles of the brain.

Circle of Willis Anastomoses of the right and left internal carotid arteries and the basilar artery which form a special cerebral circulation at the base of the brain.

Coccygeal nerves A pair of spinal nerves that arise from the coccygeal section of the spinal column and are annotated Co1.

Consciousness A state of awareness of oneself and one's surroundings.

Corpus callosum A band of white matter that connects the two cerebral hemispheres.

Cranial nerves A set of 12 nerves arising from within the brain and forming part of the peripheral nervous system, each nerve is named in accordance with its function and is identified numerically by the use of Roman numerals.

Cranium The section of the skull that encloses the brain.

CSF Cerebrospinal fluid.

Decerebrate One of two types of extensor motor response.

Decorticate One of two types of extensor motor response.

Demyelination The loss or destruction of myelin.

Dendrites Projections from the cell body of the neurone that increase the surface area of the cell membrane making it easier to connect with other neurones, bringing information to the cell body.

Dendritic spines Small hair-like projections on the dendrites that maximise the surface area of the dendrites.

Depolarisation The first phase of an action potential where the membrane potential changes from negative to positive due to the influx of sodium ions.

Dermatome A map of the parts of the body that are innervated by spinal nerves.

Diencephalon Located below the cerebrum, made up of the *thalamus*, *hypothalamus* and *epithalamus*.

Dopamine A neurotransmitter within the central and peripheral nervous systems.

Dorsal horns Section of the spinal cord, comprised of grey matter and containing sensory axons, also called the **posterior horns**.

Dura mater Outer layer of the meninges.

Efferent neurone An alternative name for a motor neurone, information is transmitted from the brain towards the periphery.

Endorphins A neuropeptide neurotransmitter, also described as an opioid-peptide, functions as a natural analgesic by binding to opiate receptors within the central nervous system.

Ependymal cells A single layer of cells that line the ventricles of the brain and the central canal of the spinal cord, they form the blood–CSF barrier to control substances entering the CSF.

Epinephrine A neurotransmitter of the sympathetic nervous system, also a catecholamine and a hormone, used to be called adrenaline.

Epithalamus Region of the diencephalon comprising the pineal gland and the habenular nuclei.

Expressive aphasia Patients are capable of thought but incapable of speech.

Facial nerve VIIth cranial nerve, sensory and motor control for closing eyes, crying, smiling, grimacing, taste and salivation.

Fissures Deep grooves between the gyri of the cerebral hemispheres.

Flexion A motor response where the limbs move towards the body in response to a pain stimulus.

Ganglion A cluster of neurone cell bodies within the peripheral nervous system.

Glasgow Coma Scale An assessment tool for assessing consciousness.

Glial cells Also known as neuroglia, the dominant cell structure within the central nervous system, cells that support neurones.

Glossopharyngeal nerve IXth cranial nerve, sensory and motor control of tongue and pharynx.

Grey matter Outer layer of the cerebral hemispheres, mainly made of neurone cell bodies, dendrites, unmyelinated axons and neuroglia. Also found within the spinal cord where it is arranged in an H shape and divided into regions called horns.

Guillain–Barré syndrome An acute demyelinating disease of the peripheral nervous system, also called acute inflammatory demyelinating polyradiculoneuropathy (AIDP).

Gyri The pleural of gyrus.

Gyrus Fold on the surface of the cerebral hemispheres which increase the surface area of the brain.

Habenular nuclei Located within the epithalamus, have an integrative role linking smell and emotion, for example a particular smell may evoke a specific memory.

Homeostasis The maintenance of a stable internal environment irrespective of external conditions.

Hydrocephaly Increase in CSF caused by obstruction of CSF drainage.

Hypernatraemia High-serum sodium.

Hypocalcaemia Low-serum calcium.

Hypoglossal nerve XIIth cranial nerve, motor function for speech and swallowing.

Hypomagnesaemia Low-serum magnesium.

Hyponatraemia Low-serum sodium.

Hypothalamus Part of the diencephalon, situated under the thalamus, controls temperature, water metabolism, autonomic function, physical symptoms of emotion and pituitary secretions such as growth hormone. Also contains a feeding centre, a satiety centre and a thirst centre.

Initial segment The proximal portion of the axon where the action potential is generated.

Intracranial pressure The pressure within the skull.

Lumbar nerves A group of five paired spinal nerves that arise from the lumbar section of the spinal column and are annotated L1–L5.

Macroglia Large glial cells.

Medulla oblongata Part of the brainstem, contains the vasomotor centre, which regulates the heartbeat and controls the diameter of blood vessels, thereby controlling blood pressure. Responsible for the rhythmical pattern of breathing. Contains ascending sensory pathways and descending motor pathways that connect the spinal cord with other parts of the brain. Contains important protective reflexes; swallowing, coughing, vomiting, sneezing and hiccoughing, and sensory nuclei for sensations of touch, pressure and vibration, taste, balance and hearing. It is the origin of cranial nerves VIII–XII.

Meninges A collective term describing the three membranes that enclose the brain and spinal cord.

Meningitis Inflammation of the meninges.

Microglia Small glial cells.

Midbrain Part of the brainstem, contains sensory and motor pathways, involved in movement of eyes, head and trunk in response to visual and auditory stimuli, also the origin of cranial nerves III–IV.

Motor end plate The post-synaptic surface of a synapse between a nerve and a muscle fibre.

Motor neurone An alternative name for an efferent neurone, information is carried from the brain towards the periphery.

Multiple sclerosis A chronic demyelinating disease of the central nervous system, also known as MS.

Muscarinic receptor A type of receptor within the parasympathetic nervous system that responds to the neurotransmitter acetylcholine.

Myasthenia gravis An autoimmune degenerative disease in which acetylcholine receptors are destroyed resulting in muscle weakness.

Myelin A lipid-based substance that is secreted by Schwann cells within the peripheral nervous system and by oligodendrocytes within the central nervous system. Myelin insulates axons and increases the speed of conduction along the axon.

Myelin sheath Up to 100 layers of myelin wrapped around an axon.

Myelinated neurone A neurone whose axon is wrapped in myelin.

Nerve A bundle of many hundreds of axons, together with their blood vessels and connective tissue. They only occur within the peripheral nervous system.

Nerve impulse The transmission of an electrical signal along a bundle of axons within the peripheral nervous system.

Neuroglia Cells that support neurones, the dominant cell structure within the central nervous system.

Neurolemma The outer layer of a myelin sheath containing the nucleus of the Schwann cell, only found in the peripheral nervous system.

Neuromuscular junction A synapse between a neurone and a muscle fibre.

Neurones Cells within the nervous system that are capable of generating an action potential.

Neurotransmitters Chemicals within the nervous system that are released from terminal boutons and diffuse across the synapse to excite or inhibit post-synaptic structures.

Nicotinic receptor A type of receptor within the parasympathetic nervous system that responds to the neurotransmitter acetylcholine.

Nissl bodies Rough endoplasmic reticulum within the cell body of the neurone, also called Nissl granules.

Nodes of Ranvier Gaps between sections of myelin where action potentials can jump along the axon in a process known as saltatory conduction. Nodes of Ranvier are more prevalent within the peripheral nervous system.

Nuclei Clusters of neurone cell bodies within the central nervous system.

Oculomotor nerve IIIrd cranial nerve, motor control of eye movement, upper eyelid control and pupil constriction.

Olfactory nerve Ist cranial nerve, sensory function for sense of smell.

Oligodendrocytes A type of glial cell which produces myelin within the CNS.

Optic nerve IInd cranial nerve, sensory interpretation of sight.

Osmoreceptors Sensory neurones in the hypothalamus that are stimulated by a change in the osmotic pressure of the blood and trigger the sensation of thirst.

Paraplegia Partial or complete loss of motor and sensory function from the thoracic region downwards.

Parasympathetic nervous system A branch of the autonomic nervous system, involuntary and as a generalisation counteracts the action of the sympathetic nervous system, it restores the body to its resting state and is needed for relaxation and sleep.

Parkinson's disease A chronic disease caused by inadequate levels of dopamine with a consequent imbalance in the ratio of dopamine to acetylcholine.

Peripheral nervous system A subdivision of the nervous system comprising the cranial nerves, spinal nerves and their branches, often referred to as the PNS.

Photophobia Intolerance of light.

Pia mater Innermost layer of the meninges.

Pineal gland Part of the epithalamus, secretes the hormone melatonin, considered an endocrine gland.

Pneumotaxic area Located within the pons, influences breathing.

Pons Part of the brainstem, contains sensory and motor pathways, a relay station between the cerebral cortex and the cerebellum, contains the apneustic and pneumotaxic areas which influence breathing. The pons is the origin of cranial nerves V–VIII.

Posterior horns Section of the spinal cord, comprised of grey matter and containing sensory axons.

Primary motor area A highly specialised area of the cerebral cortex located immediately anterior to the primary somatosensory area, in the posterior section of the frontal lobe, immediately anterior to the central sulcus, important motor control of complex, skilled or delicate movements.

Primary somatosensory area A highly specialised area of the cerebral cortex located in the anterior portion of each parietal lobe immediately posterior to the central sulci, important for perception of sensations including touch, tickle, itch, pain, temperature and joint posture.

Quadriplegia Partial or complete loss of sensation and motor function from the neck down.

Receptive aphasia Inability to put words together coherently.

Repolarisation A phase within the action potential where the membrane potential changes from positive to negative by the efflux of potassium ions and returns to its resting state.

Sacral nerves A group of five paired spinal nerves which arise from the sacral section of the spinal column and are annotated S1–S5.

Saltatory conduction The term used to describe an action potential that jumps from one node of Ranvier to another. This only occurs in myelinated axons.

Schwann cells A type of glial cell responsible for myelin production within the peripheral nervous system.

Sensory receptors Nerve endings that detect information internally and externally.

Somatic nervous system A subdivision of the peripheral nervous system.

Spinal accessory nerve XIth cranial nerve, motor control of shoulder and head movement.

Spinal cord An extension of the brainstem that runs from the medulla oblongata to the top of the second lumbar vertebra.

Spinal cord injury Damage to the spinal cord that results in loss of mobility or sensation, also known as SCI.

Spinal nerves Part of the peripheral nervous system, a group of 31 pairs of spinal nerves that exit the spinal column between each vertebra.

Stress response Activation of the sympathetic nervous system by an environmental or physiological stressor.

Subarachnoid haemorrhage Haemorrhage into the subarachnoid space.

Subarachnoid space The space between the arachnoid mater and the pia mater.

Substance P A neuropeptide neurotransmitter released by neurones in the peripheral nervous system that are responsible for the transmission of pain information to the central nervous system.

Sulci The pleural of sulcus.

Sulcus Shallow groove between the gyri of the cerebral hemispheres.

Sympathetic nervous system A division of the autonomic nervous system that is involuntary, controls the 'fight and flight' response and maintains the body in a state of alertness.

Synapse A collective term that describes the interface between a terminal bouton and another tissue structure, which may be another nerve but could also be a blood vessel, a muscle, an organ or a gland. Synapses can be electrical or chemical.

Synaptic cleft The space between the presynaptic surface and the post-synaptic surface.

Terminal boutons 'Button-like' terminals at the ends of the axon branches, containing synaptic vesicles where neurotransmitters are stored.

Tetany Muscle spasms caused by low-serum calcium.

Thalamus A pair of oval-shaped structures within the diencephalon, comprised of grey matter and usually joined by a bridge of grey matter. A relay station between the cerebral cortex and the spinal cord, also relays information between different areas of the cerebrum and between the cerebrum and the cerebellum. The thalamus is involved with consciousness.

Thoracic nerves A group of 12 paired spinal nerves that arise from the thoracic section of the spinal column and are annotated T1–T12.

Transient ischaemic attacks Brief episodes of altered consciousness caused by temporary obstruction of the arterial blood supply to the brain, also known as a TIA.

Trigeminal nerve Vth cranial nerve, sensory and motor control of face, scalp, nose and mouth.

Trochlear nerve IVth cranial nerve, motor control of eye movement.

Unconsciousness Lack of awareness of oneself and one's surroundings.

Unmyelinated neurone A neurone whose axon is not wrapped in myelin.

Vagus nerve Xth cranial nerve, motor and sensory control of pharynx, larynx, heart, lungs, gut, viscera.

Vasomotor centre Located within the brainstem, regulates the heartbeat and controls the diameter of blood vessels, thereby controlling blood pressure, also called the cardiovascular centre.

Ventriculitis Inflammation of the ventricles within the brain.

Vestibulocochlear nerve VIIIth cranial nerve, sensory control of hearing and balance.

Wernicke's area Located within the left temporal and parietal lobes, interprets speech by recognising spoken words and translating them into thoughts.

White matter Inner area of the cerebral hemisphere, mainly comprised of myelinated axons. Also found within the spinal cord where it is divided into regions called columns: anterior, posterior and lateral white columns.

Test yourself

1 The autonomic nervous system is a division of:
   a. the central nervous system
   b. the peripheral nervous system

2 A cluster of neurone cell bodies within the CNS is called:
   a. a ganglion
   b. a nucleus

3 Which type of glial cell forms part of the blood–brain barrier?
   a. ependymal cells
   b. oligodendrocytes
   c. astrocytes
   d. microglia

4 Guillain–Barré syndrome is a disease of the
   a. central nervous system
   b. peripheral nervous system

5 Which of the following neurotransmitters are classified as catecholamines:
   a. acetylcholine
   b. norepinephrine
   c. dopamine
   d. substance P

6 CSF is produced from:
   a. the medulla oblongata
   b. the subarachnoid membrane
   c. the choroid plexus
   d. the cerebral cortex

7 The vasomotor centre is responsible for:
   a. temperature regulation
   b. respiratory rate regulation
   c. blood pressure regulation
   d. heart rate regulation

8 Cranial nerves are part of the:

a. central nervous system

b. peripheral nervous system

9 The neurotransmitter of the parasympathetic nervous system is:

a. acetylcholine

b. noradrenaline

c. dopamine

d. endorphins

10 Which type of sympathetic receptor is found in the heart?

a. α_1

b. β_1

c. α_2

d. β_2

e. β_2

References

Bradley, W. G., Daroff, R. B., Fenichel, G. M. and Jankovic, J. (2004) *Pocket Companion to Neurology in Clinical Practice*, 4th edn. Philadelphia: Elsevier.

Diringer, M. N., Reaven, N. L., Funk, S. E. and Uman, G. C. (2004) Elevated body temperature independently contributes to increased length of stay in neurologic intensive care unit patients. *Critical Care Medicine* 32 (7), 1489–95.

Hickey, J. V. (2009) *The Clinical Practice of Neurological and Neurosurgical Nursing*, 6th edn. Philadelphia: Lippincott, Williams & Wilkins.

Lowenstein, D. H. and Alldredge, B. K. (1998) Status epilepticus. *New England Journal of Medicine* 338 (14), 970–6.

Markus, H., Pereira, A. and Cloud, G. (2010) *Stroke Medicine Oxford Specialist Handbooks in Neurology*. Oxford: Oxford University Press.

NHS (2011) *Stroke – Act F.A.S.T.* Available from http://www.nhs.uk/actfast/Pages/stroke.aspx, last accessed 19 June 2011.

National Institute for Health and Clinical Excellence (2010) *Quality Standards Programme – Stroke*. Available from http//www.nice.org.uk/media/7EC/67/StrokeQualityStandard.pdf, last accessed 11 June 2011.

National Institute for Health and Clinical Excellence (2007) *Head Injury: Triage, assessment, investigation and early management of head injury in infants, children and adults. Clinical Guideline 56*. Available from http://www.nice.org.uk/nicemedia/live/11836/36259/36259.pdf, last accessed 11 June 2011.

National Institute for Clinical Excellence (2004) *Type 1 Diabetes: Diagnosis and management of type 1 diabetes in adults. Clinical Guideline 15. Quick reference guide*. London: NICE. Available from http://www.nice.org.uk/nicemedia/live/10944/29391/29391.pdf, last accessed 8 May 2011.

Nursing and Midwifery Council (2010) *Standards for Pre-registration Nursing Education*. Available from http://standards.nmc-uk.org/PublishedDocuments/Standards%20for%20pre-registration%20nursing%20education%2016082010.pdf.

Nursing and Midwifery Council (2008) *The Code*. London: NMC.

Office for National Statistics (2011) Available from http://www.statistics.gov.uk/cci/nugget.asp?id=6, last accessed 6 May 2011.

Resuscitation Council (UK) (2010) *Adult Basic Life Support*. Available from http://www.resus.org.uk/pages/bls.pdf, last accessed 5 June 2011.

Royal College of Physicians (2008) *Concise Guidance to Good Practice Number 9. Chronic spinal cord injury: Management of patients in acute hospital settings. National guidelines*. London: Royal College of Physicians.

Smith, G. (2003) *ALERT Acute Life-threatening Events Recognition and Treatment*. 2nd edn. Portsmouth: The eLearning Centre, DCQE University of Portsmouth.

Tortora, G. J. and Derrickson, B. H. (2009) *Principles of Anatomy and Physiology*, 12th edn. Hoboken, NJ: Wiley.

Further reading

Department of Health (2008) *National Service Framework for Long-term Neurological Conditions: National support for local implementation 2008*. London: Department of Health.

National Council for Palliative Care (2006) *Neurological Conditions: From diagnosis to death*. London: National Council for Palliative Care.

Siddiqi, J. (2008) *Neurosurgical Intensive Care*. New York: Thieme.

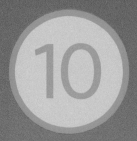

The patient with acute gastrointestinal problems

Julian Howard and Angela Morgan

Aims

The aim of this chapter is to identify key functions of the gastrointestinal system. This includes providing an insight into how disordered physiology can cause a medical emergency, and the nurse's role in recognising and responding appropriately to patients with acute gastrointestinal problems.

Objectives

At the end of this chapter you will be able to:

→ Describe the major structures of the gastrointestinal system

→ Identify the main roles of the stomach, pancreas, liver and bowel, relating this to problems arising from disordered pathophysiology

→ Identify the common gastrointestinal emergencies and differentiate between patient presentations

→ Describe the nurse's role in undertaking an assessment of the abdomen

→ Describe the nurse's role in undertaking an assessment of fluid balance in relation to gastrointestinal emergencies

→ Identify interventions which maximise gastrointestinal status

Introduction

The gastrointestinal (GI) system can be affected primarily by specific disorders and also secondarily as a consequence of pathology elsewhere in the body. Both types of disturbance can result in a medical emergency. The nurse has an important role in assessing and monitoring the patient with gastrointestinal signs and symptoms in order to identify the potential for the patient to deteriorate, either as a result of the altered pathophysiological processes or because of life-threatening complications such as infection or hypovolaemia.

Applied physiology

Overview of gastrointestinal (GI) tract

The GI tract (alimentary canal) consists of a continuous tube commencing at the mouth and ending at the anus. The organs forming this system include the mouth, most of the pharynx, oesophagus, stomach, small intestine and large intestine. The accessory organs contributing to this tract are the teeth, tongue, salivary glands, liver, gallbladder and pancreas.

The GI tract processes food from the time it is eaten until it is digested, absorbed or eliminated and in summary performs six processes:

- *Ingestion* – taking food and liquids into the mouth by eating and drinking.
- *Secretion* – the cells within the GI tract and accessory organs secrete water, acid, buffers and enzymes (total approximately 8Litres/day) into the tract lumen.
- *Mixing and propulsion* – alternating contraction and relaxation of the smooth muscle in the walls of the GI tract mixes the food and secretions: this peristaltic action promotes forward movement through the system.
- *Digestion* – food is digested mechanically by the teeth while in the mouth and is subsequently digested chemically, commencing within the stomach.
- *Absorption* – following chemical digestion the resulting products composed of small molecules are absorbed by the epithelial cells lining the GI tract. These then pass into the blood to be circulated systemically.
- *Defaecation* – material consisting of wastes, indigestible substances, bacteria and cells from the lining of the GI tract is excreted in the form of faeces.

The oesophagus

The oesophagus is a hollow muscular tube which secretes mucus and transports food into the stomach, but does not produce any digestive enzymes. The oesophagus joins the stomach at the oesophagogastric junction, and although not actually a valve, has been referred to as the 'cardiac sphincter' or lower oesophageal sphincter. If this sphincter becomes incompetent, the highly acidic contents of the stomach can reflux into the oesophagus causing inflammation, erosion and ulceration. Excessive pressure due to vomiting can also cause damage (e.g. Mallory-Weiss syndrome). Both of these situations may present as haematemesis. Another common cause of haematemesis is related directly to the gastro-oesophageal junction in the form of a variceal bleed. Oesophageal and gastric varices form (and may rupture) as a result of high pressure in the venous circulation to the liver (hepatic portal vein) arising from chronic liver damage.

The stomach

The stomach sits in the left side of the abdominal cavity under the diaphragm. It is divided into four regions: the cardiac region around the lower oesophageal sphincter, the fundus, the body and the pylorus (see Figure 10.1). The pylorus has two parts, the pyloric antrum connecting to the body of the stomach and the pyloric canal leading into the duodenum. The pyloric sphincter is located at the junction of the stomach and duodenum. The stomach acts as a temporary holding area for food that arrives from the oesophagus.

The functions of the stomach include mixing saliva, food and gastric juice to form chyme, which then passes through the pyloric sphincter into the duodenum. It secretes gastric juice which contains hydrochloric acid (HCl), pepsin, intrinsic factor and gastric lipase. The stomach mixes HCl and intrinsic factor (from parietal cells), pepsinogen (from chief cells) and mucus and bicarbonate (from mucus cells). The HCl originates from H^+ and Cl^- ions being secreted separately by the parietal cells into the stomach lining. Proton pumps, powered by H^+/K^+ ATPases, actively transport H^+ into the lumen whilst Cl^- diffuses into the stomach lining through Cl^- channels.

The secretory actions of the parietal cells keep the stomach contents acidic (pH 1.5–2.0) which enables four important functions:

1 bactericidal activity;
2 denaturing of proteins;
3 conversion of pepsinogen into an active form, pepsin, which initiates protein hydrolysis;
4 the breakdown of plant walls and connective tissue in meat.

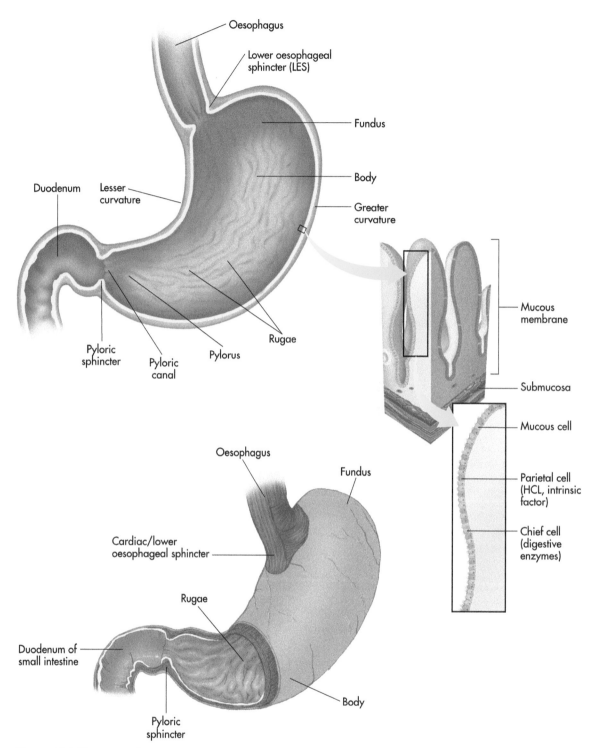

Figure 10.1 The stomach

Intrinsic factor binds with vitamin B12 (ingested mainly with dietary protein) to facilitate its absorption in the terminal ileum. Vitamin B12 cannot be absorbed in the absence of intrinsic factor. In pernicious anaemia, intrinsic factor is not secreted due to auto antibodies against parietal cells and B12 deficiency therefore occurs in this condition. B12 deficiency can also be due to an abnormal ileal mucosa. Because some intestinal bacteria need B12 for growth they can compete with gut cells for this substance if the normal pattern of flora is disturbed and B12 deficiency may result. 'Blind loop syndrome' occurs when a section of gut becomes bypassed so that digested food slows or stops moving through the intestines, leading to overgrowth of bacteria and problems in absorbing nutrients such as B12. Mucus secretion generally acts as a barrier to acid and pepsinogen which are the primary products capable of inducing injury to the mucosa.

The pancreas

The pancreas (Greek 'all flesh') is a retroperitoneal gland approximately 12–15cm long and 2.5cm thick. With respect to its location, the pancreas has been variously described as 'the finger of the liver' and 'the hermit of the abdomen' (Gavaghan 2002). It is connected by the pancreatic duct to the common bile duct which in turn empties into the duodenum. Structurally, the pancreas is composed of clustered epithelial cells, about 99% of which constitute the exocrine portion of the organ. They secrete approximately 1200–1500mL daily of pancreatic juice consisting of water, salts, sodium bicarbonate and several enzymes. It is the bicarbonate component, being alkaline (pH 8.3), that performs the function of neutralising the acidic contents of the stomach that it mixes with in the duodenum. The enzymes include a carbohydrate-digesting enzyme (pancreatic amylase), protein-digesting enzymes (trypsin, chymotrypsin and carboxypeptidase), a triglyceride-digesting enzyme (elastase) and nucleic acid-digesting enzymes (ribonuclease and deoxyribonuclease). The protein-digesting enzymes are secreted initially within the structure of the pancreas in an inactive form (trypsinogen), as the active form would damage the pancreas itself. This process is assisted also by the production of trypsin inhibitor that combines with any trypsin formed accidentally, blocking its enzymatic activity. When trypsinogen reaches the duodenum it meets with another enzyme (enterokinase) which splits off part of the tripsinogen molecule to form trypsin. In turn, trypsin acts on the inactive precursors chymotrypsinogen, procarboxypeptidase and proelastase, to produce chymotrypsin, carboxypeptidase and elastase.

The remaining 1% of the cells are organised into pancreatic islets (islets of Langerhans) which have an endocrine function. These cells secrete hormones such as glucagon, insulin, somatostatin and pancreatic polypeptide (see the section on diabetic emergencies in Chapter 11).

The duodenum

The major processes of digestion and absorption of nutrients occur in the small intestine. Its length of approximately three metres provides a large surface area for these functions, which are further enhanced by the presence of circular folds, villi and microvilli. The circular folds aid absorption, not only by increasing surface area, but by causing the chyme to spiral rather than move in a straight line as it passes through the small intestine (see Figure 10.2).

The small intestine is divided into three regions: the duodenum (25cm) commencing at the pyloric sphincter of the stomach, the jejunum (100cm) and finally the ileum (200cm). The duodenum is a C-shaped tube which curves around the head of the pancreas and secretes bicarbonate to neutralise gastric acid. It can increase bicarbonate production in response to raised acidity. The close proximity of the duodenum to the stomach, however, makes it prone to ulceration as a result of the acidity of the stomach contents.

Intestinal juice is a clear yellow, alkaline fluid (1–2litres/day) containing water and mucus. Pancreatic and intestinal juices together provide an environment that facilitates the absorption of the substances in chyme as they come into contact with the villi. The endothelial cells synthesise several digestive enzymes (brushborder enzymes) which are inserted in the plasma membrane of the microvilli. This results in some of the enzymatic digestion occurring at the surface of the endothelial cells that line the villi, rather than in the lumen itself.

Following enzymatic digestion, the resulting nutrients are absorbed through the endothelial cells. These include monosaccharides, amino acids, lipids, electrolytes and vitamins. In addition to these elemental nutrients, the small intestine absorbs water. Approximately 10 litres of water a day enter the small intestine (two litres as ingested fluids and eight litres as various gastrointestinal secretions) most of which is reabsorbed by osmosis. The remainder passes into the large intestine.

There are two types of movement in the small intestine: first, segmentations which are localised contractions that occur in areas distended by chyme and mix the chyme and enzymes together. Second, this process is followed by peristalsis whereby chyme is moved forward as a result of waves of muscular contractions. In total, the chyme is present in the small intestine for between three and five hours.

The liver (and gallbladder)

The liver is the second-largest organ in the body (after the skin), weighs approximately 1.4kg and is positioned inferiorly to the diaphragm on the right side (see Figure 10.3).

The liver is divided into two principal lobes – a large right lobe and smaller left lobe. These lobes are composed of many functional units termed lobules, each of which consists of hexagonal specialised epithelial cells called hepatocytes. The hepatocytes are arranged around a central vein. Instead of capillaries, the liver has large endothelium-lined spaces (sinusoids) through which blood passes. The sinusoids also contain fixed phagocytes called stellate reticuloendothelial (Kupffer) cells which perform several functions including the breakdown of effete red blood cells, bacteria and other foreign matter which can then pass into the venous circulation.

Bile (secreted by hepatocytes) enters into the small bile canaliculi and drains subsequently into the bile ductules and bile ducts, which eventually become the right and left hepatic ducts merging into the common hepatic duct. Having left the liver, the bile is stored in the gallbladder,

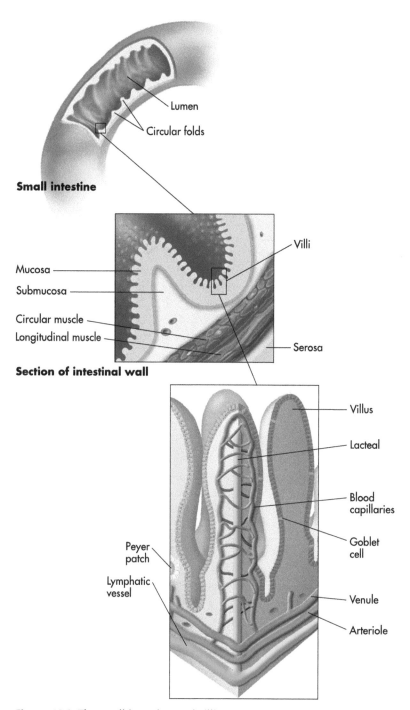

Figure 10.2 The small intestine and villi

which acts as a reservoir. This is a pear-shaped sac (7–10cm) long, located in a depression of the posterior visceral surface of the liver. The gallbladder is divided into a fundus, body and neck. The cystic duct joins the common hepatic duct which in turn merges into the common bile duct. Bile contains water, bile salts, bile pigments and electrolytes and from the common bile duct, bile is emptied into the duodenum where the bile salts emulsify fat.

The liver receives blood from two sources: the hepatic artery carries oxygenated blood (30% of liver blood flow) and the hepatic portal vein carries deoxygenated blood (70% of blood flow). The venous blood from the hepatic portal vein contains newly absorbed nutrients, drugs, microbes and toxins from the gastrointestinal tract. Branches of both of these blood vessels carry blood into the liver sinusoids where oxygen, most of the nutrients and some toxic substances are processed by the hepatocytes. The resulting venous blood drains into the hepatic vein to return to the systemic venous circulation.

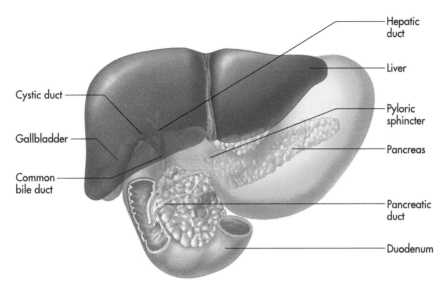

Figure 10.3 The liver

The portal vein carries approximately 1500mL/min of blood from the intestines, spleen and stomach to the liver. Obstruction to this blood flow (whatever the aetiology) will result in elevated portal venous pressure. This in turn causes distension of the proximal veins and an increase in the intracapillary pressure in the organs drained by the obstructed veins. Particularly vulnerable to this increase in pressure is the gastro-oesophageal junction where varices can develop and sometimes rupture, resulting in haemorrhage and haematemesis. Varices are portosystemic anastamoses, communications between the two systems, formed when the direct drainage routes are blocked. The typical site of varices is the lower third of the oesophagus between the lower oesophageal veins and the short gastric veins.

Functions of the liver

These are also summarised in Figure 10.4.

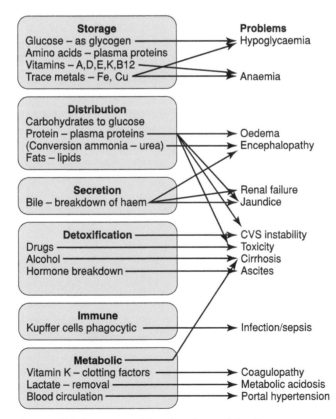

Figure 10.4 Summary of the functions of the liver

Storage

1 *Glucose* – The liver plays a major role in replenishing the blood's supply of glucose when the concentration falls below normal. Liver cells are highly permeable to glucose (digested carbohydrate) and will absorb 75% of the excess glucose in the circulation. This is accomplished by the enzyme glucokinase (regulated by blood insulin levels) which accelerates the rate of glucose uptake by the liver cell. The absorbed glucose is stored in the liver as glycogen.

2 *Amino acids* – The amino acids derived from protein digestion travel to the liver by way of the portal vein. Intracellular enzymes in the parenchymal cells of the liver convert the excess amino acids into cellular proteins. These proteins are then stored in the liver and released as required to maintain equilibrium between the body's cellular and plasma proteins.

3 *Fat-soluble vitamins (A, D, E + K)* – Vitamin K is absorbed from the GI tract and this is dependent in turn upon the liver's ability to secrete bile into the intestinal tract. More importantly, vitamin K is a vital coenzyme in the liver's ability to produce the plasma proteins, prothrombin (factor II) and some other clotting factors (e.g. VII, IX, X), and it activates enzymes in the clotting cascade. In addition to the vitamin K-dependent clotting factors (II, VII, IX, X), the liver produces clotting factors I, V, XI, XII and XIII. Vitamin B12 is also stored by the liver, but is not fat soluble.

4 *The trace metals iron (Fe) and copper (Cu)* – are stored in the liver with an excess resulting in haemochromatosis and Wilson's disease respectively.

Conversion

The liver plays an active role in the conversion of carbohydrates, proteins and fatty acids into energy (in the form of ATP) which is required for all chemical reactions to occur at a cellular level.

1 *Carbohydrates* – in the form of glucose are the main source of energy for the body. The liver responds to low plasma glucose levels (and accompanying low plasma insulin levels) by both inhibiting the uptake of circulating glucose and by breaking down stored glycogen (glycogenolysis) to make more glucose available in the circulation.

2 *Protein* – the end products of protein digestion circulate in the blood as amino acids which are resynthesised by the liver to form three plasma proteins (albumin, fibrinogen and globulins). Albumin is essential to maintain the colloid osmotic pressure, fibrinogen vital for the coagulation process and globulins are required for antibody formation. Of these, the liver produces all of the body's albumin and fibrinogen and 50% of the globulins. In addition the liver, in conjunction with vitamin K, synthesises all of the body's prothrombin (factor II) and factors VII, IX and X, essential for fibrinogen activation.

Amino acids (from protein) are also utilised for gluconeogenesis, resulting in the formation of ammonia as a by-product. The liver converts this metabolically generated ammonia into urea. Ammonia produced by bacteria in the intestines is also removed from portal blood for urea synthesis. The liver therefore converts ammonia, a potential toxin, into urea, a compound that can be excreted in the urine.

3 *Fatty acids* – triglycerides, phospholipids and cholesterol are the principle lipids which become the body's source of energy when glucose is not available. Triglycerides are broken down to fatty acids and glycerol, then to acetyl COA, then to ATP, CO_2 and H_2O for cellular energy. The additional processing of fatty acids into ketone bodies occurs primarily when the availability of glucose for metabolism is limited, such as during starvation or in uncontrolled diabetes. Under some conditions lipids may accumulate in the hepatocytes and result in a 'fatty liver', for example in alcohol excess.

Secretion

The only substance actually secreted by the liver is bile. Bile solution contains bile salts, cholesterol, bilirubin, fatty acids and plasma electrolytes. A litre a day is produced, but is concentrated in the gallbladder: 80% of bilirubin is derived from haem following the breakdown of haemoglobin in the liver, spleen and bone marrow. It is not water soluble and is carried in the plasma bound to albumin. In the liver it is transported into the hepatocytes, conjugated with glucronic acid and excreted by active transport into the bile. In the terminal ileum and colon, bacteria reduce bilirubin to stercobilirubin, and thence further to stercobilin, which is excreted in the stool. A small amount is reabsorbed and excreted in the urine as urobilinogen.

Detoxification

1 *Drugs* – the detoxification process that occurs in the liver protects the body from many harmful substances that enter the bloodstream. The liver absorbs most drugs that enter the bloodstream, usually modified and excreted. Most of these are fat soluble and their conversion by the liver into water-soluble substances facilitates excretion in bile or urine.

2 *Alcohol* – ethanol is oxidised to acetaldehyde, but as this is unstable it is further metabolised to acetic acid utilising the enzyme alcohol dehydrogenase. This in

turn collaborates with a further enzyme (ACSS2) to form Acetyl-CoA which is then available for cellular metabolism.

3 *Hormone breakdown* – e.g. oestrogen.

Immune function

The Kupffer cells are phagocytic and are very efficient in digesting bacteria, viruses and other foreign matter. These cells are particularly important because they destroy bacteria that are constantly entering the portal blood flow directly from the GI Tract. The main functions of Kupffer cells are phagocytosis of bacteria, debris and other foreign matter in hepatic blood, and a defence mechanism when bacterial translocation occurs.

Other

1 *Acid-base balance* – the liver is metabolically active, both producing and consuming H^+ ions. It consumes about 20% of the body's O_2 production and produces about 20% of the CO_2 which is excreted via the lungs. The liver normally removes 70% of lactate and there can be decreased hepatic clearance in either poor perfusion of the liver (e.g. severe shock) or liver disease resulting in a metabolic acidosis.

2 *Heat production* – the liver is second only to muscle tissue in the production of heat by its continuous cellular activity (thermogenesis). Under normal resting conditions, the liver is responsible for most of the body heat.

It acts also as a blood reservoir, containing about 10% of the circulating blood volume. The liver is essential for life. A total hepatectomy would always be fatal, death occurring in less than 24 hours from hypoglycaemia.

The jejunum and ileum

The jejunum is the middle section of the small intestine. It has longer villi than the duodenum to provide an increased surface area from which to absorb nutrients such as glucose, amino acids and vitamins. The section following the jejunum is the ileum, whose function is to absorb Vitamin B12, bile salts and other substances not taken up by the jejunum.

The large bowel

The large intestine is the terminal section of the GI tract and is approximately 1.5m long. The appendix is a vestigial (redundant) structure situated near the junction of the ileum (small bowel) and the caecum (large bowel). The caecum merges with a long tube called the colon and this is divided anatomically into four areas (ascending colon, transverse colon, descending colon and sigmoid colon) before terminating in the rectum and anus.

The wall of the large intestine differs from that of the small intestine in that there are no circular folds or villi. Instead, the mucosa consists of simple columnar epithelium, connective tissue and smooth muscle. The cells absorb further water (approx 700mL daily) and secrete mucus to lubricate the passage of the colonic contents.

Immune function of the gut

Protection against harmful organisms is a responsibility shared between several components of the gastrointestinal system. The epithelial cells lining the gut prevent migration of organisms and the mucosa itself acts as a physical barrier. The intestinal walls contain lymphocytes and macrophages, with the mesentery hosting regional lymph nodes. Intraluminal Peyers patches secrete immunoglobulin A (IgA) to prevent adherence of bacteria to the mucosal cells. These gut actions supplement the activities of the Kupffer cells in the liver and the spleen's role in trapping and phagocytosing bacteria. The acutely ill patient may thus suffer bacterial translocation if these functions are compromised as a result of altered permeability of the gut wall secondary to hypovolaemia, ischaemia or sepsis. Problems may occur also as a result of immunosuppression or increased bacterial growth in the gut secondary to overgrowth (e.g. blind loop syndrome) or intestinal stasis.

Acute problems/emergencies

Acute gastrointestinal bleeding

Acute stress ulceration is a potential complication associated with any critically ill patient, with lesions ranging from mild erosion to acute ulceration and perforation. Although the exact mechanism for this is not well understood, it is likely that hypoxia and hypoperfusion of the gastroduodenal mucosa are the most important factors. According to Sung (2009) prophylactic treatment should be reserved for high-risk patients, i.e. the critically ill in intensive care, but even when indicated there is little consensus among critical care experts in the choice of prophylactic treatment used (Lam *et al.* 1999).

Gastrointestinal bleeding is a major cause of morbidity and mortality with 80% of cases being from the upper GI tract and 20% the lower GI tract. There are many causes of GI bleeding, the most common of which is peptic ulcer disease. In particular, bleeding resulting from ruptured oesophageal or gastric varices has a high mortality rate. Acute variceal bleeding is a serious complication of portal hypertension which is in turn a sequelae of chronic liver disease (as opposed to acute liver failure). Haematemesis and melaena are the most common presentations of acute upper GI bleeding, with fresh blood from the rectum indicative usually of lower GI bleeding. A massive GI bleed will lead to the signs and symptoms associated with hypovolaemic shock (e.g. tachycardia, hypotension, pallor, sweating, cyanosis, mental confusion and oliguria). (See later, in Table 10.4.)

The principles of immediate management centre on the aims:

- to resuscitate (with blood transfusion and fluids);
- to control active bleeding and;
- to prevent recurrence of haemorrhage.

> **Remember!**
> By the time that the patient has changes in their observations they will have already lost at least 20% of their circulating volume.

Patients with non-variceal bleeding (e.g. peptic ulceration) will require blood and plasma expanders via large-bore cannulae and close monitoring of cardiovascular and fluid balance status. Once the patient is stable, early endoscopic intervention is required to identify the source of bleeding with subsequent endoscopic therapy or surgery if the bleeding continues (SIGN 2008). Patients with peptic ulcer bleeding should be tested for *Helicobacter pylori* and this should take place prior to instigation of proton-pump inhibitor therapy (SIGN 2008).

Patients with a variceal bleed are more likely to need further intervention due to a high risk of recurrent bleeding. There is a 70% risk of rebleeding and 30% of these will be fatal (Allen and Tham 2009). In addition to fluid resuscitation and close monitoring, the patient with a variceal bleed is likely to require any of the following interventions:

- pharmacological control with terlipressin (SIGN 2008) (possibly in combination with GTN) to reduce portal blood pressure;
- endoscopic variceal ligation which involves rubber bands placed so that they strangulate the bleeding varices;
- endoscopic sclerotherapy whereby sclerosants are injected directly into the variceal columns or into the adjacent mucosa;
- balloon tamponade (Sengstaken–Blakemore tube): this is used if endoscopy fails to control bleeding. It is based on the principle of inflating balloon(s) so that they exert pressure upon the bleeding varices;
- transjugular intrahepatic portosystemic shunt (TIPS) which is a procedure whereby a catheter is inserted into

the portal vein (under radiological guidance) and a stent then inserted between the portal vein and the systemic circulation, thereby reducing portal blood pressure. This last intervention is reserved for patients with recurrent bleeding (SIGN 2008). Further information regarding the rationale for these interventions is available from the World Gastroenterology Organisation (2008).

Lower gastrointestinal bleeding is more common in the elderly. Its presentation can range from minor bleeding to a life-threatening haemorrhage with an associated mortality of 5% (Tham *et al.* 2008). Most cases of lower GI bleeding are self-limiting, responsive usually to resuscitative approaches including fluid and blood administration. Close observation and monitoring of cardiovascular and fluid balance status will need to continue, and once the patient is stable the cause of the bleeding can be investigated and managed as appropriate. The management of both acute upper and lower gastrointestinal bleeding is summarised in the *National Clinical Guideline* (2008) by the Scottish Intercollegiate Network, the principles of which have been adopted nationally.

Acute pancreatitis

Its close proximity to the gallbladder and common bile duct make the pancreas particularly vulnerable to inflammation when these are diseased, with one of the most common causes of acute pancreatitis being gallstones or biliary tract obstruction. The inflamed pancreas then either releases trypsin, (instead of trypsinogen), and/or insufficient amounts of trypsin inhibitor, resulting in trypsin digesting the pancreatic cells.

The second most common cause of acute pancreatitis is alcohol abuse. The underlying pathophysiology for this is unclear, but may be due to irritation (particularly at the sphincter of Oddi) causing spasm and obstructing the flow of secretions, trapping enzymes within the pancreas. Other, rarer, causes of acute pancreatitis are included in Table 10.1.

Most patients with pancreatitis have a mild episode, but 10–20% of cases are of sufficient severity to cause a systemic inflammatory response syndrome (SIRS). Acute pancreatitis can be complicated by pancreatic necrosis, sepsis and ultimately multi-organ failure (MOF). The early recognition of infection/sepsis and hypovolaemia (due to sequestration of fluid around the inflamed pancreas) is paramount to reducing morbidity and mortality. In view of this, it is recommended that patients with severe acute pancreatitis should be managed in a high-dependency unit or intensive therapy unit with full

Table 10.1 Common causes of pancreatitis

Common causes (accounts for 80% of cases)	
Obstructive	• Gallstones (most frequently females)
Toxins	• Alcohol (most frequently males 30–45 yrs)

Rare causes	
Obstructive	• Tumours
Toxins	• Scorpion venom • Organophosphates (insecticides)
Drugs	• Definite association: azothiaprine, oestrogens, metronidazole, frusemide, sulphonamides, cimetidine, ranitidine • Possible: thiazides
Metabolic	• Hypertrigliceridaemia • Hypercalcaemia • End stage renal disease
Trauma	• Accidental: blunt abdominal injury • Iatrogenic: postoperative, post ERCP
Infections	• Parasites • Viral: mumps, rubella, hepatitis B, varicella, HIV • Bacterial: tuberculosis, legionella, campylobacter, salmonella
Vascular	• Ischaemic: hypoperfusion • Vasculitis: systemic lupus erythematosus
Idiopathic	• Biliary microlithiasis (gallbladder sludge)
Miscellaneous	• Peptic ulcer (penetrating) • Crohn's disease (of duodenum) • Pregnancy associated

monitoring and systems support (UK Working Party on Acute Pancreatitis 2005).

The main symptom of acute pancreatitis is dull upper abdominal pain which may radiate through the back and is usually worse when supine. Other symptoms include nausea, vomiting, loss of appetite, diarrhoea, pyrexia and in some cases, jaundice (see patient assessment). A diagnosis of acute pancreatitis should include at least two of the following features: acute abdominal pain typical for pancreatitis, elevated lipase or amylase (3 × normal), characteristic findings on CT scan (Hasibeder et al. 2009).

The goals of management include supportive care, limitation of systemic complications and prevention of infection if necrosis is present. All patients will need close monitoring, intravenous hydration and analgesia, with nasogastric suction being indicated for relief of nausea, vomiting and ileus. Drugs that 'rest' the pancreas such as somatostatin, calcitonin and enzyme inhibitors have not been shown to reduce morbidity or mortality. Other

controversial management strategies include the use of prophylactic antibiotics and the choice of route for administration of feeding (UK Working Party on Acute Pancreatitis 2005). If fed artificially, there is no difference in mortality between enteral (nasogastric) and TPN, however enteral feeding for pancreatitis is associated with reduced rates of infection and hospital stay. Also under debate currently is whether enteral feeding for pancreatitis should be nasogastric or nasojejunal. All patients, whether fed enterally or parenterally, require a protocol ensuring strict glycaemic control (Wyncoll 2009).

> Unfortunately, patients with pancreatitis or liver failure can be stigmatised by a public misconception that these conditions are linked exclusively to high levels of alcohol consumption.

Liver failure

O'Grady et al. (1993) classified acute hepatic dysfunction according to the time interval between the onset of jaundice and encephalopathy, with hyperacute being less than 7 days, acute being 8–28 days and subacute being 29 days–12 weeks. Additionally patients may have stable chronic liver disease that decompensates acutely. The most common causes of acute liver failure are drug induced (e.g. paracetamol) and acute viral hepatitis. Other causes are included in Table 10.2.

The main manifestations and problems of liver failure are summarised in Table 10.3 and Figure 10.4.

Table 10.2 Common causes of acute liver failure

Viral	• Hepatitis, A, B, C, D and E • Herpes virus • Adenovirus • Epstein–Barr virus • Cytomegalovirus
Drug-induced	• Paracetamol (acetaminophen)
Toxins	• Amanita (deathcap) mushrooms • Organic solvents • Phosphorus poisoning
Metabolic disorders	• Acute fatty liver of pregnancy • Reye syndrome
Vascular	• Acute circulatory failure (shock) • Budd–Chiari syndrome • Veno-occlusive disease
Miscellaneous	• Wilson's disease (Cu accumulation) • Autoimmune hepatitis

Table 10.3 Summary of main manifestations and problems of liver failure

Hepatic encephalopathy	The cause of hepatic encephalopathy is unclear, but the patient will present with alteration in conscious level resulting from a raised ICP due to cerebral oedema. The level of reduction in conscious level is classified as follows: • Grade I: altered mood, impaired intellect, reduced ability to concentrate, and impaired psychomotor function, but rousable and coherent • Grade II: inappropriate behaviour, increased drowsiness and confusion, but rousable (may have asterixis – liver flap – and dysarthria) • Grade III: stuperous, somnolent, but rousable, often disorientated, agitated and aggressive • Grade IV: coma, unresponsive to painful stimuli • In extremis, the patient may have fixed, dilated pupils and exhibit manifestations of brain herniation
Coagulopathy	Liver failure will result in a coagulopathy due to reduced levels of fibrinogen, vitamin K and clotting factors
Cardiovascular instability	Patients may become cardiovascularly unstable (hypotensive and tachycardic) due to endotoxaemia which causes vasodilation and a compensatory increase in cardiac output
Increased risk of infection	This is due to suppression of immune function, and impaired neutrophil and Kupffer cell functions
Renal failure	Deteriorating liver function can affect the circulation to the kidney, resulting in renal failure. The mechanism behind hepatorenal syndrome is poorly understood, but it is believed that the vasoconstriction in the kidney causes this rather than structural tissue damage
Hypoglycaemia	The liver plays an important in blood glucose control, and in impairment, glycogen will not be broken down into glucose and the production of new glucose will not occur
Acid base and electrolyte disturbance	Hypokalaemia, hypomagnesaemia, hyponatraemia, hypophosphataemia and hypocalcaemia can all occur in relation to liver failure. A metabolic alkalosis can result from vomiting, or the patient may have a metabolic acidosis if secondary to paracetamol overdose or lactic acid excess

Liver function tests

The patient in liver failure will also have abnormal blood results which are summarised as follows:

1 *Indicators of liver function* – abnormal clotting, pro-thrombin time e.g. prolonged (PT) or increased INR. Clotting factors are synthesised in the liver and there is a reduction in circulating clotting factors with the degree of prolongation of PT being used as a prognosticator. Serial tests need to be analysed with platelets and FFP being administered only if bleeding actively.

2 *Assessment of damage* – liver enzymes are raised. These exist normally within liver cells but will leak into the plasma when damaged) e.g. AST (aspartate transaminase) and ALT (alanine aminotransferase) (most specific for liver damage).

3 *Excretory capacity* – bilirubin is increased in obstruction (direct/conjugated) or erythrocyte breakdown (indirect/unconjugated). At a level above 50umol/L jaundice will be apparent.

4 *Other* – gamma GT is an inducible enzyme resulting from cell damage (often due to alcohol). ALP (alkaline phosphatase) can be increased in obstructive jaundice reflecting cholestasis.

Intestinal obstruction

Obstruction can occur in either the small or large bowel and if untreated can lead to perforation and peritonitis. Mechanical obstruction can be caused by tumours, impacted foreign bodies, impacted faeces or gallstones, or by strictures. Additionally, it may be caused volvulus, intussusceptions, adhesions or hernias. Clinical presentation depends on the level of obstruction. Proximal

---

Assessing liver function

A shortcut to assessing liver function is to look at the clotting (INR, PT) as abnormalities will indicate a coagulopathy (clotting problem) which in turn implies impaired liver function.

The degree to which these are deranged (e.g. extended INR) will signify the extent of the liver dysfunction.

A comprehensive analysis of LFTs will add insight into other functions of the liver. It is also important to study a series of LFTs to ascertain trends.

A low albumin level can be a contributory cause of generalised oedema or ascites as albumin (and other plasma proteins) provide an oncotic pressure, keeping fluid in the circulation. Low levels of circulating plasma proteins will tend towards fluid remaining in the tissues rather than being drawn back into the intravascular space.

obstructions tend to cause colicky abdominal pain and early vomiting, whereas in distal obstructions, abdominal distension and constipation are more common. In either case, patients may present with manifestations of hypovolaemia as fluid is sequestered into the gut.

Nursing assessment

A systematic approach to assessment is essential in order to identify quickly any problems in the deteriorating patient. Using ABCDE provides a sound basis for prioritising issues and these should be managed as they arise. The airway should be assessed for patency, patients with acute liver failure, pancreatitis or severe bleeding may have a deteriorating level of consciousness and airway protection may be required. Patients with persistent vomiting are at risk from aspiration or upper airway obstruction. Respiratory assessment is important to identify signs of compromise, for example the patient with a

gastrointestinal emergency may present with hypoxaemia and tachypnoea requiring supplemental oxygen administration. Gastrointestinal emergencies are also associated with hypovolaemia as evidenced by a combination of cold peripheries, reduced capillary refill time, tachycardia, weak pulse, hypotension, oliguria etc. Gaining intravenous access is a priority to enable rapid fluid administration as necessary. These interventions should be initiated prior to proceeding to the next assessment in the sequence. Disability assessment includes level of consciousness as well as determining blood glucose level. Exposure review involves assessment of the abdomen and interpreting blood results to help ascertain the cause of an acute deterioration. Early warning scores guide the nurse as to the appropriate care escalation required. See Table 10.4 for a summary of patient assessment findings related to specific gastrointestinal emergencies.

The most common GI symptoms are abdominal pain, heartburn, nausea and vomiting, altered bowel habits, GI bleeding and jaundice. Additional symptoms may include dysphagia, anorexia, weight loss and fatigue.

Table 10.4 Patient assessment utilising an ABCDE approach

	Variable	GI bleed	Pancreatitis	Acute liver failure	Bowel emergency (inflammation, perforation, obstruction)
A/B	• Airway patency • Respiratory rate and pattern • O_2 saturations	• Risk of airway obstruction with haematemesis • Tachypnoea due to hypoxia	• Tachypnoea and dyspnoea due to pain and proximity of pancreas to diaphragm	• Tachypnoea, shallow breathing due to respiratory compromise secondary to discomfort affecting diaphragm. Possibly secondary to a metabolic acidosis	• Tachypnoea, shallow breathing due to respiratory compromise secondary to pain affecting diaphragm
C	• BP • Pulse • Capillary refill time (CRT) • Skin • CVP • Temperature • Urine output	• Hypovolaemia due to haemorrhage (hypotension, tachycardia, cool and clammy, oliguria)	• Hypovolaemia due to sequestration of fluid around inflamed pancreas (hypotension, tachycardia, cool and clammy, oliguria) • ST segment changes on ECG • Pyrexia due to inflammatory processes or infection	• 'Vasodilatory' shock due to endotoxins and/ or sepsis hypotension, tachycardia, warm to touch, oliguria) • Oliguria may also be due to acute kidney injury (AKI) secondary to liver failure	• Evidence of hypovolaemia (hypotension, tachycardia, cool and clammy, oliguria) if ongoing diarrhoea and vomiting (D&V)
D	• GCS pain assessment	• Reduced level of consciousness if severe haemorrhage	• Severe abdominal pain, worse on lying down	• Reduced level of consciousness (LOC) due to encephalopathy	• Pain may be constant in inflammation or perforation leading to peritonitis, or colicky in nature with intestinal obstruction

Table 10.4 Patient assessment utilising an ABCDE approach (*continued*)

E1	• GI assessment	• Haematemesis with upper GI bleed • Melaena with lower GI bleed	• Distended abdomen • Possible bruising on flanks (Turners' sign), umbilicus (Cullens' sign) or groin (Fox sign)	• Distended abdomen with tender, palpable liver due to enlargement	• Distended (and taut) abdomen. Bowel sounds may at first be high-pitched 'tinkling' and later be absent • Vomiting and/or diarrhoea/ constipation • Fresh blood in stool from lower GI bleed, melaena
E2	• Blood results	• Drop in Hb	• Elevated serum amylase and lipase • Hyperglycaemia • Hypocalcaemia due to saponification of fats • Hypomagnesaemia in alcoholic pancreatitis • Hyperkalaemia due to metabolic acidosis and renal failure (AKI) • Lactate ↑ and metabolic acidosis on ABGs due to necrotic tissue • ↑ Bilirubin and jaundice due to effects on common bile duct • ↓ Prothrombin due to malabsorption of fats • Coagulopathy and abnormal LFTs if liver involvement	• Deranged LFTs: elevated enzymes (AST and ALT) • Low albumin • Deranged clotting • Elevated lactate (and metabolic acidosis) • Hypoglycaemia • Elevated Cr and urea if AKI developing • Low levels of potassium, magnesium, sodium, phosphates and calcium may occur • Jaundice due to elevated bilirubin levels	• Elevated lactate and metabolic acidosis on ABGs if ischaemic bowel present
E3	• Other medical scoring systems	• Use Rockall Numerical Risk Scoring System (a prognostic score utilising age, degree of shock, and co-morbidities)	• Use Atlanta Classification, Pancreatitis Outcome Prediction Score (POP) (or Ranson's criteria if alcohol-induced pancreatitis) for scoring severity of pancreatitis	• Use Child Pugh Scoring or MELD for severity of liver failure • Use King's criteria for indications for liver transplant	

Abdominal pain

Abdominal pain can be due to a wide range of causes (see Table 10.5). Pain may originate from inflammation of the peritoneum (peritonitis), inflammation of the bowel (e.g. gastroenteritis), dilatation of the bowel (e.g. gastroenteritis) or inflammation of any organ within the abdomen (e.g. pancreatitis, cholecystitis etc). Additionally, pain may be initiated by other body areas in the form of referred pain (thorax, spine, genitalia), metabolic conditions (diabetes, uraemia, hypercalcaemia) or neurogenic disorders (herpes zoster). Finally, abdominal pain may be psychogenic in origin.

The acute abdomen

The term 'acute abdomen' describes a syndrome of acute abdominal pain with accompanying signs and symptoms that focus attention on the abdomen. There are many causes of an acute abdomen, both abdominal and extra abdominal. These can be classified into:

Table 10.5 Abdominal pain by location

Right upper quadrant	Epigastric	Left upper quadrant
Cholecystitis Cholangitis Pneumonia Hepatitis Subphrenic abscess	Peptic ulcer Gastritis Pancreatitis Myocardial infarction Pericarditis Oesophagitis Ruptured aortic aneurysm	Splenic rupture Splenic abscess Gastritis Gastric ulcer Pancreatitis Subphrenic abscess
Right lower quadrant	**Periumbilical**	**Left lower quadrant**
Appendicitis Salpingitis Inguinal hernia Ectopic pregnancy Inflammatory bowel disease	Appendicitis (early) Gastroenteritis Bowel obstruction Ruptured aortic aneurysm	Diverticulitis Salpingitis Inguinal hernia Ectopic pregnancy Inflammatory bowel disease
Non-localised pain		
Gastroenteritis Mesenteric ischaemia Bowel obstruction	Irritable bowel syndrome (IBS) Peritonitis Metabolic disease	Diabetes Malaria Psychiatric disease

1 *Infective/inflammatory* – specific organs may be inflamed, for example as in acute cholecystitis, acute pancreatitis, acute appendicitis or pelvic inflammatory disease. Peritonitis is defined as inflammation of the peritoneal membrane. Causes include physical damage, chemical irritation and bacterial invasion, for example following perforation of the bowel. Peritonitis can be a complication of any surgery in which the peritoneal cavity is breached or any disease that perforates the walls of the stomach or intestines. Continued inflammation will be associated with guarding and rebound tenderness. The spread of infection throughout the abdominal cavity will lead to generalised abdominal wall rigidity and manifestations of sepsis.

2 *Obstructive* – this occurs when a hollow lumen has a blockage which interferes with its normal motility pattern. For example, biliary colic, when the cystic duct is blocked by a gallstone, or renal colic due to an obstructing ureteric calculus. Intestinal obstruction will result in abdominal colic, vomiting and progressive constipation. If neglected, it will lead to perforation, peritonitis and signs of an acute abdomen.

3 *Haemorrhagic* – this is not the commonest cause of acute abdominal pain, but is frequently serious. The

pain will be due to the presence of blood in the peritoneal cavity.

4 *Other causes* – abdominal pain may be present in a variety of other conditions, e.g. pneumonia (arising from parietal pleura), subphrenic abscess, myocardial ischaemia, diabetic ketoacidosis, hypercalcaemia, porphyria or psychogenic factors.

Look, listen and feel (inspection, auscultation, palpation of) the acute abdomen

Look (inspection)
A patient with an acute abdomen often exhibits pallor and anxiety, is sweating, and tachypnoeic. The patient should be assessed for pyrexia and signs of shock (hypovolaemic or septic). With colic, the patient will be restless. In acute pancreatitis, bruising may be present in the flanks (Grey–Turner's sign) and/or around the umbilicus (Cullen's sign). Inspection would also include the noting of striae (stretch marks) and surgical scars.

Apart from obesity, a distended abdomen might suggest ascites or intestinal obstruction. In obesity, the abdomen will be enlarged but not be tense, whereas ascites or intestinal obstruction will result in the skin over the abdomen being taut. In extremis, this can result in abdominal compartment syndrome (ACS) whereby the intra-abdominal pressure is so high that it compresses the kidneys and other abdominal structures and may impact on the diaphragm, compromising breathing. If the high pressure progresses renal function may be compromised. It is possible to measure intra-abdominal pressure, however, this practice is usually only carried out in the intensive care unit.

Listen (auscultation)
Bowel sounds (borborygmi) may be high pitched in intestinal obstruction, or absent in the presence of an ileus or peritonitis. Ileus is a failure of peristalsis. The presence or absence of bowel sounds should be interpreted with caution as it is possible to have sounds present with poor gut functioning and vice versa. Bowel sounds should therefore be interpreted in context with other indicators of bowel function such as distension, pain, gastric aspirate, vomiting and diarrhoea.

Feel (palpation)
Local areas of tenderness may be identified on palpation, with rebound tenderness or guarding present as underlying pathology worsens. A palpable mass may indicate a neoplasm or hernia, and if in the right iliac fossa may indicate Crohn's disease or an appendix abscess. A pulsatile mass may be identified in the presence of an abdominal aortic aneurysm.

CASE STUDY 10.1 Mr Harvey, a patient with haematemesis – Part 1

INITIAL ASSESSMENT

Mr Harvey is 60 years old and has been admitted to the admissions ward via A&E where he presented following a haematemesis at home. He has a history of chronic liver failure secondary to cirrhosis of the liver (caused by hepatitis C). He has not vomited any more blood since admission and is awaiting endoscopy.

Airway/breathing

On arrival on the ward, the nurse documents that Mr Harvey has a respiratory rate of 28 breaths per minute, however he states that his breathing is comfortable and 'normal' for him. The nurse observes his breathing to be shallow, but that he is not using any accessory muscles of respiration, and considers that his respiratory pattern may be due to anxiety. He has a fixed performance oxygen mask *in situ* (40%) and his saturations are 95%. Although he is anxious about having vomited blood, he is able to talk in whole sentences and is cooperative in answering questions. The nurse checks that the suction equipment is working as there is a risk that Mr Harvey could rebleed.

On auscultation, he has clear, bilateral air entry to both bases with no additional sounds.

Circulation

Mr Harvey has a pulse of 110 beats per minute which is regular and strong, BP 112/60mmhg, and a capillary refill time of three seconds. He is apyrexial and has warm peripheries. He has two large-bore peripheral cannula (sited in A&E) and is receiving 100mL/hour of Hartmann's solution (as he is nil by mouth). Two cannulae have been placed as a precaution in case Mr Harvey needs urgent fluid administration. He has passed 150mL of urine (using a bottle) over the past three hours.

> It is good practice to site a second cannula in a patient who may need intravenous (IV) fluids in an emergency: 'One to use and one to lose.'

Disability

Mr Harvey has a GCS of 15/15, is fully cooperative and states that he has no pain. However, as an altered conscious level is associated with liver disease (hepatic encephalopathy) he is commenced on 4-hourly neurological observations. His blood sugar on admission is 5mmol/L.

Exposure

Mr Harvey appears underweight, but he has a distended abdomen. In view of Mr Harvey's history of chronic liver

failure, it is likely that this is due to ascites (collection of fluid in the abdominal cavity), which may be contributing to his tachypnoea as the fluid collection may compromise diaphragmatic function.

Mr Harvey is weighed and this is documented carefully as daily weights in a patient with ascites can provide a guide to increased fluid formation or retention. In respect to Mr Harvey being underweight, the nurse calculates his BMI to be 18 and notes that a referral to a dietician should be made. The nurse is also aware that chronic poor nutritional status may impact adversely on prognosis.

The nurse notes that although Mr Harvey's skin is intact, it has a slight yellow tinge. This may be due to jaundice and the bilirubin level should therefore be checked when blood results are available.

A large-bore nasogastric tube is *in situ*. This has been placed to determine whether (a) active bleeding is still evident and (b) to empty blood from the stomach prior to endoscopy.

DIAGNOSIS

Given Mr Harvey's history and presentation, a provisional diagnosis is made that the haematemesis is due to ruptured oesophageal varices. This is a complication of chronic liver disease, as is ascites. There is a high risk of Mr Harvey rebleeding and therefore he has been booked for an endoscopy and intervention as relevant. It is possible also that his chronic liver disease has become 'decompensated', i.e. 'acute on chronic'. If this is substantiated, he is at even greater risk of rebleeding from his varices due to a coagulopathy. The nurse will therefore check Mr Harvey's liver function tests (LFTs), clotting profile and full blood count when they are available.

Mr Harvey appears 'stable' at present, but the nurse is aware that he has the potential to deteriorate rapidly. A modified early warning score (MEWS) at this stage would have given a tally of three points (see later). She informs the nurse in charge as per the EWS protocol. She knows that there might not be significant changes in his observations until he has lost at least 20% of his circulating volume and therefore observational trends require timely intervention (see Table 10.6). The nurse commences half-hourly observations and instigates a fluid balance chart. Mr Harvey has stated that he is worried about the bleeding recurring so the nurse provides him with a vomit bowl, tissues and call bell. She reassures him that she will be monitoring his condition closely.

CASE STUDY 10.1 Mr Harvey, a patient with haematemesis – Part 1 (*continued*)

Modified early warning score

Score	3	2	1	0	1	2	3
Systolic BP	< 70	71–80	81–100	**101–199**		> 200	
Heart rate		< 40	41–50	51–100	**101–110**	111–129	> 130
Respiratory rate		< 9		9–14	15–20	**21–29**	> 30
Temperature		< 35		**35–38.4**		> 38.5	
AVPU				A	V	P	U

Maximising GI status

Monitoring of fluid balance

The most important nursing intervention in relation to gastrointestinal emergencies is monitoring fluid balance because most of these situations will result in hypovolaemia. The early identification of fluid losses and timely administration of appropriate fluid replacement will prevent the deteriorating patient from developing hypovolaemic shock. Nurses are responsible directly with regard to monitoring patients of all ages for actual or potential fluid and/or electrolyte disturbance, and the NMC (2010) requires these assessments to be performed accurately by nurses using appropriate diagnostic and decision-making skills.

In the case of haemorrhage (e.g. from a variceal bleed), there must be an awareness that when the patient has changes in their observations, they will have suffered a blood loss of at least 20% of their circulating volume, equating to a litre of blood (see Table 10.6).

> If the patient is pyrexial, they will have increased insensible fluid losses which will further exacerbate hypovolaemia. These additional fluid losses need to be taken into consideration when calculating fluid replacement.

In total, approximately eight litres of gastrointestinal fluids are secreted (in addition to two litres ingested) with most of this volume being reabsorbed (see Table 10.7). Although there is a general consensus that we secrete around eight litres of fluid per day, a wide range of volumes are cited for the individual juices, as identified in Table 10.7. Impaired, or lack of, reabsorption (e.g. vomiting and diarrhoea) will result in fluids being lost from the body, leading to hypovolaemia. Fluids may also be lost via drains (e.g. biliary drains and nasogastric tubes on free drainage) or due to the disease process (e.g. sequestration of fluid in pancreatitis).

> Although we should drink approximately 2 litres of fluid daily, most hospitalised patients will not achieve this due to change in normal habits, lack of available fluids, general malaise, nausea, vomiting and diarrhoea. Additionally, many GI patients will also be nil by mouth. The importance of keeping accurate fluid balance charts *cannot* be overemphasised.

Table 10.6 Blood losses

	Minimal	Mild	Moderate	Severe
%	10%	20%	30%	40%+
Volume lost	500mL	1000mL	1500mL	2000mL+
HR	Normal	100–120	120–140	140+
BP systolic	Normal	Postural drop	<100	<80
Urine output	Normal	20–30mls/hr	10–20mls/hr	Anuric
Mental status	Normal	Normal	Restless	Impaired LOC
Peripheral	Normal	Cool/pale	Cool/pale	Cold/clammy

Table 10.7 Gastrointestinal daily secretions

Secretion	Volume daily	Estimated range	pH
Saliva	1500mL	1000–1500mL	6.0–7.0
Gastric juice	2500mL	2000–2500mls	1.0–3.0
Bile	500mL	500–700mL	7.8
Pancreatic juice	700mL	700–1500mL	7.0–8.3
Intestinal	3000mL	2000–3000mL	7.5–8.0

CASE STUDY 10.2 Mr Harvey, a patient with haematemesis – Part 2

Mr Harvey has a history of chronic liver failure secondary to cirrhosis of the liver. He has had a haematemesis at home. He has not vomited any further, but has a trend of a rising heart and respiratory rate and an early warning score of three. Blood results are reviewed.

Recognising early deterioration
Mr Harvey's blood results including LFTs are available and are as follows:

	Result	Normal range
INR	2	1
Prothrombin time	30 secs	12–14 seconds
Platelets	62 10⁹/L	130–450 10⁹/L
Hb	8.1g/dL	13–16g/dL in men
WBC	13.9 10⁹/L	4.4–10 10⁹/L
Sodium (Na)	130mmol/L	135–145mmol/L
Potassium (K)	3.8mmol/L	3.5–5.0mmol/L
Bilirubin	60umol/L	5–17umol/L
AST	133U/L	5–40U/L
ALP	89U/L	5–40U/L
Albumin	22g/L	35–50g/L
Urea	17mmol/L	3–6mmol/L
Creatinine	170umol/L	60–120umol/L

Commentary re blood results: Mr Harvey's clotting profile indicates abnormal liver function as evidenced by a thrombocytopenia (low platelets), extended prothrombin time and INR. These indicate collectively a coagulopathy which would make a variceal bleed even more difficult to manage. He is anaemic due to his haematemesis and six units of packed cells have been cross-matched and are ready for transfusion when prescribed. Clotting products will be administered (in addition to the blood) if bleeding actively.

White blood cells (WBC) are elevated and this may be as a result of haemorrhage and/or may indicate infection. The electrolytes (Na⁺ and K⁺) are low due to increased levels of antidiuretic hormone (ADH) causing fluid retention in response to systemic vasodilation. Bilirubin levels are elevated due to the liver being unable to process bilirubin, resulting in it remaining in the circulation and manifesting as jaundice. Liver enzymes (AST and ALP) are moderately elevated as a result of liver cell damage. Serum albumin is low due to the inability of the liver to process proteins into plasma proteins (resulting in oedema and ascites). Finally, the elevated urea and creatinine suggest renal dysfunction which may be pre-existing or due to hepatorenal syndrome.

Half-hourly observations continue, but two hours later he deteriorates. His respiratory rate is 32 breaths per minute and his oxygen saturations are 91%. The nurse increases his oxygen to 60% fixed performance oxygen in accordance with the sequence in the following table:

Oxygen administration

- Non-fixed performance: Hudson mask, nasal cannulae and all humidified systems
- Fixed performance: Venturi mask giving 24%, 28%, 35%, 40%, 60% O₂
- 15L via non-rebreathe mask is believed to give 85% O₂ and bag valve mask (BVM) believed to give between 85% and 100% O₂
- It is only possible to be certain of administering 100% O₂ when the patient is intubated

Mr Harvey's pulse has increased to 130 beats per minute (regular, but thready) and his BP is 88/55mm/hg. His peripheries feel cold and his temperature is 36°C. Mr Harvey says that he feels very nauseous and has a metallic taste in his mouth. The nausea could be due to accumulating blood in the stomach and hypotension. Mr Harvey's MEWS Score (which was previously three) has now increased to seven (see below).

The nurse informs the doctor of the changes as per MEWS protocol, she is aware that the trend in his observations (in conjunction with the nausea) indicates that he is bleeding.

Modified early warning score

Score	3	2	1	0	1	2	3
Systolic BP	< 70	71–80	81–100	101–199		> 200	
Heart rate		< 40	**41–50**	51–100	101–110	111–129	**> 130**
Respiratory rate		< 9		9–14	15–20	21–29	**> 30**
Temperature		< 35		**35–38.4**		> 38.5	
AVPU				A	V	P	U

Nausea and vomiting

Acute nausea, with or without vomiting, is a common symptom. Nausea is described as a sensation of imminent vomiting and vomiting (emesis) is the forcible expulsion of the stomach contents through the mouth. The strongest triggers are irritation (gastritis, infection or presence of blood) and also distension of the stomach, with many causes (see Table 10.8). The act of vomiting is initiated in the vomiting centre in the medulla, or the chemoreceptor trigger zone (CTZ) in the floor of the fourth ventricle via a mix of motor and autonomic response. This is why many neurological conditions and raised intracranial pressure (ICP) can include nausea and vomiting as a sign or symptom.

Nasogastric aspirate

There is no definitive level at which the amount of aspirate indicates a problem with gut function, however, 200mL (at four hours) is generally taken as a cut-off point for making a decision in regard to the commencement or continuation of feeding.

Mendelson's syndrome

This is a chemical pneumonitis caused by aspiration of gastric contents. It was first described by Mendelson in 1946 in relation to obstetric anaesthesia. It is considered that as little as 25mL of gastric contents can cause significant damage.

Table 10.8 Common causes of acute vomiting

GI tract	Peritonitis
	Bowel obstruction
	Acute pancreatitis
	Acute cholecystitis
	Acute appendicitis
	Mesenteric ischaemia
CNS	Raised intracranial pressure
	CNS tumours
	Meningitis
	Vestibular disorders/travel (motion sickness)
	Cerebral abscess
	Subarachnoid haemorrhage
	Head injury
	Migraine
Drugs	Chemotherapy
	Antibiotics/antivirals
	Narcotics
	Analgesics
Infections	Gastroenteritis (food poisoning, e.g. salmonella)
	Epidemic, e.g. Norwalk virus
	Hepatitis viruses
	Non-GI tract infections
Endocrine	Diabetic ketoacidosis
	Adrenal insufficiency
	Hypercalcaemia
	Uraemia
Miscellaneous	Ethanol abuse
	Recreational drug abuse
	Radiotherapy
	Pregnancy (hyperemesis gravidarum)
	Post-myocardial infarction/CCF
	Carcinoma
	Postoperative

Aspiration of stomach contents

Aspiration pneumonia occurs if stomach contents are aspirated into the lungs. This can result in an acute lung injury, which may be fatal. There is an increased risk of aspiration associated with a reduced level of consciousness, absent cough/gag reflexes, delayed gastric emptying, paralytic ileus or by simply having an enteral feeding tube *in situ*. Strategies to minimise the risk of aspiration include monitoring nasogastric aspirates, nursing patients upright (45%) and confirming and monitoring tube positioning. The National Patient Safety Agency provides guidelines on checking the position of nasogastric tubes and reducing harm caused by misplaced tubes (NPSA 2011).

> **A 'never event'**
>
> It should *never happen* that a patient is fed via a misplaced nasogastric tube, as correct tube position should always be checked prior to commencing feeding. The gold standard for confirming tube position is CXR and the use of pH testing strips.

Diarrhoea

This is defined as a reduced consistency (or increased liquidity) of the faeces. Physiologically this will be due to inadequate reabsorption of water by the bowel (and/or increased mucus secretion) as the contents transit. There is an extensive differential diagnosis however, including infective (bacterial, viral, parasitic, and toxins), inflammatory bowel disease (e.g. Crohn's, ulcerative colitis), drugs (antibiotics, ACE inhibitors, chemotherapy, laxatives), faecal impaction with overflow and in the critically ill altered gut motility and paralytic ileus.

Nursing management should focus upon close monitoring of cardiovascular and fluid balance status (early recognition of hypovolaemia) and a fresh stool sample sent for culture and sensitivity (in particular to exclude *Clostridium difficile* enterotoxin which is one of the most common nosocomial infections).

Administration of stress ulceration medication

- *H2 receptor antagonists* – e.g. Ranitidine. These drugs suppress acid secretion by competing for the histamine receptor on the parietal cell.
- *Proton-pump inhibitors* – e.g. Omeprazole or Lansoprazole. These are acid-suppressing agents as they block the final pathway of acid secretion by the parietal cell, i.e. the proton pump. These are indicated for patients with major peptic ulcer bleeding following endoscopic intervention according to SIGN (2008).
- *Sucruflate* – this increases mucus secretion, mucosal blood flow and local prostaglandin production. These effects protect the mucosa against damage by acid or pepsin. It forms a protective barrier over the gastric mucosa (but does not alter gastric pH. It is given via nasogastric (NG) tube (1g every 4–6 hours).
- *Antacids* – given hourly via NG tube can maintain gastric alkalinisation. These can contain magnesium, aluminium, calcium or sodium with problems resulted from excessive intake. They are rarely used now.

Administration of anti-emetics

- *Ondansetron* – a serotonin 5-HT3 receptor antagonist (IV, IM or orally administered).
- *Prochlorperazine (Stemetil)* – this is antidopaminergic and is particularly useful for vestibular vomiting. Administered IM.
- *Cyclizine* – this is a histamine H1 receptor antagonist and is effective for motion sickness and vestibular causes and where there is a contraindication to Prochlorperazine, e.g. Parkinson's disease. Side effects include tachycardia.
- *Domperidone* – this is a dopamine receptor antagonist useful for a wide range of causes of nausea and vomiting.

Nutritional support

According to NICE Guidelines (2006) nutritional support should be considered in people who are malnourished or are at risk of malnutrition. This is also emphasised by ESPEN Guidelines (2009) which state that insufficient provision of nutrients is likely to result in undernutrition with 8–12 days following surgery (or ICU admission). This principle can be transposed to all acutely ill patients and particularly those with gastrointestinal disorders in whom feeding by normal methods is challenging (e.g. during gastrointestinal emergencies). A degree of malnutrition is *extremely common* in most hospitalised patients. It is estimated that 40% of hospitalised patients are malnourished and that this is frequently undiagnosed (British Dietetic Association 2006). Poor nutritional status will also affect mortality, morbidity and overall prognosis adversely, for example the patient with chronic liver failure and cachexia is likely to fare less well when undergoing liver

Table 10.9 Comparison of enteral and parenteral routes

	Enteral nutrition (EN)	Parenteral nutrition (PN)
Advantages	• As it uses the natural route, is considered more physiologically normal • It is relatively cheap (and simple) • Does not require vascular access • Preserves gut mucosal integrity • Stimulates immune barrier function • May prevent bacterial translocation	Greater potential for successful absorption of nutrients
Disadvantages	• Associated with diarrhoea • Inadequate feeding if interrupted for procedures or if patient not absorbing • Increased risk of nosocomial pneumonia • Not all patients will be capable of absorbing feed	• Relatively expensive • Requires vascular access • Needs individualised calculations for constitution of feed
Complications	• The tube may become knotted or blocked • Aspiration • Incorrect placement • Nasopharyngeal erosions and discomfort • Sinusitis • Oesophagitis • Tracheo-oesophageal fistula • Abdominal distention • Ruptured oesophageal varices • May cause nausea and vomiting • Risk of aspiration • Diarrhoea • Abdominal distension and cramping • Constipation • Hyperglycaemia • Hypercapnia (due to high level of carbohydrate) • Electrolyte and trace element abnormalities	Risks associated with central line placement (pneumothorax, catheter misplacement etc.) • Infection • Metabolic complications such as hyperglycaemia, hypoglycaemia and hyperlipidaemia • Hepatic dysfunction • Acid base disturbance • Electrolyte disturbance • Risk of 'refeeding syndrome'

transplantation than a patient with liver failure who is well nourished.

Nutrition may be administered artificially either enterally or parenterally. Both routes are compared and contrasted in Table 10.9.

Enteral nutrition (EN)

Enteral feeding tubes can be placed into the stomach, duodenum or jejunum. Enteral feeding guidelines have shown evidence in favour of early institution of feeding and the continuing delivery of food via the GI tract to be efficacious in the majority of the hospital population.

Parenteral nutrition (PN)

Although enteral nutrition is favoured, PN is an alternative when it is not possible to use other routes, or enteral nutrition has failed. ESPEN Guidelines on parenteral nutrition: Intensive care (2009) recommend that all patients receiving less than their targeted enteral feeding after two days

should be considered for PN, which should be administered in the form of a complete 'all in one bag'. For a comparison of enteral and parenteral routes see Table 10.9.

Conclusion

An insight into the common gastrointestinal emergencies will assist the nurse in recognising and responding to the deteriorating patient with these problems. In particular, an understanding of the disordered pathophysiology will support the nurse in a systematic assessment of the patient and an appreciation of the rationale for the patient's presentation, signs and symptoms. Gastrointestinal emergencies often result in increased fluid losses and disruption to the normal secretion and reabsorption of bodily fluids, culminating in hypovolaemia and hypovolaemic shock. Therefore fluid balance assessment is of paramount importance and a vital role for the nurse in caring for these patients.

Glossary

Ascites Excess fluid that has accumulated in the peritoneal cavity. Comes from the Greek *askites*, 'bag-like'. It can also be called hydroperitoneum.

Asterixis This is the term for hepatic flap (of the hands). The word comes from 'without fixed position'. When the patient with hepatic encephalopathy stretches out their hands, they have jerky irregular flexion/extension of the wrist. It is thought to be due to the interference with the inflow of joint position sense to the brainstem. Although characteristic of liver failure, it can also occur in cardiac, respiratory and renal failure.

Bacterial translocation of the gut Passage of indigenous bacteria from the GI tract to the systemic circulation. This can be due to a breach of mucosal barrier, impaired immune defence mechanisms and/or bacterial overgrowth.

Bile Bile (or gall) is fluid produced by the liver (and stored in the gall bladder) that is used to digest fats in the duodenum.

Chyme From Greek *khymos* meaning 'juice'. This is semi-fluid, partly digested food expelled by the stomach into the duodenum.

Cirrhosis From Greek *kirrhos* meaning 'yellowish or tawny' which is the colour of the diseased liver. Cirrhosis is the consequence of chronic liver disease whereby the liver tissue is replaced by fibrosis and scar tissue.

Endocrine From Greek *endo* meaning inside, and *crinis*, to secrete. The endocrine system secretes hormones into the circulation to elicit a response in target organs.

Exocrine Exocrine glands secrete their products into ducts, e.g. stomach, pancreas or liver.

Haematemesis Vomiting of blood ('haem' is blood and 'emesis' vomiting).

Melaena This is the black, tarry faeces associated with gastrointestinal haemorrhage. The black ('melan') colour is caused by the oxidation of iron in the haemoglobin during the passage through the ileum and colon.

Pancreatitis Inflammation of the pancreas that may either be acute or chronic.

Paralytic ileus Disruption in the normal propulsive ability of the gastrointestinal tract.

Peristalsis Contraction and relaxation of muscles which propagates in a wave down a muscular tube. From Greek *peristallein* (to wrap around) from *peri* (around) and *stallein* (to place).

Peritonitis Inflammation of the peritoneum – the membrane which lines part of the abdominal cavity and viscera.

Sengstaken–Blakemore tube This is used in upper GI tract bleeding. It consists of a tube with two balloons, one of which is inflated against the walls of the oesophagus, and the other in the stomach, the purpose of which is to apply pressure to bleeding points.

Varices Varices are distended veins. From the Latin *varix* meaning twisted veins.

Venturi masks These oxygen masks are so named because they utilise a Venturi effect, which is to entrain air to mix with piped oxygen to achieve a specified oxygen percentage being delivered to the patient (fixed performance oxygen).

Test yourself

1 Reflux of gastric contents into the oesophagus can cause ulceration because gastric contents are:

   a. acidic
   b. alkaline

2 In liver failure, low levels of plasma proteins can predispose to:

   a. oedema
   b. ascites
   c. jaundice
   d. infection

3 The most common causes of pancreatitis are _____ and _____

4 Liver function tests include:

   a. clotting profile
   b. AST

   c. electrolytes
   d. bilirubin

5 The vomiting centre is in the:

   a. medulla
   b. frontal lobe

6 A necrotic pancreas may be evidenced by:

   a. a high white blood cell count
   b. a low haemoglobin
   c. a metabolic acidosis
   d. pyrexia

7 Epigastric pain may typically be due to:

   a. gastritis
   b. ectopic pregnancy
   c. myocardial infarction
   d. inguinal hernia

8 Approximately how many mL of gastric juice is secreted daily?

9 Patients with diarrhoea should always have a sample sent for culture and sensitivity (C&S)

in case they have which common nosocomial infection?

10 The correct term for vomiting blood is _____ and coughing blood is _____

References

Allen, P. and Tham, T. (2009) Approach to upper gastrointestinal bleeding. In Tham, T., Collins, J. and Soetikno, R. (2008) *Gastrointestinal Emergencies*, 2nd edn. Oxford: Wiley-Blackwell, pp. 11–18.

British Dietetic Association (2005). Website: www.bda.uk.com.

ESPEN (European Society for Clinical Nutrition and Metabolism) (2009) ESPEN Guidelines on parenteral nutrition: Intensive care. *Clinical Nutrition* 28 (4), 1–14.

Gavaghan, M. (2002) The pancreas – hermit of the abdomen. *AORN* 75 (6), 1109–38.

Hasibeder, W., Torgersen, C., Reiger, M. and Dunser, M. (2009) Critical care of the patient with acute pancreatitis. *Anaesthesia and Intensive Care* 37, 190–206.

Lam, N. P., Le, P. D., Crawford, S. Y., and Patel, S. (1999) National survey of stress ulcer prophylaxis. *Critical Care Medicine* 27, 98–103.

NICE (2006) *Nutritional Support in Adults. February 2006 Clinical Guideline 32*. London: National Institute for Clinical Excellence.

NPSA (2011) Checking placement of nasogastric feeding tubes in adults (interpretation of x-ray images): Summary of a safety report from the National Patient Safety Agency. *British Medical Journal* 342, d2586.

NMC (Nursing and Midwifery Council) (2010) *Standards for Pre-registration Nursing Education*. Available from http://standards.nmc-uk.org/PublishedDocuments/Standards%20for%20pre-registration%20nursing%20education%2016082010.pdf.

O'Grady, J., Schalm, S. and Williams, R. (1993) Acute liver failure: Redefining the syndromes. *Lancet* 342, 273–5.

SIGN (Scottish Intercollegiate Guidelines Network) NHS Quality Improvement Scotland (2008) *Management of Acute Upper and Lower Gastrointestinal Bleeding. A National Clinical Guideline September 2008*. Edinburgh: SIGN.

Sung, J. (2009) Acute gastrointestinal bleeding. In Bersten, A. and Soni, N. (2009) *Oh's Intensive Care Manual*, 6th edn. Philadelphia: Butterworth Heinemann.

Tham, T., Collins, J. and Soetikno, R. (2008) *Gastrointestinal Emergencies*, 2nd edn. Oxford: Wiley-Blackwell.

UK Working Party on Acute Pancreatitis (2005) UK Guidelines for the management of acute pancreatitis. *Gut* 54, 1–9.

World Gastroenterology Organisation (2008) *Practice Guidelines Esophageal Varices*.

Wyncoll, D. (2009) Severe acute pancreatitis. In Bersten, A. and Soni, N. (2009) *Oh's Intensive Care Manual*, 6th edn. Butterworth Heinemann.

Further reading

Mills, A. (2011) *Gastrointestinal Emergencies*. London: Saunders.

Norton, C. (2008) *Oxford Handbook of Gastrointestinal Nursing*. Oxford: Oxford University Press.

Tham, T. C. K., Collins, J. S. A. and Soetikno, R. (2008) *Gastrointestinal Emergencies*, 2nd edn. Oxford: Wiley-Blackwell.

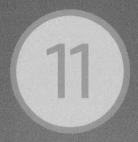

The patient with acute endocrine problems

Angela Morgan, Julian Howard and Margaret Kirkby

Aims

The aim of this chapter is to identify key roles and functions of the endocrine system, to appreciate how disordered physiology can disrupt homeostasis and cause a medical emergency, and define the nurse's role in recognising and responding appropriately to patients with acute endocrine problems.

Objectives

After reading this chapter you will be able to:

→ Describe the major organs and tissues involved in endocrine function

→ Identify the roles of the liver and pancreas in glucose metabolism

→ Identify the common endocrine emergencies and differentiate between patient presentations

→ Relate the principles underlying diabetic emergencies to disorders of fluid and electrolyte balance

→ Identify interventions that maximise endocrine status

→ Describe the responsibilities of the nurse in monitoring blood glucose and administering insulin

Introduction

Although most endocrine emergencies occur rarely, diabetic emergencies are witnessed by most nurses caring for patients within the hospital setting. It is important therefore that nurses have insight into glucose metabolism and control and into their responsibilities in monitoring and managing this aspect of patient care. These principles are paramount not only in regard to an emergency situation, but routinely, as the monitoring and control of blood glucose is frequently part of patient management.

Uncommon presentations of endocrine malfunction that can occur acutely include thyrotoxicosis, acute adrenal insufficiency and the seldom witnessed catecholamine crisis. All these can present with severe patient deterioration, so a basic understanding of the endocrine system and associated hormones is required.

Applied physiology

Overview of the endocrine system

The endocrine system includes all the organs and tissues of the body that produce hormones or cytokines. Endocrine glands, which are ductless, secrete these directly into the circulation, whereas exocrine glands discharge their products, via ducts, into the external environment. Hormones are chemical messengers that are released by tissue (glands) in low concentrations into the circulation acting on specific protein receptors on cells in other tissues, whereas cytokines (also chemical messengers) usually have a more localised effect within the tissue.

The endocrine glands can be divided into three groups:

● the pituitary gland, which secretes hormones that exercise control and influence much of the rest of the endocrine system. This gland is controlled mainly by the hypothalamus;
● endocrine glands affecting metabolism;
● endocrine glands affecting the reproductive system.

Figure 11.1 identifies the position of the major endocrine glands and the hormones they produce.

Hormones have a wide variety of functions and their effects can last for minutes, hours or even days. Hormones are composed predominantly from amino acids, or sometimes cholesterol, as with the steroid hormones. They affect organs that have hormone-specific receptors and these are known as target cells for that hormone. The target cell's receptors are situated either outside the cell, as for amino acid-based hormones, or inside the cell for the highly lipid-soluble steroid hormones. Those hormones whose target receptors are outside the cell are used as first messengers that activate second messengers located inside the cell, exerting the hormonal specific actions within the cytoplasm. Circulating hormones activate the target cells directly and the degree of response is related to total blood concentration. The more hormone circulating the greater the target cell activity. Some hormones can have powerful effects at a very low concentration. Hormones are broken down rapidly either within their target cells or by the liver and kidney.

The endocrine glands and their hormones

The hypothalamus

The hypothalamus, located in the diencephalon, is an important link between the nervous system and the endocrine system. It is involved in many of the normal physiological mechanisms that contribute to homeostasis such as temperature control, thirst and hunger reflexes. The hypothalamus controls the pituitary gland, which in its turn regulates most of the other glands in the endocrine system. Figure 11.2 demonstrates the extensive influence of the hypothalamus, the anterior and posterior pituitary gland and their target organs.

The pituitary

The pituitary gland has an important role in the control of other glands. It has two lobes, anterior and posterior, producing eight hormones in total: these are summarised in Table 11.1.

The **anterior pituitary** is under the control of the hypothalamus but also acts independently. The hormones most likely to be related to a medical emergency are:

● Adrenocorticotrophic hormone (ACTH)
● Thyroid stimulating hormone (TSH).

The anterior pituitary gland produces adrenocorticotrophic hormone (ACTH) in response to corticotrophin-releasing hormone (CRH) released by the hypothalamus under the neural influence of the sympathetic nervous system. ACTH causes the adrenal cortex to secrete glucocorticoid hormones such as cortisol (hydrocortisone). Glucocorticoid receptors are widely present in most body tissues. The major functions of cortisol are:

● increased gluconeogenesis;
● inhibition of glucose utilisation;
● fatty acid mobilisation and catabolism by muscle cells;
● modification of the body's response to injury.

These represent a metabolic response to stress and oppose the action of insulin.

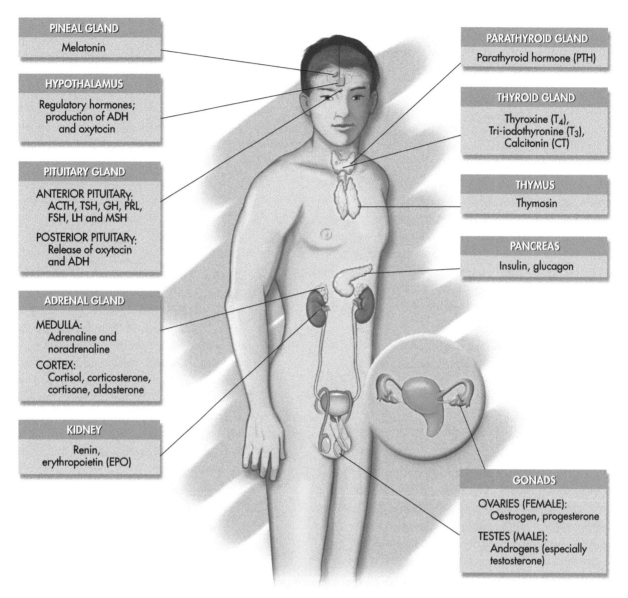

PINEAL GLAND
Melatonin

HYPOTHALAMUS
Regulatory hormones;
production of ADH
and oxytocin

PITUITARY GLAND
ANTERIOR PITUITARY:
ACTH, TSH, GH, PRL,
FSH, LH and MSH

POSTERIOR PITUITARY:
Release of oxytocin
and ADH

ADRENAL GLAND
MEDULLA:
Adrenaline and
noradrenaline
CORTEX:
Cortisol, corticosterone,
cortisone, aldosterone

KIDNEY
Renin,
erythropoietin (EPO)

PARATHYROID GLAND
Parathyroid hormone (PTH)

THYROID GLAND
Thyroxine (T_4),
Tri-iodothyronine (T_3),
Calcitonin (CT)

THYMUS
Thymosin

PANCREAS
Insulin, glucagon

GONADS
OVARIES (FEMALE):
Oestrogen, progesterone

TESTES (MALE):
Androgens (especially
testosterone)

Figure 11.1 The position of the major endocrine glands and the hormones they produce

The anterior pituitary produces thyroid-stimulating hormone (TSH) in response to thyrotropin-releasing hormone (TRH) from the hypothalamus. TSH targets the thyroid gland resulting in rising levels of thyroid hormones (T4 thyroxine, T3 triiodothyronine). Thyroid hormones control cell metabolism and growth.

The posterior lobe of the pituitary is an extension of the hypothalamus, and contains hypothalamic neurones that are specialised to secrete hormones rather than neurotransmitters. The hormone most likely to be related to a medical emergency is antidiuretic hormone (ADH).

Antidiuretic hormone (ADH), also known as vasopressin, is made by the hypothalamus, but is actually secreted from the posterior pituitary. It is released in response to several different stimuli, but most importantly to a change in the solute concentration of the blood, or a change in blood pressure. Osmoreceptors are situated in the hypothalamus and respond to the changes in tonicity (effective osmolality) of extracellular fluid. If the tonicity rises then ADH release is stimulated and the kidneys will increase reabsorption of water, resulting in concentrated urine. If the extracellular fluid tonicity falls then ADH release is inhibited, leading to reduced water reabsorption resulting in dilute urine. Osmoreceptors will respond to a change in tonicity of around 2%. Baroreceptors are situated in the right atrium and carotid sinus. They respond to changes in intravascular volume. A reduced circulating volume will result in increased ADH release and an increased circulating volume will inhibit ADH release. Baroreceptors require a 10% change in circulating volume before they respond. In some circumstances, baroreceptors can override osmoreceptors

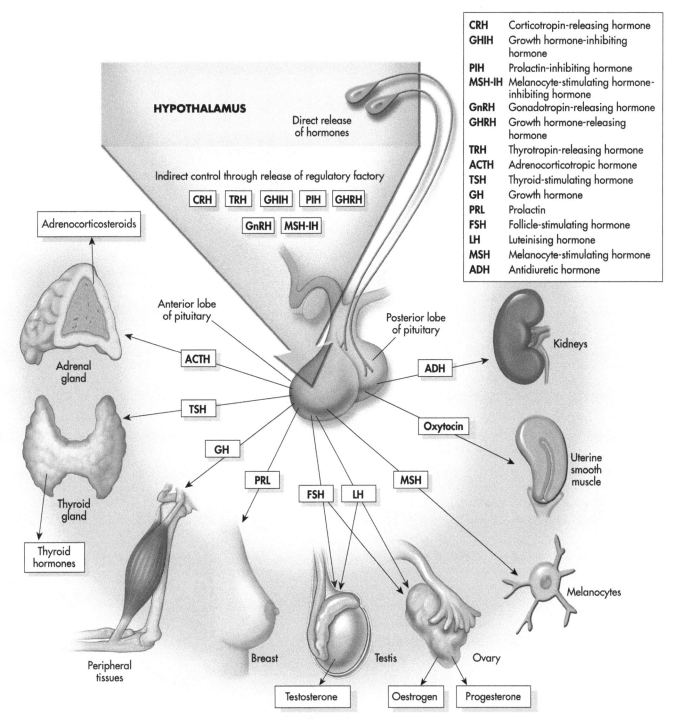

CRH	Corticotropin-releasing hormone
GHIH	Growth hormone-inhibiting hormone
PIH	Prolactin-inhibiting hormone
MSH-IH	Melanocyte-stimulating hormone-inhibiting hormone
GnRH	Gonadotropin-releasing hormone
GHRH	Growth hormone-releasing hormone
TRH	Thyrotropin-releasing hormone
ACTH	Adrenocorticotropic hormone
TSH	Thyroid-stimulating hormone
GH	Growth hormone
PRL	Prolactin
FSH	Follicle-stimulating hormone
LH	Luteinising hormone
MSH	Melanocyte-stimulating hormone
ADH	Antidiuretic hormone

HYPOTHALAMUS

Direct release of hormones

Indirect control through release of regulatory factory

CRH TRH GHIH PIH GHRH

GnRH MSH-IH

Adrenocorticosteroids

Anterior lobe of pituitary

Posterior lobe of pituitary

Kidneys

Adrenal gland

ACTH

ADH

TSH

GH

Oxytocin

Uterine smooth muscle

Thyroid gland

PRL

FSH   LH

MSH

Thyroid hormones

Melanocytes

Peripheral tissues

Breast

Testis

Ovary

Testosterone

Oestrogen   Progesterone

Figure 11.2 The hypothalamus, anterior and posterior pituitary glands, their targets and associated hormones

because the control mechanism will attempt to maintain intravascular volume at the expense of normal extracellular fluid osmolality.

ADH and alcohol

Alcohol inhibits ADH production. The more alcohol you drink, the more ADH is inhibited and the more urine you pass. Thus dehydration contributes to the symptoms of a hangover.

ADH also causes vasoconstriction of the peripheral vessels, which helps elevate blood pressure. Because of this action, a vasopressin infusion is used sometimes in critical care situations to maintain mean arterial blood pressure.

The thyroid gland

The thyroid gland is composed of two lobes joined by an isthmus. It is located in the lower part of the neck anterior to the trachea, inferior to the thyroid cartilage (see

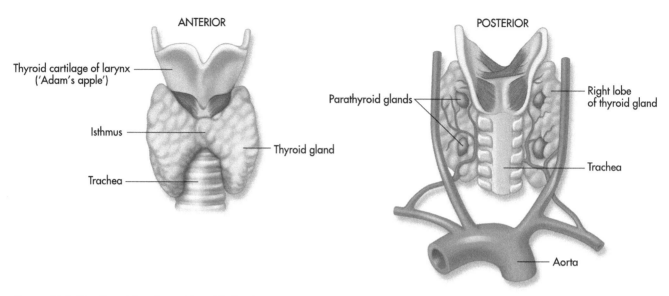

Figure 11.3 The thyroid and parathyroid glands

Figure 11.3) and has an extensive arterial blood supply. When viewed under the microscope the thyroid gland is composed of closely packed follicles which comprise epithelial cells enclosing a colloid filled space. These functional units synthesise, store and secrete thyroid hormones. Thyroid cells form the wall of each follicle and these cells enlarge as their metabolic activity increases. This accounts for the gland becoming visible (goitre) in certain thyroid disorders. In addition to supporting cells, the thyroid also contains C cells which synthesise calcitonin.

Two pairs of parathyroid glands are embedded in the posterior surface of the thyroid gland.

The thyroid makes and stores thyroid hormones (T3 and T4), it is able to hold up to 100 days' supply. Iodine is necessary for the creation of thyroid hormone. Thyroid hormones affect virtually every organ in the body and increase metabolic rate. The parathyroid glands produce parathyroid hormone (PTH) which regulates serum calcium levels. PTH secretion is stimulated when ionised serum calcium falls. This hormone influences the bones and the kidneys, leading to restoration of normal calcium levels (bone resorption and increased renal tubular calcium reabsorption respectively).

Effects of thyroxine include:

- stimulates basal metabolic rate resulting in increased oxygen consumption and heat production (thermogenesis);
- CNS and cardiovascular sensitivity to catecholamines, e.g. increased heart rate and contractility;
- enzyme synthesis which promotes protein, fat and carbohydrate metabolism;
- growth and development, e.g. of the nervous system.

PTH is one of the principal hormones that control mineral metabolism, the others being vitamin D and calcitonin. It is important that a constant ionised calcium concentration is maintained in the extracellular fluid as key physiological functions, e.g. bone mineralisation, neuromuscular excitability, blood coagulation and cell membrane integrity, are reliant upon this state.

Most hormone production is affected by negative feedback loops, whereby the initial hormone producer reacts to subsequent levels of hormones produced by the target organ. The regulation of the production of thyroid hormone is a good example of a negative feedback loop (see Figure 11.4).

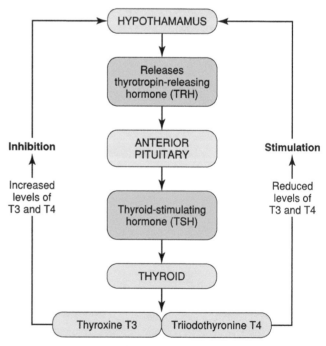

Figure 11.4 Example of a negative feedback loop

Steroids

For example prednisolone, hydrocortisone, dexamethasone

Used to treat inflammation, immune system disorders, and prevent rejection of transplanted organs. Side effects include:

- weight gain (truncal obesity);
- hair growth (hirsutism);
- delayed wound healing;
- diabetes;
- muscle weakness and wasting;
- bone thinning and osteoporosis;
- fluid retention (oedema);
- gastric ulceration;
- skin thinning, acne and stretch marks;
- suppression of all inflammatory processes and generalised reactions of inflammation (can mask signs of underlying pathology, e.g. acute abdomen);
- increased susceptibility to infections.

Steroids must not be withdrawn suddenly, as the adrenal glands need time to increase their own production of corticosteroids.

Adrenal glands

The adrenal glands are a pair of small glands situated on top of the kidneys. There are split into two regions:

- Adrenal cortex
- Adrenal medulla.

The adrenal cortex secretes many steroid hormones, collectively known as corticosteroids. In addition to the glucocorticoids (e.g. cortisol) the other major groups of adrenocortical hormones include mineralocorticoids (e.g. aldosterone) and androgenic hormones (e.g. dehydro-epiandrosterone – DHEA). Production of cortisol and androgen precursors is controlled by ACTH. The androgen precursors are converted in peripheral tissues to oestrogen and testosterone. Aldosterone production is regulated by angiotensin and potassium. This hormone is the principal sodium-retaining steroid hormone and maintains normal fluid balance and circulating volume.

The adrenal medulla is both a part of the autonomic nervous system and endocrine system. On response to sympathetic stimulation two hormones, adrenaline and noradrenaline, are released. Adrenal medulla cells can be considered as neuronal cells which function as an endocrine gland.

Noradrenaline is a both a neurotransmitter of the sympathetic nervous system and a hormone, when released from the adrenal medulla. As noradrenaline and adrenaline enter the bloodstream, heart rate, blood pressure and respiratory rate increase, sweat glands become more active, the mouth becomes dry, glycogen breakdown increases and blood glucose levels increase.

If the adrenal glands are destroyed or removed, appropriate steroid replacement will be required, including glucocorticoids and mineralocorticoids as these are essential for life. Interestingly, medullary catecholamine replacement is not required because the sympathetic nervous system can independently produce noradrenaline, which acts on adrenergic receptors producing the characteristic sympathetic effects.

We have reviewed the function of the endocrine organs that may be involved in a medical emergency. A summary of the main elements involved in the endocrine system have been included (see Table 11.1). The discussion will now move on to the role of the liver and pancreas in glucose homeostasis.

Glucose homeostasis

Maintenance of plasma glucose levels within certain limits is of vital importance because the central nervous system, including the retina, depends upon an uninterrupted supply for normal functioning, the brain being an obligate glucose user (exclusive utilisation of glucose as oppose to free fatty acids or amino acids). Variation from the normal range (both excess and deficit) will cause neurological dysfunction, adversely affect other body systems, and may prove fatal. There are, however, many mechanisms in place that operate both to increase and decrease circulating glucose as necessary to maintain homeostasis.

Dietary sources of glucose

The two main sources of glucose are intestinal absorption of dietary glucose and its precursors and release of glucose from the liver. Plasma glucose levels increase with meals, rising slightly and then returning to basal levels after around two hours, therefore both of these mechanisms are necessary for normal daily functioning.

The most direct pathway for the formation of glucose is as a result of carbohydrate metabolism. As there is very little pure glucose in the diet, this results predominantly from the breakdown of disaccharides and polysaccharides. The former are hydrolysed and absorbed rapidly, causing a prompt increase in plasma glucose concentration (high glycaemic index), whereas the latter enter the bloodstream more slowly, therefore having a low glycaemic index.

Proteins are metabolised to amino acids with some able to donate their carbon atoms for glucose formation. Glucose generation from protein or any other non-glucose source is called gluconeogenesis. With regard to fat metabolism, triglycerides release glycerol which can be converted readily to glucose by the liver, but this accounts only for approximately 10% of the carbon atoms available

Table 11.1 Summary of the hormones of the endocrine system and their effects

Tissue	Hormones	Target/effect/function
Hypothalamus	TRH thyrotropin-releasing hormone	• Stimulates TSH (thyroid-stimulating hormone) release from the anterior pituitary • Stimulates prolactin release from the anterior pituitary
	DA dopamine (or prolactin-inhibiting hormone)	• Inhibits prolactin release from anterior pituitary
	GHRH growth hormone-releasing hormone	• Stimulates GH (growth hormone) release from the anterior pituitary
	SS somatostatin (or GHIH growth-hormone inhibiting hormone)	• Inhibits GH release from the anterior pituitary • Inhibits TSH being released by the anterior pituitary
	GnRH gonadotropin-releasing hormone	• Stimulates FSH (follicle-stimulating hormone) release from the anterior pituitary • Stimulates LH (luteinising hormone) release from the anterior pituitary
	CRH corticotrophin-releasing hormone	• Stimulates ACTH (adrenocorticotrophic hormone) release from the anterior pituitary
Pituitary gland: anterior lobe	ACTH (adrenocorticotrophic hormone)	• Stimulates the adrenal cortex – specifically targets cells that produce glucocorticoids which influence glucose metabolism
	TSH (thyroid-stimulating hormone)	• Targets the thyroid gland with subsequent release of thyroid hormones T4 (thyroxine) and T3 (triiodothyronine)
	GH (growth hormone)	• Stimulates cell growth and replication
	FSH (follicle-stimulating hormone)	• Affects follicle development in females – stimulates oestrogens by ovarian cells • Stimulates cells in tubules where sperm differentiate
	LH (luteinising hormone)	• Induces ovulation in females and androgens including testosterone in males
	Prolactin	• Stimulates milk production by the mammary glands
Pituitary gland: posterior lobe	ADH (antidiuretic hormone)	• Increases the absorption of water in the distal tubule and collecting duct in the kidney
	Oxytocin	• Stimulates smooth muscle in the wall of the uterus promoting labour and delivery
Pineal gland	Melatonin	• Control of 'biological clock'
Thyroid gland	T4 (thyroxine) T3 (triiodothyronine)	• Directly affect the mitochondria in cells and therefore metabolic rate
	Calcitonin	• Regulation of calcium concentration in body fluids
Parathyroid	PTH (parathyroid hormone)	• Regulation of calcium concentration in body fluids
Heart	Natriuretic peptides: (ANP and BNP – atrial natriuretic peptide and brain natriuretic peptide)	• If there is an increase in pressure/stretch in the atria or ventricles, natriuretic peptides will promote water and sodium loss at the kidneys
Thymus	Thymosins	• Role in immunity
Kidney	EPO (erythropoietin)	• In response to low oxygen levels in the kidneys, EPO stimulates the production of red blood cells by the bone marrow
	Calcitriol (1,25 dihydroxycholecalciferol)	• This is the active form of vitamin D and stimulates calcium and phosphate ion absorption in the digestive system

Table 11.1 (*continued*)

Tissue	Hormones	Target/effect/function
Adrenal glands	Adrenal medulla: • Adrenaline • Noradrenaline	• Stimulation of alpha and beta receptors in the blood vessels and myocardium to cause either vasoconstriction or vasodilation as required • Also accelerates the utilisation of cellular energy and mobilisation of energy reserves
	Adrenal cortex: • Mineralocorticoids • Glucocorticoids • Sex hormones	• Mineralocorticoids, e.g. aldosterone secretion targets cells that regulate the sodium and potassium ions in excreted fluids • Glucocorticoids, e.g. cortisol regulates metabolism of fat, protein and carbohydrates • Sex hormones: androgens, oestrogens and progesterone influence reproductive functioning
Pancreatic islets	Insulin	• Lowers blood glucose levels by increasing the rate of glucose uptake and utilisation by cells
	Glucagon	• Raises blood glucose levels by increasing rates of glycogen breakdown and glucose release by the liver
	Somatostatin	• Inhibits insulin and glucagon release by the pancreas • Also suppresses exocrine secretion by the pancreas
	Pancreatic polypetides (PP)	• Self-regulates endocrine and exocrine pancreatic activity
Digestive tract	Ghrelin	• Released by the stomach and upper intestine prior to eating and falls in direct relation to calorie intake, thus playing a role in body weight regulation
	Peptide YY	• Released by the distal gut following food ingestion in direct relation to calorie intake, thus playing a role in body weight regulation
	Glucagon-like peptide-1 (GLP-1) Oxyntomodulin (OXM) Cholecystokinin (CCK) Pancreatic polypeptide (PP)	• These are all released in response to food intake and play a role in signalling satiety and the consequent inhibition of food intake. There are many other substances that are unresearched. No deficiency syndromes have been identified, but their role is unclear
Adipose tissue	Leptin	• Satiation and regulation of appetite
Gonads	Male testes: androgens	• Affects reproductive functioning
	Female ovaries: oestrogens	• Secondary sexual characteristics

from triglycerides, and thus has only a minor role in gluconeogenesis.

The role of the pancreas in glucose homeostasis

The endocrine component of the pancreas consists of the islets of Langerhans, which contain hormone-secreting cells. Alpha cells secrete glucagon; beta cells, insulin; delta cells, somatostatin and gamma cells, pancreatic polypeptides. It is the alpha, beta and delta cells that have the primary role in blood glucose homeostasis. The plasma glucose level is the most important determinant of the rate of insulin release from the beta cells or glucagon from the alpha cells. High levels of glucose trigger insulin secretion and low plasma glucose leads to glucagon secretion which in turn promotes glycogenolysis by the liver. Thus insulin may

be considered an anabolic hormone whereas glucagon is catabolic in nature. Insulin and glucagon have an inhibitory effect on each other and both can be inhibited by somatostatin: thus there is complex interplay between the three hormones. Figure 11.5 gives a summary of the control of blood glucose by pancreatic enzymes and the liver.

Glucagon

In an emergency, glucagon can be administered intravenously to a patient who is hypoglycaemic, but unable to take glucose orally.

• Blood glucose will rise by inhibiting the secretion of insulin by the pancreas stimulating the liver to breakdown glycogen into glucose (glycogenolysis).

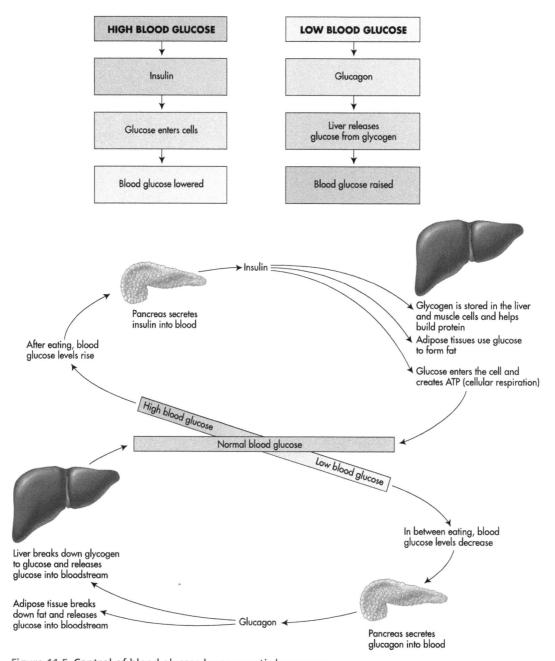

Figure 11.5 Control of blood glucose by pancreatic hormones

Insulin secretion can also be triggered by an increase in amino acids (e.g. a high protein meal) and ingestion of food as a result of hormones released by the gastrointestinal mucosa. Type I diabetes: insulin-dependents diabetes mellitus (IDDM) is the result of a primary defect in the ability of the pancreatic islet tissue to respond to glucose with a release of insulin.

Insulin performs many important functions, including:

- *Facilitating the transport of glucose into cells.*
- *Promoting glycogen storage in the liver and muscles* – by activating enzymes to enable the storage of glucose.

- *Converting glucose into fat* – Excess glucose is initially used to form glycogen, but a surplus will be converted into fat by the liver and then later released for storage in fat tissues.
- *Inhibiting fat metabolism* – Cells exploit glucose preferentially for energy facilitated by insulin. The presence of the insulin inhibits fat metabolism while glucose is utilised. In the absence of insulin (either due to low glucose levels or inadequate circulating levels of insulin) fat metabolism is increased and free fatty acids released into the circulation. These are used as an alternative energy source as the cells are unable to take up glucose due to the lack of insulin. It is this mechanism

that accounts for the weight loss exhibited by new Type I diabetics.

- *Promoting protein deposition in cells and tissue growth* – A lack of insulin will also lead to protein being used as alternative energy by cells. It is the utilisation by the cells of amino acids (protein) and free fatty acids that results in ketoacidosis.

The role of the liver in glucose homeostasis

The greatest amount of glucose input during the periods between meals and during the overnight fast comes from the contribution by the liver. The liver plays such an important role in glucose production that a total hepatectomy will result in death within 24 hours due to hypoglycaemia. The liver donates glucose to the plasma by two general mechanisms:

- the breakdown of stored glycogen (glycogenolysis);
- the formation of glucose from non glucose precursors (gluconeogenesis).

If dietary glucose is available, the liver increases its store of glycogen, but this is limited to 75–100g. The minimum required by the body daily is 125–150g in order to supply the brain, for which glucose is a mandatory requirement. During fasting, the initial source of glucose is from stored glycogen, but as this is restricted, amino acids (released from tissue protein) contribute about 75g of glucose daily via gluconeogenesis. This is mostly muscle protein, but there is a degree of protein breakdown from most organs. Glycerol (released from adipose tissue) can be converted to glucose by the liver, providing a further source of glucose, but can only contribute about 20g. Finally, lactate (produced from muscle) can also be metabolised by the liver for gluconeogenesis and thus additional glucose.

> ### Catecholamines in the acutely ill
>
> An increase in adrenaline or noradrenaline levels due to stress of critical illness (sympathetic nervous system stimulation) or via infusion to manage hypotension, can result in hyperglycaemia.
>
> Catecholamines stimulate glycogen breakdown into glucose by the liver (glycogenolysis) and inhibit insulin secretion by the pancreas. A patient may therefore require an insulin infusion *temporarily* to control the high blood sugar.

The liver is responsive to plasma glucose levels, with low levels resulting in a release of glucose (by glycogenolysis) and high levels leading to glucose uptake. However, the liver also very sensitive to levels of insulin (and glucagon) as glycogenolysis will continue to occur even in the face of a high plasma glucose level (as in the diabetic without insulin) identifying the importance of the hormonal influence. In the presence of insulin however, glycogenolysis is inhibited whereas glucagon will have the opposite effect. The role of the liver in glucose metabolism is summarised in Figure 11.6.

The role of the kidney in glucose homeostasis

No glucose is excreted by the kidney under normal conditions. Glucose is filtered into the glomerular fluid, and is reabsorbed, but in hyperglycaemia some of the glucose will be present in the urine (glycosuria). The presence of the glucose in the distal tubules raises the osmotic pressure of the urine and reduces the amount of water reabsorbed by the proximal tubule, thus resulting in an increase in urine output (polyuria) and subsequent hypovolaemia (triggering thirst – polydipsia). This accounts for these symptoms being predominant in the presentation of diabetes mellitus. Sustained hyperglycaemia will result in dehydration with fluids and electrolytes lost from the body as a result of an osmotic diuresis.

Utilisation of glucose

All tissues utilise plasma glucose, with some being obligatory users that cannot mobilise alternative substances when glucose is unavailable. Nervous tissue is unable to utilise free fatty acids (FFA) which are a major circulating fuel, hence the serious neurological sequelae of hypoglycaemia. Other tissues that require exclusively glucose include red blood cells, the intestinal mucosa and the renal medulla. The remaining tissues are facultative users of glucose. When FFA levels are high and glucose and insulin levels low, they will switch to use FFA as their primary metabolic fuel.

Insulin facilitates the entry of glucose into cells. Type II diabetes: non-insulin-dependent diabetes mellitus (NIDDM) manifests as a relative insensitivity of the tissues to plasma insulin. The rate of glucose uptake by the cells is multifactorial and is influenced by:

- *Plasma glucose levels* – Raised plasma glucose levels will result in an increase in the rate of cellular uptake. This is maximised in the presence of insulin.
- *Presence of free fatty acids* – In the fasting state, elevation of FFA levels will inhibit glucose utilisation by the peripheral tissues, helping to conserve the limited supply of glucose required for the brain to function.
- *Muscular work* – The rate of glucose uptake into skeletal and cardiac muscle is enhanced by muscular contraction; hence insulin-dependent diabetics reduce their insulin requirements when anticipating vigorous exercise.

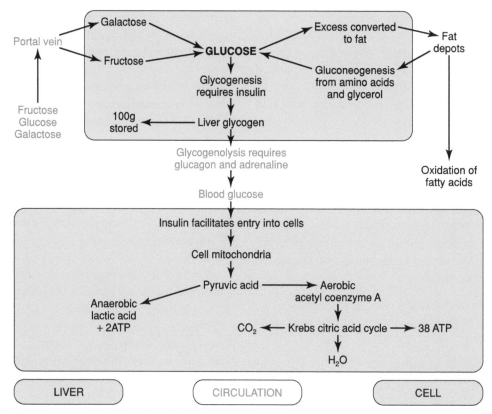

Figure 11.6 The role of the liver in glucose metabolism

- *Hormonal effects* – Insulin is the most important hormone controlling rates of glucose removal from the plasma. However, increased levels of catecholamines (adrenaline and noradrenaline) will reduce cellular glucose uptake (and increase rate of glycogenolysis by the liver) with the net effect of increasing plasma glucose levels.

A summary of the characteristics of diabetes is shown in Table 11.2.

Acute endocrine problems and emergencies

Thyroid storm/crisis

Hyperthyroidism results from an excess of thyroid hormones (T3 and T4), with an exaggerated form being a thyroid crisis. A thyroid crisis (or storm) can be triggered by infection, surgery, trauma or any other acute episode

Table 11.2 Summary of diabetes

Insulin-dependent diabetes mellitus (IDDM)	Non-insulin-dependent diabetes mellitus (NIDDM)
Type I diabetes	Type II diabetes
• Less common (10% of diabetics)	• Increasingly common (90% of diabetics)
• Sudden onset at any age, but mostly affecting young persons. Usually underweight or normal weight at diagnosis	• Gradual onset, mostly in adults. Usually overweight at diagnosis
• Characterised by a deficiency of insulin being produced by the beta cells in the islets of Langerhans in the pancreas. This is thought to be immune induced in most cases	• Characterised by an insulin resistance (cause unknown) which may be combined with a relative reduction in insulin production
• Managed by insulin administration	• Managed by dietary control and oral hypoglycaemic medications

Gestational diabetes

This is diabetes occurring during pregnancy (2–5% of pregnancies) and most closely resembles type II diabetes. This often self-corrects post-delivery but affected mothers have a predisposition to develop type II diabetes later in life.

(e.g. myocardial infarction, stroke and eclampsia), but fortunately is very rare. An over-secretion of thyroid hormones will lead to a hypermetabolic state resulting in hyperpyrexia, tachycardia, hypertension, agitation and tremors. The management is aimed essentially at reducing the effects of these hormones until the patient is stable. Drug therapy will include the use of beta-blockers, sedatives, hydrocortisone and specific anti-thyroid drugs such as Lugol's iodine or carbimazole.

> **Pharmacology for hyperthyroidism**
>
> **Carbimazole** is converted to thiamazole (methimazole) which inhibits enzymes that play a role in T3 and T4 production.
>
> **Lugol's iodine:**
>
> - Named after French physician J Lugol; first made in 1829 as a solution of iodine and potassium iodide to be used as an antiseptic and disinfectant.
> - More recently is used to inhibit thyroxine release and treat some forms of hyperthyroidism. Certain autoimmune causes of hyperthyroidism are contraindicated as Lugol's iodine may result in such effective blockade that hypothyroidism may result.

Myxoedema coma

Myxoedema results from decreased thyroid hormone secretion, with signs such as bradycardia and slow mental functioning being representative of the hypometabolic state. A myxoedema coma (rare, but with a high mortality) can occur in a patient with a chronic condition who is challenged by additional stress such as trauma. The extreme hypometabolic condition will result in bradycardia leading to hypotension and poor tissue perfusion which in turn can result in a metabolic acidosis. Hypoventilation may result from the decreased conscious level leading to hypercarbia and hypoxia. Other manifestations that may occur include fatigue, paralytic ileus, reduced cardiac output and an increased sensitivity to drugs, e.g. opiates. The coma itself is likely to have been caused by multiple contributory factors including the primary hypometabolism and secondary hypothermia, hypoxia, hypercarbia and hypoglycaemia. Management strategies are focused upon organ support and addressing the causative emergency, i.e. by administration of thyroxine.

Adrenal insufficiency

Addison's disease is a chronic deficiency of cortical hormones, with symptoms reflecting the lack of cortisol (muscle weakness, fatigue, hypoglycaemia, ileus, reduced immunity to infection, low cardiac output), aldosterone (polyuria, dehydration, thirst, hypovolaemia, hyponatraemia, hyperkalaemia, postural hypotension, arrhythmias) and androgens (loss of libido and body hair). The condition is controlled by lifelong hormone replacement therapy.

In times of stress (e.g. surgery, trauma, infection) where the increased demand for cortisol cannot be met, a patient may develop an Addisonian crisis or acute adrenal insufficiency. The immediate management of this life-threatening emergency will include urgent rehydration and correction of the hypoglycaemia. Cortisol will need to be administered, e.g. in the form of intravenous hydrocortisone, and the trigger for the crisis (e.g. infection) addressed.

> **Causes of acute adrenal insufficiency:**
>
> - abrupt withdrawal of steroid therapy;
> - stress, trauma, infection, surgery;
> - addison's disease;
> - pituitary or hypothalamic damage.

Phaeochromocytoma or catecholamine crisis

A phaechromocytoma is a (very rare) tumour of the adrenal medulla whereby abnormally high levels of adrenaline and noradrenaline are secreted into the systemic circulation. The release of these catecholamines is intermittent, but results in headaches, tachycardia, hyperglycaemia, blurred vision, bowel disturbances and very severe hypertension. Following blood pressure stabilisation (usually with alpha- and beta-blockers) a phaechromocytoma will require surgical removal.

Diabetes insipidus (DI)

This is due to an insufficiency of ADH (antidiuretic hormone) being produced by the posterior pituitary. This can be precipitated by neuropathology affecting the hypothalamus or pituitary, or rarely, by an insensitivity of the kidney to ADH (nephrogenic diabetes insipidus). It results in excessive water loss (polyuria) and if untreated the patient will become profoundly hypovolaemic and hypernatraemic (as water is lost in excess of sodium). This situation is managed by the administration of desmopressin (DDAVP).

Syndrome of inappropriate antidiuretic hormone hypersecretion (SIADH)

This is characterised by excessive antidiuretic hormone (ADH) being secreted by the posterior pituitary gland. Its aetiology includes neuropathology (e.g. head injury, subarachnoid haemorrhage) or some carcinomas or infections. SIADH causes water retention (potential fluid overload) and haemodilution of solutes resulting in hyponatraemia. Initial management necessitates fluid restriction with some situations including the administration of saline, but extreme care must be taken not to increase the plasma sodium by more than 12mmol/L per 24 hours (i.e. 0.5mmol per hour). It is important that SIADH is differentiated from other conditions causing hyponatraemia (e.g. cerebral salt-wasting syndrome) in which there is an accompanying hypovolaemia, as opposed to hypervolaemia, with its corresponding implications for fluid management strategies.

Diabetic emergencies

Endocrine emergencies account for about 1.5% of medical emergency admissions in England, and the majority are related to diabetes (Kearney and Dang 2007). Early recognition and treatment of possible problems, with an understanding of glucose management, is essential for the nurse caring for patients with diabetes. The most common problems are:

- hypoglycaemia;
- hyperglycaemia either due to diabetic ketoacidosis (DKA) or hyperglycaemic hyperosmolar syndrome (HHS).

Hypoglycaemia
Hypoglycaemia is a biochemical diagnosis based on a blood glucose of less than 3mmol/L. The patient who is hypoglycaemic will exhibit autonomic symptoms such as sweating, warmth sensation, anxiety, nausea and palpitations as a result of sympathetic nervous system stimulation. Other symptoms (e.g. tiredness, poor coordination, visual disturbances, drowsiness, confusion, coma, seizures) are due to the effects of low glucose levels upon the nervous system (neuroglycopenia). The autonomic symptoms usually occur first, with neuroglycopenia more evident with a blood glucose of less than 2.5mmol/L.

> Once a patient has had a severe episode of hypoglycaemia, they may have impaired recognition of hypoglycaemia symptoms over the subsequent 24 hours.

Mild episodes can be treated by consuming refined carbohydrates, such as dextrose tablets, followed by long-acting carbohydrates, e.g. biscuits. Otherwise patients may be treated with 'hypostop' (30% glucose) which is a gel that is applied to the buccal mucosa. In unconscious patients 1mg of glucagon can be given, intramuscular (IM) or

intravenous (IV). Hospitalised patients may be treated with 250mL of 10% dextrose (IV) administered over a few minutes, and followed by a continuous infusion depending upon local hospital guidelines. If no IV access is available, glucagon may be given intramuscularly. The administration of high concentrations of dextrose intravenously carries the risk of thrombophlebitis, therefore cannulae insertion sites should be monitored closely.

> **Iatrogenic hypoglycaemia**
> One cause of hypoglycaemia that can be prevented is iatrogenic, i.e. caused by health care professionals. An example of this would be stopping artificial feeding (enteral or total parenteral nutrition) e.g. for procedures such as CT scan, but leaving an insulin infusion running!

Severe hypoglycaemia (blood glucose less than 1mmol/L) is a medical emergency and if prolonged for more than a few minutes is likely to damage the brain.

Hyperglycaemia: diabetic ketoacidosis (DKA) and hyperglycaemic hyperosmolar syndrome (HHS)
Most cases of DKA occur in patients with diabetes, most commonly type I diabetes, but occasionally type II. DKA is a triad of hyperglycaemia, ketosis and acidaemia. Both DKA and HHS are triggered commonly by infection, but may be secondary to trauma, myocardial infarction and non-compliance with diabetes management. These emergencies may occur also in previously undiagnosed diabetics, thus being a first presentation of diabetes mellitus. Some of the similarities and differences between DKA and HHS are presented in Table 11.3.

DKA and HHS are caused by an absolute or relative deficiency of effective circulating insulin with associated increased levels of glucagon, catecholamines, cortisol

> **Ketoacidosis**
> A metabolic condition associated with an accumulation of ketone bodies. Ketones (acetoacetic acid and beta hydroxybutyrate) result from the breakdown of free fatty acids and deamination of amino acids. Ketones can be smelt on the breath (like fruit or nail polish remover) due to acetone (from acetoacetic acid).
>
> **Differential diagnosis:**
> - *diabetic ketoacidosis* – known history of diabetes;
> - *alcoholic ketoacidosis* – usually known history of alcohol abuse (no hyperglycaemia).
>
> Starvation: ketosis (rather than ketoacidosis) (no hyperglycaemia).

Table 11.3 Comparisons and contrasts between DKA and HHS

	Diabetic ketoacidosis (DKA)	Hyperglycaemic hyperosmolar syndrome (HHS)
Definitions (American Diabetic Association)	• Blood glucose > 13.8mmol/L • PH < 7.30 • Bicarbonate < 18mmol/L • Anion gap > 10 • Ketonaemia	• Blood glucose > 33.3mmol/L • Ph < 7.30 • Bicarbonate > 15mmol/L • Serum osmolality > 320osmol/kg
Demographics	• Most commonly younger, slimmer patients with type I diabetes • Mortality less than 5% – most common cause of death in young people with diabetes	• More commonly older, obese patients with type II diabetes • Mortality 15%
Presentation	• Rapid onset (< 24 hours) • Vomiting, polyuria, polydipsia, weight loss plus abdominal pain	• Insidious onset (several days – weeks) • Vomiting, polyuria, polydipsia, weight loss
Physical signs	• As per hypovolaemia: tachycardia, hypotension, low CVP • Confusion is rare	• As per hypovolaemia: tachycardia, hypotension, low CVP • Confusion more common
Biochemistry	• Blood glucose rarely greater than 40mmol/L • Ketones in urine	• Blood glucose often greater than 50mmol/L • No ketones in the urine

and growth hormone. These result in increased glycogenolysis by the liver, generating hyperglycaemia. In DKA, the deficiency of insulin and increased counter-regulatory hormones lead to increased lipolysis and production of ketone bodies, with a resulting metabolic acidosis. The disturbed acid-base balance due to the metabolic acidosis is due to the dissociation of the H^+ ion from the ketone body acetoacetic acid. Patients with HSS do not develop ketoacidosis, but the mechanism for this is unclear.

Both DKA and HHS present with vomiting, and a history of polyuria, polydipsia and weight loss. Patients with DKA can additionally have abdominal pain, although the underlying pathophysiology for this is unclear. Confusion is more common in HHS and believed to be related to the increase in serum osmolality rather than the hyperglycaemia.

Physical signs include those associated with hypovolaemia (see patient assessment) resulting from the polyuria. This has been estimated to reach 5–8 litres in DKA and 8–10 litres in HHS (Kearney and Dang 2007). The excessive urine output leads to depletion in sodium, potassium, magnesium and phosphates.

The main aims for treating both DKA and HHS are to correct dehydration, decrease the blood glucose level, correct electrolyte abnormalities and treat any precipitating causes, such as infection. These principles are discussed under 'Maximising endocrine status'. Some patients with DKA or HHS will require initial management in the intensive care unit.

Hypovolaemia and urine output

Although patients with DKA or HHS will develop hypovolaemia (as a result of polyuria) they will still be passing urine. This is in contrast to patients who are hypovolaemic from other (non-diabetic) causes (e.g. haemorrhage) who will be oliguric or even anuric.

Assessment and physical examination

A systematic ABCDE approach to patient assessment is essential in order to identify problems and initiate appropriate and timely interventions. Patients with DKA may have airway problems due to deteriorating levels of consciousness. Respiratory assessment may reveal signs of hypoxaemia and respiratory distress if a chest infection is the cause of the disruption in glucose homeostasis. Tachypnoea, with deep sighing respirations, can occur as a result of respiratory compensation for the metabolic acidosis arising from their ketoacidosis. Those with DKA or HHS may be cardiovascularly unstable as a result of hyperglycaemia because their urine output may be inappropriately high (due to excreting excess glucose accompanied by water), resulting in severe hypovolaemia and dehydration with associated tachycardia, hypotension and hypothermia. The hypoglycaemic patient is often clammy or sweaty, whereas the patient with hyperglycaemia typically appears warm and dry, hence touching the patient may be informative. Disability assessment (including blood glucose measurement) will reveal hypo- or hyperglycaemia and may demonstrate altered neurological function (confusion, weakness and reduced level of consciousness) caused by altered glucose levels. Abnormal observations should always be reported immediately (NMC 2010), particularly adverse changes in neurological status. Finally, measurement of the blood glucose, biochemistry and electrolytes will assist in identifying the underlying cause of the endocrine dysfunction. Table 11.4 gives an account of assessment findings of people with abnormal blood glucose levels.

Table 11.4 Summary of examination and assessment

	Variable	Hypoglycaemia	DKA	HHS
A/B	• Airway patency • Respiratory rate pattern • O$_2$ saturations	• Most commonly: normal respiratory rate and pattern	• Tachypnoea • **Kussmaul breathing** (rapid, deep laboured) due to respiratory compensation for a metabolic acidosis	• Most commonly: normal respiratory rate and pattern
C	• BP • Pulse • Capillary refill time (CRT) • Skin • CVP • Temperature • Urine output	• Sweating • Palpitations due to sympathetic nervous system (SNS) stimulation	• Tachycardia, hypotension, low CVP due to hypovolaemia • Increased CRT • Dysrhythmias due to electrolyte imbalance • Often hypothermic • Urine output may be inappropriately high due to hyperglycaemia	• Tachycardia, hypotension, low CVP due to hypovolaemia • Increased CRT • Dysrhythmias due to electrolyte imbalance • Often hypothermic • Urine output may be inappropriately high due to hyperglycaemia
D	• GCS pain assessment	• Anxiety (due to SNS stimulation) • Tiredness, poor coordination, visual disturbances, drowsiness, confusion, coma, seizures are due to the effects of low glucose levels upon the nervous system (neuroglycopenia) • Reduced level of consciousness due to neuroglycopenia • Low GCS	• Confusion, lethargy, reduced level of consciousness	• Confusion (thought to be due to increased serum osmolality)
E1	• Blood results	• Blood glucose < 3mmol/L	• Blood glucose > 13.8mmol/L • PH < 7.30 • Bicarbonate < 18mmol/L • Anion gap > 10 • Ketonaemia • Hyponatraemia • Hypo/hyperkalaemia • Hypomagnesaemia • Hypo- or hyperphosphataemia	• Blood glucose > 33.3mmol/L • Ph < 7.30 • Bicarbonate > 15mmol/L • Serum osmolality > 320osmols/kg • Small amount (or no) ketones • Hyponatraemia • Hypo/hyperkalaemia • Hypomagnesaemia • Hypo- or hyperphosphataemia
E2	• Other	• Nausea (due to SNS stimulation)	• Nausea, vomiting • Abdominal pain • Acetone smell on breath due to ketones	

CASE STUDY 11.1 Mr Richards, type I diabetic: hypoglycaemic secondary to chest sepsis – Part 1

INITIAL ASSESSMENT

Mr Richards, 61 years old, is brought to A&E with shortness of breath and a temperature. He has a past medical history of type I diabetes. He is a coach driver and appears overweight.

Airway/breathing

On assessment, his nurse notes he is able to speak a sentence but is very short of breath. He is drowsy and says he feels unwell. He has a respiratory rate of 23/minute on 4L oxygen via a non-fixed-performance Hudson mask with oxygen saturations of 93%, suggesting he is hypoxic as this is below his target saturation of 94–98%. The nurse requests an arterial blood gas sample. He is using accessory muscles with poor respiratory excursion. He has bilateral air entry with coarse crackles at the lung bases and is expectorating thick yellow secretions with difficulty. She checks that the bedside suction equipment is working as he may need help clearing secretions.

Circulation

His temperature is 38°C, with hot peripheries. He feels thirsty. He has a capillary refill time of less than two seconds. His pulse is 99 beats per minute and is regular and bounding. These observations all suggest he is vasodilated as a result of systemic infection. His manual BP is 110/40mmHg. He has two peripheral lines inserted as there is concern that he may become more unstable. He has intravenous fluid prescribed to prevent dehydration because of high insensible losses due to pyrexia and tachypnoea. He has not passed urine since admission. A fluid balance chart is started.

Disability

His GCS is 15/15 and blood glucose is 17mmol/L (normal 4–10mmol/L). This suggests catecholamines have stimulated glycogen breakdown (glycogenolysis) into glucose and inhibited insulin production to meet the increased energy demands of a raised metabolic rate secondary to infection. His nurse discusses his normal insulin regime. He is on twice daily subcutaneous (SC) insulin with meals (in addition to a daily long-acting insulin). It is now 1800h. He has his evening dose and she checks he eats supper.

Exposure

Mr Richards looks flushed and feels clammy. The nurse reads his notes and finds that his BMI is 40, confirming obesity. His abdomen is large but soft. He is splinting his diaphragm which will contribute to his shortness of breath, so she sits him up. He has bowel sounds, is not constipated and is pain free. His nurse notices nicotine stains on his fingers and asks if he smokes. He says he has smoked about 20 cigarettes a day for the last 45 years.

Diagnosis

Given his history and presentation, a provisional diagnosis is made of sepsis secondary to a chest infection.

> Sepsis kills more people in the UK annually than lung cancer or bowel and breast cancer combined. The international *Surviving Sepsis Campaign* guideline (2008) suggests *sepsis* can be diagnosed when patients have two or more specific signs and symptoms present with a history suggestive of a new infection: temperature > 38.3°C or < 36°C, pulse > 90 beats per minute, respiratory rate > 20/min, white blood cells < 4 or > 12 × 10⁹/L acutely altered mental status and hyperglycaemia (glucose > 6mmol/L unless diabetic).

Mr Richards is tachypnoeic, dyspnoeic and hypoxaemic. His nurse is aware that he has the potential to deteriorate rapidly. A modified early warning score (MEWS) at this stage would have given a score of two points (see below).

Modified early warning score

Score	3	2	1	0	1	2	3
Systolic BP	< 70	71–80	81–100	101–199		> 200	
Heart rate		< 40	41–50	51–100	101–110	111–129	> 130
Respiratory rate		< 9		9–14	15–20	21–29	> 30
Temperature		< 35		35–38.4		> 38.5	
AVPU				A	V	P	U

He has a productive cough, is pyrexial and a smoker which are all suggestive of infection. Doctors request a portable chest X-ray (CXR), arterial blood gas, routine bloods, 12-lead ECG, sputum sample for MCS, urinary catheter and blood cultures. Following the septic screen he is commenced on IV antibiotics. A urinary dipstick is performed, which being normal further supports the notion that his chest is the likely source of sepsis. He is prescribed SC Tinzeparin and anti-thrombolytic stockings as he has a high risk of thrombus formation secondary to high BMI, smoking history and reduced mobility. An elective CTPA scan is performed and a pulmonary embolus excluded. He is transferred to the medical assessment unit for ongoing care.

> GCS measures responsiveness (eye movement, verbal response and limb movement). Always describe the score in detail, e.g. a GCS score of 13/15 being E: 3 V: 4 M: 6. A GCS score of 8/15 or less is potentially life threatening as the patient may not be able to maintain or protect their airway so request urgent expert medical help in accordance with your local escalation algorithm for the *Acutely Ill Patients in Hospital* (NICE 2007). Hypoglycaemia is a common cause of a reduced GCS on the wards and can present with drowsiness, confusion or coma due to its effect on the nervous system (neuroglycopenia). Always check a blood glucose if a patient's GCS drops.

Maximising endocrine status

Insulin administration

Insulin treatment will increase glucose utilisation in peripheral tissues and also decrease glucose production by the liver. It also decreases the formation of ketones and inhibits the release of free fatty acids (FFAs), thereby correcting the metabolic acidosis. The use of low-dose insulin (initially six units/hour) is standard for DKA and HHS with an ultimate aim of a blood glucose between 10–15mmol/L over 24–48 hours. The use of insulin may lead to hypokalaemia, as it facilitates movement of potassium into cells. Close electrolyte monitoring is therefore essential and replacement administered to maintain serum potassium between 4–5mmol/L.

> **National Patient Safety Agency (NPSA) insulin safety guidance (2010)**
>
> Recommendations to reduce the number of wrong dose incidents involving insulin:
>
> - All insulin bolus doses should be measured and administered using an insulin syringe (not intravenous syringe).
> - The term 'units' should be used at all times (not u or iu).
> - Training programmes should be in place for all health care professionals involved in the administration of insulin.

The transition from insulin infusion to the subcutaneous route is challenging, but should be attempted once the patient is stable and is able to eat and drink. The American Diabetic Association (2004) suggests criteria such as: blood glucose less than 11mmol/L, bicarbonate greater than 18mmol/L and pH greater than 7.30.

Glycaemic control

Normal fasting blood glucose levels are 3.5–5.5mmol/L, fluctuating to 7–9mmol/L following a meal. Insulin infusions are titrated against a sliding scale of blood sugars, aiming usually for a blood sugar within the 'normal range'. It is well recognised that hyperglycaemia is toxic: Falciglia *et al.* (2009) demonstrated an increase in mortality of ICU patients with a blood glucose of greater than 6.1mmol/L which was unrelated to illness severity. However, such tight control over blood sugar brings logistical challenges with the frequency of monitoring of blood glucose, and more importantly, a risk of iatrogenic hypoglycaemia which can be harmful. A blood glucose of 2.2mmol/L is associated with a sixfold increase in mortality, and lower levels could be fatal. Hence local recommendations are

to maintain a blood glucose between 4 and 10mmol/L rather than strictly between 4 and 6mmol/L in the critical care setting (see NICE-SUGAR Study 2009). Medications should be administered as prescribed, with relevant monitoring of levels, electrolytes and vital signs as indicated for each medication (NMC 2010).

> **NICE-SUGAR Study (2009) – a large randomised controlled trial**
>
> On admission to intensive care, patients were randomised to:
>
> - either maintain intensive glucose control of between 4.5–6.0mmol/L;
> - or conventional glucose control – less than 10mmol/L.
>
> Although there was no difference between the two groups regarding length of stay on intensive care, the conclusion of this large multi-centre international trial was that intensive glucose control increased mortality among adults in intensive care.
>
> There were also significantly more episodes of severe hypoglycaemia (less than 2.2mmol/L) in the group with intensive glycaemic control (6.8% versus 0.5%) and increased morbidity.

Fluid and electrolyte management

Fluid administration for hypovolaemic patients (DKA and HHS) commonly includes using isotonic/normal saline (0.9% NaCl), but hypernatraemic patients may need half normal saline (0.45%NaCl). Correcting the fluid deficit will increase the intravascular volume and lower the plasma osmolality and blood glucose levels by dilution. The infusion rate will depend upon the circumstances, but the initial aim would be to correct the hypovolaemia within 24 hours. Hyponatraemia should be corrected cautiously as rapid increases in serum sodium levels can precipitate severe neurological problems, e.g.

> **Hyperglycaemia and serum sodium**
>
> Measured serum sodium needs to be recalculated in hyperglycaemia to obtain a 'true sodium level'. This is because extracellular osmolality rises in the presence of excess glucose (as slower to enter cells if relative lack of insulin) with water accompanying the glucose into the extracellular fluid. As the extracellular fluid is diluted, the sodium concentration falls. This is described as a translational hyponatraemia because there is no change in total body water. The sodium level will not need to be treated as this will correct itself as the glucose level normalises.
>
> A formula for correcting the sodium:
>
> measured sodium + 1/3 × blood glucose = approximate sodium
>
> e.g. measured sodium 140mmol/L + 1/3 glucose 60mmol = sodium 160mmol/L (approximately)

cerebral oedema. The chronicity of the situation should be considered with acute hyponatraemia (< 48 hours) being more amenable to a faster correction than a long-standing condition, however plasma sodium levels should not be increased faster than 12mmol per 24 hours.

Hypokalaemia will need correction, particularly with respect to patients receiving insulin, to attain levels between 4–5mmol/L. Patients who are hypokalaemic due to polyuria are at risk of having their hypokalaemia exacerbated iatrogenically when large fluid volumes are administered as they will be haemodiluted. Fluid administration in these circumstances should therefore include a potassium supplement. Phosphate depletion is common in DKA, but replacement is seldom required.

Pharmacological interventions

Oral hypoglycaemics include:

- *Sulphonylureas* – e.g. glibencamide, gliclazide, chlorpro-pamide, tolbutamide. These drugs lower blood glucose

levels by increasing insulin production by the pancreas. They may also increase the sensitivity of the tissues to insulin. Drug interactions may include NSAIDs (including aspirin) enhancing the effect and thiazide diuretics reducing efficacy.

- *Metformin* – this belongs to a group of chemicals called biguanides. The mechanism of action is not understood fully, but it may stimulate uptake of glucose into muscle and reduce glucose release from the liver. It is most commonly prescribed in conjunction with a sulphonylurea if a patient is not responding to the latter alone.

- *Thiazolidinediones* – e.g. pioglitazone, rosiglitazone which belong to chemicals called glitazones. They appear to reduce tissue resistance to insulin and are usually administered alongside a sulphonylurea or metformin.

- *Prandial (relating to a meal) glucose regulators* – nateglinide and repaglinide have differing mechanisms of action but both are unique in that they act postprandially (after eating) to stimulate insulin release by the pancreas.

CASE STUDY 11.2 Mr Richards, type I diabetic: hypoglycaemic secondary to chest sepsis – Part 2

RECOGNISING EARLY DETERIORATION

The A&E nurse hands over using an SBAR framework (situation, background, assessment and recommendations). Recommendations include continuous cardiac and oxygen saturation monitoring, hourly manual observations and blood glucose measurements, 40% fixed performance oxygen, regular saline nebulisers, physiotherapist referral and appropriate pressure-relieving mattress. Doctors review his arterial blood gas and blood results and discuss their implications with the nurses caring for Mr Richards.

Blood results

	Result	Normal range
Hb	13.2g/dL	13–16g/dL in men
WBC	17.5 10⁹/L	4.4–10 10⁹/L
C-reactive protein (CRP)	210mg/L	0–5mg/L
Urea	13mmol/L	3–6mmol/L
Creatinine	100umol/L	60–120umol/L

COMMENTARY

Mr Richards' haemoglobin is normal. This was checked to exclude anaemia as a cause of reduced oxygen saturations and tachypnoea. In the hypoxaemic patient (paO$_2$ < 8kpa on air), it is common to maintain haemoglobin levels at least 10g/L to facilitate oxygen delivery (DO$_2$). (DO$_2$ depends

upon cardiac output, haemoglobin and oxygen saturation.) His white blood cell (leukocyte) count and CRP levels are both raised. A WBC count will rise with a new infection as additional leukocytes are produced to attack bacteria. Increased levels of CRP are produced by macrophages due to the presence of bacteria and so act as a 'marker' of infection. His urea and creatinine are checked to assess renal function and guide his IV fluid regime. He is pyrexial and tachypnoeic with a productive cough. He is at greater risk of 'pre-renal' renal failure secondary to dehydration. His elevated urea in the presence of a normal range creatinine demonstrates this. In view of the dehydration 500mL of IV colloid is given stat, and maintenance IV fluids are increased to 1litre/2 hours.

Arterial blood gas

	Result	Normal range
pH	7.32	7.35–7.45
PaCO$_2$	4.5	4.5–6.1kpa
PaO$_2$	9.5	11–13.5kpa
HCO$_3^-$	21	24–26mmol/L
BE	–4	–2 to +2
SaO$_2$	94%	96–100%
Inspired oxygen	40% fixed performance	
Serum lactate	4.1	< 2mmol/L

CASE STUDY 11.2 Mr Richards, type I diabetic: hypoglycaemic secondary to chest sepsis – Part 2 (*continued*)

Commentary

His arterial blood gas shows a metabolic acidosis
(pH low = acidosis, CO_2 normal = not respiratory, HCO_3 low
= metabolic) with a type I respiratory failure (hypoxaemia
without raised CO_2). His serum lactate is elevated. Serum
lactate levels rise in the presence of cellular hypoxia and
as such are a 'marker' of the switch from normal aerobic
to abnormal anaerobic metabolism. This occurs when
oxygen delivery to cells is either reduced (e.g. with severe
hypoxaemia) or cannot meet demand (e.g. secondary to
a raised metabolic rate in sepsis). His inspired oxygen is
increased to 60% in response to the hypoxaemia and
reduced oxygen saturations. His CXR is reviewed and shows
bilateral basal consolidation supporting the likelihood of a
chest infection.

The nurse returns to Mr Richards to assess vital signs and
finds him unresponsive, but he is breathing and has a pulse
(cardiac output). The nurse calls for assistance and a cardiac
arrest call is put out as he is peri-arrest in accordance with
the local escalation algorithm for the *Acutely Ill Patients
in Hospital* (NICE 2007). Meanwhile, with help from a
colleague, he is put in the recovery position and reassessed
(A/B: patent airway, RR 26 breaths per minute, SpO$_2$
94%, C: HR 120 beats per minute, BP 100/45mmHg,
D Unresponsive). The team arrive and reassess Mr Richards.
He is put onto the cardiac monitor via defibrillator pads as
he may deteriorate. In addition to the above observations,
he is hot and sweating profusely with a temperature of
38.8°C, his GCS is 5/15 (E 1 V1 M3), pupils are equal and
reactive to light (3mm) and blood glucose is 2.4mmol/L.

The international *Surviving Sepsis Campaign* guidelines
(2008) suggest *severe sepsis* is present if any of the
following (plus others) are present:

- systolic blood pressure < 90mmHg or mean < 65mmHg
- new or increased oxygen requirement to maintain SpO$_2$
  > 90%
- urine output < 0.5mL/kg/hrfor 2 hours
- lactate > 2mmol/L.

The *Sepsis six* interventions should be implemented within
the first hour of diagnosis:

1 85% fixed performance oxygen
2 Blood cultures
3 IV antibiotics
4 Fluid challenge
5 Arterial blood gasses and lactate
6 Fluid balance chart and monitor urine output

(Dellinger *et al.* 2008)

At this stage, a modified early warning score (MEWS)
would have given a score of 10 points (see below).

Modified early warning score

Score	3	2	1	0	1	2	3
Systolic BP	< 70	71–80	**81–100**	101–199		> 200	
Heart rate		< 40	41–50	51–100	101–110	**111–129**	> 130
Respiratory Rate		< 9		9–14	15–20	21–29	> 30
Temperature		< 35		35–38.4		**> 38.5**	
AVPU				A	V	P	U

Doctors diagnose a reduced GCS secondary to profound
hypoglycaemia (< 2.5mmol/L) caused by sepsis. Causes of
hypoglycaemia in sepsis are thought to be multifactorial but
may include depleted glucagon stores in the liver, impaired
gluconeogenesis and increased cellular utilisation of glucose.
It is an increasingly common medical emergency. Mr Richards
is given 250mL 10% dextrose IV in 50mL incremental doses
as priority with blood glucose checks every 5 minutes. His
blood glucose rises to 7.5mmol/L and he becomes responsive
with a GCS of 13/15, soon improving to 15/15. A 10%
dextrose infusion is commenced to keep the blood glucose
between 4 and 10mmol/L.

On reassessment following these interventions, his MEWS score
reduces from 10 to 6 as his systolic BP has risen from 100 to
110mmHg and he is now awake. As he is still tachypnoeic,
tachycardic and pyrexial, he remains at risk of deterioration
and therefore continues on half-hourly observations and
glucose monitoring. His insulin and fluid regime is reviewed
and he is to be referred to the diabetic team in the morning.

Modified early warning score

Score	3	2	1	0	1	2	3
Systolic BP	< 70	71–80	**81–100**	101–199		> 200	
Heart rate		< 40	41–50	51–100	101–110	**111–129**	> 130
Respiratory rate		< 9		9–14	15–20	**21–29**	> 30
Temperature		< 35		35–38.4		**> 38.5**	
AVPU				A	V	P	U

Common treatment choices for hypoglycaemia

1 If conscious/not nil by mouth/has feeding tube: Lucozade
Original 100mL plus long-acting source carbohydrate,
e.g. slice of bread or 100mL nasogastric feed.
2 If conscious/nil by mouth/IV access: give 50mL boluses
(up to 250mL) of 10% dextrose IV immediately then
10% dextrose infusion (Resuscitation Council 2011).
3 If unconscious/no feeding tube/no IV access: cardiac
arrest call as he is peri-arrest, 1mg glucagon IM,
insert IV access and give 10% dextrose infusion.

All: identify source of hypoglycaemia/review insulin regime/
inform diabetic team.

The *Sepsis six* interventions are then implemented and
microbiologists are consulted. Mr Richards remains under
close observation on medical admissions unit.

Conclusion

In the hospital setting, it is claimed by Kearney and Dang (2007) that with improved care and early detection, DKA and HHS can be prevented entirely. Certainly awareness and prompt recognition of these conditions will promote better outcomes in such patients (Kisiel and Marsons 2009). Fortunately, DKA and HHS are relatively uncommon, however the diabetic emergency of hypoglycaemia is more frequently encountered, so this situation requires particular insight and awareness by nurses into the importance of their role, as many hypoglycaemic episodes are iatrogenic in causation and are associated with increased morbidity and mortality.

Glossary

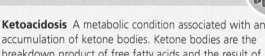

Endocrine From Greek *endo* inside and *crine* to secrete. The secretion of hormones via ductless glands directly into the bloodstream.

Exocrine *Exo* = outside. Secretion of chemicals via glands with ducts.

Gluconeogenesis Metabolic pathway resulting in the generation of glucose from non-carbohydrate sources such as lactate, glycerol and glucogenic amino acids.

Glycogenolysis Conversion of stored glycogen to glucose by the liver.

Glycosuria Presence of glucose in the urine.

Ketoacidosis A metabolic condition associated with an accumulation of ketone bodies. Ketone bodies are the breakdown product of free fatty acids and the result of deamination of amino acids.

Kussmaul breathing Rapid, deep, laboured breathing due to respiratory compensation for a severe metabolic acidosis. This can arise from either ketoacidosis or renal failure. Named after Adolf Kussmaul, a nineteenth-century German doctor.

Neuroglycopenia A deficiency of glucose in the brain as a result of hypoglycaemia. This adversely affects the functioning of neurones.

Test yourself

1 Antidiuretic hormone is produced by the:

   a. anterior pituitary
   b. posterior pituitary

2 Glucagon is secreted by:

   a. alpha cells in the pancreas
   b. beta cells in the pancreas

3 The newly diagnosed person with type I diabetes may have presented with:

   a. polydipsia
   b. polyuria
   c. cough
   d. recurrent infections

4 The maximum rate of correcting serum sodium in the hyponatraemic patient is _____ mmoL/hour.

5 Ketoacidosis may occur in:

   a. HHS
   b. DKA

6 The effect of hypoglycaemia on the nervous system is known as _____

7 Catecholamines stimulate glycogen breakdown by the liver, this process being called _____ and results in _____ blood glucose levels.

8 Patients who are hypoglycaemic may present with:

   a. sweating
   b. anxiety
   c. abdominal pain
   d. palpitations

9 Glucose in the urine is called _____

10 HHS is more common in:

   a. type I diabetics
   b. type II diabetics

References

American Diabetic Association (2004) Management of diabetes and hyperglycaemia in hospitals. *Diabetes Care* 27(2), 553–91.

Dellinger, R., Leuy, M. and Carlet, J. (2008) Surviving Sepsis Campaign: International guidelines for the management of severe sepsis and septic shock. *Intensive Care Medicine* 34, 17–60.

Falciglia, M., Freyberg, R. and Almenoff, P. (2009) Hyperglycaemia-related mortality in critically patients varies with admission diagnosis. *Critical Care Medicine* 37, 3001–3009.

Kearney, T. and Dang, C. (2007) Diabetic and endocrine emergencies. *Postgraduate Medical Journal* 83, 79–86.

Kisiel, M. and Marsons, L. (2009) Recognising and responding to hyperglycaemic emergencies. *British Journal of Nursing* 18 (18), 1094–98.

NICE (National Institute For Health and Clinical Excellence) (2007) *Acutely Ill Patients in Hospital: Recognition of and response to acute illness in adults in hospital.* Guideline 50. London: NICE.

NICE-SUGAR Study (2009) Intensive versus conventional glucose control in critically ill patients. *New England Journal of Medicine* 360, 1283–97.

NPSA (National Patient safety Agency) (2010) *New Insulin Safety Guidance Issued to Reduce Wrong Dosages*, 17 June 2010, Available from www.npsa.nhs.uk.

NMC (Nursing and Midwifery Council) (2010) *Standards for Pre-registration Nursing Education.* Available from http://standards.nmc-uk.org/PublishedDocuments/Standards%20for%20pre-registration%20nursing%20education%2016082010.pdf.

Resuscitation Council UK (2010) *Resuscitation Guidelines.* Available from www.resus.org.uk.

Surviving Sepsis Campaign (2008) www.survivingsepsis.org.

Further reading

Diabetes UK, www.diabetes.org.uk.

Hinson, J., Raven, P. and Chew, S. L. (2010) *The Endocrine System*, 2nd edn. Edinburgh: Churchill Livingstone.

International Diabetes Federation, www.idf.org.

Molina, P. E. (2010) *Endocrine Physiology.* New York: McGraw-Hill.

Scottish Intercollegiate Guidelines (SIGN) (2010) *Management of Diabetes.* www.sign.ac.uk.

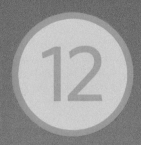

The immune and lymphatic systems, infection and sepsis

Andrea Blay, Jacqui Finch and Helen Dutton

Aims

The aim of this chapter is to provide you with insight and understanding of the immune and lymphatic systems, as well as understanding the nurse's role in the recognition and management of patients who are at risk of acute deterioration due to altered immunity and sepsis.

Objectives

After reading this chapter you will be able to:

→ Review the components and function of the lymphatic and immune systems and outline their purpose

→ Review the types of infective microorganisms, methods of infection transmission and infection control strategies, considering the nurse's role in reducing infection

→ Describe the pathophysiology and immediate management of allergy and anaphylaxis

→ Review the pathophysiology of sepsis and understand the contribution of the Surviving Sepsis Campaign to the current evidenced guidelines and care-bundle approach for sepsis and sepsis management

→ Understand the nurse's role in the systematic assessment of the patient who has problems with immunity and/or sepsis

→ Consider management and supportive interventions in order to maximise recovery from immunity and sepsis-related illnesses.

Introduction

This chapter will review the important cellular and chemical components that seek and destroy invading microorganisms in order to protect the body from infection. This coordinated response is the role of the immune and complement systems and in combination with the body's natural defences protects from a multitude of microbes. The body's response to infection will be explored, reviewing the pathophysiology of fever, the activation of the inflammatory response and problems of allergy and anaphylaxis. The spread of microbes and the role of health care professionals in actively preventing the spread of health care associated infections (HCAIs) will also be discussed. The role of the nurse is crucial in recognising the early signs of infection and in the delivery of evidence-based care to those who experience acute deterioration from problems related to immunity and infection.

Applied anatomy and physiology

The body contains a remarkable array of cells, proteins and complex networks of interrelated hormones and chemicals which provide constant surveillance of our body for any signs of invasion from microbial or other organic substances, e.g. pollen, that might cause harm. This array is collectively known as the immune system. It alerts our defence systems when microorganisms are breaching our natural defences and provides the first line of defence. For the immune system to function rapidly and effectively, it must have a transport network that delivers the immune response to its target location: that system is called the lymphatic system.

The lymphatic system

The lymphatic system is sometimes neglected and underestimated, silently going about its functions. It is closely linked to the cardiovascular system, providing an open-ended comprehensive network of drainage, defence and the storage of white cells.

The lymphatic system consists of lymphatic (lymphoid) tissue, capillaries and vessels, lymph nodes and collecting ducts. The organs of the lymphatic system are the spleen, thymus and the tonsils, which are located in the posterior aspect of the oral cavity and nasopharynx and are the smallest lymphoid organs (see Figure 12.1). All are interconnected by lymph capillaries which run alongside blood capillaries, reabsorbing any excess interstitial fluid and escaped plasma proteins into the lymph fluid and back into the venous system. This is important in maintaining fluid balance between the interstitial and vascular fluid compartments.

The lymphatic system recycles approximately 2–4L per day of interstitial fluid back into the bloodstream (Marieb and Hoehn 2010). Lymphatic vessels, like peripheral veins, contain valves which ensure the one-way movement of lymph back into the venous system. Lymph fluid drains into collecting vessels, then into several lymphatic trunks and finally into two main collecting ducts:

- the right lymphatic duct;
- the thoracic duct.

The right lymphatic duct drains the right upper arm, the right side of the head, thorax, subclavian and jugular regions and opens into the right subclavian vein. The larger thoracic duct drains into the left subclavian vein. Over two-thirds of lymph from the body drains into this duct via the right lymphatic duct.

Thus circulation of lymph fluid follows the pattern given in Colbert *et al.* (2009):

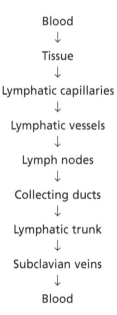

Blood
↓
Tissue
↓
Lymphatic capillaries
↓
Lymphatic vessels
↓
Lymph nodes
↓
Collecting ducts
↓
Lymphatic trunk
↓
Subclavian veins
↓
Blood

Lymphocytes

Lymphocytes are the cells of the lymphatic system: produced in the bone marrow, they form part of the cell-mediated response to antigens. As their name suggests they spend most of their life cycle, which is about 2–4 years, within the lymphoid tissues. There are different types and sizes of lymphocytes, T cells and B cells. T cells are produced in the bone marrow but are matured (or become immunocompetent) within the thymus. B cells are also produced in the bone marrow but remain there to

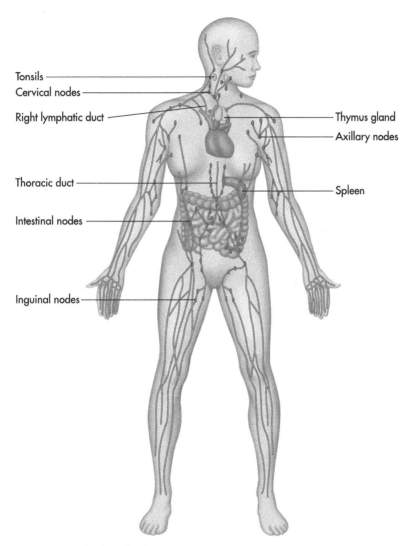

Tonsils

Cervical nodes

Right lymphatic duct

Thymus gland

Axillary nodes

Thoracic duct

Spleen

Intestinal nodes

Inguinal nodes

Figure 12.1 The lymphatic system

mature and become immunocompetent (see Figure 12.2). The T and B cells are exposed to antigens, normally in the lymphoid tissue, where they differentiate and mature. Within the T and B cell population there are a range of cells with differing functions. B cells mediate the humoral or antibody response and T cells mediate the cellular immune response.

Lymphoid tissue
Lymphoid tissue is composed of reticular connective tissue which provides support for lymphocytes and macrophages. These lymphocytes and macrophages can quickly squeeze through the capillary walls to circulate in the blood. This recirculation of lymphocytes between the blood, lymphatic tissues and organs is vitally important in exposing many lymphocytes to an invading pathogen or antigen. Depending on the route of entry the antigen will be conveyed from the site of infection to the lymphatic tissues, where antigen-presenting cells, e.g. dendritic cells of lymphoid tissue and macrophages, are waiting to

phagocytose the microbes and present the microbial antigen on their surface for antibodies to respond to. Antigens causing a tissue infection will be conveyed to the appropriate draining lymph nodes: the lymph node effectively closes down to retain the antigen-specific cells within the lymph node, thereby containing the infection within a small area (Stewart 2007). This causes swollen, painful lymph nodes as experienced with an infection within the tonsils (tonsillitis). Cancerous cells can also be trapped within the lymph node: the node may become swollen but not painful which is a useful sign in differentiating between infection and cancer.

Within the small intestine are collections of lymphoid tissues or nodules called Peyer's patches. Similar nodules are also found within the appendix, they are well situated to detect and destroy any pathogenic bacteria found within the intestine, preventing these bacteria from translocating or crossing the gastrointestinal wall. These tissues or nodules are collectively called mucosa-associated lymphatic tissue (MALT), and along with the tonsils and

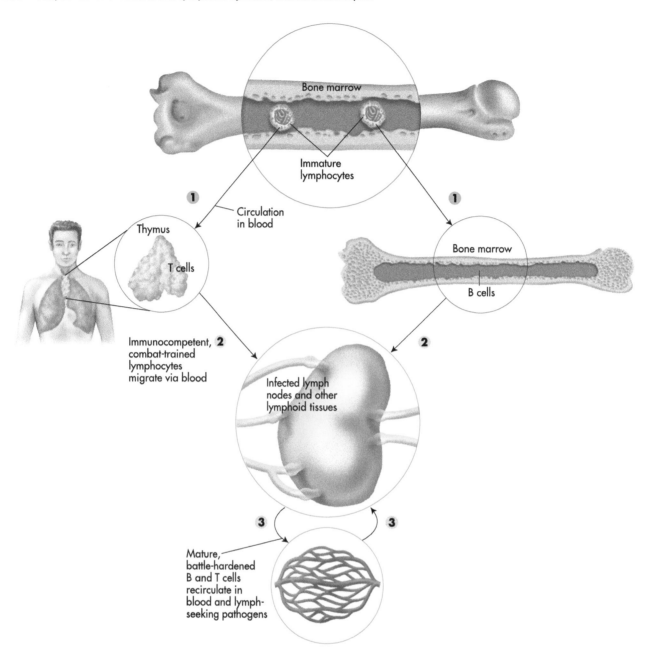

Bone marrow

Immature
lymphocytes

1

1

Circulation
in blood

Thymus

T cells

Bone marrow

B cells

Immunocompetent, **2**
combat-trained
lymphocytes
migrate via blood

2

Infected lymph
nodes and other
lymphoid tissues

3

3

Mature,
battle-hardened
B and T cells
recirculate in
blood and lymph-
seeking pathogens

KEY:

1 Site of lymphocyte origin: some lymphocytes are sent to the thymus where they become T cells, while others remain in the bone marrow to become B cells. These cells are now much like soldiers in bootcamp that have learned their combat training but have yet to face the real enemy.

2 Sites of development of immunocompetence as B or T cells: an infection occurs and these cells are now given their marching orders to travel to the site of need. This is usually in the lymphoid tissue where the antigen challenge (the enemy has arrived) and the lymphocytes get placed into actual battle.

3 Site of antigen challenge and final differentiation to mature B and T cells: now the battle-hardened lymphocytes can competently patrol the rest of the body through the blood and lymph system, seeking out the enemy.

Figure 12.2 Lymphocyte differentiation and activation

nodules within the bronchi protect the respiratory and digestive systems from a continuous barrage of pathogens.

Lymph nodes

Lymph nodes range from the size of a pinhead to a small grape; they are strategically placed in vulnerable regions such as the digestive, respiratory and reproductive areas. Loaded with lymphocytes, they are ready to destroy harmful pathogens. Lymph nodes act like sieves, filtering the fluid and returning it cleansed of harmful microbes back into the lymphatic and circulatory systems. The lymph nodes are found mainly in the neck (cervical) under the armpits (axillary), in the groin (inguinal), within the pelvis, abdominal and thoracic cavities (see Figure12.1) (Colbert *et al.* 2009).

The spleen

The spleen is located just under the diaphragm in the upper left quadrant of the abdominal cavity, curving around the anterior aspect of the stomach; it is supplied by the splenic artery which enters at the hilus. The main functions of the largest lymphoid organ are:

- surveillance for infection;
- lymphocyte propagation;
- filtering and cleaning of the blood from blood-borne pathogens and toxins;
- storage of platelets and removal of ageing, faulty platelets and red blood cells and the extraction and storage of iron for the production of haemoglobin.

> **Ruptured or damaged spleen**
>
> If the spleen is damaged it must be removed as haemorrhage from the splenic artery is life threatening.
>
> Post-splenectomy (asplenism) the patient is at risk of developing serious life-threatening infections.
>
> The main infectious organisms to cause death are:
>
> - Pneumococcus
> - Haemophilus influenzae
> - Meningococcus.
>
> Vaccines exist to protect against these organisms, and these with regular boosters and health education are essential to reduce the risk of serious infection.

The spleen is made up of areas of white and red pulp. The white pulp regions congregate around the splenic artery and blood sinuses and are primarily concerned with the immune surveillance function and the production of lymphocytes when required. The red pulp region removes worn-out blood cells, platelets and pathogens. The spleen has a very thin outer capsule and any blunt trauma may cause the spleen to rupture, potentially leading to life-threatening haemorrhage. If the spleen is removed (splenectomy) its function is taken over by the liver and bone marrow.

The thymus

The thymus is located in front of the aortic arch behind the sternum. In children the thymus is very large as it is very active fending off many new infections, but with increasing age the immune system matures and the thymus shrinks or may even disappear. The cells of the thymus are primarily lymphocytes. The primary function of the thymus is to secrete thymosin and thymopoietin which bring about the maturing and immunocompetence of T cell lymphocytes.

Immunity

There are two types of immune defence system:

- innate or natural immunity;
- adaptive or acquired immunity which is specific to each person.

Immunity and natural defences

We are born with our own inherent immune system or innate immunity, which is made up of passive immunity and natural defences.

Passive immunity

Passive immunity is part of the innate immunity or non-specific immunity and has no memory; it can recognise our own cells (self) or antigens but cannot recognise a pathogen that has previously invaded the body. The foetus acquires some immunity via the placenta: this is called passive immunity and lasts for about 3–6 months; the main antibody which is able to cross the placenta is immunoglobulin IgG. Although the time period for providing this passive immunity is limited, it is important at a time when the immune system is immature. After about six months infants are more prone to respiratory and gastric infections, and this is in part due to the loss of fetal antibodies before the B and T lymphocytes are fully immunocompetent.

> The Respiratory Syncytial Virus (RSV) causes croup and bronchiolitis in the first few months of the infants' life despite the presence of IgG from the mother.

Natural defences

One of the natural defences of the body is the skin; the largest impermeable organ in the body, it provides our

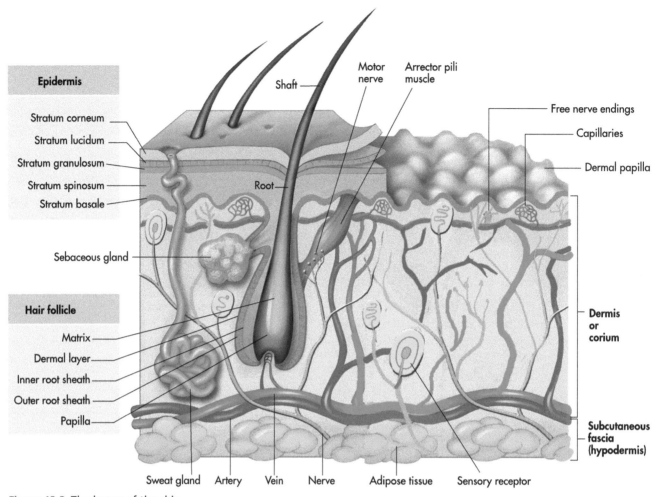

Figure 12.3 The layers of the skin

first line of protection against a barrage of potentially harmful microorganisms. It contains three layers – the epidermis, dermis and hypodermis – in which there are motor and sensory nerves, hair follicles and sweat glands (see Figure 12.3). The epidermis is heavily keratinised; keratin is a protein that is resistant to bacterial toxins and enzymes (Stewart 2007). The dermis also produces sweat and sebum from sebaceous glands which contain lactic and fatty acids (Stewart 2007). The epidermis also contains Langerhans cells that are involved in the natural defences. The low pH of between three and five is acidic and inhibits the growth and survival of non-commensal bacteria. An exception to this is *Staphylococcus aureus*, a salt-resistant gram-positive organism and opportunistic skin pathogen. *Staph. aureus* is found in the nose in about 30% of healthy people (Humphreys 2007). The cocci exist in clusters, causing many soft tissue infections by invading hair follicles and sebaceous glands. This can manifest as surgical wound infections, abscesses or boils. They can also produce pneumonia. *Staph. aureus* can also release enterotoxins which when ingested cause food poisoning, and other toxin-mediated diseases such as toxic shock

syndrome and scaled skin syndrome. Some strains of *Staphylococcus aureus* are resistant to many of the antibiotics used to eradicate the bacterium. MRSA infections are a particular problem in large hospitals, where stringent hygiene measures are needed to prevent it spreading between patients.

Methicillin-resistant staphylococcus aureus (MRSA)

S. aureus began to develop resistance to penicillin in the early 1950s, since then it has developed resistance to gentamicin and vancomycin (VRSA). Globally there have been many worldwide outbreaks of MRSA. Those most at risk are:

- the critically ill;
- those on dialysis;
- oncology patients;
- immunocompromised patients;
- patients with prosthetic heart valves;
- patients with indwelling venous catheters.

The incidence of MRSA bacteraemia is monitored at the Department of Health (DH); each NHS organisation must declare its annual MRSA bacteraemia rates. There are financial penalties for exceeding the target, which is associated with quality of care and cleanliness.

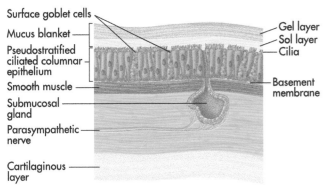

Surface goblet cells
Mucus blanket
Pseudostratified
ciliated columnar
epithelium
Smooth muscle
Submucosal
gland
Parasympathetic
nerve
Cartilaginous
layer

Gel layer
Sol layer
Cilia

Basement
membrane

Figure 12.4 The mucociliary escalator

All openings into the body are protected by mucus membranes which secrete acids, enzymes and sticky fluids to protect the tissues underneath from microorganisms. The respiratory tract is protected by several naturally occurring mechanisms; the columnar cells in the nasal passages project 200–250 cilia which beat up to 1500 times per minute, humidifying, filtering and trapping particles and dust in a gel-like substance (see Figure 12.4). The mucociliary escalator constantly expels debris forward to the nose, this mechanism is assisted by the physical act of coughing and sneezing, expelling debris (sputum) from the deeper areas of the lungs into the upper airways where it can be coughed out or swallowed.

Eyes are protected by the lacrimal fluids or tears which contain the enzyme lysozyme, also found in saliva. Both fluids neutralise bacteria, especially gram-positive organisms inhibiting bacterial growth. Saliva also contains IgA antibodies and defensins which act as a local antibiotic and stimulate the release of neutrophils if the oral mucosa is damaged. Lysozyme is secreted by leucocytes and is also found in the genito-urinary tract. Combined with the regular flushing of urine this protects the urinary tract from pathogens.

> **Defensins** are a group of small antimicrobial peptides occurring in neutrophils and macrophages.

The stomach is protected by the production of hydrochloric acid (HCl) from parietal cells, the acidity or pH of the gastric juices is about 1.5–3.5, which kills many ingested pathogens. The opposite occurs in the small intestine, where the pH is very high (pH 8–9). This alkaline state again destroys most pathogens with the exception of typhoid and cholera (Gould and Brooker 2000).

Vaginal secretions produce lactobacilli which can form lactic acid, creating an acidic environment within the vagina. The vaginal secretions have a pH of 4–5. Semen also contains chemicals that protect from invasion.

Humans are host reservoirs for a number of commensal microorganisms, for example *Escherichia coli* (*E. coli*) and natural flora that exist either in the gastrointestinal system or on the skin. There is a fine balance between host and commensal organisms and this relationship is important to maintain health. When an imbalance occurs or the commensal enters into an area where it is not usually present, such as *E. coli* entering into the urinary tract, an infection can occur. These organisms, called opportunistic pathogens, can pose serious consequences for those who have undergone surgical treatments such as joint replacement or those who are immunocompromised.

In essence any natural opening has several mechanisms to protect the delicate membranes from invasion. The natural defence systems combined with our complex molecular and chemical immunity largely protect from infection. When the natural defences are breached a complex range of components are released to counteract invasion. The blood components of immunity and how they become activated will now be considered.

Major groups of leucocytes

Once the natural barriers have been breached the innate system is instantly activated, targeting the source of infection with a barrage of white cells or leucocytes. Leucocytes are formed in the bone marrow and make up the white cells that comprise the white cell differential. White cells are activated when they come in to contact with damaged cells and tissues, complement proteins, antibodies and chemicals released by bacterial cells.

> **Normal serum values for white blood cell count (WBCC) and white blood cell count differential**
> - WBCC 4–11 × 10⁹/L
> - Neutrophils 2–7.5 × 10⁹/L
> - Lymphocytes 1.5–4 × 10⁹/L
> - Monocytes 0.2–0.8 × 10⁹/L
> - Eosinophils 0.04–0.4 × 10⁹/L
> - Basophils 01–0.1 × 10⁹/L.

Figure 12.5 shows the five major leucocytes or white blood cell groups:

1 Neutrophils
2 Eosinophils
3 Basophils
4 Monocytes
5 Lymphocytes.

Neutrophils

Neutrophils, eosinophils and basophils are polymorphonuclear granulocytes (i.e. they contain cytoplasmic granules), of which the most abundant are neutrophils. They are the first cells to arrive at the scene of infection or tissue damage. Their primary function is phagocytosis; that is, they act as scavengers engulfing and destroying microbes. On ingestion of the microbe the phagocytes cytotoxic enzymes digest the organism (Marieb and Hoehn 2010). Neutrophils clump together around sites of tissue injury releasing chemicals (cytokines) which stimulate other immune cells to be activated. This stimulation causes local inflammation. A more severe inflammatory response during a bacterial infection may cause the death of the neutrophils; this cell debris forms pus or a wound infection which occurs at the site of tissue injury. A full blood count is performed as part of the clinical assessment to diagnose the presence of infection; leucocytosis or elevated white count confirms the presence of infection. Alternatively a low white cell count or leucopenia can be seen in immunocompromised patients, those with cancer or those with a very severe infection.

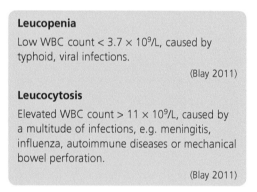

Leucopenia

Low WBC count $< 3.7 \times 10^9$/L, caused by typhoid, viral infections.

(Blay 2011)

Leucocytosis

Elevated WBC count $> 11 \times 10^9$/L, caused by a multitude of infections, e.g. meningitis, influenza, autoimmune diseases or mechanical bowel perforation.

(Blay 2011)

Basophils

The main function of basophils (see Figure 12.5) is to promote inflammation, but they are also involved in anaphylactic reactions. Basophils can leave the bloodstream to enter sites of tissue damage: when they do this they transform into mast cells. Mast cells are found in connective tissue and in the mucosa and release histamine and heparin. Histamine is a vasoactive amine causing vasodilation of the arteriole/capillary vascular bed and enlargement of the intracellular pores in the capillary membrane. This increases pooling of blood in the area of tissue damage. The systemic vascular resistance is lowered which manifests as hypotension or low blood pressure if a significant area of capillary bed is affected. In response to this the patient develops a tachycardia. In anaphylactic reactions, histamine release increases vascular capillary permeability, causing local oedema which may exacerbate breathing problems and potentially cause obstruction of the airway.

Eosinophils

Eosinophils are phagocytic in nature; they counteract the chemical effects of histamine to reduce the effects of the inflammatory response. They have a role in fighting parasitic worm invasion. Both basophils and eosinophils have low cell counts unless activated by pathogens (see Figure 12.5).

Mononuclear cells

There are two main types of mononuclear cell (agranulocytes): monocytes and lymphocytes (see Figure 12.5), they have very little granular matter. The mature form of the monocyte that has left the bone marrow is a macrophage. Macrophages can survive for many months; they are phagocytic in nature and leave the bloodstream to enter tissues in later stages of infection. Macrophages release chemicals such as prostaglandins, complement,

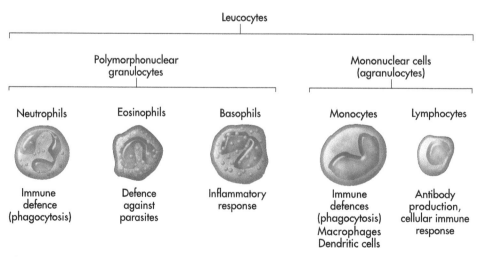

Figure 12.5 Major leucocytes

interferon and cytokines such as tumour necrosis factor (TNF) which are important in stimulating T and B lymphocytes as part of the innate immune response.

> **Macrophage** from Greek: *macro* = big, *phage* = eat.

Dendritic cells

These are modified phagocytic monocytes or antigen-presenting cells (APCs). They, with similarly acting white cells, form the link between the innate and adaptive immune systems. They have an important function in ingesting pathogens and then placing the foreign antigens into their own cell membrane. This process triggers the adaptive immune system, when they enter the lymph nodes searching for the lymphocytes that match the antigen.

Natural killer cells

These are large granular lymphocytes, belonging to the natural defences and innate immunity; their origin is unknown and they have no memory, they constitute < 1% of the total leucocyte count and are activated by interferon and cytokines (Gould and Brooker 2000). Natural Killer (NK) cells are like vigilantes, killing indiscriminately by releasing chemicals and enzymes that target the invader cell membranes, damaging the membrane and causing holes to appear. They naturally kill all manner of cells from cancer cells, viruses and even body cells if the host's cell is infected with a virus. Natural killer cells also stimulate the inflammatory response by releasing chemicals.

Interferons

Interferons were first discovered in 1957. There are three types of these naturally occurring antiviral agents, α-interferon (IFN-α) β-interferon (IFN-β) and γ-interferon (INF-γ). They belong to the family of cytokines and are produced in response to viral infections by T cells. Interferons have myriad complex actions that ultimately inhibit viral replication and transcription phases, alter the production of proteins and cell functions and mediate other immune responses.

The complement system

The complement system is part of the innate and adaptive immune response; it is involved in the destruction (lysis) of bacteria, caused by the combination of antibody and protein activation in the blood. Like all cascade systems, it provides a rapid and augmented response. The proteins are inactive until triggered by pathogens. There are at least 20 proteins involved in the complement system. Some of them are labelled as follows; C1–C9, factors B, D and P. There are other proteins included in the system, e.g. regulatory proteins that are not usually specifically identified (Colbert *et al.* 2009). There are two pathways: the classical pathway which is activated by forming an antigen–antibody complex as previously described. Once this has formed one of the proteins from the complement system attaches itself to the complex, this is called complement fixation (Colbert *et al.* 2009). The alternative pathway is the interaction between bacterial membrane surfaces and factors B, D and P. The complement pathway is a sequential cascade system amplifying the immune response to bring about a variety of mechanisms with the aim to cause bacterial death or lysis. The following mechanisms also assist with this process:

- The process of *opsonisation* prepares the bacteria by coating the antigen with opsonin; this enables phagocytic cells to attach more quickly to begin the process of phagocytosis.
- The release of chemicals or *chemotaxis* by white blood cells and microorganisms attracts macrophages and other phagocytes to the pathogens, like bees to a honeypot.
- Inducing localised and in severe cases systemic *inflammation* is essential to activate and convey white blood cells and platelets to the area so that the process of removing pathogens and cell debris can begin.

There are several causes that trigger the inflammatory response: see Figure 12.6 to review the aetiologies. Inflammation is part of our innate immunity response, playing an important part in our adaptive immunity.

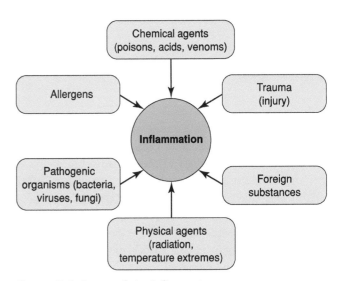

Figure 12.6 Causes of the inflammatory response

C-reactive protein (CRP)

C-reactive protein (CRP) is a blood protein and member of the class of acute phase proteins (Goering *et al.* 2008). It increases dramatically during inflammation and is therefore one of the inflammatory markers used to identify sepsis and infection. CRP is synthesised by the liver and therefore its production is reduced in liver disease. The normal serum value is less than 10mg/L. The level can be raised to between 40–200mg/L in the presence of active bacterial infection and inflammation. In severe infections the levels can be more than 200mg/L. Some types of bacterium, dying or dead cell release a substance called phosphocholine, CRP binds to this so that the complement system can be activated. It also enhances macrophage phagocytosis and opsonisation processes as previously described.

Activation of the immune system

The way in which the body responds to infection varies and is related to several factors such as our own genetic disposition, previous exposure to antigens and the pathogenicity or virulence of the organism. Inflammatory responses also vary: some individuals may exhibit an excessive immunological response which can cause many problems and in some cases may actually lead to death, such as in anaphylaxis or hypersensitivity to allergens. Inflammation is another innate immune response and is described below.

Inflammatory response

The inflammatory response is a natural and well-documented tissue response to a number of agents (see Figure 12.6). Inflammation is characterised by the following clinical signs:

- redness of the skin or erythema;
- swelling;
- heat;
- pain;
- loss of movement or reduced function.

Pathophysiology of inflammation

On exposure to one of the causative agents capillaries surrounding damaged tissues and cells become increasingly permeable due to a variety of mechanisms. IgE mediates histamine release from basophils or mast cells and other chemical mediators such as 5-hdroxytryptamine, bradykinins from neutrophils and prostaglandins released by the injured tissues increase capillary vascular permeability, ultimately causing arteriolar vasodilation. This increased blood supply to the damaged area and chemoattractants released by tissue damage, encourage neutrophils and other cells to the site to begin the process of phagocytosis (Gould and Brooker 2000). The metabolic activity of the inflammatory cells increases the temperature within the tissue creating heat; as the inflammatory process evolves redness (erythema) or hyperaemia and swelling caused by oedema from the increased leakage of vascular fluid develops. Swelling and pain caused by the interaction of bradykinin and prostaglandins result in loss of movement or function. Toxins are diluted by the increase in fluid in the area, and combined with the effect of complement proteins, lymphocytes and macrophages; microbes are contained and removed from affected tissues. Chemotaxis encourages more leucocytes into the area to neutralise and engulf pathogens and remove debris: as this progresses a fibrin mesh is created to contain the spread of infection. Coating the antigens with opsonins and the effects of complement proteins enables macrophages to identify intruders for phagocytosis.

The acute inflammatory process can result in either the complete resolution of the infection and the return of normal function or the acute phase moves into a chronic phase with resistant infections, colonisation, scarring and pus-producing abscesses that become difficult to treat, often due to their inaccessibility.

Pathophysiology of fever

Fever or pyrexia is derived from the latin word *febris* or febrile. Fever occurs when the body temporarily fails to maintain the temperature within normal limits. Fever accelerates tissue metabolism and the activity of defences (Martini and Ober 2011). The set-point is elevated by 1–2°C and is a symptom of many medical conditions and one of the oldest indicators of disease. In response to a stimulus, such as inflammation or the release of endotoxins from bacteria, leucocytes release endogenous pyrogens, 'fire starters', or cytokines into the bloodstream. These chemicals act directly on the thermostat or 'set-point' in the hypothalamus, causing the release of prostaglandin and elevating or resetting the hypothalamic set-point to a higher level.

> **Normal body temperature**
>
> Temperature has a narrow range: between 35.6–37.8°C despite changes in air temperature.
>
> Body temperature fluctuates 1°C in 24 hours, being at the lowest in the early morning and highest in the early evening.

Fever or pyrexia can be defined as the following:

- Low grade: 38–39°C
- Moderate: 39–40°C
- High grade: more than 40°C.

Hyperpyrexia is defined as a temperature greater than 42°C and is classed as a medical emergency. A temperature above 41°C can result in convulsions or seizures; the upper limit for human life is 43°C and at this point proteins and cells denature and are unable to function normally.

Fever has several functions. Its primary aim is to increase the basal metabolic rate so that bacterial growth is inhibited; most organisms cannot tolerate extremes of temperature or temperatures in excess of 37°C. Raised temperature increases the rate of elimination of toxins and tissue repair is heightened, all of which assist the body's defence mechanisms to fight invading pathogens. Eating is inhibited and proteins are denatured at higher temperatures, which can result in irreversible brain damage. An increase in temperature increases enzymatic reactions; thereby each rise in temperature of 1°C can result in a 10% increase in cellular chemical reactions, an increase the heart rate by 10 beats/minute and an increase in the respiratory rate.

The stages of fever

There are three stages in the life cycle of a fever;

- *Stage 1* – the cold or 'chilly' heat-generating stage.
- *Stage 2* – heat maintaining.
- *Stage 3* – the defervescence stage where the thermostat has been reset to a lower level and the body now attempts to lose heat.

During the cold phase heat-production mechanisms such as shivering and vasoconstriction are activated and conserve body heat. This may last for 10–40 minutes causing a rapid, steady rise in temperature. The basal metabolic rate (BMR), heart and respiratory rates are also increased. The patient can feel chilly and experience goose bumps and sweating ceases.

The second stage is heat maintaining, the length of time spent in this phase depends on how long it takes to eradicate the pyrogen. Patients with severe infections and/or resistant microorganisms may remain in this phase for several weeks. The body now attempts to balance heat loss and heat-production mechanisms. The patient is flushed, hot, tachycardic, thirsty and possibly tachypnoeic. They may complain of headache and loss of appetite. Some patients may have a seizure. The hot stage ends when the cause of the fever has been eliminated, resulting in a decrease in the hypothalamic set-point to normal.

The final stage is the defervescence or heat-dissipating stage; this is when the hypothalamic set-point is returning to normal. The body now employs the heat-loss mechanisms of vasodilation, sweating and inhibition of heat-producing mechanisms to lower the temperature. The patient usually feels hot during this phase.

Causes of fever

There are many causes of fever:

- infection, e.g. bacterial, viral, fungal or protozoan;
- autoimmune diseases such as lupus erythaematous;
- inflammatory bowel disease;
- the breakdown of red blood cells or haemolysis from surgery can induce a temperature postoperatively;
- myocardial infarction;
- crush syndrome as a result of rhabdomyolysis;
- drugs can also cause a 'drug fever' either as a direct consequence of the drug or as an adverse reaction to the drug (e.g. allergic reaction to antibiotics). Discontinuation of some drugs, for example heroin withdrawal, can induce a fever.

Adaptive immunity

Adaptive or specific immunity is the second line of defence. Once the natural defences have been breached or failed to control the invasion, the immune system attempts to instigate containment and control by limiting the spread of infection and ultimately destroying the pathogens. The cells involved in providing this defence are lymphocytes and macrophages which contain the body's memory bank. Adaptive immunity is long-lasting, but can be affected by the ability of microorganisms to change and adapt so that they are not recognised by the immune system. It is important to appreciate that the response of the immune system depends on the nature of the infection or antigen, the route of entry into the body and the individual response, which varies between individuals and populations. The response can be systemic or localised to one region, organ or tissue. For the purposes of clarity the humoral and cell-mediated branches of the adaptive immune system will be considered separately.

> **Antibodies** are the substances that bind to the antigens.
>
> **Antigens** are substances that stimulate the host's lymphoid cells and tissues to mount a specific direct response to the antigen and not to an unrelated substance.

Antibodies

The memory of previous pathogens or antigens is contained within antibodies which have specific sites that recognise past exposure to an antigen. Antibodies are soluble gamma globulin proteins that are classed as immunoglobulins. Their function is to hold the 'memory' of previously experienced pathogens and to recognise them.

Antibodies are large proteins produced by B lymphocytes of which there are five classes: IgD, IgM, IgG, IgA,

Table 12.1 Immunoglobin classes

Class	Generalised structure	Where found	Biological function
IgD		Virtually always attached to B cell	Believed to be cell surface receptor of immunocompetent B cell; important in activation of B cell
IgM	J chain	Attached to B cell; free in plasma	When bound to B cell membrane, serves as antigen receptor; first Ig class *released* to plasma by plasma cells during primary response; potent agglutinating agent; fixes complement
IgG		Most abundant antibody in plasma; represents 75% to 85% of circulating antibodies	Main antibody of both primary and secondary responses; crosses placenta and provides passive immunity to fetus; fixes complement
IgA	J chain	Some (monomer) in plasma; dimer in secretions such as saliva, tears, intestinal juice and milk	Bathes and protects mucosal surfaces from attachment of pathogens
IgE		Secreted by plasma cells in skin, mucosae of gastrointestinal and respiratory tracts, and tonsils	Binds to mast cells and basophils, and triggers release of histamine and other chemicals that mediate inflammation and certain allergic responses

IgE. All have different functions, are slightly different in structure and are found in different parts of the body. They are stimulated in response to foreign antigens. The most abundant is IgG and the largest is IgM (see Table 12.1).

Humoral immunity

B cells or B lymphocytes are responsible for humoral or antibody-mediated immunity and form part of the adaptive immune response. There are two types of B cell:

- plasma cells which produce antibodies, the primary response;
- memory B cells, stored in lymph nodes, remember pathogens, allowing a much faster response to a second or subsequent exposure to the pathogen, the secondary response (see Figure 12.7) (Colbert *et al.* 2009).

When an antigen or 'foreign' substance is detected, B cells or plasma cells (found in lymphoid tissue) are

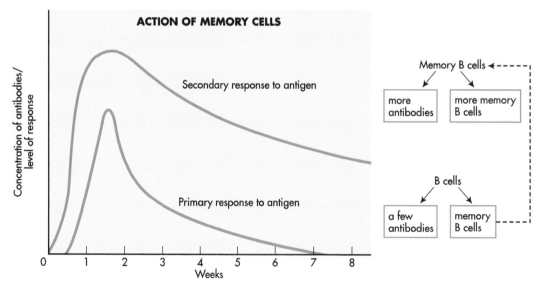

Figure 12.7 Primary and secondary responses to antigen

stimulated to secrete large quantities of antibodies which bind to specific antigens, forming the antigen–antibody complex. Each antibody has a specific adapter site, epitope or 'lock' that fits a particular antigen or 'key'. Each antibody recognises the shape of the antigen to which they are programmed to bind.

Antibodies or immunoglobulins have a number of functions and effects:

- on activation they bind to the pathogen, causing clumping or agglutination;
- once bound they act as opsonins, identifying or signalling that particular antigen for phagocytosis;
- binding triggers the production of identical plasma cells or clones which all produce the same antibody: this is called clonal expansion;
- phagocytosis and the complement cascade system are also activated.

Antibodies are unable to enter cells, therefore in viral infections they can be ineffective, especially against viruses that spread directly from cell to cell. Antibodies can bind to the surface of infected host cells via epitopes, which may affect the viral replication processes. Antibodies can also block the virus attaching to the host cell; this reduces the likelihood of penetration and accumulation of the virus and limits infection spread. If the virus is conveyed via the bloodstream then the virus can be neutralised before it reaches its target organ, e.g. poliovirus (Stewart 2007). The common cold (coryza) virus targets the respiratory mucosa. Antibodies are ineffective against the virus as they are not present in the mucosa membranes and secretions.

Experiencing a childhood disease such as chickenpox, caused by the *Varicella zoster* virus, produces antibodies and renders the body immune to chicken pox via the humoral immunity system. Unfortunately, there is no immunity from the common cold as we do not possess an antibody to this virus.

Cell-mediated immunity
T cells are produced by the red bone marrow and matured in the thymus gland. The four main types of differentiated T cell are:

- T helper inducer T cells (T4)
- Cytotoxic T cells (T8)
- Memory T cells
- Suppressor (or regulatory)T cells (T8) (Martini and Ober 2011).

T cells make up about 80% of all lymphocytes and are activated when an antigen binds to the T cell surface receptor site. They then undergo rapid proliferation and

differentiation into one of the following, depending on the nature of the antigen:

- T helper cells respond by secretion of interleukins or messenger proteins promoting the proliferation of B lymphocytes, other T lymphocytes and natural killer cells to phagocytose (Jones and Shelton 2009).
- T helper cells also promote the maturation of B cells and T lymphocytes once interleukins have been released.
- Cytotoxic T cells recognise and destroy cells infected by viruses and cells altered by cancer.
- Memory cells continue to exist after an infection has resolved. They remember antigens and quickly expand if the infection is encountered again.
- T suppressor or regulatory cells downregulate the immune response when the objective has been achieved.

Autoimmunity
The immune system is a complex and dynamic system in which the ability to recognise 'self', i.e. the body's own cells and tissues, is hugely important. Failures in this mechanism which are multifactorial can lead to the development of autoimmune diseases such as systemic lupus erythematosus (SLE). Other abnormal responses mediated by the immune system are allergic reactions to blood products, antibiotics and other allergens. The suppression of the immune system post tissue and organ transplantation is essential in order to prevent rejection of 'foreign' tissue. With age the immune system is less efficient and therefore older people become more prone to cancer and other diseases. This may be one of the reasons why there is an increase in malignancy as we get older. The role of the immune system in the development of malignancy is part of ongoing research into cancer.

Microorganisms

There are several organisms that can cause serious illness and even death. Understanding and appreciating the properties of microorganisms can only enhance knowledge and assist practitioners in understanding how hospital-acquired infections (HAI) may occur and our role as nurses in reducing the risk to patients.

Even though humans have daily contact with millions of bacteria and viruses, the effectiveness of natural defences and immunity systems results in very few serious infections or diseases. To understand the nature of infection and sepsis it is important to have some understanding of the important bacteria, viruses, fungi and protozoa that affect patients. It must be remembered that the influence of foreign travel will also predispose travellers to other infections that are not common to Western Europe. This section is designed to give a brief overview of common organisms seen in UK hospitals and not the vast array of other microbes seen around the world.

Commonly used definitions

It is helpful to review definition of commonly used terms related to microbiology and infection.

- *Infection* – presence of a microorganism in the tissues that causes a host response (Fraise and Bradley 2009).
- *Pathogenicity* – the capacity of an organism to cause disease (Bannister *et al.* 2006).
- *Virulence* – the ability of an organism to cause disease. This is dependent on how large the inoculation dose is and the ability of the mircoorganism to invade the host's defences (Gould and Brooker 2000).
- *Colonisation* – presence of multiplying organisms in the tissue producing no or only minimal host response (Fraise and Bradley 2009).
- *Contamination* – soiling of inanimate objects or living material, e.g. medical equipment, with potentially harmful infectious matter (Fraise and Bradley 2009). Wounds are considered contaminated if there are organisms on the surface of the wound bed but there is no replication or host response.
- *Hospital* or *'nosocomial' infection* – is an infection acquired by patients or hospital staff in a hospital setting, or health care-associated or acquired infection (HCAI) an infection associated with the delivery of health care in a variety of settings (Fraise and Bradley 2009).
- *Cross-* or *exogenous infection* – means acquired from staff, patients or even relatives (Fraise and Bradley 2009).
- *Self-* or *endogenous* – infection caused by microbes that the patient carries, our own normal bacterial flora (Fraise and Bradley 2009).
- *Source* – a place where pathogenic organisms are growing, e.g. food poisoning from contaminated food or a collection of pus within a cavity or tissues (Fraise and Bradley 2009).
- *Reservoir* – a place where pathogens can survive and then be transferred to patients directly or indirectly, e.g. blood pressure cuffs that have been inadequately cleaned prior to use on patients (Fraise and Bradley 2009).

Classification of microorgansims

Microorganisms are classified according to their structure and shape or morphology, spore-forming or slime-producing properties. The main classes of microorganisms that are associated with or are medically important

to humans are viruses, bacteria, protozoa, fungi and moulds and parasitic worms. Although not microscopic the last group come under the general heading of microbiology.

A group of infectious proteins called prions are also included because of their microscopic and infectious nature. The proteins remain controversial but are implicated in a number of encephalopathies such as variant Creutzfeldt–Jakob disease (see Table 12.2).

Gram staining to aid identification

Bacteria are classified in a number of different ways. In the laboratory they are stained using a Gram stain; Gram-positive organisms will retain the dye and stain a deep violet colour, Gram-negative organisms lose the violet stain but appear pink as they take up a red counter stain as part of the gram-staining process. The staining process is useful because the Gram-positive and Gram-negative organisms respond to different antibiotics.

Vulnerability to infection

Normally the immune system's complex mechanisms are extremely effective at maintaining health by destroying invading pathogens. However, there are a number of factors that increase vulnerability to infections, and these high-risk groups required close monitoring to detect early signs of infection. Risk relates to both the patient and to treatment-related factors (see Table 12.3). These vulnerable groups are at high risk from developing infection both in the community and in the hospital setting.

Health care-associated infection (HCAI)

It is estimated that about 1 in 10 patients develops an infection during a stay in a hospital in the UK (National HCAI Research Network 2011). The consequences of this for the patient are unpleasant, increasing their length of stay, causing pain, distress, loss of earnings and reducing their chances of a completely successful recovery. Whilst not all HCAI can be avoided, it has been estimated that 15–30% could be with everyone in health care having a role to play in infection reduction.

A particular challenge for England is *C. difficile* and MRSA. Government strategy is focused on these infections, however, effective infection control measures should reduce all HCAIs (DH 2008). The EPIC 2 guidelines (Pratt *et al.* 2007) consider standard principles for infection prevention focusing on four areas:

1 Hospital environmental hygiene
2 Hand hygiene
3 Personal protective equipment
4 Safe disposal of sharps.

Table 12.2 Microorganisms: structure and examples

Microorganism	Structure/characteristics	Examples and diseases
Viruses	• Smaller than bacteria and can only be seen under an electron microscope, varying in size from 10–300nm • Contain a strand of nucleic acid, either DNA or RNA, which is enclosed in a protein coat or capsid • Viruses replicate inside the host cell and contain few enzymes	*Herpes viridae* family causes: • herpes simplex • *varicella zoster* (chickenpox and shingles) • cytomegalovirus • hepatitis B virus • papovaviruses associated with malignancy (cervical cancer) • chlamydia, sexually transmitted disease • retroviruses which cause HIV (HTLV-1) causing AIDS Some of the most serious infections known to man are caused by filovirus which causes ebola and Marburg viruses
Bacteria	Bacteria are classified according to four main properties: their shape, which is divided into the following: • Cocci (spherical) • Bacilli (rod-shaped) • Coccobacilli (short rods) • Spiral-shaped (spirochetes) Other determinants include: • Whether they require oxygen (obligate aerobes) • Not requiring oxygen (obligate anaerobes) Gram stain and presence of spores Acid-fast bacilli, Gram-positive, aerobic organisms e.g. *Mycobacterium* of which the most important human pathogen is *M. tuberculosis* or TB	• *Staphylococcus aureus* (Gram positive), causes superficial and deep tissue infections • *Streptococci pneumoniae* causes meningitis, pneumonia, septicaemia • *Clostridium spp.* is a Gram-positive bacilli producing spores and are anaerobic, cause gas gangrene and muscle infections, tetany Important Gram negatives: • *Pseudomonas aeruginosa* (pneumonia in CF), opportunistic infection producing blue-green distinctive pus • *Escherichia coli* Gram-negative bacillus causing meningitis, septicaemia and commonly urinary tract infections (UTI) • *Shigella* causes mild dysentery • *Klebsiella* causes UTI wounds infections
Protozoa	Unicellular animals	e.g. *Plasmodium spp.* which causes malaria
Fungi	Classification is based on reproductive and morphology characteristics	• Immunocompromised patients are very susceptible to *Candida albicans* (thrush) • *Aspergillus* can cause a serious lung infection • *Cryptococcus* is associated with HIV infections
Prions	Proteins without their own nucleic acid, resistant to heat and chemical disinfectants	Transmissible spongiform encephalopathies (TSE) are rare neurological degenerative conditions causing dementia and destruction of brain tissue, e.g. the fatal Creutzfeldt–Jakob disease (CJD), related to bovine spongiform encephalopathy (BSE)

Table 12.3 Risk factors for infection and sepsis

Patient-related factors	Treatment-related factors
• Extremes of age • Chronic illness such as diabetes, cancer, COPD • Nutritional status • History of infections • Immunosupressed status • Neutropenia • Drug or alcohol abuse • Splenectomy	• Recent surgery • Use of invasive catheters • Trauma • Invasive diagnostic procedures • Drug therapy, steroids, antibiotics, cytotoxic agents • Hospital inpatients

Source: Johnson, K. and Henry, K. (2009) Shock, systemic inflammatory response syndrome and multiple organ dysfunction syndrome in Morton, P. and Fontaine, D. (eds) *Critical Care Nursing: A Holistic Approach*, 9th edn. London: Lippincott, Williams and Wilkins, reproduced with permission.

Evidence of contamination of the hospital environment, with pathogens of the same strain of microorganisms colonising patients, clearly indicates the importance of hospital environmental hygiene. Shared clinical equipment such as stethoscopes and commodes are all potential sources for contamination, so it is essential that equipment is washed thoroughly with detergent and water, or, if in an outbreak situation, hypochlorite should be considered (Pellowe and Loveday 2007). While actual evidence of transmission of infection from the environment is not strong, it is logical to surmise that hand

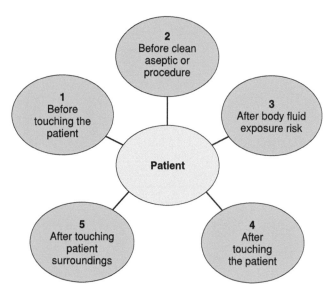

Figure 12.8 WHO 5 moments for hand hygiene

Source: Adapted from WHO (2009).

contamination from the environment will increase the spread of microorganisms.

Hand hygiene, with seemingly simple basic measures such as hand-washing, is widely regarded as one of the most effective ways of reducing HCAI (Gould 2010), but audit demonstrates that poor hand-washing frequency and technique is often practised by health care professionals (Gould *et al.* 2008). The World Health Organisation's '5 moments for hand hygiene' (WHO 2009) indicates moments where hand hygiene should occur for all health care professionals involved in direct patient contact (see Figure 12.8). Clear guidance for the procedures of hand washing and use of hand rub have been devised by the WHO (2009) and can be accessed at http://www.who.int/gpsc/tools/GPSC-HandRub-Wash.pdf.

The use of personal protective equipment such as gloves has been shown to reduce the transmission of microorganisms. It must be remembered though that contamination is still possible, especially during glove removal, so good hand-washing technique is still essential to prevent infection transmission (Pellowe and Loveday 2007). Gloves are single-use items and are changed between caring for different patients. Plastic aprons are also used for a single episode of care, and disposed of as clinical waste.

Safe disposal of sharps is essential to prevent risk of blood-borne viruses such as:

- Hepatitis B virus
- Hepatitis C virus
- Human immunodeficiency virus (HIV).

Saving lives, high-impact interventions (HII) (DH 2011)

High-impact interventions (HII) are an evidence-based approach to key clinical procedures or care processes that can reduce the risk of infection. Specific clinical activities in the form of care bundles have been developed to guide and audit areas of practice. A care bundle is a group of critical elements in a care process: when all elements are performed this is associated with an improved outcome. Current HIIs related to infection control have been developed (and are available at http://hcai.dh.gov.uk/whatdoido/high-impact-interventions/) include:

- peripheral intravenous cannula (insertion and ongoing);
- central venous catheter care (insertion and ongoing);
- urinary catheter care (insertion and ongoing);
- *Clostridium difficile* infection;
- blood cultures.

The central venous catheter care (ongoing care) bundle is shown in Figure 12.9, and is paired with a central line insertion care bundle. Each element of the bundle needs to be completed, and this can be audited to evaluate compliance. Bloodstream infections associated with central venous catheters are a major cause of morbidity (DH 2011), with 42.3% of bloodstream infections being central line-related. The care bundle is based on the EPIC guidelines (Pratt *et al.* 2007), and when all the elements of the bundle are performed the risk of infection is reduced (DH 2011). Compliance with care bundles involves all health care disciplines, and a cohesive consistent approach is required to reduce the burden of infection.

Acute problems related to the immune system

Hypersensitivity or allergic reactions

An allergen is defined as an antigen that causes an allergic reaction. The reaction maybe immediate (within minutes

Table 12.4 Central venous catheter bundle, ongoing care (DH 2011)

1 Hand hygeine	• Hands are decontaminated immediately before and after each episode of patient contact using the correct hand hygiene technique (Use of the World Health Organizations '5 moments of hand hygiene' or the NPSA 'Clean your hands campaign' is recommended)
2 Site inspection	• Site is inspected daily for signs of infection and is noted in the patient's record
3 Dressing	• An intact, dry, adherent transparent dressing is present • Insertion site should be cleaned with 2% chlorhexidine gluconate in 70% isopropyl alcohol prior to dressing change
4 Catheter injection ports	• Injection ports are covered by caps or valved connectors
5 Catheter access	• Aseptic techniques are used for all access to the line • Ports or hubs are cleaned with 2% chlorhexidine gluconate in 70% isopropyl alcohol prior to catheter access • Flush line with 0.9% sodium chloride for lumens in frequent use
6 Administration set replacement	• Set is replaced immediately after administration of blood/blood products • Set is replaced after 24 hours following total parenteral nutrition (if it contains lipids) • Set is replaced within 72 hours of all other fluid sets
7 Catheter replacement	• Catheter is removed if no longer required or decision not to remove is recorded • Details of removal are documented in the records (including date, location, and signature and name of operator undertaking removal)

Source: Department of Health (2011), High Impact Intervention: Central venous catheter care bundle, London: DH, pp. 2–3. Available at http://hcai.dh.gov.uk/files/2011/03/2011-03-14-HII.

of exposure) or delayed, depending on previous exposure, and the type of allergen, for example snake venom or insect stings. If left untreated it can cause severe shock and circulatory collapse within 10–15 minutes. According to the Resuscitation Council there are approximately 20 deaths in the UK per annum from anaphylaxis (RCUK 2011).

There are four types of hypersensitivity reaction: types I, II, III are mediated by antibodies and are classified as below (Weston 2008), and type IV by T cells:

● Type I (anaphylaxis, asthma and eczema).
● Type II involves IgM and IgG – caused by cytotoxic reactions which damage cells and tissues of the host (Weston 2008), e.g. a blood transfusion reaction.
● Type III hypersensitivity reactions occur when the antibody–antigen complexes of IgM and or IgG cause inflammatory reactions within the tissues or bloodstream.
● Type IV hypersensitivity reactions are mediated by T cells and may occur over a number of hours after exposure to the allergen, e.g. eczema skin reactions occur over a number of days.

The response to an allergen is mediated by the immunoglobulin IgE, during the primary exposure plasma cells produce large quantities of IgE which binds to mast cells. On subsequent exposure the allergen attaches itself to the IgE antibodies on the mast cell surface; this causes the mast cells to degranulate releasing histamine and triggering

the hypersensitivity reaction, inducing a variety of effects such as allergic rhinitis or a runny nose (see Figure 12.9).

The most severe form and medical emergency is anaphylaxis – 'a severe life-threatening, generalised or systemic hypersensitivity reaction' (Resuscitation Council 2011). There are multiple triggers ranging from antibiotics and muscle relaxants, to peanuts and other foods, insect stings and venom from snake bites. In children, food allergies tend to be the most common culprits. Health care practitioners who administer blood transfusions, human albumin solutions or gelatins (e.g. gelofusine), X-ray contrast media and intravenous (IV) antibiotics should be alert to the early signs of anaphylaxis as the IV route is the fastest trigger, causing reactions within seconds.

Other culprits especially in the elderly are aspirin and non-steroidal anti-inflammatory drugs (NSAIDs). Many cases are not mediated by IgE and are termed idiopathic, i.e. the causative allergen is not identified (RCUK 2011).

Clinical signs and symptoms

Not all patients who have an allergic reaction will go on to develop anaphylaxis and not all reactions are detected. Skin reactions such as urticaria (raised lumps or hives) and erythema (reddening of the skin caused by increased capillary blood flow) are common in about 80% of reactions; gastrointestinal symptoms may also be present such as vomiting and abdominal pain (RCUK 2011).

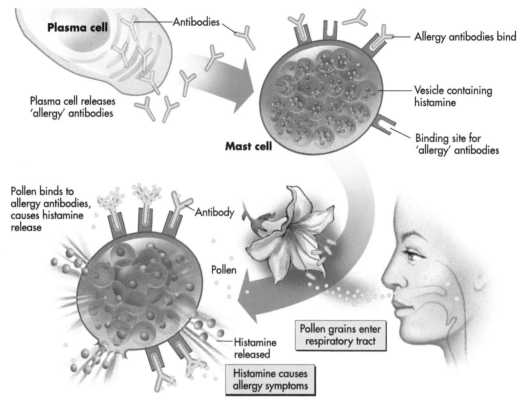

Figure 12.9 An example of local allergic reaction, allergic rhinitis

Anaphylaxis is likely when all three of the following conditions are present together and the onset of symptoms is within a few minutes of exposure:

- sudden onset and rapid progression of symptoms;
- life-threatening airway and/or breathing and/or circulation problems;
- skin and/or mucosal changes (flushing, urticaria, angioedema).

The patient will start to complain of feeling very unwell, they may become agitated and restless and may state that they have a feeling of an impending sense of doom, the symptoms if left untreated may rapidly progress to respiratory and cardiac arrest and death.

Rapid assessment

The patient should be rapidly assessed using the ABCDE approach. Questions should be direct and closed-ended if the patient can only answer in short sentences or singular words, the purpose is to elicit the nature of the problem, the allergen if known, if they have an adrenaline auto-injector or previous history of allergic reactions and how severely they may manifest. The preceding events or causative event is crucial in establishing the allergen. However, life-saving treatment such as oxygen, the administration of adrenaline and other anti-inflammatory drugs should not be delayed.

Signs and symptoms of anaphylaxis

- Airway swelling
- Hoarse voice
- Stridor
- Increased respiratory rate
- Wheeze
- Confusion (hypoxia)
- Central cyanosis (late sign)
- Respiratory arrest
- Pale or flushed
- Clammy
- Tachycardic
- Hypotensive
- Dizziness/loss of consciousness
- Cardiac arrest
- Erythmema
- Urticaria
- Angioeodema.

Airway patency can be compromised due to rapidly swelling deep tissues of the mucus membranes and lips known as angio-oedema. Swelling of the tongue associated with oropharyngeal and laryngeal oedema may also threaten the airway. The patient's ability to swallow their own saliva should be assessed and the development of a hoarse voice indicates partial airway obstruction. High-pitched inspiratory noise or stridor is caused by upper airway obstruction and should be immediately recognised and dealt with by summoning help via the peri-arrest or cardiac arrest call systems. Under the direction of the medical team intramuscular adrenaline and other pharmacology agents should be urgently administered. Worsening signs of airway obstruction include:

- Swelling of tongue and lips
- Hoarseness
- Oropharyngeal swelling.

Breathing assessment will reveal shortness of breath and respiratory difficulties. Bronchoconstriction causes wheezing, increasing the work of breathing resulting in greater respiratory distress. Central cyanosis may be evident although this is a late sign, the patient may become confused with the development of cerebral hypoxia. As the patient tires respiratory arrest is possible.

Circulation. The cardiovascular system should be assessed for the following clinical signs:

- tachycardia, with or with out associated myocardial ischaemia (chest pain);
- profound hypotension and dizziness due to peripheral vasodilation;
- clammy, sweaty skin, flushed or pale skin depending on the reaction.

Remembering the processes for the inflammatory response, there will be increased capillary permeability leading to the sequestering of fluids in the tissues giving rise to swelling and oedema. If left untreated, the patient may go on to develop cardiac arrest.

Disability. The neurological assessment under disability involves rapid assessment for confusion, agitation and reduced, or loss of, consciousness. An unconscious patient should already have been identified through the ABC assessment. A blood glucose should be checked *but* should not delay or distract from more urgent life-saving treatment, e.g. administration of adrenaline.

Exposure of the patient is important especially in allergic reactions, as there is a combination of both skin and mucosal changes in over 80% of reactions. The patient may complain of itchiness or urticaria from hives or raised red lumps or weals.

The diagnosis and treatment of anaphylaxis
The priority for all health care practitioners is to recognise the early signs of allergy; know and institute the UK Resuscitation Council's anaphylaxis algorithm (2008) (see Figure 12.10) and begin aggressive treatment to prevent development of the complications of anaphylaxis.

If possible the patient should be in a comfortable position, supine if hypotensive, or sitting up if experiencing breathing difficulties. The trigger if known should be removed or stopped but this may not always be possible. Intramuscular (IM) adrenaline 1:1000 (0.5mL or 500mcgs), is the drug of choice. The best injection site is the outer aspect of the middle third of the thigh muscle, or the anterolateral aspect. Adrenaline is an alpha-receptor agonist reversing the vasodilation, reducing oedema and dilating the bronchioles due to its beta-receptor agonist properties. Adrenaline also suppresses the release

of histamine, thus reducing the vasodilatory effects. IM adrenaline can be administered if required every 5 minutes; the patient's response should be continuously monitored (RCUK 2011).

High-flow oxygen therapy, intravenous access and full cardiac monitoring should be established. The administration of a bolus of 500mL IV fluids and second line treatment of antihistamines such as chlorphenamine and steroids such as hydrocortisone which shorten the reaction, should be given. Other considerations are treating for asthma-like symptoms that may involve the administration of nebulised salbutamol and ipratropium. Once the patient has stabilised they need to be monitored closely in a critical care area for a period of time.

The nurse's role may be very varied depending on experience. For the senior student or newly qualified nurse it will be a supportive role, getting equipment and drugs, recording observations or importantly remaining with the patient and supporting and reassuring them. A more experienced nurse may cannulate the patient, prepare and administer intravenous fluids, administer the intramuscular adrenaline and perform many other functions.

Infection, sepsis, severe sepsis and septic shock

Incidence
Sepsis has an annual incidence of 3.0 cases per 1000 of the population. Over 18 million people are affected worldwide every year and this accounts for an international total of approximately 1400 deaths per day (Garry *et al.* 2009). In 2005, in the United Kingdom alone, there were said to be 36,800 deaths attributed to severe sepsis and this figure is thought to be rising by 1.5% every year, possibly due to the increased age of patients and the existence of co-morbidities (Peel 2008, Steen 2009). Sepsis presents a major challenge for all nursing and medical personnel, both in terms of recognising and diagnosing infection early and in the optimal management of the condition with the health care resources available to them.

Definition
Sepsis is a complex syndrome that as it progresses affects all body systems, eventually leading to multiple organ failure. Historically, there has been some confusion regarding the definition and classification of the phenomenon, but since 1991 experts from around the world have worked collaboratively to produce the internationally agreed terminology we now have today (see Table 12.5) (Peel 2008, Steen 2009). This consensus of opinion regarding the stages of sepsis has been an invaluable guide to clinical practice, research and education, providing

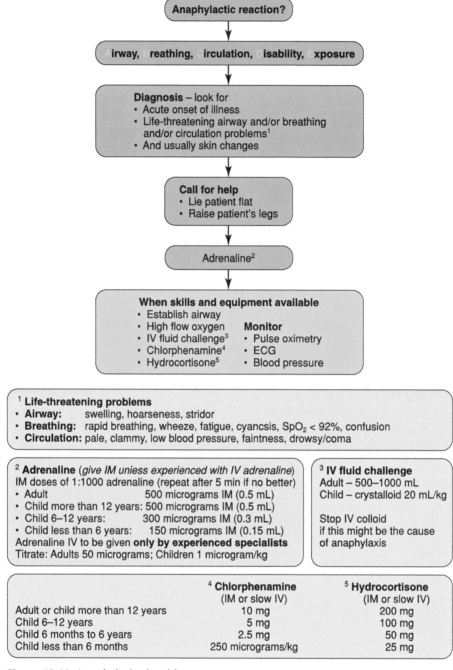

Anaphylactic reaction?

↓

Airway, **B**reathing, **C**irculation, **D**isability, **E**xposure

↓

Diagnosis – look for
- Acute onset of illness
- Life-threatening airway and/or breathing and/or circulation problems[1]
- And usually skin changes

↓

Call for help
- Lie patient flat
- Raise patient's legs

↓

Adrenaline[2]

↓

When skills and equipment available
- Establish airway
- High flow oxygen   **Monitor**
- IV fluid challenge[3]   • Pulse oximetry
- Chlorphenamine[4]   • ECG
- Hydrocortisone[5]   • Blood pressure

[1] **Life-threatening problems**
- **Airway:** swelling, hoarseness, stridor
- **Breathing:** rapid breathing, wheeze, fatigue, cyancsis, $SpO_2 < 92\%$, confusion
- **Circulation:** pale, clammy, low blood pressure, faintness, drowsy/coma

[2] **Adrenaline** (*give IM unless experienced with IV adrenaline*)
IM doses of 1:1000 adrenaline (repeat after 5 min if no better)
- Adult   500 micrograms IM (0.5 mL)
- Child more than 12 years: 500 micrograms IM (0.5 mL)
- Child 6–12 years: 300 micrograms IM (0.3 mL)
- Child less than 6 years: 150 micrograms IM (0.15 mL)
Adrenaline IV to be given **only by experienced specialists**
Titrate: Adults 50 micrograms; Children 1 microgram/kg

[3] **IV fluid challenge**
Adult – 500–1000 mL
Child – crystalloid 20 mL/kg

Stop IV colloid
if this might be the cause
of anaphylaxis

	[4] **Chlorphenamine** (IM or slow IV)	[5] **Hydrocortisone** (IM or slow IV)
Adult or child more than 12 years	10 mg	200 mg
Child 6–12 years	5 mg	100 mg
Child 6 months to 6 years	2.5 mg	50 mg
Child less than 6 months	250 micrograms/kg	25 mg

Figure 12.10 Anaphylaxis algorithm

Source: Resuscitation Council UK (2008) *Emergency Treatment of Anaphylactic Reactions: Guidelines for Healthcare Providers*, Figure 3, p. 20. Reproduced with the kind permission of the Resuscitation Council (UK).

the foundation for effective diagnosis and therapeutic intervention.

Stages of sepsis: clinical presentation and patient assessment

The body is constantly at risk from infection, thus several mechanisms for preventing invasion by pathogens have evolved; the protective covering of the skin, the pH of body fluids, the mucociliary escalator of the respiratory tract and the enzyme lysosome found in tears are amongst the host defences against infection. Together with the immune system these fight off a variety of Gram-negative and Gram-positive bacteria, viruses and fungi. If, however, these homeostatic processes become overwhelmed, a complex chain of events is set in motion.

Stages 1 and 2: exposure to the infective organism and the onset of systemic inflammatory response syndrome (SIRS)

The site of the infection may be anywhere in the body with wound sites, the lungs, the urinary tract and the

Table 12.5 Classification of sepsis

Systemic inflammatory response syndrome (SIRS)	This may be precipitated by an infection or, in some circumstances, damage to tissue such as ischaemia. In all cases two or more of the following will be present: • Temperature > 38°C or < 36°C • Heart rate > 90 beats per minute (unless taking medication that will affect the rate such as beta-blockers) • Respiratory rate > 20 breaths per minute or $PaCO_2$ < 4.3kpa • White blood cell count > 12 × 10^9/l or < 4 × 10^9/l
Sepsis	SIRS, plus a known or suspected infection
Severe sepsis	Sepsis associated with organ dysfunction. Hypoperfusion results in tissue hypoxia and eventually organ failure manifest by: • Hypotension: systolic blood pressure < 90mmHg, mean arterial pressure (MAP) < 65mmHg or a reduction of > 40mmHg from usual reading • Lactate > 4mmol/L • Altered mental state • Hyperglycaemia in the absence of diabetes mellitus • Hypoxaemia, with oxygen saturation < 93% • Urine output < 0.5ml/kg/hr and/or a raised urea or creatinine • Coagulopathy, international normalised ratio (INR) > 1.5
Septic shock	Presence of severe, unresolved sepsis, with: • Hypotension or raised lactate that does not improve with adequate fluid resuscitation
Multiple organ dysfunction syndrome	Failure of more than one organ requiring therapeutic intervention to maintain homeostasis

gastrointestinal system being commonly affected areas. As discussed earlier in the chapter, there is an initial humoral response to an invading organism and antibodies will stick to bacteria, thus marking them for destruction by macrophages. Neutrophils in particular have a key role to play in this process, furthermore they will also initiate the release of cytokines. The activation of these non-antibody proteins has two key effects: first, it contributes to the inflammatory changes that are occurring such as the vasodilatation, the increased blood flow, the swelling, the redness and the heat. Second, as the inflammation progresses, cytokine action leads to the activation of many proinflammatory agents made from monocytes and macrophages, the most significant of which are tumour necrosis factor, interleukins 1, 6 and 8, interferon-γ and tissue factor (see Table 12.6). These are important substances because they contribute to changes in the vascular endothelium, causing further permeability and the promotion of blood clot formation. Initially this process is beneficial, isolating pathogens and preventing them from entering the systemic circulation: the clots that are being formed are then broken down by normal fibrinolysis and therefore coagulation is controlled. However, if inflammation and increased permeability persist, a marked reduction in blood flow occurs and this exacerbates the procoagulant state. The body tries to regulate this process by releasing counter-inflammatory agents

such as interleukins 4 and 10 and transforming growth factor-β (TGF β) (see Table 12.6), but for some patients the inflammation and ensuing endothelial changes become overwhelming and are no longer localised or controlled (Balk *et al.* 2001, Johnson and Henry 2009, Steen 2009).

In such cases, a systemic response to the infection has begun and the patient is known or thought to be septic. In accordance with the SIRS criteria, changes to the patient's vital signs will also be evident. Using a track and trigger system the nurse will be able to identify and report early deterioration by calculating the early warning score (EWS) and noting the point at which the patient triggers. During assessment of the airway they will determine the degree to which the patient is able to speak and if any obstruction is apparent: secretions may lead to gurgling noises and there may be evidence of wheezing or stridor. It is important to remember that a reduction in the circulating volume will quickly impair cerebral perfusion and this can have a major impact on the patient's ability to maintain their airway. Level of consciousness may also swiftly be impaired by decreased cerebral oxygenation and increased cerebral acidosis.

Similarly, while assessing the patient's breathing, the nurse will be aware that inadequate tissue perfusion with worsening cellular hypoxia will lead to an accumulation of metabolic acid in all body fluids. At the bedside, even before any blood tests are taken, the nurse may observe an

Table 12.6 Some of the many pro and counter inflammatory mediators released in sepsis

Proinflammatory mediators	Clinical effect
Tumour necrosis factor (TNF)	Hypotension, tachycardia, tachypnoea, hyperglycaemia, metabolic acidosis, third spacing
Interleukin-1 (IL-1)	Fever, increased white blood cells, released amino acids from skeletal muscle, decreased systemic vascular resistance
Interleukin-6 (IL-6)	Fever, antibody secretion
Interleukin-8 (IL-8)	Stimulates neutrophil function and attracts inflammatory cells to site of infection/injury
Tissue factor	Initiates blood clotting
Interferon-γ	Macrophage activation
Counter-inflammatory mediators	**Clinical effect**
Interleukin-4 (IL-4)	T cell inhibition, suppression of TNF and IL-1, plus regulation of IgE and IgG secretion
Interleukin-10 (IL-10)	Suppresses procoagulant activity
Transforming growth factor-β (TGF β)	Promotes cell development and repair

increase in the patient's respiratory rate. Hyperventilation may occur in an attempt to reduce the acid load and this will be evident when calculating the EWS. Without obvious exertion, an increase in respiration over 12 breaths per minute warrants investigation and, if over 20, a sign of underlying pathology. Jevon and Ewens (2007) stress that a rise in the respiratory rate is a key indicator of patient deterioration and, for this reason, accurate counting of the respiratory rate for a full minute is required. At this time it is also important to look for any corresponding changes in the oxygen saturation reading (SpO_2), as this will deteriorate as the cellular hypoxia worsens.

Other factors increasing the EWS that the nurse should observe for will include the changes to the patient's circulation. First, owing to the vasodilatation and a relative hypovolaemia (the latter due to the increased capillary permeability) the heart, stimulated by the sympathetic autonomic nervous system, must pump faster and harder to maintain the cardiac output and the blood pressure. Second, the patient's temperature may rise or fall in response to the infection, but it should be remembered

that both hyperthermia and hypothermia will impact on the patient's metabolic rate and therefore oxygen delivery to the tissues. Finally, in the early stages of sepsis changes in the patient's white cell count may occur: the patient may produce an increased number of white cells to fight the infection or in some cases present with a neutropenia where white cell function is deficient.

Stage 3: severe sepsis – the systemic response
As the endothelial damage advances nitric oxide synthase, a potent vasodilator, is released from the endothelium and now widespread vasodilatation and persistently leaking blood vessels lead to a gross maldistribution of the circulating volume. This together with the intravascular micro-thrombi formation causes a further decrease in perfusion and a greater imbalance between oxygen demand and oxygen supply to the tissues. As a result, the septic patient will now begin to exhibit a complex array of systemic signs and symptoms. Further changes in respiratory, cardiac, renal, neurological and metabolic function may develop swiftly in response to the tissue hypoxia that is occurring and the nurse needs to be diligent during the assessment process in order to detect a worsening of the patient's condition. The NMC (2010) stresses the importance of the nurse possessing in-depth knowledge and having the ability to carry out an accurate assessment of a patient with complex problems, using appropriate diagnostic and decision-making skills.

Again using a systematic approach to patient assessment, the nurse will observe for changes to the patient's Glasgow Coma Score. With increasing cerebral acidosis the GCS may soon drop to eight or below, requiring endotracheal intubation to protect the airway. The patient's breathing will also become increasingly compromised. An arterial blood gas taken at this time would reveal a metabolic acidosis and serum lactate levels would be elevated owing to ongoing tissue ischaemia. The patient who is already hyperventilating because of the increasing acidosis must now also be observed for evidence of respiratory distress, for example, use of the accessory muscles of respiration indicating that the work of breathing has increased. A chest X-ray will aid medical diagnosis and may reveal areas of patchy consolidation consistent with deteriorating lung function. As the patient's respiratory function worsens and acute lung injury (ALI) progresses to acute respiratory distress syndrome (ARDS) the patient may start to hypoventilate. Widespread bronchoconstriction with poor lung compliance, a non-cardiogenic pulmonary oedema (evident on chest auscultation and through observation of frothy sputum) and a ventilation/perfusion mismatch all contribute to a refractory hypoxaemia requiring mechanical ventilation (Leach 2009).

Signs of severe sepsis

- Confusion/drowsiness
- Hypoxaemia
- Tachypnoea
- Hypotension
- Tachycardia
- Abnormal capillary refill
- Metabolic acidosis
- Low CVP
- Oedema
- Low urine output
- Pyrexia or hypothermia
- Flushed appearance/cyanosed
- High blood glucose.

With ongoing vasodilatation and loss of circulating volume the patient may exhibit further cardiovascular changes, many of which will increase the EWS score significantly. There may be marked hypotension, tachycardia with a bounding pulse and an impaired capillary refill; the last may be rapid at first and then reduced as peripheral perfusion worsens. It should be noted that in the early phase of sepsis, as the heart tries to compensate for the persistently low systemic vascular resistance, the cardiac output may be high. Unfortunately for the deteriorating patient, this will not achieve an increase in tissue perfusion owing to the circulation of substances like Myocardial Depressant Factor, synthesised in shock by ischaemic pancreatic tissue and directly impairing myocardial contractility.

With reduced arterial blood pressure perfusion to the kidneys will also be affected. The patient will have a falling urine output, with less than 0.5mL per kg per hour produced and this will be secondary to a reduced glomerular filtration rate. Normal homeostatic processes like the renin–angiotensin–aldosterone system and the sympathetic autonomic nervous system will have been activated early in the septic process in an attempt to restore perfusion by fluid retention and vasoconstriction, but the numerous powerful inflammatory mediators will counteract all compensatory mechanisms by maintaining dilatation of blood vessels.

The patient may now appear flushed due to the ongoing vasodilatation and be hot to the touch if pyrexial or cold if hypothermic. They may also appear cyanosed due to poor oxygenation, have mottled skin or be oedematous, the last due to fluid leaking from the capillary bed into the interstitium. Disturbances of the albumin and electrolyte levels may also be apparent as normal fluid and electrolyte balance is disrupted. Finally, as the prothrombotic state advances and the coagulation system is inappropriately activated, the clotting factors become depleted as a result of forming multiple clots in the capillary bed. This has two physiological effects: first, it puts the patient at risk from spontaneous bleeding and, second, because of the number of clots forming, it also increases the chance of thrombosis occurring. Furthermore, the latter is exacerbated by the rapid consumption of the normal regulators of clotting like protein C and by the release of plasminogen activator inhibitor, preventing fibrinolysis. These changes

herald the onset of disseminated intravascular coagulation syndrome (DIC), a common feature of advanced sepsis (Dellinger et al. 2008, Johnson and Henry 2009, Leach 2009). Lastly, decreased cerebral oxygenation and increasing acidosis will further impair neurological function. The ongoing vasodilatation will lead to a rise in intracranial pressure and the formation of further oedema which, if not alleviated by rapid intervention, will cause irreparable damage to neurones.

The blood glucose, essential for neurological function, will also rise as a result of sympathetic stimulation, with increased gluconeogenesis and increased glycogenolysis occurring in an effort to provide energy for cellular function. Ultimately, this too will not be of benefit to the patient, as the glucose will rise too high (circulating adrenaline indirectly leading to insulin resistance) and this will trigger further inflammatory action from neutrophils (Burdett and Rinsky 2010).

Stage 4: septic shock and progression to multiple organ dysfunction syndrome (MODS)

With advancing sepsis and worsening anaerobic metabolism, adenosine triphosphate production will decline and organs will eventually fail. The damage is determined by the extent to which the patient's hypotension and raised lactate levels respond to volume loading with crystalloid and colloid infusion. Refractory clinical states (those which are unresponsive to treatment) herald the risk of multiple organ dysfunction syndrome and finally death.

Management of severe sepsis and septic shock

All nurses managing septic patients should remember the well-known adage 'prevention is better than cure'. Earlier in the chapter, we discussed how nurses have a major role in maintaining asepsis and reducing the incidence of cross-infection in health care settings. Preventing contamination of vulnerable patients by ensuring invasive catheters are removed promptly when no longer required and providing optimal respiratory management for patients who are unable to fully mobilise are just two ways in which infection can be minimised (Steen 2009).

To avoid the progression of the continuum from infection and sepsis to death, comprehensive assessment skills noting key clinical indicators and timely interventions are required by the health care team. These have been summarised in Figure 12.11, followed by a detailed discussion of sepsis management.

It is of course not possible to eradicate all sources of infection that the patient may be exposed to, and for this reason a comprehensive international strategy to manage sepsis has been developed. Rivers et al. (2001) first described goal-directed therapy in treating patients with

CASE STUDY 12.1 Simon – Part 1

Simon, a previously fit, healthy 37-year-old presented in A&E for removal of a foreign body from his penis. He appears anxious, and in some discomfort but has no relevant past medical history.

After the foreign body has been removed the nurse checks to see that he is comfortable, but notices he looks unsettled. He denies any pain, but feels hot and uncomfortable, and so the nurse decides to complete an ABCDE assessment.

Airway

10.00h: His airway is clear and Simon is able to respond appropriately to the nurse's questions, but appears distracted and fidgety. He is able to demonstrate an effective cough, and there are no sounds of stridor or wheezing.

Breathing

When assessing his respiratory status Simon shows no signs of central or peripheral cyanosis, but appears slightly flushed. His respiratory rate is 22 breaths per minute, and his oxygen saturations are 95% on room air, which is within his target range of 94–98% set by the medical staff. There are no adventitious sounds on lung auscultation, and his chest is expanding equally with each breath. The respiratory rate triggers on the early warning score used in the department.

Circulatory

Assessment reveals that he has warm peripheries and a central temperature of 38.1°C. He is mildly tachycardic at 95 beats per minute, his pulse pressure is strong, and the rhythm regular. His blood pressure is recorded at 90/60mmHg, the pulse pressure calculated at 30mmHg. The blood pressure is lower than his admission reading of 110/80mmHg. He has not passed urine since the removal of the object. The temperature triggers on the EWS, and the nurse wonders if he might be developing an infection, which may lead to sepsis. He knows there is a sepsis protocol used in the trust, and decides to refer to it after completing his assessment.

Disability

Assessment records that he is alert on the AVPU scale, and that his blood glucose is within normal limits.

Exposure

The nurse asks Simon's permission to check the rest of his body for any new signs. The penis and scrotal area look oedematous and swollen, but have not changed markedly since admission.

The nurse totals the EWS score, one for each of temperature, blood pressure and respiratory rate, a total of three which requires that a doctor attends the patient. He gathers the notes and observation chart, tells Simon that he is going to ask the doctor to come and see him, as his temperature is raised and he may need some antibiotics. The nurse uses SBAR to guide his discussion with the doctor, who will attend as soon as she has finished clerking her patient on the surgical ward.

The nurse, concerned that Simon may be developing an infection, refers to the sepsis protocol used in the trust. The protocol is based on the care-bundle approach described by Dellinger *et al.* (2008): Simon's temperature, tachypnoea and tachycardia, along with the clinical suspicion of infection, means that he fulfils the criteria for sepsis. He decides to gain peripheral vascular access whilst waiting for the doctor to arrive.

Sepsis protocol

1 Unstable patient: Is the patient infected?		
Known, or strongly suspected infection?	yes/no	Details Possibly: 2 hours after removal of foreign body
And any *two* of these • Fever or hypothermia: (T > 38°C or < 36°C) • Tachycardia: (HR > 90/min) • Tachypnoea: (RR > 20, or spontaneous PaCO$_2$ < 4.3kPa) • WBC > 12,000/mm³ or < 4,000/mm³	Tick ✓ ✓ ✓	
Or clinical suspicion	yes/no	Details: Foreign object removed 2 hours ago

sepsis, and in 2002 the Surviving Sepsis Campaign (SSC) was launched. The aim of this campaign was to reduce mortality from sepsis and since its inception it has produced a series of explicit and detailed guidelines on the recognition and treatment of septic patients (Peel 2008). The 'care bundle' the campaign has produced outlines,

first, the resuscitation interventions that should be carried out within the first six hours and, second, the sepsis management actions that need to be addressed within the first 24 hours (Dellinger *et al.* 2008). Listed in Table 12.7 are the resuscitation bundle elements together with an explanation of each component.

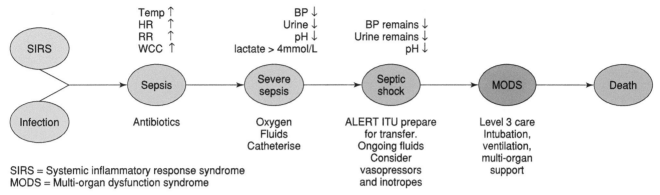

Figure 12.11 The spectrum of sepsis: clinical indicators and key interventions

Table 12.7 Sepsis resuscitation bundle: the first six hours

Bundle element 1: measure the serum lactate
• A blood sample for measuring lactate should be taken. When the level is greater than 4mmol/L treatment for severe sepsis should commence
Bundle element 2: blood cultures to be taken prior to antibiotic administration and source of infection to be identified
• Blood cultures should be taken prior to any antibiotic administration. At least two sets of cultures (one of which should be percutaneous) should be taken and all central lines that have been *in situ* for more than 48 hours should be cultured. Waiting for the results of the blood cultures should not delay treatment • Cultures of sputum, urine and material from any existing wound sites should also be taken so that any specific anatomical sites of infection can be located rapidly • Remove intravascular access devices and other invasive catheters if potentially infected
Bundle element 3: administer antibiotic therapy
• Intravenous broad-spectrum antibiotics should be given within the *first hour*. This is because each hour of delay significantly increases the risk of mortality
Bundle element 4: fluid resuscitation for hypotension and elevated lactate
As soon as hypoperfusion is identified, fluid administration should be commenced. Fluid administration should initially be delivered according to the following regime: • 20mL/kg of crystalloid; for a 70kg patient this would mean a fluid challenge of around 1500ml of crystalloid or 5.75mL/kg of colloid; for a 70kg patient this would mean a fluid challenge of around 500ml of colloid. This should be given in the first 10 minutes. In total, the patient may require 6–10 litres of fluid in the first 24 hours (Peel 2008). Dellinger *et al.* (2008) note that if there is evidence of cardiac insufficiency the volume of fluid should be reduced or administered with caution • A mean arterial pressure of > 65mmHg should be aimed for. If fluid administration alone cannot achieve this, a vasopressor in the form of norepinephrine should be administered via the central line. Dopamine may also be administered and at higher doses it can increase the systemic vascular resistance. If the cardiac output remains low in spite of fluid and vasopressor therapy, dobutamine will need to be commenced (Dellinger *et al.* 2008, Garry *et al.* 2009)
Bundle element 5: maintain adequate central venous pressure and central venous oxygen saturation
• A central line should be inserted and fluid resuscitation should achieve a central venous pressure of 8–12mmHg (unless mechanically ventilated, in which case a higher CVP target will be set to reflect the changes in intrathoracic pressure) • In the presence of persistent hypotension and a raised lactate level achieve a central venous oxygen saturation ($ScvO_2$) > 70% or a mixed venous oxygen saturation (SvO_2) > 65%. These are surrogate markers of tissue oxygenation, if their values drop it is an indication that the oxygen delivery (DO_2) is insufficient to maintain demand (Garry *et al.* 2009) • If there is difficulty in achieving a central venous oxygen saturation > 70% in the first six hours blood products should be given. The goal is to maintain the haemoglobin between 7.0–9.0g/dL (Dellinger *et al.* 2008)

Table 12.8 Sepsis six: the first hour of sepsis management

Administer oxygen therapy	• All patients should receive high-dose oxygen therapy via a non-rebreathing mask to achieve an SpO_2 reading of 94–98%
	• Medical staff may request central or mixed central venous blood samples to gain further information about tissue oxygenation
Take blood cultures	• Locate source of infection quickly
	• Pyrexial patients may require antipyretic therapy
Give intravenous antibiotics	• Administer broad spectrum antibiotics within *1 hour* according to local protocol
Commence intravenous fluid resuscitation	• Administer Hartmann's or equivalent
	• Once central line is inserted monitor central venous pressure as part of ongoing patient assessment
Check lactate level	• Increasing levels will indicate worsening tissue hypoxia
Hourly urine output measurement	• Consider urinary catheterisation if an indwelling catheter is not already *in situ*

In 2007, the SSC introduced 'Survive Sepsis', an initiative targeted at ward staff and designed to focus attention on the six key areas of treatment required by the septic patient in the *first hour*. These are known as the 'Sepsis six' and the current 2010 version produced by 'Survive Sepsis' is outlined in Table 12.8. Failure to observe the recommended timing of treatment will result in further patient deterioration, and the nurse has a key role in coordinating interprofessional intervention to ensure that this does not happen. Nurses should always provide leadership in managing adult nursing care, identifying the priorities and ensuring that time and resources are used effectively (NMC 2010).

Ongoing management

Patients developing septic shock will be transferred to the intensive care unit where they will receive ongoing support of their organ dysfunction. For most patients this will entail mechanical ventilation, additional inotropic support for cardiac function, haemofiltration for renal impairment and further haematological support for coagulopathy. They will also be nursed in an upright position to prevent any additional pulmonary infection and be commenced on prophylactic therapy for stress ulcer formation and deep vein thrombosis (Dellinger *et al.* 2008).

The SSC has also specified another three bundle elements to be accomplished within the first 24 hours of a septic shock presentation. These will also be implemented in the intensive care unit, depending on the assessment findings of the individual patient. They are:

• The administration of low-dose steroids to support adrenal function if fluid therapy and vasopressor agents have proved unsuccessful in treating hypotension.
• Glycaemic control to maintain blood glucose at a normal limit and no greater than 10mmol/L.
• Use of a 'lung protective' strategy for mechanically ventilated patients to regulate inspiratory plateau pressures and deliver tidal volumes at no greater than 6mL/kg.

CASE STUDY 12.2 Simon – Part 2

Simon has become unwell two hours after having a foreign body removed. The sepsis protocol is being used to guide treatment as infection and sepsis is suspected.

The nurse looks at the second question on the sepsis protocol while he is waiting for the doctor to attend. The systolic BP of 90mmHg could be indicative of organ hypoperfusion. The nurse is now concerned that Simon may be deteriorating and developing severe sepsis, and is aware that this is associated with the risk of developing septic shock. The doctor arrives and examines Simon, noting the observation chart showing tachypnoea, tachycardia and pyrexia which are all indicators of sepsis (Dellinger *et al.*

CASE STUDY 12.2 Simon – Part 2 (*continued*)

2008). She follows up the blood results taken earlier, which show a normal white cell count but a raised C-reactive protein. This indicates an early stage of infection.

Sepsis protocol

2 Is there evidence of hypoperfusion or organ failure?		
Any *one* of these	yes/no	
Systolic BP < 90 or MAP < 70 1 hour or more	Tick ✓	
Urine output < 0.5mL/kg/hr for 1 hour or more	tick	
Deteriorating conscious level Not due to sedation or CNS disease	tick	
Metabolic acidosis: pH < 7.30 + Base deficit > 5mmol or lactate > 4mmol/L	tick	Unknown at 10.35
If criteria 1 and 2 fulfilled: yes **Severe sepsis diagnosis made**	**Start time**	Document the time: 10 30am Start the clock

This is a medical emergency. Inform the SpR or consultant. Yes 10.35am.

The doctor consults the microbiologist regarding appropriate antibiotic therapy, and asks the nurse to repeat his observations in 30 minutes. At 10.30h the repeated observations reveal a further deterioration in Simon's condition, with his oxygen saturations decreasing to 93%, and respiratory rate rising to 26 breaths per minute. His blood pressure is now 87/50mmHg systolic, with a tachycardia of 105 beats per minute, but he is still warm and peripherally dilated. The pulse pressure has increased from 30 to 37mmHg, which is consistent with the vasodilation of sepsis. The EWS is scoring four as the raised heart rate gives an additional score of one. The evidence of hypoperfusion is now clear, so a diagnosis of severe sepsis is made, and the time filled in on the sepsis protocol. Severe sepsis is considered a medical emergency and a number of actions need to be taken within the next hour in order to maximise Simon's prospect of a speedy recovery. The nurse is aware from attending a recent study day, of the 'Sepsis six' advocated by 'Survive Sepsis', and realises this strategy is consistent with the Trust protocol for sepsis management.

3 First hour from start time: ward actions				
Action		Initials	Grade	Variation (give reason)
100% oxygen via non-rebreathe oxygen mask	time 10.35	RR	Band 6	
Early resuscitation: gelofusine or crystalloid	time 10.50	RR		
Blood culture taken (consider also sputum, urine, line tips etc.)	time 10.40	RR	Band 6	
Broad-spectrum antibiotic prescribed	Time 10.40	DT	FY2	
Broad spectrum antibiotic *given*	time 10.45	DT	FY2	
Urinary catheterisation	time	No		Passed small amount of urine
Lactate sample taken	time 10.40	NT	FY2	
One hour time check – all steps done?	Yes/ no	Lactate result 4.2mmol/L		

The nurse places Simon on high-flow oxygen at 15 litres via a non-rebreathe mask to try and increase his oxygen saturations back to within the target range. Blood cultures are taken: one from the newly inserted venflon and one percutaneously. The nurse is unable to obtain a sputum sample, but Simon is able to pass a small amount of bloodstained urine, which is sent for culture and sensitivity. The doctor informs the SpR about the change in Simon's condition. Gentamycin 80mg is prescribed (usual dose 5–7mgs/kg) as advised by the microbiologist. This, along with paracetamol 1 gram, is given intravenously by the doctor.

A sample of blood for lactate and an arterial blood gas is taken. An infusion of 500mL of intravenous gelofusine is prescribed to run over 15 minutes, as per protocol. Dellinger *et al.* (2008) stresses the importance of lactate in severe sepsis as a marker of anaerobic metabolism. A lactate of above 4mmol/L would suggest that fluid resuscitation was necessary to improve blood pressure and tissue perfusion.

At 11.00h the nurse repeats Simon's observations to assess his response to the fluid challenge. There are some signs of

CASE STUDY 12.2 Simon – Part 2 (*continued*)

improvement with the heart rate decreasing to 100 beats per minute, and the blood pressure increasing back to 90mmHg. Oxygen saturations are 98% on 10L of oxygen, and Simon's respiratory rate is reduced at 24 breaths per minute.

Arterial blood gases and lactate results return and are as follows

- pH 7.32
- $PaCO_2$ 3.5kPa
- PaO_2 10.2kPa
- HCO_3^- 19mmol/L
- BE −3.5mmol/L
- Lactate 4.2mmol/L.

Simon's oxygenation is adequate, and the flow of oxygen is reduced to 8 litres. The lowered pH indicates an acidosis, and paired with the negative base excess and lowered bicarbonate, is consistent with a metabolic acidosis. The increased respiratory rate has reduced Simon's carbon dioxide levels, and partially compensated for the metabolic acidosis. The lactate is above 4mmol/L and further confirms the diagnosis of severe sepsis. On discussion with the medical team the possibility of placing a central line is discussed, along with the insertion of a urethral catheter to allow close monitoring of urine output. The doctors decide to see if Simon continues to respond to fluid therapy and

the antibiotics over the next hour. If he does not then further interventions may be required.

Another 500mL of gelofusine is prescribed and given rapidly over 15 minutes.

At 11.35h the nurse checks that all the requirements of the 'Sepsis six' and the trust sepsis protocol have been adhered to, as the first hour has passed. He also evaluates Simon's response to the second 500mLs of gelofusin. The nurse is pleased to observe that Simon is more chatty, saying that he feels more comfortable. He shows no sign of respiratory distress, with his SpO_2 maintained at 98%, and respiratory rate now reduced to 20 breaths per minute. His temperature has reduced to 37.4°C, his heart rate 95, and his blood pressure is now 100/60mmHg. Simon asks the nurse for a bottle, and passes 400mL of urine, which looks clear, but with a slightly pink tinge. His hands feel a little cooler with the reduced temperature. The EWS has now reduced to one (respiratory rate) but the nurse still decides to record hourly observations, so that any clinical change will be detected early. The medical staff are pleased with Simon's prompt response to treatment. He is commenced on 500mL of Hartmann's to run over four hours, but required no additional intervention at this stage, just close monitoring so that early intervention is possible should his clinical condition change.

Conclusion

A fully functioning immune system is vital for the maintenance of good health. An overview of applied physiology of this system has been given, and the clinical problems that may lead to a medical emergency of anaphylaxis and sepsis have been explored. Lack of recognition and appropriate intervention of these problems may lead swiftly to cardiac arrest, multiple organ dysfunction and death.

Infections, health care-associated infections and the spectrum of sepsis increase mortality, but there is consensus in the literature that early recognition of the deteriorating, septic patient and timely instigation of therapeutic management is key to mortality reduction. The nurse, at the bedside, has a major role to play in this and by working collaboratively with other members of the multidisciplinary team they can ensure the delivery of quality care to patients facing problems with their immune system, infection and sepsis.

Glossary

Abscess A collection of pus accumulation in a cavity.

Aetiology The causes or origin of a disease.

Anaphylaxis An acute multi-system severe type I hypersensitivity allergic reaction.

Angioedema Swelling of the deeper layers of the skin, this is often severe and is caused by a build-up of fluid.

Asepsis The absence of pathogenic organisms.

Basal metabolic rate The base rate at which the body consumes calories for basic metabolic functions such as maintaining internal temperature and repairing cells.

Commensal Living on or within another organism and deriving benefit without harming or benefiting the host.

Croup A respiratory condition that is usually triggered by an acute viral infection of the upper airway.

Enterotoxin A protein toxin released by a microorganism in the intestine.

Enzyme Proteins that catalyse chemical reactions.

Fibrin A fibrous protein involved in the clotting of blood.

Haemolysis The breaking down of erythrocytes.

Heparin An injectable anticoagulant.

Histamine A chemical that is released in the body as part of an allergic reaction.

Immunoglobulin Also known as an antibody.

Innate Existing since birth.

Microbes Tiny organisms that cannot be seen by the naked eye.

Microthrombi Small thrombus located in a capillary or other small blood vessel.

Morphology The study of the form and structure of organisms.

Pathogens An infectious agent (a germ).

Stridor A high-pitched wheezing sound resulting from turbulent air flow in the upper airway.

Toxin A poisonous substance produced within living cells or organisms.

Test yourself

1 Name the two types of immune defence system in the body.

2 List the five major white blood cell groups.

3 Identify the three main functions of the complement system.

4 What is the primary function of fever?

5 Define the following terms:
   a. antigen
   b. antibody

6 Name the four main classes of microorganism affecting humans.

7 List six key signs and symptoms of anaphylaxis.

8 Name the four physiological parameters that change during a systemic inflammatory response.

9 What is the significance of a raised serum lactate level?

10 Name the Sepsis six.

References

Balk, R., Ely, E. and Goyette, R. (2001) *Sepsis Handbook: National initiative in sepsis education* Tennessee, Vanderbilt University Medical Center.

Bannister, B., Gillespie, S. and Jones, J. (2006) *Infection Microbiology and Management*, 3rd edn. London: Blackwell Publishing.

Blay, A. (2011) Introduction to routine blood tests, normal values and relevance to clinical practice. In Phillips, S., Collins, M. and Dougherty, L. *Venepuncture and Cannulation* (*Essential Clinical Nurses*). Chichester: Wiley-Blackwell.

Burdett, D. and Rinsky, M. (2010) Systemic inflammatory response syndrome treatment and management. Available from http://emedicine.medscape.com/article/168943-treatment, last accessed August 2011.

Colbert, B., Ankney, J., Lee, K., Steggall, M. and Dingle, M. (2009) *Anatomy and Physiology for Nursing and Health Professionals*. Harlow: Pearson Education Limited.

Dellinger, R., Levy, M. and Carlet, J. (2008) Surviving Sepsis Campaign: international guidelines for the management of severe sepsis and septic shock. *Critical Care Medicine* 36 (1), 296–327.

DH (2011) *Saving Lives, High Impact Interventions*. Available from http://hcai.dh.gov.uk/whatdoido/high-impact-interventions/, last accessed August 2011.

DH (2008) *Clean Safe Care: Reducing infections and saving lives*. Available from http://www.dh.gov.uk/prod_consum_dh/groups/dh_digitalassets/documents/digitalasset/dh_081719.pdf, last accessed August 2011.

Fraise, A. and Bradley, C. (2009) *Ayliffe's Control of Health-Associated Infection*, 5th edn. London: Hodder Arnold.

Garry, P., Garry, D. and Kapila, A. (2009) Surviving sepsis – the physiology behind why we should intervene early. *Care of the Critically Ill* 25 (2), 36–39.

Goering, R., Dockrell, H., Zuckerman, M., Wakelin, D., Roitt, I., Mims, C. and Chiodini, P. (2008) *Mims' Medical Microbiology*, 4th edn. London: Elsevier Limited.

Gould, D. (2010) Auditing hand hygiene in practice. *Nursing Standard* 25 (2), 50–56.

Gould, D. and Brooker, C. (2000) *Applied Microbiology for Nurses*. London: Macmillan.

Gould, D., Drey, N., Moralejo, D. Grimshaw, J. and Chudleigh, J. (2008) Interventions to improve hand hygiene compliance in patient care. *Journal of Hospital Infection* 66 (1), 6–14.

Humphreys, H. (2007) Staphylococcus skin infections; osteomyelitis; food poisoning; foreign body infections; MRSA. In Greenwood, D., Slack, R., Peutherer, J. and Barer, M. (eds) *Medical Microbiology A Guide to Microbial Infections: Pathogenesis, immunity, laboratory diagnosis and control*, 17th edn. London: Elsevier.

Jevon, P. and Ewens, B. (2007) *Monitoring the Critically Ill Patient*, 2nd edn. Oxford: Blackwell.

Johnson, K. and Henry, K. (2009) Shock, systemic inflammatory response syndrome and multiple organ dysfunction syndrome. In Morton, P. and Fontaine, D. (eds) *Critical Care Nursing a Holistic Approach*, 9th edn. London: Lippincott, Williams & Wilkins.

Jones, K. and Shelton, B. (2009) Common immunological disorders. In Morton, P. and Fontaine, D. (eds) *Critical Care Nursing a Holistic Approach*, 9th edn. London: Lippincott, Williams & Wilkins.

Leach, R. (2009) *Acute and Critical Care Medicine*, 2nd edn. Oxford: Blackwell.

Marieb, E. and Hoehn, K. (2010) *Human Anatomy and Physiology*. San Francisco: Benjamin Cummings.

Martini, F. H. and Ober, W. C. (2011) *Martini's Atlas of the Human Body*. San Francisco: Pearson.

National HCAI Research Network (2011) *About Healthcare-associated Infections*. Available from http://www.hcainetwork.org/about%20hcai.htm, last accessed August 2011.

Nursing and Midwifery Council (2010) *Standards for Pre-registration Nursing Education*. Available from http://standards.nmc-uk.org/PublishedDocuments/Standards%20for%20pre-registration%20nursing%20education%2016082010.pdf, last accessed August 2011.

Peel, M. (2008) Care bundles: Resuscitation of patient with severe sepsis. *Nursing Standard* 23 (11), 41–46.

Pellowe, C. and Loveday, H. (2007) Epic 2: Updating Department of Health guidelines for preventing healthcare-associated infections. *Infant* 3 (2), 15–20.

Pratt, R., Pellowe, C., Wilson, J., Loveday, H., Harper, P. J., Jones, S. R. L. J., McDougall, C. and Wilcox, M. H. (2007) National evidence-based guidelines for preventing healthcare associated infections in NHS hospitals in England. *Journal of Hospital Infection* 65, S1–S64.

RCUK (Resuscitation Council UK) (2011) *Advanced Life Support*, 6th edn. RCUK.

RCUK (Resuscitation Council UK) (2008) *Emergency Treatment of Anaphylactic Reactions. Guidelines for healthcare providers*. Available from http://www.resus.org.uk/pages/reaction.pdf, last accessed August 2011.

Rivers, E., Nguyen, B., Havstad, S., Ressler, J., Muzzin, B., Bernhard, B., Knoblich, M., Peterson, E. and Tomlanovich, M. (2001) Early goal-directed therapy in the treatment of severe sepsis and septic shock. *New England Journal of Medicine* 345 (19), 1368–77.

Steen, C. (2009) Developments in the management of patients with sepsis. *Nursing Standard* 23 (48), 48–55.

Stewart, J. (2007) Innate and acquired immunity. In Greenwood, D., Slack, R., Peutherer, J. and Barer, M. (eds) *Medical Microbiology A Guide to Microbial Infections: Pathogenesis, immunity, laboratory diagnosis and control*, 17th edn. London: Elsevier, pp. 107–33.

Weston, D. (2008) *Infection Prevention and Control Theory and Practice for Healthcare Professional*. Chichester: Wiley.

WHO (2009) *WHO Guidelines on Hand Hygiene in Health Care, First Global Patient Safety Challenge Clean Care is Safer Care*. © World Health Organization 2009. Available from http://whqlibdoc.who.int/publications/2009/9789241597906_eng.pdf, last accessed August 2011.

Further reading

Daniels, R. and Nutbeam, T. (2010) *ABC of Sepsis*. Oxford: Wiley.

Kaye, K. and Moellering, R. C. (2011) Infection prevention and control in the hospital. *Infectious Disease Clinics of North America* 25 (1).

Royal College of Nursing (2011) *Infection Prevention and Control: Information and learning resources for health care staff*. London: RCN.

Wood, P. J. (2011) *Understanding Immunology*. Harlow: Prentice Hall.

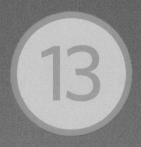

The safe transfer of acutely ill patients

Jacqui Finch

Aims

The aim of this chapter is to increase your knowledge with regard to the safe transfer of acutely ill patients.

Objectives

After reading this chapter you will be able to:

→ Differentiate between 'intra' and 'inter'-hospital transfers

→ Identify the reasons for transferring acutely ill patients

→ Debate the ethico-legal issues that arise in practice when transferring patients

→ Using the ABCDE format, describe the safe and effective preparation of the patient and the equipment prior to transfer

→ Highlight the physiological and psychological complications that the patient could sustain during the transfer process and how to manage them

→ Critically review the role of the nurse during transfer

Introduction

A patient presenting with an acute medical emergency is, at some point in their treatment, likely to require transfer from one place to another for continuity of care. Indeed, in the event of sudden deterioration they may have initially been transferred into hospital via the accident and emergency department and will then subsequently be moved to a ward, a high-dependency unit or an intensive care unit for further monitoring and management, depending on the severity of the clinical condition. Once in these designated areas, a patient may need to be moved again to other departments for medical investigations or surgery and, ultimately, transfer to another hospital for specialist or ongoing management may be necessary. It must also be noted that although thankfully not a common occurrence, transfer would also be mandatory in the event of an unforeseen emergency occurring within the clinical area, such as a fire breaking out.

It is very unlikely that an acutely ill patient will not need to be moved at all during their hospital admission; as a result, the transfer of patients between clinical areas is a key aspect of their care and one that the nurse has to be familiar with. All practitioners must possess the relevant knowledge and skills to safely and effectively transport the patients in their care from one place to another without incident. For this reason, there has been a growing focus over the last few years on the development of specialist training courses in order to better prepare clinicians for this role. To this end, this chapter will explore the preparation for transfer and the process itself, with particular regard to the physiological complications and organisational problems that may occur and how to avoid them. When considering the optimal management of acutely ill patients there are also a number of ethico-legal issues arising from the transfer procedure itself. Nurses need to be aware of the significance of these matters, particularly with regard to their own professional accountability and their duty of care to patients.

Reasons for transfer

Patients may be transferred for specific clinical reasons, they may be moved because of capacity issues in certain areas or they may leave one hospital to go to another for sociogeographic reasons, such as returning to a place nearer their home. The exact number of transfers taking place on a yearly basis within UK hospitals is not known, but it is estimated that about 1.3 million transfers are made per year for non-clinical reasons alone (West 2010). There is a lack of specific data with regard to this aspect of practice and this is because historically it has not been possible to retrieve exact figures for transfer: no national, systematic method of data collection exists. Furthermore, it has been suggested that in some places ad hoc recording of transfer events has taken place, particularly when patients are moved around within the same building. A 2009 freedom of information request approached 88 trusts for transfer data. Of the 42 trusts that responded to the survey, only six were able to provide specific information on clinical and non-clinical transfers. The key issue emerging from this exercise was that there had been considerable variation in the way the figures had been collated in different institutions, therefore making any comparison or analysis of data very difficult (West 2010).

By definition, some transfers will be intra-hospital, involving those individuals who are transported between areas within the same building, for example, from a ward to the radiology department for an investigation like a computerised tomography (CT) scan. Others will be inter-hospital involving ambulance personnel, where a patient is moved from one hospital to another for specialist treatment such as neurological surgery or to an external agency such as a rehabilitation centre for further therapy. Wherever patients are moved to, medical and nursing staff must be cognisant of the fact that the same levels of care are always required. Whether a patient is being transferred a long distance or a short one, meticulous preparation of the patient and the equipment is always necessary. As Handy and Van Zwanenberg (2009: 30) note 'a 100 yards or a 100 miles', the same principles should always be applied.

Ethico-legal issues

The decision to transfer a patient either for clinical or non-clinical reasons will be debated by the multidisciplinary team, with the ultimate responsibility lying with the consultant overseeing the patient's care. From an ethical perspective, moving from one area to another should be an act of beneficence, taken in the patient's best interests, especially as the move may cause their clinical condition

Millions of patient transfers occur every year.

Transfer of the patient should be clinically in their best interests.

to deteriorate further. As key members of the multi-disciplinary team nurses have a professional responsibility to work within recognised ethical and legal frameworks, with their first and foremost concern being the safety of the patients in their care (Nursing and Midwifery Council 2010).

Ideally, no patient should be transferred purely on the grounds of capacity, however, a pragmatic approach must be taken when dealing with the realities of clinical practice. Occasionally, workload constraints mean that transfer for a non-clinical reason such as a bed shortage does occur and all members of the multidisciplinary team must ensure that this is a safe, well-implemented and well-documented procedure. In all patient transfers the mode, timing and process of the move should be carefully planned taking clinical parameters such as the patient's condition and environmental factors like travel arrangements into consideration (Intensive Care Society 2011).

The role of the nurse in the transfer of an acutely ill patient is a challenging one, as it requires the practitioner to apply a range of knowledge and clinical skills in unfamiliar circumstances. The patient requires the delivery of a high standard of care throughout the transfer process, much of which inevitably takes place outside of the normal clinical environment. Managing a deteriorating patient in a well-known working context is easier than trying to cope in a series of places that the nurse is not accustomed to working in, such as corridors, lifts and ambulances. Problems may occur and without meticulous preparation of the accompanying staff member, the patient and the equipment being used, the results may be disastrous.

During preparation for transfer, there are four key areas to consider (Figure 13.1):

- staff training for the procedure;
- patient readiness to go;
- equipment checked and accessible;
- communication with all members of the multidisciplinary team: verbal and written.

Staff training

This is a key factor in the successful transfer of patients but, until fairly recently, there has been little formal training of nursing and medical staff in this area and this has led to an increase in patient morbidity and even mortality in some cases (Andrews *et al.* 2008). In the past, an assumption has been made that if staff members possess a level of clinical expertise within their own working environment they will be able to apply their knowledge and skills anywhere, however this is not always the case. Many practitioners may in fact be quite poorly prepared

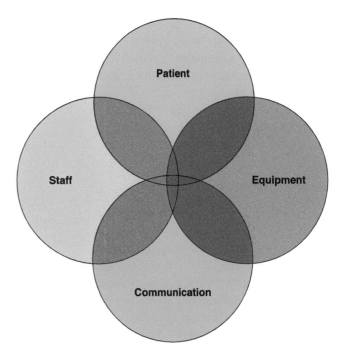

Figure 13.1 Four key areas in preparation for patient transfer

> Nurses are professionally accountable for their own actions and omissions and they must always be able to justify their decisions (Nursing and Midwifery Council 2008).

for transferring patients and the lack of specialist training for the experience exacerbates this. Added to which, it is often the junior staff who are sent to accompany patients on inter or intra-hospital transfer because the senior staff cannot leave the clinical area for managerial reasons. Cook and Allan (2008) found that the training of medical staff in the field of transfer was often haphazard and almost entirely dependent on local initiatives, there being no systematic approach to transfer education in place. This is an issue of concern for nursing staff who may look to their medical colleagues for guidance and support during the transfer process, because as Watson (2006) notes, nurses are nearly always the second attendant. Remember also that, in some cases, depending on the severity of the patient's condition, the nurse may be the only health care professional present during the transfer process.

> Specialist training in the transfer of patients is recommended for all nursing and medical staff.

All staff should therefore receive some specialist training in this area of clinical practice (Association of Anaesthetists of Great Britain and Ireland 2006) and always acknowledge their own limitations when carrying out the procedure, seeking assistance where appropriate. In addition, they must be aware of their own professional accountability and the legal implications when undertaking transfer. Nurses have a duty of care to their patients, and they must constantly maintain and update their knowledge and skills in order to enhance clinical performance and promote the delivery of safe and effective therapeutic intervention. They must also respond autonomously and confidently in unplanned as well as planned situations (Nursing and Midwifery Council 2010).

Patient preparation

Acutely ill patients have an increased risk of deterioration during transfer (Dunn *et al.* 2007), and for this reason the nurse should adopt a systematic approach when planning to move a patient. In previous chapters, we have seen how the use of the ABCDE format for assessment, goal planning, intervention and evaluation enables clinicians to effectively manage the patients in their care. Collecting both subjective and objective data during the assessment process can assist with the generation of an early warning score. Track and trigger systems provide valuable information about the severity of a patient's condition, and will therefore assist the nurse to identify whether or not the patient is ready to be moved or requires additional clinical optimisation.

Airway
Continuous monitoring of the patient's ability to maintain an airway is required. If there is any doubt, either due to impaired consciousness or sounds of obstruction being heard such as stridor, then the airway should be secured by artificial means. Remember, tracheal intubation is mandatory prior to transport if there are any concerns of this nature.

> Before transfer patients should be assessed systematically using the ABCDE format. Remember to:
> - Look
> - Feel
> - Listen.

Breathing
Similarly, if patient assessment reveals inadequate breathing such as changes in the respiratory rate, the use of accessory muscles, evidence of poor gas exchange or the presence of adventitious breath sounds, action should be taken to improve the adequacy of ventilation before transfer – either by the administration of oxygen therapy or by initiating non-invasive or invasive mechanical means, depending on the severity of the patient's condition. It is important to note that problems with oxygenation are more likely to occur during transfer, because when a patient

is being moved on a trolley, a bed or maybe even in a vehicle like an ambulance, the body is exposed to gravitational forces, the main hazard of which is acceleration. In health, physiological compensatory mechanisms enable the individual to cope with these forces as long as they are not too severe or too prolonged, but in acute illness the patient's ability to do so is insufficient and deleterious effects will occur. To illustrate this, in the lungs changes in the distribution of blood flow would result quite quickly in a mismatch between alveolar ventilation and perfusion. Poor gas exchange would ensue and the patient's oxygen saturation would drop significantly (Lawler 2000). Constant monitoring of all respiratory parameters is therefore required.

Furthermore, the identification of specific respiratory problems such as the presence of a pneumothorax must be addressed immediately, with chest drain insertion occurring prior to departure. Every action must be taken to avoid deterioration of the patient's condition during transfer, and if physiological problems are evident from the outset these have to be addressed as a priority.

Circulation
A thorough assessment of the patient's cardiovascular status is essential before departure. As noted in previous chapters, information needs to be gathered regarding general appearance, perfusion and capillary refill, skin temperature, skin sensation to touch and the degree of hydration. The transferring team should proceed only when confident that the patient's condition, and in particular the vital signs, have been rendered as stable as possible. If there are any concerns regarding the heart rate, blood pressure or fluid status, the patient should not, under any circumstances, be moved until the problems have been resolved (Intensive Care Society 2011). Similarly, knowledge of the patient's haematological status is crucial prior to departure, with problems such anaemia or a coagulopathy being addressed as a matter of urgency.

Of particular concern is hypovolaemia, which can occur for a number of reasons, including haemorrhage secondary to trauma, dehydration and sepsis. Volume depleted patients do not tolerate being transported very well. As noted earlier, acceleratory forces alter blood flow distribution and this can be exacerbated if a patient is fluid-depleted. Movement towards the head (such as a trolley being pushed forwards), will result in blood moving suddenly towards the feet and pooling there. In contrast, during acceleration towards the feet, blood rushes towards the head. The net effect of these forces is to render the patient hypotensive, with poor cardiac output, because the more volume depleted they are, the more scope for volume movement within the body.

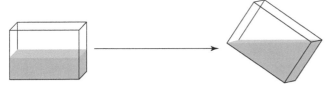

Transport in hypovolaemia: there is rapid movement of fluid in an underfilled patient

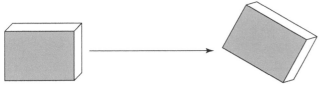

Transport in normovolaemia: less movement of fluid occurs

Figure 13.2 Treating hypovolaemia reduces the physiological effect of gravitational forces on blood flow

Source: Reproduced with kind permission from Dr J. Handy, NWL Critical Care Network.

In Figure 13.2, we can see how a vessel that is only partially full allows room for movement of the fluid within it during transport. In contrast, when a vessel is completely full with fluid, the fluid cannot be rapidly shifted from one end to another because there is no empty space for it to move in to. The same principle applies to patients: if they are normovolaemic, with a good circulating volume, they are less likely to suffer from the effects of gravity on blood flow. One maxim to remember that summarises this issue very well is that 'full patients travel better' (Handy and van Zwanenberg 2009: 10).

> Gravitational forces will be poorly tolerated if the patient is hypovolaemic. Remember 'full patients travel better'.

Always ensure therefore that a patient is haemodynamically stable and any fluid deficits addressed before moving them. Acutely ill patients should have cardiac monitoring in place, non-invasive blood pressure recording (if not invasive), intravenous access *in situ* and SpO_2. If hypovolaemia is identified, intravenous fluid replacement should be administered promptly, although caution must be taken not to 'overfill' as this will lead to further problems in the form of pulmonary oedema. Remember patients may also have been receiving volume via enteral sources and these should be stopped and tubes left on free drainage during transfer. Free drainage is important because the gut will be exposed to the same gravitational forces as other organs and will not function well, leading to poor absorption and an increased risk of aspiration.

> During transfer acutely ill patients must have at least:
> - cardiac monitoring;
> - non-invasive blood pressure monitoring;
> - intravenous access;
> - SpO_2 monitoring.

Constant observation of fluid status is therefore required, another key factor is urinary output monitored by hourly measurements if the patient is catheterised. When a patient is already well-filled with fluid, further therapy in the form of inotropes for additional cardiovascular support may be commenced. Anti-arrhythmic agents such as amiodarone might also be prescribed if patients are not monitoring in sinus rhythm or are experiencing ectopic beats. Remember, too, that blood chemistry such as urea, electrolyte and blood glucose levels should all be checked prior to moving a patient, so that complications in transit arising from abnormal values can be avoided wherever possible.

> All blood results should be checked before departure, so that abnormalities can be corrected.

Disability

Neurological assessment is another crucial aspect of patient preparation. All patients should be kept fully informed regarding the transfer and, if conscious, given the opportunity to ask questions and participate in the decision-making process where possible. It is almost inevitable that informing a conscious patient that they are to be moved will provoke some anxiety and in some cases maybe even anger. The nurse therefore has a responsibility to work in partnership with service users and their families, using effective communication and interpersonal skills to deliver compassionate, empathetic care (Nursing and Midwifery Council 2010). Keeping people informed as to what is happening can allay their fears and concerns, whilst simultaneously reducing their sense of powerlessness when faced with the stressful circumstances invariably accompanying critical illness. Gustard *et al.* (2008) found in their study of 249 patients who were being transferred that when nursing staff gave repeated information at regular intervals about proceedings it lessened the patients' anxiety.

For unconscious patients or those with a reduced level of consciousness constant monitoring with the Glasgow Coma Scale (GCS), together with pupillary assessment, is essential. The nurse must observe the patient's ability to maintain an airway and self-ventilate, the degree to which they have normal verbal and motor function and any changes to pupil size and reaction. It is also important to continuously note vital signs: these may be affected if the intracranial pressure is rising and hypotension can exacerbate this owing to a reduction in cerebral perfusion pressure (Glover and Murphy 2009). Should any deterioration be noted, prompt action will be required to stabilise the patient before transferring. For some patients, however, the move may be related to a primary neurological disorder such as an intracranial bleed and this would require specialist surgical intervention at another hospital. In such cases the airway should be secured first, in fact any patient with a Glasgow Coma Score of eight or below will require immediate intubation and mechanical ventilation.

> A patient with a GCS of eight or below requires endotracheal intubation before transfer.

For all patients, clinicians should be aware that the aforementioned gravitational changes in blood flow can severely compromise neurological status, especially if blood rushes to the patient's head during a manoeuvre. A patient with raised intracranial pressure would not be able to tolerate this haemodynamic instability: changes to intracranial blood flow could precipitate cerebral oedema, ischaemia and acidosis, risking further neuronal injury. To reduce the chance of this occurring, patients should be positioned 'head up', as this will limit positive and negative acceleratory forces (Handy and van Zwanenberg 2009). Always remember that cervical spine injury (a particular risk for trauma patients) must be excluded before moving the patient from a supine position. A protective hard collar should be worn at all times, until radiological investigation confirms that neck immobilisation is no longer necessary. Permanent spinal cord damage may be sustained if the patient's neck is moved prematurely (Leach 2009).

> Cervical spine injury must be excluded or a protective hard collar worn by the patient before transfer commences, otherwise permanent injury may occur.

If a patient requires intubation and mechanical ventilation they will be sedated and might have intravenous analgesia in progress. These measures are necessary to safely facilitate therapeutic intervention and promote patient comfort. Many patients however are transferred whilst fully conscious and self-ventilating, and the nurse should be aware that these individuals might experience pain and discomfort when being prepared for transfer and during the actual process itself. Ischaemia, surgical wound sites, fractures or tissue damage amongst other causes may be present and often the patient will be immobilised on a trolley of some description. They may also find other forms of sensory disturbance, such as bright lighting or unfamiliar noises occurring as they are being moved, distressing. Levels of pain and discomfort should always be assessed by the nurse either by verbal or visual means, such as pain scoring charts or by careful observation. While unable to verbalise their feelings a semi-conscious

patient may grimace or display tachycardia, hypertension and sweating if upset and in pain (Jevon and Ewens 2007). Should it be required, analgesia should be prescribed and administered before moving the patient and consideration given to continuous pain management during the transfer process.

> Ensure the patient is pain free before and during the transfer process.

Exposure

When preparing a patient for transfer the nurse should remember that corridors and vehicles can be cold places and the patient will soon lose body heat if exposed to a low temperature. Hypothermia is when the core temperature drops below 35°C, and this can lead to repetitive skeletal muscle contraction in the form of shivering. Hormonal release from the adrenal and thyroid glands also occurs with a low core temperature and the net effect of all these physiological responses is for the metabolic rate to increase and oxygen consumption to increase with it. This in turn may lead to other problems such as cardiac arrhythmias, electrolyte imbalance and hyperglycaemia (Jevon and Ewens 2007).

> Ensure the patient is warm enough, as hypothermia can induce a stress response.

Pyrexia may be an alternative complication and one that is a pre-existing feature of the patient's clinical condition. This will also increase the metabolic rate and subsequently oxygen consumption, therefore also leading to cardiovascular instability (Jevon and Ewens 2007). Finally, wounds may be present and, apart from being a source of pain for the patient, may serve as access points for infection and should therefore be well protected and securely dressed. Similarly varying types of intravenous cannula may be *in situ* during transfer and these also require continuous stabilisation and monitoring.

Equipment preparation

Every effort must be made not just to prepare the patient prior to transfer but also the equipment that will be used, and this is why a 'transfer bag' is recommended. It is not appropriate or safe practice for the nurse to be gathering items when the patient's move is imminent, especially if it is an emergency situation. All equipment should be checked and well maintained, ready to use and secured in one place so that it can be collected prior to departure, with clinicians confident that all necessary kit is present for monitoring and managing the patient during transfer.

There is nothing worse than not having the necessary tools or finding out that they do not work when they are most needed, this obviously endangers patient safety but is also very stressful for the staff involved. Circumstances like these could also raise concerns regarding professional and legal accountability, all practitioners having a duty of care to the patient. This means that when an intervention is proposed the level of risk and the potential harm that may occur to a patient through carrying it out is taken into account. Failure to do this may result in patients or their relatives challenging standards of care where there is a perception of negligence (Bell 2008, Hurley 2011).

> All transfer equipment must be checked and ready to go.

Assembly and maintenance of the transfer bag requires a checklist, itemising all requisite components. The contents of the bag need to be monitored and signed for by a registered nursing practitioner on a daily basis, even if they have not been used. In addition, other larger items than will not fit into the bag such as an oxygen cylinder and a portable monitor need to be readily accessible and fully functioning. Transfer equipment should be treated the same as any other emergency equipment, always there and always ready for use. The Nursing and Midwifery Council (2010) stresses in its documentation on competency acquisition for entry to the register the importance of nurses being familiar with the use of technology in health care (including all medical devices) and taking prompt steps to rectify any problems with it.

Specific recommendations have been made with regard to the equipment that should be taken on a patient transfer (Intensive Care Society 2002, North West London Critical Care Network 2011). Table 13.1 is an example of a transfer equipment checklist for an acutely ill, unstable (but, in this case, non-ventilated) patient. All of the items identified should be placed in the transfer bag or, if too large, be placed on or attached to the trolley/bed that the patient is being moved on.

Communication and documentation

The NMC (2010) stresses the importance of nurses using a full range of communication methods; demonstrating verbal, non-verbal and written skills. They must also be able to work effectively as part of the multidisciplinary team, providing leadership and coordinating interprofessional care. In short, they have an integral role in the delivery of quality patient care in a variety of clinical circumstances.

> Good communication and teamwork is essential for successful transfer.

Often, when problems occur during the transfer of a patient from one area to another, it is because there has been 'systems failure': organisational issues have occurred and these have compromised the safety of the patient. Ineffectual communication with other clinical teams, poor preparation of staff, inadequate stabilisation of the patient and insufficient checking of equipment have all contributed to unsafe practice. The completion of a designated transfer form outlining the key areas to be addressed when transporting patients is one of the ways in which these problems can be minimised. Although not currently existent across the whole of the National Health Service and independent sector, it is recommended that these forms be completed so that there is a detailed record of all transfer events taking place (Association of Anaesthetists of Great Britain and Ireland 2006). Whatever the design of the form, certain requisite information should be included, as illustrated in Figure 13.3.

Whilst all clinicians must be professionally accountable for their own actions or omissions, it is imperative that one person takes overall responsibility for procedures like transfer and the nurse is often the best team member to do this (Handy and van Zwanenberg 2009). The nurse has close proximity to the patient and can effectively liaise with other team members that may be based in different departments or indeed different hospitals. The transfer process spans a range of activities that the nurse should coordinate, as outlined in Table 13.2.

The preparation process the nurse should adhere to when transferring a patient is illustrated by the following case study.

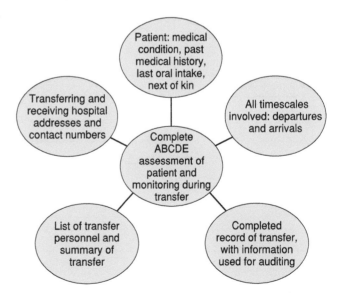

Figure 13.3 Information to be included in a transfer form

Table 13.1 Transfer equipment checklist

Item	Checked	Item	Checked
Airway:		**Circulation:**	
A selection of face masks		Venous access: 14–22 gauge cannulae	
Guedal airways sizes 2, 3 and 4		A variety of needles and syringes	
Naso pharyngeal airways, sizes 6 and 7		Scalpel	
Bag valve mask with reservoir		2 silk sutures, sizes 0 or greater	
2 laryngoscopes with size 3 and 4 blades with functioning bulbs (plus spare bulbs)		Sterile scissors	
Endotracheal tubes (ET) sizes 6–9mm		Forceps	
Tracheostomy tubes sizes 6–9mm with obturators		20mL lignocaine 2% with Adrenaline	
Tracheostomy dilator		Selection of giving sets and burrettes	
2 laryngeal masks sizes 3 and 4		2–4 litres of colloid	
Bougie		2–4 litres of Hartmann's solution	
Lubricant		2 × 50mL 50% Glucose	
Magill's forceps		200mL 8.4% Bicarbonate	
10mL syringe to inflate endotracheal cuff		250mL 20% Mannitol	
Endotracheal tape to secure tube		Portable intravenous infusion stand	
Catheter mount		Glucometer	
Cricothyroidotomy kit		Emergency drugs: • Atropine 1mg/10mL • Atropine 3mg/10mL • Epinephrine 1:10,000/10mL • Amiodarone 300mg/10mL	
Portable suction equipment			
Yankeur sucker			
Suction catheters of different sizes			
Breathing:			
Oxygen cylinder: with sufficient amount of oxygen for a return journey, plus a 100% or one-hour reserve – whichever is greater		Mains and battery-powered monitor with ECG and non-invasive blood pressure capability. Battery to be fully charged and spare available	
SpO$_2$ monitoring		Syringe drivers for all infusions with at least one spare	
Chest drain equipment: **Heimlich** valves		Direct current defibrillator (depending on the severity of the patient's condition)	
Aminophylline 25mg/mL (10mL)		**Disability:**	
		Working pen torch and spare battery	
		Diazemul 5mg/mL (2mL)	
		Exposure:	
		Core and peripheral temperature monitoring	
		Warming blankets	
		Wound dressings	
		Name and signature:	**Date and time:**

Table 13.2 Nursing responsibilities during the transfer process

Action	Rationale
Effectively communicating the decision to transfer to all concerned parties	All staff members at the transferring and receiving ends need to be fully informed that the patient is being moved and why the move is necessary. The patient's family also needs to be informed
Informing all staff involved of the timescales to be observed	All staff members need to know the time of departure and the anticipated time of arrival, so that the process runs smoothly without delays. If ambulance personnel are involved, they must be contacted in advance and everything in place for their arrival time
Preparing the patient, staff and equipment for the move	The patient should be fully assessed and prepared for transfer: • The transfer bag, plus any additional equipment required, should be ready for use • The staff accompanying the patient should be suitably prepared to go in terms of personal readiness, for example, possessing a mobile phone, being appropriately dressed and having money to hand. All necessary as there may be delays or on an intra-hospital transfer they may have to find their own way back to their workplace. Remember ambulances are not taxis – they can be called away to another clinical incident
Executing the move safely and efficiently	All accompanying medical and nursing personnel must constantly monitor the patient in transit and record any problems encountered
Giving a detailed handover to receiving nursing staff	While medical staff will liaise with each other regarding the patient's condition, a thorough nursing handover must be given to nursing colleagues and this should include the following information about the patient: • present medical and nursing problems including the reason for transfer • past medical history • any known allergies • current medication • any known source of infection (for example, methicillin-resistant *Staphylococcus aureus*: MRSA) • therapy delivered during transit and any problems encountered • social circumstances (next of kin) and all relevant contact numbers It is recommended that the SBAR tool (situation, background, assessment and recommendation) be used in order to deliver a systematic report (as discussed in Chapter 1)
Producing documentation to support the verbal handover	For legal and professional reasons there must be clear, legible and accurate nursing documentation accompanying the handover discussion. Good record keeping is essential (Nursing and Midwifery Council 2010). Nursing staff must also ensure that all other relevant clinical information pertaining to the patient is transferred with them, for example, medical notes and chest X-rays
Liaising with the doctor to complete a transfer form	Both the transferring and receiving clinical teams keep copies of this multidisciplinary documentation
Auditing of the transfer process	Auditing of all transfer events is important so that problems that may have occurred anywhere in the procedure can be identified and acted upon quickly in order to prevent repetition Auditing can also contribute to the collection of national data

CASE STUDY 13.1 An intra-hospital transfer

Mrs Khan, a 60-year-old retired teacher, has been admitted to the high-dependency unit with a diagnosis of acute pancreatitis and she is clinically unstable. The consultant has requested an urgent CT scan of her abdomen, because cyst formation, a common feature of the disease, is suspected. It is now 08.00hrs and the nurses on the day shift have just come on duty: during the handover they are informed that the scan is booked for 11.00hrs in the radiology department. The porter has already been called and asked to arrive at 10.45hrs, so that there will be sufficient time to transport the patient to the ground floor where the scanner is.

The nurse allocated to care for Mrs Khan conducts an initial assessment of her condition in order to effectively plan the transfer procedure.

Airway
Mrs Khan is fully conscious, speaking and able to maintain her own airway.

Breathing
She is sitting in an upright position at a 30° angle but complaining of feeling breathless. Her respiratory rate is assessed for a full minute and found to be 28 breaths per minute, although no use of accessory muscles of respiration is observed. She is receiving 5 litres of oxygen per minute via a face mask and her SpO_2 reading is currently 90% saturation. On chest auscultation, no adventitious breath sounds are heard, but she does have a productive cough and a sputum sample has already been sent to the microbiology department by the night staff for culture and sensitivity. An arterial blood gas taken during the night has also revealed the following information:

pH 7.32
PaO_2 8.0kpa
$PaCO_2$ 4.5kpa
HCO_3^- 18mmol/L
BE – 6mmol/L.

The nurse interprets this as a metabolic acidosis with evidence of hypoxaemia, and attributes this finding to the anaerobic metabolism that is occurring secondary to sepsis and hypovolaemia.

Circulation
Mrs Khan appears well perfused, with no sign of central or peripheral cyanosis, but her skin is warm and dry to the touch and her capillary refill is prolonged at four seconds. Her vital signs have been recorded hourly and are currently as follows: arterial blood pressure: 90/50mmHg, heart rate: 110 beats per minute, sinus rhythm and a central venous

pressure reading of 5mmHg via a catheter inserted into the right internal jugular vein. She is currently receiving intravenous colloid in the form of gelofusine and has a urinary output of 25–30mL hour, which at an estimated body weight of 85 kilograms is insufficient. The nurse concludes that in spite of the fluid replacement in progress the patient remains volume depleted, owing to the sepsis and accompanying hypovolaemia. She is nil by mouth and has a nasogastric tube *in situ* on free drainage and 200mL of bile-stained fluid is present in the bag. Blood tests taken on admission to hospital confirm that she has an elevated white cell count, serum amylase, serum lipase and blood glucose. She is receiving a sliding scale insulin infusion for the latter.

Disability
The Glasgow Coma Score is calculated at 15: E4/V5/M6 as Mrs Khan is alert, orientated and able to hold a coherent conversation with the nurse. He asks her if she currently has any pain, noting that during the night she graded her pain as 9/10; this was using a numerical scoring system, where 0 equalled no pain and 10 equalled very severe pain. Patient-controlled analgesia (PCA) was commenced by the night staff and the nurse is pleased to hear Mrs Khan say that she is now comfortable.

Exposure
Mrs Khan's temperature is 38.5°C, for which blood cultures have been taken and intravenous antibiotics commenced. She has no wounds or broken areas to her skin, but does have peripheral and central venous access. Both cannulae sites are well secured and the surrounding skin does not appear inflamed.

NURSING GOAL AND INTERVENTIONS
The nurse's goal is the safe transfer of the patient, avoiding any complications en route, as these will be more difficult to remedy outside the high-dependency department than in it. He concludes from his preliminary assessment that Mrs Khan is acutely unwell, with a risk of deterioration; her immediate problems being increasing hypoxaemia and hypovolaemia of septic origin. He calculates her early warning score (EWS) according to trust documentation, with the following findings:

A temperature between 38 and 38.5°C = **1**
A systolic blood pressure between 81 and 100 mm Hg = **1**
A heart rate between 101 and 110 beats per minute = **1**
A respiratory rate between 21 and 29 beats per minute = **2**
A urine output less than 35mL per hour = **1**

Total EWS score = **6**

CASE STUDY 13.1 An intra-hospital transfer *(continued)*

The trigger point is **4**, therefore validating the nurse's initial concern regarding the patient's condition. In spite of the short time frame and the urgency of the investigation, Mrs Khan must be stabilised prior to transfer or her condition will deteriorate further. As cardiorespiratory instability in particular can be exacerbated by the gravitational forces experienced during transfer, the nurse contacts the specialist registrar and discusses the need for additional oxygen therapy and fluid resuscitation. This is duly prescribed and the oxygen is increased to 8 litres per minute and another 1000mL of gelofusine is commenced to run over the next two hours. Following this, the nurse continues with his preparation for the transfer, as follows:

- fully informing Mrs Khan of the transfer procedure;
- collection of the transfer equipment he will require – the unit keeps a bag stocked at all times with the items necessary for the safe mobilisation of patients;
- collection of a portable suction unit in case of airway occlusion;
- collection of a full oxygen tank (size F: 1360L) which will allow for a 2-hour journey;
- checking that the infusion pumps are fully charged and the collection of a spare battery-operated pump in case the one in use fails;
- preparation of spare insulin and the patient-controlled analgesic infusions in case the current ones run out;

- attachment of a portable intravenous infusion stand to the bed Mrs Khan will be transferred on, which the patient-controlled analgesic pump and intravenous infusions can be secured upon;
- collection of all of the patient's notes and the chest X-rays: these are important as the radiologist will want to refer to them;
- informing the unit team when the transfer is imminent and contacting the radiology department when Mrs Khan is fully prepared and ready to be moved.

EVALUATION

Mrs Khan's clinical condition was effectively stabilised prior to departure. Her blood pressure increased to 110/70mmHg, her heart rate decreased to 86 beats per minute and her SpO_2 increased to 97%.

She could therefore be transferred at the allotted time to the radiology department, without any delay occurring. As the nurse had fully prepared the patient prior to departure, collected all the necessary equipment and communicated effectively with other members of the multidisciplinary team, the procedure went smoothly without any complications occurring. On return to the high-dependency unit, a transfer form recalling details of the event and the fact that it took place without incident was duly completed and sent to the unit manager.

Conclusion

In this chapter we have discussed the intra and inter-hospital transfer of patients, a procedure that takes place frequently on a daily basis throughout the United Kingdom. Even if a patient is only being transferred a short distance, the procedure is potentially hazardous and requires meticulous planning so that physiological and organisational complications can be avoided: the key areas of concern are the stabilisation of the patient and the preparation of staff and equipment.

To effectively and safely mobilise patients from one clinical area to another without incident, a systematic, coordinated approach is required. With appropriate training in the role, the nurse is well placed to act as a team leader in this situation and ensure that all patient transfers are conducted in a safe and professional manner.

Glossary

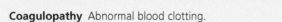

Coagulopathy Abnormal blood clotting.

Cricothyroidotomy Cannula insertion into the cricothyroid membrane to facilitate ventilation.

Gravitational forces Forces generated by gravity.

Heimlich valve A type of portable chest drain.

Hypovolaemia Reduced circulating volume.

Inter-hospital transfer Moving a patient from one hospital to another.

Intra-hospital transfer Moving a patient from one area to another within the same hospital.

Pneumothorax A collapsed lung.

Stridor A high-pitched sound heard on inspiration indicating airway obstruction.

Transfer bag A bag that contains all the necessary transfer equipment. This is checked on a daily basis by the nurse.

Transfer equipment checklist A checklist of transfer bag equipment.

Transfer for clinical reasons Moving a patient because she requires treatment.

Transfer for non-clinical reasons Moving a patient because there are capacity issues or they are transferring to a hospital nearer to home.

Transfer form A record of the transfer event documenting any problems that occurred.

Test yourself

1 Name the two types of transfer that take place.

   _____

   _____

2 Identify two reasons for transferring a patient.

   _____

   _____

3 Name two physiological problems that may occur as a result of the gravitational forces experienced during transfer.

   _____

   _____

4 If a patient is prescribed oxygen therapy, how much should be taken on a transfer?

   _____

5 At what point on the Glasgow Coma Scale does a patient require endotracheal intubation?

   _____

6 Why should enteral feeding be stopped before transfer?

   _____

7 Name the four therapeutic interventions that must be used for the transfer of an acutely ill patient.

   _____

   _____

   _____

8 List the eight responsibilities of the nurse prior to and during transfer.

   _____

   _____

   _____

   _____

   _____

   _____

   _____

   _____

9 What must be done if a critical incident occurs during the transfer of a patient?

10 The decision to transfer the patient is the responsibility of whom?

References

Andrews, S., Catlin, S., Lamb, N. and Christensen, M. (2008) A dedicated retrieval and transfer service: The QUARTS Project. *Nursing in Critical Care* 13 (3), 162–8.

Association of Anaesthetists of Great Britain and Ireland (2006) *Recommendations for the Safe Transfer of Patients with Brain Injury*. Available from http://www.nasgbi.org.uk/resources/1/Documents/braininjury.pdf.

Bell, D. (2008) The Mental Capacity Act 2005 – rights, responsibilities, regulation and redress. *Care of the Critically Ill* 24 (1), 17–22.

Cook, C. and Allan, C. (2008) Are trainees equipped to transfer critically ill patients? *Journal of the Intensive Care Society* 9 (2), 145–7.

Dunn, M., Gwinnuitt, C. and Gray, A. (2007) Critical care in the emergency department: Patient transfer. *Emergency Medicine Journal* 24, 40–44.

Glover, G. and Murphy, P. (2009) Inter-hospital transfer of patients with severe traumatic brain injury. *Care of the Critically Ill* 25 (1), 7–14.

Gustard, T., Chabover, W. and Wallis, M. (2008) *Intensive Care Patients Transfer Anxiety: A prospective cohort study*. Available from http:www.ncbi.n/m.nih.gov/pubmed/18805700.

Handy, J. and van Zwanenberg, G. (2009) North West London Critical Care Network Transfer Handbook; 1–42. Based on the pre-proof of 'Secondary transfer of the critically ill patient' (2007). *Current Anaesthesia and Critical Care* (18), 303–10.

Hurley, C. (2011) A model to support the ethical elements of decisions made by advanced levels practitioners. *Nursing in Critical Care* 16 (2), 53–4.

Intensive Care Society (2011) *Guidelines for the Transport of the Critically Ill Adult*, 3rd edn. Available from http://www.ics.ac.uk/intensive_care_professional/standards_and_guidelines/transport_3_3_.

Jevon, P. and Ewens, B. (2007) *Monitoring the Critically Ill Patient*, 2nd edn. Oxford: Blackwell.

Lawler, P. (2000) Transfer of critically ill patients: Part 1 Physiological concepts. *Care of the Critically Ill* 16 (2), 61–8.

Leach, R. (2009) *Acute and Critical Care Medicine at a Glance*, 2nd edn. Oxford: Blackwell.

North West London Critical Care Network (2002) *Adult Critical Care Record of Transfer*. Available from www.nwlcritcarenetwork.nhs.uk.

Nursing and Midwifery Council (2010) *Standards for Pre-registration Nursing Education*. Available from http://standards.nmc-uk.org/PublishedDocuments/Standards%20for%20pre-registration%20nursing%20education%2016082010.pdf.

Nursing and Midwifery Council (2008) *The Code: Standards of conduct, performance and ethics for nurses and midwives*. Available from www.nmc.org/.

West, D. (2010) *Half of Hospital Trusts Cannot Report Patient Transfer*. Available from http://www.nursingtimes.net/specialist_news/half_of_hospital_trusts_ cannot_report-patient_transfer_data/5019996.article.

Further reading

Dalton, A. (2012) *EMPACT. Emergency medical patients: Assessment, care and transport*. Boston, MA: Pearson.

Department of Health (2010) *Ready to go? Planning the discharge and the transfer of patients from hospital and intermediate care*. London: DH.

NHS Wales (2009) *Designed for Life. Welsh guidelines for the transfer of the critically ill adult*. Cardiff: NHS Wales.

Appendix: Test yourself answers

Chapter 1
1. c
2. c
3. d
4. a
5. d
6. c
7. c
8. a
9. d
10. a

Chapter 2
1. The Nursing and Midwifery Council exists to safeguard the health and well-being of the public
2. False, nurses are accountable to the patient
3. b
4. False
5. d
6. Your definition may have been similar to this – alerting someone inside or outside of your organisation or outside your immediate working environment to some kind of wrongdoing
7. c
8. d
9. True
10. d

Chapter 3
1. d
2. b
3. a
4. c
5. b
6. a
7. c
8. d
9. d
10. b

Chapter 4
1. c
2. a
3. False
4. c
5. b
6. d
7. a
8. True
9. True
10. False

Chapter 5
1. b
2. a
3. c and d
4. Medulla oblongata/carbon dioxide
5. a
6. a and d
7. b and d
8. c
9. c
10. c

Chapter 6
1. d
2. a
3. c
4. b
5. c
6. b
7. b
8. e
9. e
10. d
11. f
12. a
13. c
14. b
15. a
16. Albumin: maintains colloid oncotic pressure, binds with drugs and hormones; globulin: forms antibodies; fibrinogen: essential for blood clotting
17. a
18. c
19. c
20. c

Chapter 7
1. a
2. c
3. c
4. b
5. d
6. d
7. c
8. c
9. c
10. d

Chapter 8
1. Vasa recta
2. Tunica mucosa, tunica muscularis and tunica adventitia
3. Tubular filtration, tubular reabsorption and tubular secretion
4. Blood and albumin
5. 125ml per minute
6. Vasopressin, the antidiuretic hormone (ADH)
7. Oliguria
8. Creatinine
9. Weak, dilute urine
10. Intravenous dextrose and insulin in combination and intravenous or nebulised salbutamol

Chapter 9
1. b
2. b
3. c
4. b
5. b and c
6. c
7. c and d
8. b
9. a
10. b

Chapter 10
1. a
2. a, b, d
3. Gallstones and alcohol
4. a, b, d
5. a
6. a, c, d
7. a, c
8. 2000–2500mL/daily
9. *Clostridium difficile*
10. Haematemesis, haemoptysis

Chapter 11

1. b
2. a
3. a, b, d
4. 0.5mmoL/hour
5. b
6. Neuroglycopenia
7. Glycogenolysis, higher/raised
8. a, b, d
9. Glycosuria
10. b

Chapter 12

1. Innate or natural immunity and adaptive or acquired immunity, specific to each individual
2. Neutrophils, lymphocytes, monocytes, eosinophils and basophils
3. Opsonisation, chemotaxis and Inflammation
4. To increase metabolic rate and therefore inhibit bacterial growth
5. An *antigen* is a foreign substance that the host's lymphoid cells and tissues mount a direct response to. An *antibody* is a soluble protein that holds the memory of a previous pathogen and binds to the surface of an antigen
6. Bacteria, viruses, fungi and protozoa
7. Airway swelling, stridor, wheezing, hypotension, tachycardia and erythema
8. Temperature, heart rate, respiratory rate and white cell count
9. A raised level indicates tissue hypoxia and the presence of metabolic acidosis
10. Administer oxygen therapy, take blood cultures, give intravenous antibiotics, commence intravenous fluid resuscitation, check the lactate level and monitor urine output hourly

Chapter 13

1. Intra- and inter-hospital transfers
2. Transfer to a specialist centre for treatment and transfer to the radiology department for an investigation
3. Hypoxaemia and hypotension
4. There should be a 100% or one-hour reserve, whichever is greater
5. When the Glasgow Coma Score is 8 or below
6. The feed will be poorly absorbed because of reduced blood flow to the gut and there will be a risk of aspiration
7. The patient must have at least: cardiac monitoring, non-invasive blood pressure monitoring, intravenous access and SpO_2 monitoring
8. The eight responsibilities of the nurse are:
   - effective communication with the multidisciplinary team
   - informing all parties of the timescale involved
   - preparing the patient, staff and equipment
   - safely executing the move with colleagues
   - giving a detailed nursing handover
   - producing accurate documentation
   - completion of a transfer form if one is available
   - auditing of the transfer process
9. The patient must be made safe, safety of staff attending must be secured, all relevant personnel must be made aware of the incident, the patient's relative must be made aware of the incident, an incident form must be completed, lessons must learnt to prevent reoccurrence. Local policy must be adhered to
10. The patient's consultant

Glossary

α_1 **receptor** Receptor within the sympathetic nervous system located on the post-synaptic surface, responds to epinephrine creating a physiological effect, e.g. vasocostriction.

α_2 **receptor** Receptor within the sympathetic nervous system located on the pre-synaptic surface, detects unused or surplus epinephrine and inhibits further epinephrine secretion.

Abducens VIth cranial nerve, motor control of eye movements.

Abscess A collection of pus accumulation in a cavity.

Acetylcholine A neurotransmitter of the parasympathetic nervous system released by many neurones within the peripheral nervous system and by a few neurones in the central nervous system.

Acetylcholinesterase inhibitors Drugs that block the production of the enzyme acetylcholinesterase, e.g. pyridostigmine.

Acetylcholinesterase The enzyme that destroys the neurotransmitter acetylcholine.

Action potential An electrical signal that travels along the surface of a neurone, the signal is propagated by the movement of ions across the cell membrane of the neurone.

Action potential An event in which the electrical membrane potential of a cell rapidly changes due to ionic movement in and out of the cell. In the cardiac cell, this starts the wave of depolarisation giving rise to the PQRS complex.

Active transport Any movement of substances across a membrane that requires the input of energy.

Active transport Using energy in the form of adenosine triphosphate (ATP) to move fluid and solutes between cellular compartments.

Acute coronary syndrome (ACS) An umbrella term encompassing unstable angina, NSTEMI and STEMI.

Acute kidney injury An abrupt reduction in kidney function characterised by a rising serum creatinine level and a reduction in the urine output.

Adenosine triphosphate Usually abbreviated to ATP, this is a molecule that stores and provides energy for the metabolic activity of cells.

Adrenaline Naturally occurring hormone, also known as epinephrine, given during cardiac arrest to increase coronary and cerebral perfusion.

Adrenaline Now called epinephrine, neurotransmitter of the sympathetic nervous system.

Adrenergic receptors Receptors of the sympathetic nervous system, subdivided into alpha beta 1 and beta 2.

Aetiology The causes or origin of a disease.

Afferent neurone An alternative name for a sensory neurone, carries information towards the brain.

Afterload The load the (normally left) ventricle has to work against to open the aortic valve and eject its stroke volume. It can also be seen as ventricular wall stress in systole.

Aggregated weighted track and trigger system (AWTTS) AWTTS allocate points in a weighted manner (e.g. the more the parameter has deviated from normal, the higher the score generated) and these points are added to generate the early warning score. AWTTS allow the generation of low-, medium- and high-risk categories as recommended by NICE (2007).

Agonal breathing Deep sighing, irregular gasping breathing, also known as Cheyne–Stokes breathing, which occurs at the end of life.

Aldosterone A hormone produced by the adrenal cortex. Aldosterone increases sodium and water reabsorption from the distal convoluted tubule in the kidney and increases potassium excretion.

Algorithm Step-by-step procedure for problem-solving, often expressed as diagram or flow chart.

Alpha receptor Receptor of the sympathetic nervous system mainly located in the peripheral vasculature.

Amino acid The building blocks of proteins.

Anaemia A lower than normal number of red blood cells which depletes the ability to transport oxygen.

Anaphylaxis An acute multi-system severe type I hypersensitivity allergic reaction.

Angioedema Swelling of the deeper layers of the skin, this is often severe and is caused by a build-up of fluid.

Angiotensin-converting enzyme inhibitors (ACEI) A hormone necessary for the conversion of angiotensin 1 to angiotensin 2.

Anion A negatively charged electrolyte.

Anterior horns Section of the spinal cord, comprised of grey matter and containing motor axons.

Anticonvulsants Drugs used to control seizures.

Antidiuretic hormone (ADH) Also known as vasopressin, ADH is a hormone secreted from the posterior pituitary which promotes reabsorption of water back into the circulation via the collecting ducts of the kidney. It also causes widespread constriction of arterioles, which leads to increased arterial pressure.

Anuria Less than 100ml of urine in 24 hours.

Apathy Lack of interest or concern.

Aphasia Absence of speech.

Apneustic centre Located within the pons, controls breathing in conjunction with the pneumotaxic centre and the medulla.

Apnoea Temporary cessation of breathing, usually self-terminating, more prevalent following brainstem injury.

Aqueous Pertaining to water or water-based environments.

Arachnoid mater Middle layer of the meninges.

Arrhythmia Any electrical activity in the heart that differs from the normal.

Ascites Excess fluid that has accumulated in the peritoneal cavity. Comes from the Greek *askites*, 'bag-like'. It can also be called hydroperitoneum.

Asepsis The absence of pathogenic organisms.

Asterixis This is the term for hepatic flap (of the hands). The word comes from 'without fixed position'. When the patient with hepatic encephalopathy stretches out their hands, they have jerky irregular flexion/extension of the wrist. It is thought to be due to the interference with the inflow of joint position sense to the brainstem. Although characteristic of liver failure, it can also occur in cardiac, respiratory and renal failure.

Astrocyte A type of glial cell within the central nervous system, star-like in appearance, with multiple processes extending from the cell body, some of which end in foot processes that interface with cerebral blood vessels forming part of the blood–brain barrier.

Asystole Complete absence of electrical and mechanical activity in the heart.

Atherosclerosis Disease of large and medium-sized muscular arteries where the lumen of the vessel is narrowed by build-up of lipid, cholesterol and calcium. This build-up results in plaque formation, abnormalities of blood flow and eventually diminished oxygen delivery.

Atrial fibrillation Common cardiac arrhythmia in which multiple ectopic foci in the atria cause them to fibrillate, rather than contracting in a coordinated manner. AF is characterised by an irregular pulse and lack of p waves on the ECG.

Atrial flutter Cardiac arrhythmia in which a single ectopic focus in the atria fires rapidly causing abnormal atrial conduction. Atrial flutter is normally regular (or regularly irregular) and is characterised by 'saw tooth' waves replacing the P wave on the ECG.

Atrioventricular node The conduit of the electrical impulse from the atria to the ventricles.

Automaticity The capacity of a cell to initiate an impulse without an external stimulus, i.e. to spontaneously generate an impulse.

Autonomic dysreflexia Extreme autonomic response that can occur in patients with spinal cord injury above the level of T6.

Autonomic nervous system Branch of the peripheral nervous system containing two major subdivisions; the sympathetic and parasympathetic nervous systems.

Autonomic nervous system The nervous system is divided into the somatic (voluntary) and autonomic (involuntary). The autonomic regulates individual organ function and homeostasis.

Autonomy The right of patients to make decisions about their health care without the health care provider trying to influence the decision.

Axon The section of the neurone that extends away from the cell body.

β_1 receptors Part of the sympathetic nervous system, adrenergic receptors located within the heart muscle, stimulation causes increase in heart rate and contractility.

β_2 receptors Part of the sympathetic nervous system, adrenergic receptors with widespread activity including vasodilation and bronchodilation.

β_3 receptors Part of the sympathetic nervous system, adrenergic receptors located in brown adipose tissue, stimulation causes thermogenesis.

Bacterial translocation of the gut Passage of indigenous bacteria from the GI tract to the systemic circulation. This can be due to a breach of mucosal barrier, impaired immune defence mechanisms and/or bacterial overgrowth.

Bag valve mask A device used to provide artificial ventilation which consists of a manual compressible chamber with an oxygen reservoir at one end and a one-way valve and mask at the other.

Baroreceptors Sensory nerve endings in the carotid bodies and aortic arch that detect stretch and therefore blood pressure changes.

Basal metabolic rate The base rate at which the body consumes calories for basic metabolic functions such as maintaining internal temperature and repairing cells.

Basic life support See cardiopulmonary resuscitation.

Basophil A type of white blood cell that contains histamine and heparin.

Beta adrenergic receptor A receptor of the sympathetic nervous system subtypes; beta 1 (in myocardium) and beta 2 (in smooth muscle).

Bile Bile (or gall) is fluid produced by the liver (and stored in the gall bladder) that is used to digest fats in the duodenum.

Blood–brain barrier An important structure that prevents harmful substances from entering the brain tissue. The blood–brain barrier has two main components; a thick capillary basement membrane and tight junctions between the endothelial cells of the capillaries.

Brainstem An essential structure within the brain containing the *midbrain*, the *pons* and the *medulla oblongata*.

Broca's speech area Motor control of speech within the cerebral cortex, motor neurones connect Broca's speech area with the larynx, pharynx, mouth and respiratory muscles to enable coordination of talking, breathing and swallowing.

Capillary The smallest of the body's blood vessels.

Cardiac output The amount of blood ejected by the ventricle in one minute:

$$CO = SV \times HR$$

Cardiopulmonary arrest The sudden cessation of breathing and effective cardiac output.

Cardiopulmonary resuscitation (CPR) Emergency procedures to be undertaken in the event of cardiopulmonary arrest aimed at preventing irreversible brain damage caused by lack of oxygen. CPR consists of rescue breathing and cardiac compressions. CPR is also known as basic life support (BLS).

Cardiovascular centre An area in the medulla of the brain that regulates the cardiovascular system. It responds to sensory information from the autonomic nervous system, and acts to maintain cardiac output via the sympathetic and parasympathetic nerves.

Care escalation Care moved forward in order that a set of timely appropriate interventions prescribed by clinicians with competence in critical care, aimed at treating/preventing acute deterioration, are commenced. May involve advice from critical care outreach, ITU, and transfer to a higher level of care.

Cation A positively charged electrolyte.

Cauda equina A collection of lumbar, sacral and coccygeal nerve roots within the spinal canal below the height of L2.

Cell body The main part of the neurone containing cytoplasm and organelles.

Cell The basic structural unit of living organisms.

Central nervous system A subdivision of the nervous system comprising the brain and spinal cord often referred to as the CNS.

Centrifuge A device that separates the components of a liquid, by spinning the liquid at a high speed.

Centriole Rod-like structures in the centrosome that are responsible for the production of the mitotic spindle.

Centrosome An area near the nucleus that contains the centrioles and is involved in mitosis.

Cerebellum Part of the brain that lies beneath the cerebral hemispheres and posterior to the brainstem, regulates posture and balance, important for the coordinated contraction of skeletal muscle.

Cerebral cortex Outer rim of grey matter that forms part of the cerebral hemispheres.

Cerebral dominance The development of one cerebral hemisphere more than the other.

Cerebral hemispheres The two halves of the cerebrum.

Cerebral oedema Swelling of the brain.

Cerebral perfusion pressure Or CPP, calculated from the mean arterial blood pressure minus the ICP, the pressure of the blood perfusing the brain.

Cerebrospinal fluid Also called CSF, a colourless, clear liquid that circulates around the brain and spinal cord, produced by a network of capillaries in the cerebral ventricles called the choroid plexus.

Cerebrum The largest part of the brain, divided into two parts by the *great longitudinal fissure*, each half is called a *cerebral hemisphere*.

Cervical nerves A group of eight spinal nerves that arise from the cervical section of the spinal column and are annotated C1–C8.

Cholinergic receptors Receptors within the sympathetic nervous system, divided into two subtypes; nicotinic receptors and muscarinic receptors.

Choroid plexus A network of capillaries in the walls of all four ventricles of the brain.

Chyme From Greek *khymos* meaning 'juice'. This is semi-fluid, partly digested food expelled by the stomach into the duodenum.

Circle of Willis Anastomoses of the right and left internal carotid arteries and the basilar artery which form a special cerebral circulation at the base of the brain.

Cirrhosis From Greek *kirrhos* meaning 'yellowish or tawny' which is the colour of the diseased liver. Cirrhosis is the consequence of chronic liver disease whereby the liver tissue is replaced by fibrosis and scar tissue.

Clinical governance A framework through which organisations are accountable for continually improving the quality of services and safeguarding high standards of care.

Coagulopathy Abnormal blood clotting.

Coccygeal nerves A pair of spinal nerves that arise from the coccygeal section of the spinal column and are annotated Co1.

Coercion Applying either physical or moral force to another.

Colloid oncotic pressure The pressure exerted by plasma proteins that pulls water back into capillaries.

Colloid A solution with large insoluble molecules that can generate an osmotic pressure and expand the plasma compartment.

Commensal Living on or within another organism and deriving benefit without harming or benefiting the host.

Compliance When referring to the heart: the ease with which the ventricle expands or stretches to accommodate ventricular filling.

Computerised tomography (CT) scan A specialised X-ray where pictures are taken from a multidimensional perspective.

Conduction system Specialised conducting tissue of the heart which transmits an electrical wave across the heart, causing myocardial contraction.

Consciousness A state of awareness of oneself and one's surroundings.

Contractility The ability of the myocardium to contract.

Corneocytes The outer cells of the epidermis that are flattened and contain no nucleus. These are the cells that are shed from the surface of the skin.

Coronary circulation Arterial supply for the heart, arising from behind the aortic cusps of the aortic valve.

Corpus callosum A band of white matter that connects the two cerebral hemispheres.

CPAP (continuous positive airways pressure) A respiratory support therapy in which continuous positive pressure is delivered via a face mask, nasal mask or mouth piece. Positive end-expired pressure (PEEP) is achieved through a PEEP valve. This increases the lung functional residual capacity and aids oxygenation.

CPR Cardiopulmonary resuscitation (CPR) is an emergency procedure used to manually support the circulation, thereby preserving blood flow to the brain.

Cranial nerves A set of 12 nerves arising from within the brain and forming part of the peripheral nervous system, each nerve is named in accordance with its function and is identified numerically by the use of Roman numerals.

Cranium The section of the skull that encloses the brain.

Creatinine A waste product of muscle metabolism secreted by the kidney.

Cricothyroidotomy Cannula insertion into the cricothyroid membrane to facilitate ventilation.

Critical care outreach A team, often multi-professional, that provides clinical and educational support in the recognition and treatment at the onset of deteriorating health of adult patients on general wards. It also provides for patients after a period of critical illness when they are discharged back to a lower level of care on the general wards.

Croup A respiratory condition that is usually triggered by an acute viral infection of the upper airway.

Crystalloid An aqueous solution that contains mineral salts and other water soluble molecules.

CSF Cerebrospinal fluid.

Cytoplasm The contents of a cell inside the plasma membrane excluding the nucleus.

Cytoskeleton An array of connective tissue within the cell which helps to give the cell shape and to act as an attachment for organelles and inclusions.

Cytosol The viscous liquid component of the cytoplasm of cells in which organelles and inclusions are suspended.

Decerebrate One of two types of extensor motor response.

Decorticate One of two types of extensor motor response.

Defibrillation The reversal of fibrillation (inefficient and non-rhythmic contraction) by the delivery of a controlled electric shock.

Delirium Acute confusional state.

Demyelination The loss or destruction of myelin.

Dendrites Projections from the cell body of the neurone that increase the surface area of the cell membrane making it easier to connect with other neurones, bringing information to the cell body.

Dendritic spines Small hair-like projections on the dendrites that maximise the surface area of the dendrites.

Depolarisation A rapid movement of ions across the cell membrane causing a change in voltage, that leads to the action potential. In cardiac muscle this initiates myocardial contraction.

Depolarisation The first phase of an action potential where the membrane potential changes from negative to positive due to the influx of sodium ions.

Dermatome A map of the parts of the body that are innervated by spinal nerves.

Diastole The resting phase of the cardiac cycle in which ventricular filling occurs.

Diastolic pressure The pressure exerted (usually in the vessels) during the relaxation phase of the cardiac cycle.

Diencephalon Located below the cerebrum, made up of the *thalamus*, *hypothalamus* and *epithalamus*.

Diffusion The movement of solutes from a state of higher concentration to that of lower concentration.

Dignity Providing dignity in care focuses on three integral aspects: respect, compassion and sensitivity.

Discrimination This can be direct or indirect and is associated with treating a person or a group of people less favourably than others in the same situation.

Disempowerment Processes that lead to a reduction of the power which individuals have to make their own choices and shape their own lives as well making decisions about their own health care and health care needs.

Diuretic A drug that elevates the rate of urine production.

Diuretic A drug that increases urine output.

Dopamine A neurotransmitter within the central and peripheral nervous systems.

Dorsal horns Section of the spinal cord, comprised of grey matter and containing sensory axons, also called the **posterior horns**.

Dura mater Outer layer of the meninges.

Early warning system (EWS) A scoring system that detects early deterioration in the patient's condition.

Efferent neurone An alternative name for a motor neurone, information is transmitted from the brain towards the periphery.

Effusion Excess accumulation of fluid in a space.

Ejection fraction The amount of blood ejected from the ventricle in systole, divided by the amount of blood that was in the ventricle at the end of diastole.

Electrolyte A solution containing solutes that can conduct an electrical charge.

Electrolytes Atoms or molecules in an aqueous solution that have an electrical charge produced by the gaining or losing of an electron and can therefore conduct electricity.

Embolism Circulating foreign object such as air, fat or a blood clot which can lodge in and block a vessel.

End diastolic volume The amount of blood in the ventricle at the end of diastole.

Endocarditis An infection, usually caused by bacteria, of the inner lining of the heart which can damage the cardiac valves.

Endocardium The innermost layer of the heart.

Endocrine From Greek *endo* inside and *crine* to secrete. The secretion of hormones via ductless glands directly into the bloodstream.

Endocytosis A process whereby molecules too large to pass across the cell membrane can enter the cell. This is achieved by pinching off of a small section of the plasma membrane and forming a vesicle that can then pass into the cell. Water can be transported this way (pinocytosis) as can cell debris and microorganisms (phagocytosis).

Endoplasmic reticulum The array of tubes and discs in the cell that is responsible for production and processing of a variety of molecules in the cell. It has two forms: rough, which has ribosomes attached, and smooth which does not.

Endorphins A neuropeptide neurotransmitter, also described as an opioid-peptide, functions as a natural analgesic by binding to opiate receptors within the central nervous system.

Endothelium A thin layer of cells that lines the blood vessels.

Enterotoxin A protein toxin released by a microorganism in the intestine.

Enzyme Proteins causing chemical reactions.

Enzyme Proteins that catalyse chemical reactions.

Eosinphils Type of white blood cell so called because they can be stained with a dye called eosin.

Ependymal cells A single layer of cells that line the ventricles of the brain and the central canal of the spinal cord, they form the blood–CSF barrier to control substances entering the CSF.

Epinephrine A neurotransmitter of the sympathetic nervous system, also a catecholamine and a hormone, used to be called adrenaline.

Epithalamus Region of the diencephalon comprising the pineal gland and the habenular nuclei.

Erythrocyte A red blood cell.

Erythropoietin A hormone produced in the kidney that promotes erythrogenesis in the bone marrow.

Ethics A system of moral principles, rules of conduct.

EWS (early warning score/system) *System*: a process by which objective criteria are used to generate a score, which is used as an indicator for 'calling for help'. *Score*: each of six physiological variables generates a number as it deviates from acceptable ranges. The EWS is the sum of those numbers.

Exocrine *Exo* = outside. Secretion of chemicals via glands with ducts.

Exocrine Exocrine glands secrete their products into ducts, e.g. stomach, pancreas or liver.

Exocytosis This is the reverse of endocytosis and involves a vesicle formed in the interior of the cell joining the cell membrane and expelling its contents into the interstitial space.

Expressive aphasia Patients are capable of thought but incapable of speech.

Extracellular matrix The fluid and connective tissue that fills the space between cells in the body.

Extracellular Relating to the internal areas of the body that are not cellular. The extracellular space is usually divided into interstitial and vascular space.

Facial nerve VIIth cranial nerve, sensory and motor control for closing eyes, crying, smiling, grimacing, taste and salivation.

Fibrin A fibrous protein involved in the clotting of blood.

Fibrinogen A substance in the plasma activated by thrombin to produce fibrin, necessary for clot formation.

Fibrinolysis The breakdown of a clot also know as thrombolysis.

Filtration (renal) The forcing of blood and the substances in it through the glomerular-capsular membrane under arterial pressure.

Filtration The movement of dissolved substances across a membrane. The term implies that some molecules, protein and other insoluble substances will not be filtered.

First heart sound Heard as 'lub', this is the sound of the atrioventricular valves closing in the onset of systole.

Fissures Deep grooves between the gyri of the cerebral hemispheres.

Fistulae An abnormal connection or passageway between two epithelium-lined organs or vessels that do not usually connect.

Flexion A motor response where the limbs move towards the body in response to a pain stimulus.

Foam cells Foam cells are found in atheromatous plaques and are made up from both macrophages and smooth muscle.

Fraud A crime associated with deception deliberately practised in order to secure unfair or unlawful gain.

Ganglion A cluster of neurone cell bodies within the peripheral nervous system.

Glasgow Coma Scale An assessment tool for assessing consciousness.

Glial cells Also known as neuroglia, the dominant cell structure within the central nervous system, cells that support neurones.

Glomerular filtration rate (GFR) The rate at which substances pass through the filtration membrane and enter the proximal convuluted tubule.

Glomerulonephritis Inflammation of the glomerulus.

Glomerulus The part of the nephron where the blood is filtered as the first step of urine production.

Glossopharyngeal nerve IXth cranial nerve, sensory and motor control of tongue and pharynx.

Gluconeogenesis Metabolic pathway resulting in the generation of glucose from non-carbohydrate sources such as lactate, glycerol and glucogenic amino acids.

Glycogenolysis Conversion of stored glycogen to glucose by the liver.

Glycoproteins Molecules that are composed of elements of carbohydrates and proteins.

Glycosuria Presence of glucose in the urine.

Golgi apparatus A series of flattened discs that are involved in finishing molecular production in the cell.

Gravitational forces Forces generated by gravity.

Grey matter Outer layer of the cerebral hemispheres, mainly made of neurone cell bodies, dendrites, unmyelinated axons and neuroglia. Also found within the spinal cord where it is arranged in an H shape and divided into regions called horns.

Guillain–Barré syndrome An acute demyelinating disease of the peripheral nervous system, also called acute inflammatory demyelinating polyradiculoneuropathy (AIDP).

Gyri The pleural of gyrus.

Gyrus Fold on the surface of the cerebral hemispheres which increase the surface area of the brain.

Habenular nuclei Located within the epithalamus, have an integrative role linking smell and emotion, for example a particular smell may evoke a specific memory.

Haematemesis Vomiting of blood ('haem' is blood and 'emesis' vomiting).

Haematuria The presence of blood in the urine.

Haemoglobin A red pigment present in red blood cells made of haem, a molecule containing iron and globin, a protein with oxygen-carrying properties.

Haemolysis The breaking down of erythrocytes.

Haemolytic Destruction of red blood cells.

Haemopoesis Production of red blood cells and platelets from the bone marrow.

Haemostasis The stoppage of bleeding following the formation of a clot.

Harassment Any unwanted or uninvited behaviour which is offensive, embarrassing, intimidating or humiliating.

Health Service Ombudsman Exists to provide a service to the public by undertaking independent investigations into complaints about health services that have not acted properly or fairly or have provided a poor service.

Heimlich valve A type of portable chest drain.

Heparin An injectable anticoagulant.

Histamine A chemical that is released in the body as part of an allergic reaction.

Histocompatability This is the term used to describe the body's identification system and is usually based on molecules attached to the surface of cells identifying that the cell belongs to the particular person.

Homeostasis The maintenance of a stable internal environment irrespective of external conditions.

Hydrocephaly Increase in CSF caused by obstruction of CSF drainage.

Hydrophillic Any substance that interacts with water.

Hydrophobic Any substance that does not interact with water.

Hyperkaleamia High level of potassium in the blood.

Hypernatraemia High-serum sodium.

Hypertension High blood pressure.

Hypocalcaemia Low-serum calcium.

Hypoglossal nerve XIIth cranial nerve, motor function for speech and swallowing.

Hypokalaemia Low level of potassium in the blood.

Hypomagnesaemia Low-serum magnesium.

Hyponatraemia Low-serum sodium.

Hypothalamus Part of the diencephalon, situated under the thalamus, controls temperature, water metabolism, autonomic function, physical symptoms of emotion and pituitary secretions such as growth hormone. Also contains a feeding centre, a satiety centre and a thirst centre.

Hypothermia Abnormally low temperature.

Hypovolaemia Low circulating blood volume.

Hypovolaemia Reduced circulating volume.

Hypoxaemia A low level of oxygen in the blood, measured by arterial blood gas analysis or by SpO_2 in pulse oximetry.

Hypoxaemia Low level of oxygen in the blood.

Hypoxia Low levels of cellular oxygen.

Ileum The final section of the small intestine.

Immunoglobulin Also known as an antibody.

Inclusions These are found in cells and are large unspecified molecules, food particles or cell debris.

Inflammation One of the body's non-specific responses to trauma or infection involving dilatation of blood vessels and movement of blood components into the interstitial space.

Initial segment The proximal portion of the axon where the action potential is generated.

Innate Existing since birth.

Inodilators A drug which has both inotropic and vasodilator properties.

Inotropic therapy Drugs that work on the contractility of the myocardium and ultimately improve cardiac performance.

Inotropic (also inotrope) Has an effect on myocardial contractility. A positive inotrope increases contractility, a negative inotrope decreases contractility.

Insomnia Inability to obtain an adequate amount or quality of sleep.

Inter-hospital transfer Moving a patient from one hospital to another.

Interstitial fluid Fluid around and between tissue cells.

Interstitial This refers to the space around cells that contains fluid (interstitial fluid) or connective tissue.

Intracellular fluid Fluid inside the cell walls.

Intracellular The contents of, or any activity that takes place inside, the cell.

Intracranial pressure The pressure within the skull.

Intra-hospital transfer Moving a patient from one area to another within the same hospital.

Intraosseous The inside of a bone.

Intravenous pyelogram (IVP) Investigation of the kidney and ureters for obstructive lesions (using contrast media).

Intravenous The inside of a vein.

Ischaemia A restriction of blood supply.

Isovolumetric ventricular contraction Phase of the cardiac cycle after ventricular depolarisation. All four valves are closed as the pressure in the ventricle is increasing, but not yet sufficient to open the aortic and pulmonic valves.

Jejunum The middle aspect of the small intestine.

Jugular venous pressure (JVP) The pressure in the jugular veins which can be seen as a pulsating column in the neck. It can be used to estimate whether cardiac filling pressures are high.

Juxta glomerular cells A group of cells situated in the afferent arteries of the nephrons in the kidney that store renin.

Ketoacidosis A metabolic condition associated with an accumulation of ketone bodies. Ketone bodies are the breakdown product of free fatty acids and the result of deamination of amino acids.

Kussmaul breathing Rapid, deep, laboured breathing due to respiratory compensation for a severe metabolic acidosis. This can arise from either ketoacidosis or renal failure. Named after Adolf Kussmaul, a nineteenth-century German doctor.

Leucocyte A white blood cell containing a nucleus but no haemoglobin.

Leukaemia A malignant disease of the blood in which large numbers of leucocytes are present.

Lumbar nerves A group of five paired spinal nerves that arise from the lumbar section of the spinal column and are annotated L1–L5.

Lymphatic system A collection of capillaries, nodes and ducts that removes excess fluid and cell debris from the interstitial spaces and returns it to the vascular system via the subclavian veins.

Lysis Destruction of a cell or the process of breaking up or destruction.

Lysosome Intracellular organelle that is involved in processing microorganisms and cell debris entering the cell through phagocytosis.

Macroglia Large glial cells.

Malar flush A high colour over the cheekbones, often with a bluish tinge. May be indicative of mitral stenosis.

Malnutrition Any condition in which the body does not receive enough nutrients for effective function. Malnutrition may range from mild to severe and life threatening.

Mean arterial pressure (MAP) The average pressure in the circulation throughout the cardiac cycle.

Medical emergency teams (MET) A team of health care professionals who have advanced life support skills, who are able to respond to patients who have abnormal physiological signs indicative of clinical deterioration. MET were first used in Australia.

Medical emergency An acute life-threatening event, usually preceded by a period of physiological deterioration and changes in vital signs.

Medulla oblongata Part of the brainstem, contains the vasomotor centre, which regulates the heartbeat and controls the diameter of blood vessels, thereby controlling blood pressure. Responsible for the rhythmical pattern of breathing. Contains ascending sensory pathways and descending motor pathways that connect the spinal cord with other parts of the brain. Contains important protective reflexes; swallowing, coughing, vomiting, sneezing and hiccoughing, and sensory nuclei for sensations of touch, pressure and vibration, taste, balance and hearing. It is the origin of cranial nerves VIII–XII.

Melaena This is the black, tarry faeces associated with gastrointestinal haemorrhage. The black ('melan') colour is caused by the oxidation of iron in the haemoglobin during the passage through the ileum and colon.

Membrane potential This is the voltage across the cell membrane created by the distribution of electrolytes. Changes in voltage across the cell membrane are important for stimulating electrical potential in nerves and muscles and also for ion pumps.

Meninges A collective term describing the three membranes that enclose the brain and spinal cord.

Meningitis Inflammation of the meninges.

Metabolism The term that describes all the chemical reactions that take place in the body.

Microbes Tiny organisms that cannot be seen by the naked eye.

Microglia Small glial cells.

Microthrombi Small thrombus located in a capillary or other small blood vessel.

Midbrain Part of the brainstem, contains sensory and motor pathways, involved in movement of eyes, head and trunk in response to visual and auditory stimuli, also the origin of cranial nerves III–IV.

Mitochondrion An intracellular organelle in which oxidative phosphorylation takes place.

Mitosis Asexual cell division involving the production of two daughter cells that are copies of the parent cell. Also known as mitotic cell division.

Mitotic cell division See Mitosis.

Mitral valve Valve which separates the left atria from the left ventricle.

Morphology The study of the form and structure of organisms.

Motor end plate The post-synaptic surface of a synapse between a nerve and a muscle fibre.

Motor neurone An alternative name for an efferent neurone, information is carried from the brain towards the periphery.

Multinucleate Cells that contain more than one nucleus.

Multi-parameter early warning system Multi-parameter systems trigger on two or more physiological variables that fall outside a predetermined range.

Multiple sclerosis A chronic demyelinating disease of the central nervous system, also known as MS.

Muscarinic receptor A type of receptor within the parasympathetic nervous system that responds to the neurotransmitter acetylcholine.

Myasthenia gravis An autoimmune degenerative disease in which acetylcholine receptors are destroyed resulting in muscle weakness.

Myelin sheath Up to 100 layers of myelin wrapped around an axon.

Myelin A lipid-based substance that is secreted by Schwann cells within the peripheral nervous system and by oligodendrocytes within the central nervous system. Myelin insulates axons and increases the speed of conduction along the axon.

Myelinated neurone A neurone whose axon is wrapped in myelin.

Myocardial infarction Death of cardiac muscle usually caused by acute lack of blood supply following blockage of coronary arteries.

Myocardium The thick muscle layer of the heart which contracts in a wave-like motion.

Neglect This is a type of abuse where a person has been remiss in their provision of care or treatment.

Nephron The functional unit of the kidney, where blood is filtered and urine is produced.

Nephrotic syndrome An inflammatory disease of the glomerulus characterised by proteinuria, hypoalbuminaemia, oedema and hyperlipidaemia.

Nerve impulse The transmission of an electrical signal along a bundle of axons within the peripheral nervous system.

Nerve A bundle of many hundreds of axons, together with their blood vessels and connective tissue. They only occur within the peripheral nervous system.

Neuroglia Cells that support neurones, the dominant cell structure within the central nervous system.

Neuroglycopenia A deficiency of glucose in the brain as a result of hypoglycaemia. This adversely affects the functioning of neurones.

Neurolemma The outer layer of a myelin sheath containing the nucleus of the Schwann cell, only found in the peripheral nervous system.

Neuromuscular junction A synapse between a neurone and a muscle fibre.

Neurones Cells within the nervous system that are capable of generating an action potential.

Neuropathic pain Pain that is generated by damaged nerves or central nervous system structures rather than in response to inflammation through pain receptors.

Neuropathy Damage to nerves.

Neurotransmitters Chemicals within the nervous system that are released from terminal boutons and diffuse across the synapse to excite or inhibit post-synaptic structures.

Neutrophil A type of white blood cell that can attack and destroy bacteria.

NHS Early Warning Score (NEWS) A proposed national early warning system to be used by the NHS, currently under development.

Nicotinic receptor A type of receptor within the parasympathetic nervous system that responds to the neurotransmitter acetylcholine.

Nissl bodies Rough endoplasmic reticulum within the cell body of the neurone, also called Nissl granules.

Node Localised swelling.

Nodes of Ranvier Gaps between sections of myelin where action potentials can jump along the axon in a process known as saltatory conduction. Nodes of Ranvier are more prevalent within the peripheral nervous system.

Non-invasive ventilation (NIV) A process that enables different pressures to be delivered during inspiration and expiration and providing ventilatory support. NIV is delivered via face or nasal mask, does not require intubation and is most commonly used for patients with type 2 respiratory failure.

Nuclei Clusters of neurone cell bodies within the central nervous system.

Oculomotor nerve IIIrd cranial nerve, motor control of eye movement, upper eyelid control and pupil constriction.

Oedema Excess fluid, above the normal, found in the interstitial spaces that is not rapidly removed.

Olfactory nerve Ist cranial nerve, sensory function for sense of smell.

Oligodendrocytes A type of glial cell which produces myelin within the CNS.

Oliguria 100–400ml of urine in 24 hours.

Optic nerve IInd cranial nerve, sensory interpretation of sight.

Organ A combination of two or more tissues adapted to carry out a specific function.

Organelles Structures within the cytosol that are the sites of specific cellular activity.

Orthopnoea Shortness of breath when lying flat.

Osmolality The concentration of solutes in a kilogram of water.

Osmoreceptors Sensory neurones in the hypothalamus that are stimulated by a change in the osmotic pressure of the blood and trigger the sensation of thirst.

Osmosis The distribution of water from a lesser area of solute concentration to an area of higher concentration.

Osmosis The movement of water from an area of high solute concentration to one of lower concentration.

Pancreatitis Inflammation of the pancreas that may either be acute or chronic.

Pancreatitis Inflammation of the pancreas.

Paralytic ileus Disruption in the normal propulsive ability of the gastrointestinal tract.

Paranoia Unfounded or exaggerated distrust of others.

Paraplegia Partial or complete loss of motor and sensory function from the thoracic region downwards.

Parasympathetic nervous system A branch of the autonomic nervous system.

Parasympathetic nervous system A branch of the autonomic nervous system, involuntary and as a generalisation counteracts the action of the sympathetic nervous system, it restores the body to its resting state and is needed for relaxation and sleep.

Parkinson's disease A chronic disease caused by inadequate levels of dopamine with a consequent imbalance in the ratio of dopamine to acetylcholine.

Pathogens An infectious agent (a germ).

Pericardiocentesis A procedure in which fluid from the pericardial sac is removed by a needles.

Pericardium Rigid sac-like structure surrounding and protecting the heart.

Peripheral cyanosis A blue tinge in fingers or extremities, due to inadequate circulation.

Peripheral nervous system A subdivision of the nervous system comprising the cranial nerves, spinal nerves and their branches, often referred to as the PNS.

Peristalsis Contraction and relaxation of muscles which propagates in a wave down a muscular tube. From Greek *peristallein* (to wrap around) from *peri* (around) and *stallein* (to place).

Peritonitis Inflammation of the peritoneum – the membrane which lines part of the abdominal cavity and viscera.

Peroxisomes Membranous sacs that are involved in intracellular detoxification.

pH A logarithmic scale representing H^+ concentration where '0' is the highest acidity and '14' is the lowest.

Phagocytosis See Endocytosis.

Phospholipid A triacylglycerol (triglyceride) fat that has one of the three fatty acid components replaced by a phosphate molecule.

Photophobia Intolerance of light.

Physiological needs Physiological needs are those required to sustain life, such as air, water, nourishment and sleep.

Physiological variable A clinical measurement such as heart rate, respiratory rate, that varies over time.

Pia mater Innermost layer of the meninges.

Pineal gland Part of the epithalamus, secretes the hormone melatonin, considered an endocrine gland.

Pinocytosis See Endocytosis.

Plasma membrane A membrane composed of phospholipids, proteins and cholesterol that surrounds cells and intracellular organelles.

Plasma protein A protein found in plasma, e.g. albumin, gamma globulin, fibrinogen.

Plasma Yellow watery liquid that makes up the fluid component of blood.

Platelet A small blood cell which multiplies rapidly following injury and encourages clotting of blood.

Pneumotaxic area Located within the pons, influences breathing.

Pneumothorax A collection of air in the pleural space (between the lung and the chest wall) resulting in collapse of the lung on the affected side.

Polyuria The passage of large amounts of urine.

Pons Part of the brainstem, contains sensory and motor pathways, a relay station between the cerebral cortex and the cerebellum, contains the apneustic and pneumotaxic areas which influence breathing. The pons is the origin of cranial nerves V–VIII.

Posterior horns Section of the spinal cord, comprised of grey matter and containing sensory axons.

Preload Left ventricular end diastolic pressure/volume. It can be thought of as the amount of blood returning to the heart from the circulation into the ventricle.

Primary motor area A highly specialised area of the cerebral cortex located immediately anterior to the primary somatosensory area, in the posterior section of the frontal lobe, immediately anterior to the central sulcus, important motor control of complex, skilled or delicate movements.

Primary somatosensory area A highly specialised area of the cerebral cortex located in the anterior portion of each parietal lobe immediately posterior to the central sulci, important for perception of sensations including touch, tickle, itch, pain, temperature and joint posture.

Proteinuria The presence of protein in the urine.

Pulmonary embolism The blockage of a pulmonary artery by a blood clot, fat or air.

Pulse pressure The difference in pressure between systole and diastole.

Pulseless electrical activity (PEA) Organised electrical cardiac activity in the absence of a pulse.

Quadriplegia Partial or complete loss of sensation and motor function from the neck down.

Racism Discrimination or prejudice based on race.

Receptive aphasia Inability to put words together coherently.

Renal calculi Stones made up of calcium and minerals that can obstruct the ureters.

Renal replacement therapy An extra-corporeal circuit used to filter excess fluid and waste products from the blood.

Renin A protein produced by the juxta glomerular apparatus that leads to the formation of angiotensin 2.

Repolarisation A phase within the action potential where the membrane potential changes from positive to negative by the efflux of potassium ions and returns to its resting state.

Repolarisation Movement of ions back across the cell membrane causing the resting potential to be re-established.

Respect To show regard or consideration for another person, respect a person's rights.

Ribosome An intracellular organelle composed of protein and ribonucleic acid which is responsible for protein production in the cell.

RSVP Reason–Story–Vital Signs–Plan System used in acute life-threatening events recognition and treatment (ALERT) course. An easy to remember tool including essential information to be used in an emergency, to enable medical staff to respond appropriately.

Sacral nerves A group of five paired spinal nerves which arise from the sacral section of the spinal column and are annotated S1–S5.

Saltatory conduction The term used to describe an action potential that jumps from one node of Ranvier to another. This only occurs in myelinated axons.

Sarcomere The basic functional unit of striated muscle made up of muscle fibres.

SBAR Situation, Background, Assessment, Recommendation. An easy to use mechanism used to structure communication, to communicate accurately what requires a clinician's immediate attention.

Schwann cells A type of glial cell responsible for myelin production within the peripheral nervous system.

Second heart sound Heard as 'dub', this is the sound of the aortic and pulmonic valves closing at the beginning of diastole.

Selectively permeable A membrane that is able to control molecules that can cross it. It is usually referred to in connection with the movement of water from an area of high solute concentration to one of lower concentration. This is also known as osmosis.

Self-esteem Central to a person's survival, the basis of our well-being, the degree of worth and competence one attributes to oneself.

Sengstaken–Blakemore tube This is used in upper GI tract bleeding. It consists of a tube with two balloons, one of which is inflated against the walls of the oesophagus, and the other in the stomach, the purpose of which is to apply pressure to bleeding points.

Sensory depravation Deprivation of adequate and appropriate interpersonal or environmental experience and deprivation of usual external stimuli and the opportunity for development.

Sensory receptors Nerve endings that detect information internally and externally.

Sepsis A life-threatening illness caused by the body overreacting to an infection.

Sexism Discrimination or prejudice based on sex.

Single-parameter early warning system Single-parameter systems trigger on one extreme physiological observation value.

Sino-atrial node The heart's primary pacemaker which spontaneously depolarises 100 times per minute.

Somatic nervous system A subdivision of the peripheral nervous system.

Specific gravity A measurement of urine osmolality.

Spinal accessory nerve XIth cranial nerve, motor control of shoulder and head movement.

Spinal cord injury Damage to the spinal cord that results in loss of mobility or sensation, also known as SCI.

Spinal cord An extension of the brainstem that runs from the medulla oblongata to the top of the second lumbar vertebra.

Spinal nerves Part of the peripheral nervous system, a group of 31 pairs of spinal nerves that exit the spinal column between each vertebra.

Splinter haemorrhages Tiny line haemorrhages that can be seen under the nails, indicative of bacterial endocarditis.

Statute A law enacted by a legislator.

Stress response Activation of the sympathetic nervous system by an environmental or physiological stressor.

Stridor A high-pitched sound heard on inspiration indicating airway obstruction.

Stridor A high-pitched wheezing sound resulting from turbulent air flow in the upper airway.

Stroke volume The amount of blood ejected by the ventricle during systole, normally about 70mL.

Subarachnoid haemorrhage Haemorrhage into the subarachnoid space.

Subarachnoid space The space between the arachnoid mater and the pia mater.

Substance P A neuropeptide neurotransmitter released by neurones in the peripheral nervous system that are responsible for the transmission of pain information to the central nervous system.

Sulci The pleural of sulcus.

Sulcus Shallow groove between the gyri of the cerebral hemispheres.

Sympathetic nervous system A branch of the autonomic nervous system.

Sympathetic nervous system A division of the autonomic nervous system that is involuntary, controls the 'fight and flight' response and maintains the body in a state of alertness.

Sympathomimetic A substance that mimics the sympathetic nervous system (used to categorise inotropic pharmacology).

Synapse A collective term that describes the interface between a terminal bouton and another tissue structure, which may be another nerve but could also be a blood vessel, a muscle, an organ or a gland. Synapses can be electrical or chemical.

Synaptic cleft The space between the presynaptic surface and the post-synaptic surface.

Systemic vascular resistance The resistance offered to the circulation by the peripheral circulation.

Systole Phase of the cardiac cycle when contraction occurs.

Systolic pressure Pressure, usually systemic, exerted on the walls of the arteries during systole.

Tamponade Compression of the heart by the accumulation of fluid in the pericardial space.

Tension pneumothorax Presence of air in the pleural space that occurs when air escapes into the pleural cavity from a bronchus but cannot regain entry into the bronchus. As a result, continuously increasing air pressure in the pleural cavity causes progressive collapse of the lung tissue.

Terminal boutons 'Button-like' terminals at the ends of the axon branches, containing synaptic vesicles where neurotransmitters are stored.

Tetany Muscle spasms caused by low-serum calcium.

Thalamus A pair of oval-shaped structures within the diencephalon, comprised of grey matter and usually joined by a bridge of grey matter. A relay station between the cerebral cortex and the spinal cord, also relays information between different areas of the cerebrum and between the cerebrum and the cerebellum. The thalamus is involved with consciousness.

Thalassaemmia A hereditary disorder that causes an abnormality in the protein component of haemoglobin.

Thoracic nerves A group of 12 paired spinal nerves that arise from the thoracic section of the spinal column and are annotated T1–T12.

Thrombin A substance which converts fibrinogen to fibrin to enable blood clotting.

Thrombocyte Another name for **platelet**.

Thrombus A blood clot.

Tissue Combination of similar cells and extracellular substances that perform a specific function.

Toxin A poisonous substance produced within living cells or organisms.

Track and trigger tool A set of predetermined objective criteria used as indicators for 'calling for help' in the management of a patient at risk of clinical deterioration.

Transfer bag A bag that contains all the necessary transfer equipment. This is checked on a daily basis by the nurse.

Transfer equipment checklist A checklist of transfer bag equipment.

Transfer for clinical reasons Moving a patient because she requires treatment.

Transfer for non-clinical reasons Moving a patient because there are capacity issues or they are transferring to a hospital nearer to home.

Transfer form A record of the transfer event documenting any problems that occurred.

Transient ischaemic attacks Brief episodes of altered consciousness caused by temporary obstruction of the arterial blood supply to the brain, also known as a TIA.

Transport molecules These are molecules attached to the surface of the cell or free-moving inside the cell that act as transport or carrier molecules for other molecules being brought into the cell or transferred from one organelle to another.

Triacylglycerol Known as triglycerides or neutral fats. These molecules are composed of a glycerol molecule joined to three fatty acid molecules.

Tricuspid valve Valve which separates the right atrium from the left ventricle.

Trigeminal nerve Vth cranial nerve, sensory and motor control of face, scalp, nose and mouth.

Trochlear nerve IVth cranial nerve, motor control of eye movement.

Tubular reabsorption Reabsorption of the filtrate back into the peritubular capillaries.

Tubular secretion Substances are filtered out of the blood into the tubular fluid for secretion.

Tumour A lump or growth of tissue made up from abnormal cells.

Ultrasound The production of an image from ultrasound waves that are created by structures within the body.

Unconsciousness Lack of awareness of oneself and one's surroundings.

Unmyelinated neurone A neurone whose axon is not wrapped in myelin.

Urea A waste product of protein metabolism.

Vagal tone The level of activity in the parasympathetic nervous system, for example the vagus nerve has an inhibitory affect on the heart rate.

Vagus nerve Xth cranial nerve, motor and sensory control of pharynx, larynx, heart, lungs, gut, viscera.

Varices Varices are distended veins. From the Latin *varix* meaning twisted veins.

Vasa recta A network of blood vessels found in the cortex and medullary regions of the kidney.

Vasomotor centre Located within the brainstem, regulates the heartbeat and controls the diameter of blood vessels, thereby controlling blood pressure, also called the cardiovascular centre.

Vasopressin Also known as the antidiuretic hormone, this polypeptide controls water reabsorption and secretion.

Vasopressor A substance (often a drug) which increases the degree of vasoconstriction of the blood vessels.

Vennule Small vessel connecting the capillary bed and vein.

Ventricular assist device (VAD) A mechanical device which can be used to assist the pumping action of the heart.

Ventricular fibrillation Disorganised electrical activity in the ventricular myocardium resulting in an absence of effective cardiac output.

Ventricular hypertophy A thickening of the muscle layer of the heart, the ventricular myocardium, usually in response to disease, high blood pressure, or problems that increase ventricular afterload.

Ventricular tachycardia Cardiac arrhythmia originating from within the ventricles characterised by rapid ventricular complexes at a rate greater than 100/min. It may or may not be associated with a pulse.

Ventriculitis Inflammation of the ventricles within the brain.

Venturi mask Type of disposable oxygen face mask which delivers a precise consistent mixture of air and oxygen regardless of the patient's inspiratory flow rate.

Venturi masks These oxygen masks are so named because they utilise a Venturi effect, which is to entrain air to mix with piped oxygen to achieve a specified oxygen percentage being delivered to the patient (fixed performance oxygen).

Venule A small blood vessel in the microcirculation.

Vesicle A small fluid-filled sac. In cellular terms it is surrounded by plasma membrane and may also contain particulate matter and a variety of metabolic intermediates and products.

Vestibulocochlear nerve VIIIth cranial nerve, sensory control of hearing and balance.

Wernicke's area Located within the left temporal and parietal lobes, interprets speech by recognising spoken words and translating them into thoughts.

White matter Inner area of the cerebral hemisphere, mainly comprised of myelinated axons. Also found within the spinal cord where it is divided into regions called columns: anterior, posterior and lateral white columns.

Xanthelesma Yellow/white fatty bumps under the skin around the eye lids, often the upper lid.

Xanthomata A bump in the skin caused by fats building up under the surface. They appear as small white, or larger yellow bumps, and may be associated with a high level of lipids in the blood.

Index